D0467196

PSYCHOPHARMACOLOGY
A Biological Approach

SERIES IN EXPERIMENTAL PSYCHOLOGY

Richard L. Solomon · Consulting Editor

EPSTEIN, KISSILEFF, AND STELLAR · *The Neuropsychology of Thirst: New Findings and Advances in Concepts*

LEVITT · *Psychopharmacology: A Biological Approach*

PSYCHOPHARMACOLOGY
A Biological Approach

Robert A. Levitt
Department of Psychology
Southern Illinois University at Carbondale

HEMISPHERE
PUBLISHING CORPORATION
Washington, D.C.

A HALSTED PRESS BOOK

JOHN WILEY & SONS
New York   London   Sydney   Toronto

To my wife, Phyllis

Copyright © 1975 by Hemisphere Publishing Corporation. All rights reserved. No part of this book may be reproduced in any form, by photostat, microform, retrieval system, or any other means, without the prior written permission of the publisher.

Hemisphere Publishing Corporation
1025 Vermont Ave., N.W., Washington, D.C. 20005

Distributed solely by Halsted Press, a Division of John Wiley & Sons, Inc., New York.

Library of Congress Cataloging in Publication Data

Levitt, Robert A
    Psychopharmacology: a biological approach.

    (Series in experimental psychology)
    Bibliography: p.
    Includes indexes.
    1. Psychopharmacology. I. Title. [DNLM: 1. Psycho-
pharmacology. QV77 L666p]
RM315.L46   615'.78   74-26749
ISBN 0-470-53149-5

Printed in the United States of America

CONTENTS

CHAPTER COAUTHORS

Patrick D. Brophy, Division of Humanities and Social Sciences, Rose-Hulman Institute of Technology, Terre Haute, Indiana

Hugh E. Criswell, Department of Psychology, Williams College, Williamstown, Massachusetts

George D. Goedel, Department of Psychology, State University of New York, Geneseo, New York

Barry J. Krikstone, Department of Psychology, Saint Michael's College, Winooski, Vermont

Daniel J. Lonowski, Department of Psychology, Southern Illinois University, Carbondale, Illinois

James Y. O'Hearn, School of Medicine, University of Illinois, Chicago, Illinois

Richard E. Wilcox, Department of Psychology, Southern Illinois University, Carbondale, Illinois

PREFACE

This book represents an attempt to create a teachable discipline out of the subject of psychopharmacology. Our purpose was to integrate the various aspects of this subject into a coherent framework specifically designed for the student of psychology. The author is a physiological psychologist and has attempted to organize the subject of psychopharmacology as a subdiscipline of psychobiology. Therefore, the book emphasizes explanations of drug-behavior interactions based on the effects of drugs on biological processes in the nervous and endocrine systems. However, the roles of past experience and present environment in determining the behavioral actions of drugs will also be discussed.

This book is written primarily for the student of psychology; it is intended to be appropriate for use by advanced undergraduate students as well as by graduate students, regardless of their specific interests or specialty area within psychology. Students in the other social and life sciences may also find this material useful. The book is not aimed at the "drug scene" course but at a higher-level course for students who have a professional or scientific interest in the topic.

We have assumed that the student has had previous courses in psychology and is thus somewhat familiar with the terminology, techniques, and concepts of this discipline. We recommend that the introductory course in psychology and also a beginning course in physiological psychology be the minimum prerequisites for a course that would use this book. Without a background in chemistry, much of the biochemistry included in this book will not be readily comprehended. However, this should not preclude the understanding of basic concepts and relationships.

We have attempted to produce a general textbook on the subject of psychopharmacology, one that would range broadly among the chemical agents that alter mood and behavior. We have discussed the individual drugs in relation to their usefulness in medicine and psychiatry and also in relation to their use in animal and human research studies. In research, drugs are sometimes used to better understand the mechanism of the drug's action and sometimes to aid in the analysis of certain behaviors. Research of both of these types is included in this text.

The book consists of twelve chapters. The first is an introduction to some of the basic concepts of pharmacology. Chapter 2 concerns the biochemical systems on which drugs act. We have not included a chapter on neuroanatomy since the student is expected to already have completed a physiological psychology course. Chapters 3 through 9 discuss the various categories of drugs whose principal mechanism of action is via the nervous system. These chapters are broad, frequently ranging into physiology and pathology. Chapter 10 is devoted to a newly emerging area of psychopharmacology research, the biochemical basis of memory and the use of drugs to investigate memory. These drugs primarily affect nervous system processes, and it seems to us that the only way to rationally review these particular drug effects is in a separate chapter on memory. Chapters 11 and 12 are concerned with drug effects on the endocrine system. Chapter 11 deals with basic endocrinology, and Chapter 12 is devoted entirely to sexual functions, a subject of special interest to psychologists. These last two chapters are broad surveys of endocrinology, since in our experience, psychology students get little exposure to this subject.

In the summer of 1971 I used my first draft of this book in a graduate seminar. Through this seminar several students became interested in the book and began working on the chapters with me. Seven of the now former graduate students have made a sufficient contribution to the book to earn first or second authorship on one or more of the chapters. Working on this book with these young men has been for me an exciting and rewarding experience. I wish to thank several other people who have made a contribution to the book. R. David Sturgeon and David Rowland contributed to earlier versions. Neil Carrier, Daniel J. Lonowski, and Barry J. Krikstone each read and criticized many of the chapters. James H. McHose and David C. Rimm each commented on one of the chapters. Connie Thelander did much of the early typing and paperwork. My wife, Phyllis Levitt, typed the complete final draft and has also provided much of the support and encouragement that sustained my efforts to complete this manuscript.

Robert A. Levitt

1
INTRODUCTION
TO PHARMACOLOGY

Daniel J. Lonowski and Robert A. Levitt

Psychopharmacology is the study of chemicals (drugs) that have the potential to alter the mood, perception, emotional state, or behavior of a subject. Since these alterations typically involve a change in mental or psychological state, substances of this type have been classified as *psychoactive*. The specific psychoactive properties of these kinds of drugs are, however, quite diverse and are determined by a number of related factors.

The effects of any drug are most basically defined by the chemical configuration and composition of that drug. These properties will affect how the drug is to be administered, how readily it will be absorbed, broken down or metabolized, and eliminated from the body. These physical aspects of drug action, however, may be modified to a great extent by the nature of the organism receiving the drug. A particular drug may have quite contrasting effects, for example, on different animal species; and too, there are individual variations in response to certain drugs within species. These variations are largely determined by biochemical and experiential factors specific to the individual. Thus, it seems safe to say that the mood- or behavior-altering properties of any psychoactive drug are the culmination of complex interactions involving the physical attributes of the chemical, physiological processes, species characteristics, and experiential factors.

The focus of this book is directed at an understanding of both the psychological (behavioral) and the physiological (biochemical) actions of psychoactive drugs. Since it is our belief that the understanding of psychoactive drug effects must be based on a consideration of biological factors, several of the most important of these determinants will be dealt with in the pages to follow. Further, it is our intent to provide a foundation of basic pharmacological principles with which the reader may critically evaluate and interpret the meaning and significance of materials presented throughout this text.

The specific areas to be included in the following overview of pharmacological principles are routes of drug administration; ways in which drugs are absorbed, distributed, metabolized, and excreted by the body; and variations in specific drug effects as they relate to individual physiological or experiential factors.

ROUTES OF ADMINISTRATION

There are a variety of methods by which drugs may be introduced into an organism. The manner of administration will affect the speed or onset of drug effects, the duration of the effects, and degree of effectiveness.

When a localized area of the body is to be influenced, as in the alleviation of superficial pain, local anesthetics such as benzocaine may be applied to the skin area. The direct application of drugs to the skin is referred to as *topical administration*, and is commonly used for temporary relief of pain or for minor surgical procedures.

When a rapid drug onset is desired and a more accurate drug dosage is required, *parenteral* (systemic action by injection) routes of administration are employed. These routes of drug delivery include *subcutaneous* (under one or more layers of skin); *intramuscular* (into the muscle); and *intravenous* (into a vein). Any number of drugs may be introduced into the body by the parenteral routes in order to achieve accurate, rapid effects.

Several other routes of administration are also available according to the specific response one wishes to achieve. Considered briefly, these include the *inhalation* method (into the lungs), often used to administer anesthetics or antiasthmatics; *intrathecal* administration (into the cerebrospinal fluid of the spinal cord), which is sometimes used to achieve a spinal block; *rectal* administration (into the rectum), employed commonly in infants as a means of achieving anesthesia, sedation, or analgesia; *intraperitoneal* administration (into the peritoneal cavity of the abdomen), which is a parenteral route employed primarily in experimental animals because of its efficiency and ease of administration. The intraperitoneal route is not usually employed for humans, however, due to the relatively high probability of bacterial introduction into the peritoneal cavity; *sublingual* administration (under the tongue) is used frequently on heart patients to achieve the rapid drug onset needed during instances of heart failure; and the *oral* route of administration (swallowed by mouth), which is perhaps the most common and widely used form of drug delivery in humans.

Although the oral route is the most prevalent and easiest means of administering a drug, it is not necessarily the most efficient. There are disadvantages to the use of this method. For instance, usually a drug's action is considerably slower when it is taken orally, the effects may be more variable, a larger amount of the drug may be needed to compensate for the digestion and excretion of the drug in the alimentary canal, and finally, some drugs are rendered inactive by exposure to the acid environment of the stomach. The advantages and disadvantages of the various routes of drug administration are a topic of importance to the student of psychoactive drugs. Students wishing additional information on routes of administration may consult Goodman and Gilman (1970) or Thompson and Schuster (1968).

DRUG ABSORPTION

Once administered, most drugs become distributed to varying degrees throughout the body. This distribution is most often accomplished via the circulatory system in the water medium or plasma of the blood. A drug may gain access to the circulatory system by being injected directly into the bloodstream or it may first be deposited in physiological depots such as the digestive system, pulmonary epithelium, or skin. If a drug is injected intravenously, it is, in essence, already absorbed by the body fluids. However, if a drug is placed in a physiological depot, as in a subcutaneous injection, it will encounter certain barriers prior to its entry into the bloodstream. These barriers are the membranes of cells.

The Cell Membrane

The topic of drug passage through membranes is an extremely important one, since the ability of a drug molecule to be absorbed into the bloodstream, and even to be taken up by specific cells and later excreted, is highly dependent on the ease with which the drug molecule can pass in and out of a cell through its membrane. It should be emphasized that drug passage across cell membranes remains remarkably similar for all types of physiological boundaries. This generally applies to single cells and cell nuclei, which both have simple plasma membranes, to more complex boundaries like intestinal epithelia, which possess single cell layers, and to skin barriers, which are usually several cells thick.

Before discussing the nature of drug passage across membranes, let us first examine the cell membrane itself (Figure 1.1). A typical cell membrane is thought to be composed almost entirely of lipids (fats) and proteins. Although evidence is not conclusive, the molecular organization of a membrane is thought to consist of three layers. The membrane appears to have a central layer of lipids, a thin outer (extracellular) layer of protein, and an inner surface (next to the cytoplasm) of polypeptides or proteins. This structural relationship renders the outer and inner surfaces of the membrane hydrophylic, or attractive to the water molecules which are found in the intracellular and extracellular spaces; while the central region of the membrane remains hydrophobic or water-fearing (not mixable or soluble with water). The ability of lipids and proteins to be readily joined into a membrane structure, despite their antagonism with respect to solubility in a water medium, is attributed to the phospholipid molecules

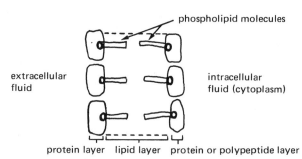

FIGURE 1.1.   Proposed structure of a cell membrane.

which lie at the base of the protein molecules and extend into the lipid layer of the membrane. The lipid portion of the phospholipid is attracted to the central lipid region while the protein end protrudes toward the surface of the membrane. In this way, phospholipid molecules hold the protein and lipid components together and form a stable membrane structure (Fox, 1972).

Active and Passive Transport

Now that we have discussed the organization of the cellular membrane, let us look at the ways in which substances or, more specifically, drugs, pass through a membrane. Drugs pass across membranes by means of two physical events, by diffusion (passive transport) and by active transport. Diffusion is based on the random movement of substances that is caused by the normal kinetic motion of matter. Stated another way, this means that as the number or concentration of drug molecules increases on the outside of a membrane, for example, the probability that those molecules will collide with each other increases, and the probability that they will strike the membrane increases as well. As this occurs, the molecules of the drug will tend to pass through the membrane and be absorbed into the cell until the molecular activity on the inside of the cell is in equilibrium with that on the outside. When this process has continued for some period of time, there will be no concentration difference across the membrane and absorption will cease (or rather no further change in concentration will occur since the number of collisions from the inside wall equals the number from the outside). The rapidity and extent to which a particular drug diffuses through a membrane are accentuated by smaller, low weight molecules, high drug concentrations, thin membranes, and large cross-sectional membranes which allow for more diffusion to take place.

Under certain conditions, drugs may pass through membranes in the absence of those properties which facilitate passive transport. This is accomplished by the process of active transport. Active transport may occur either in the same direction as a concentration gradient or in the opposite direction. In either case, an active metabolic energy-using process (not just passive diffusion) is responsible for picking up the drug molecule and carrying it across the membrane. The active transport mechanism by which a substance may pass from an area of low concentration to one of high concentration is attributed to protein or lipoprotein carriers, provided with energy, that bind with the substance on the outside of the membrane, and then transport it to the inside of the cell (or vice versa). The carrier is then thought to release the substance and return to the membrane's outer surface (in our example of carrying from the outside to the inside) in order to bind with another molecule and repeat the active transport process (Goldstein, Aronow, & Kalman, 1973).

Other Factors Determining Drug Absorption

With an understanding of the processes of diffusion and active transport that allow a drug to cross a physiological barrier such as a membrane, we may begin to consider some of the more general factors that determine the accessibility of drugs to the vascular circulation. Among those factors that determine the degree of drug absorption are the solubility of the drug and its concentration or dosage, the size of the absorbing surface within physiological depots, and the degree of blood circulation that is present at the site of absorption. If a drug is already in a dissolved state, the rate of absorption from the area of administration into the body fluids will be greatly enhanced. Thus, if a rapid response is desired, liquid drug forms are usually selected. Further, because diffusion gradients are from areas of high concentration to those of low concentration, drugs that are in solutions of high concentration are even more rapidly absorbed into the circulatory system. In a similar sense, drugs are more easily absorbed from large physiological depots such as the gastrointestinal tract. This is also because of the rich blood supply given to this depot.

DRUG DISTRIBUTION

Protein Bonding

Once a drug has entered the circulatory system it will be distributed to various regions of the body. Yet, many drugs can form reversible bonds with the plasma proteins normally found in the blood. The chemical bonds established between drug molecules and plasma proteins, however, are usually weak and easily disrupted. Once this protein bonding takes place, a significant portion of the drug molecules in the circulatory system (the ones that are bonded to proteins) will not be able to pass out of the plasma to find their way to specific target organs. The net result of this situation is that more of the drug will be found in the plasma than in or on target tissues. As a general rule, the amount of a drug that may influence target cells is but a fraction of the total drug level in the body.

By far the most important contribution to drug bonding is made by the principal protein of the plasma, albumin. Albumin represents approximately 50% of the total plasma proteins and is capable of bonding with a wide variety of drugs (different albumin molecules may bond at the same time to several different drugs). Some of these are the barbiturate sedatives, thyroxine (the major hormone of the thyroid gland), salicylate (the analgesic principle of aspirin), digitoxin (a drug to slow the heart rate), and many of the antibiotics. If any one of these drugs were given systemically to a subject, the rate of transfer of the drug molecules from the bloodstream into the tissues, by diffusion across cell membranes, would depend on the concentration gradient of the free (unbound) drug molecules. Protein bonding, therefore, can slow the disappearance of a drug from the circulation, while providing a reservoir of bound drug molecules that will not be readily metabolized or excreted (as only free drug molecules can be metabolized and excreted). Protein bonding thus works against achieving an even distribution of a drug throughout the body, and may also greatly prolong the duration of drug effects. An equilibrium tends to be reached in the circulatory system between bound and unbound drug molecules. As unbound molecules pass out of the circulatory system to influence body tissues, some more bound molecules separate from the plasma proteins and become available.

Other Factors Determining Drug Distribution

As previously stated, only free drug molecules are able to diffuse across membranes into target cells or organs. However, in the same manner that absorption of a drug into the circulation is limited by relative rates of blood flow through depots where drugs are placed, and by the concentration of the drug at these sites, so too, passage of drug molecules out of the circulation and into the cells is determined by these variables. Unless ideal conditions prevail, therefore, uneven drug distribution to tissues will result. In addition to plasma protein bonding, uneven drug distribution may occur as a result of absorptive or partitioning processes occurring at subcellular levels such as in the nuclei of cells, as well as by entrapment in the various fluid compartments found in the body.

For example, of the 40 liters of fluid normally found in the average adult male, 25 liters are located inside the cells of the body (this is called *intracellular fluid*, or *cytoplasm*) while the remaining 15 liters are distributed as extracellular fluids. The major types of extracellular fluids include blood plasma, cerebrospinal fluid, interstitial fluid (that found in the spaces between cells), and the fluids of the gastrointestinal tract. Each of these body fluids represents the water medium of distinct fluid compartments, each separated by a variety of membrane structures and other physiological boundaries, and each capable of partitioning off drug molecules from other regions of the body.

In addition, uneven distribution may be the result of selective absorption and accumulation of drug molecules by certain cells of the body. The cells of the liver, connective tissue and fat depots are especially efficient in amassing enormous quantities of some drugs. Fat, for example, may accumulate up to 70% of the lipid-soluble barbiturate anesthetic drug thiopental (Pentothal) within 3 hours after the time of injection. Thus, the liver may remove large quantities of this drug from the circulatory system, thus allowing fewer molecules to reach specific target cells. For further information on drug distribution see Holland, Klein, and Briggs (1964) or Goldstein, Aronow, and Kalman (1973).

Blood-Brain Barrier

A special consideration within the topic of drug distribution is the accessibility of drugs to the central nervous system (CNS). This topic is especially relevant to an understanding of psychoactive drugs whose principal effects are on the specialized cells (neurons) found in the brain. The brain constitutes only 2% of the weight of the human body, yet receives about one-fifth of the total heart output. It is thus most richly supplied in arterial blood. As stated previously, the amount of blood supply is of prime importance for the rapid distribution of drug molecules to the cells of the body. On the surface, one might expect, therefore, that drug exchange between blood and brain would be quite rapid, and indeed, this is so for many drugs. Many other drugs, however, enter the brain only very slowly, and some hardly ever pass into neural tissue.

One reason for this selective partitioning of certain drugs from the central nervous system may be found by examining the structural relationship between the vascular system and the specialized glial cells which are found in the brain in close proximity to nerve cells. This vascular-glial relationship in the central nervous system may be referred to as the *blood-brain barrier* (Figure 1.2) and is thought to act as a functional barrier to some drugs as they attempt to pass from blood into brain tissue (Davson, 1972). A drug molecule may pass from capillary into brain tissue only after it has been transferred through both the capillary membrane (endothelium) and the glial cell membranes. Since the capillary membrane and the glial cells are primarily composed of nonionized lipids, water-soluble and ionized drugs will not readily diffuse into the brain cells. On the other hand, lipid-soluble and nonionized drugs enter the brain cells with relative ease because they may diffuse through these lipid constituents. As a general rule, therefore, most of the psychoactive drugs are, to varying degrees, lipid-soluble, nonionized compounds.

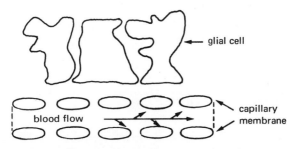

FIGURE 1.2. Representative diagram of the structural components of the blood-brain barrier.

Although the most common route by which drugs will enter the central nervous system is from blood directly to brain, an alternative route, though less probable, also exists from the blood into the cerebrospinal fluid (CSF) and then into brain tissue. (However, a blood-brain barrier also exists between CSF and neurons, since glial cells also separate this fluid system from the neurons.) Cerebrospinal fluid is manufactured by a specialized type of blood vessel system (choroid plexus) found along the walls of the large central fluid-filled chambers or ventricles of the brain. Cerebrospinal fluid flows from the choroid plexi through and around the brain in a system of channels and aqueducts, and is eventually removed from the ventricular system by the arachnoid villi to flow into venous blood. Drugs may thus enter the CSF by way of the choroid plexi. This is accomplished primarily because of the very rich supply of arterial blood given to the choroid plexi. Once in the ventricular system, drugs may diffuse directly into the brain tissue. However, since there is a relative absence of proteins in the CSF, except in certain pathological states, drug-protein bonding is infrequent in ventricles. As a result, most drugs do not remain in the CSF long enough to enter neural cells in effective quantities, but rather are filtered through the arachnoid villi and returned to the blood.

Summary

In summary, any drug that acts upon the central nervous system must have three basic properties. First, the drug should not bond readily with plasma proteins in order to insure a high level of free drug molecules. Second, the drug must exhibit low ionization at plasma pH (acidity). It should not be characterized by positively and negatively charged portions when dissolved in the plasma medium since ionic or charged compounds will not readily penetrate membranes. Third, the drug must have a high lipid-water partition coefficient, i.e., it must be more lipid soluble than it is water soluble. Considering these last two features, therefore, it should not seem surprising that highly lipid-soluble drugs like the general anesthetics, the barbiturates, or the various other psychoactive drugs like amphetamine, chlorpromazine, reserpine, and LSD are able to gain easy access into neural tissue and thereby exert powerful psychopharmacological effects. On the other hand, it follows that water-soluble compounds, such as epinephrine, serotonin, streptomycin, penicillin, and many acids which readily ionize in water, will be barred from the CNS and may not exert psychoactive effects when systemically administered.

METABOLISM AND EXCRETION OF DRUGS

Even as drugs are being absorbed and distributed throughout the body, two physiological processes are initiated which tend to reduce the overall impact of the drug. These two interlocking processes are metabolism and excretion.

Metabolism

The metabolic breakdown of drugs is accomplished in a variety of ways. However, there are four basic chemical reactions performed by the body which account for most metabolic transformations. These are oxidation, reduction, hydrolysis, and conjugation.

The *oxidation* of drugs involves the addition of an oxygen atom or the loss of a hydrogen atom from the chemical composition of the drug. Some of the more common drugs which undergo oxidation are the barbiturates and ethyl alcohol, which are metabolized by the liver. The overall effect of the oxidation process by the liver, therefore, is to transform the active drug into an inactive or water-soluble form such that it is readily excreted from the body.

The metabolism of drugs by way of *reduction* reactions involves the addition of hydrogen atoms or the loss of oxygen atoms from the active drug molecule. This process will transform many lipid-soluble compounds into inactive water-soluble forms. However, reduction reactions, in addition to inactivating various drugs, may also transform inactive compounds into pharmacologically active forms. The inactive sulfa drug, Prontosil, for example, is reduced by the body into the active chemical agent, sulfanilomide. It is true that oxidation and reduction are opposite processes and that if both acted equally on a drug molecule, the drug would remain unchanged in the system. However, in general, each particular drug is metabolized via only one of the two processes.

The *hydrolysis* of drugs typically involves the splitting of a drug compound into fragments by the addition of water (H_2O); the hydroxyl (OH^-) group becomes incorporated into one fragment and the hydrogen ion (H^+) is incorporated into another. The hydrolysis of drugs may occur in the plasma, as well as in various other tissues or organs, including the liver. Many esters and amides are metabolized in this manner, as are certain anesthetics such as procaine, and cholinergic agents such as acetylcholine.

Lastly, *conjugation* reactions take place by the joining together of two compounds to produce another compound that can be readily eliminated from the body. The majority of conjugating reactions occur in the liver and the kidney, and are responsible for the metabolism of such diverse compounds as alcohol, phenol, carboxylic acids like acetic acid (vinegar), nicotinic acid, epinephrine, norepinephrine, and salicyclic acids such as aspirin.

It should be clear from the preceding that the major organ functioning in drug metabolism is the liver. In the absence of normal liver functioning, therefore, the metabolism of drugs may result in undesirable side effects. Patients with liver disease, for example, will tend to be more sensitive to drugs. This sensitivity may result either from a failure to degrade active drug molecules or from the production of toxic compounds by the pathological liver.

Excretion

The most common mode of excretion of drugs is via the urine. However, before a drug can be processed by the kidneys and eliminated from the body, it must first be metabolized to an ionized or water-soluble form. Water-soluble drugs, therefore, are ideally suited for rapid elimination from the body, unlike the lipid-soluble drugs, which require metabolic breakdown to a water-soluble form before they can be eliminated. Further, only the protein-free or unbound drug molecules in the plasma will be passed in the urine since the kidneys are capable of constantly reabsorbing proteins. Thus, the kidneys can indirectly reabsorb drug molecules because they are bound to proteins, which are kept in the vascular circulation for a longer period of time. The physiological mechanisms by which kidney excretory processes are accomplished are, however, too complex to review here. For a detailed review of this topic see Guyton (1971).

Although the kidneys perform the major excretory function in the removal of drugs from the body, several subsidiary processes may also be involved. The liver, for example, can deposit drug metabolites into the bile, from which they are then emptied into the small intestine. From the intestinal tract, the metabolites will consequently be eliminated in the feces. The fecal excretion of drugs, however, is more usually the result of compounds taken orally which have failed to be absorbed from the gastrointestinal tract.

To a small extent, unmetabolized or lipid-soluble drugs may also be excreted from the body. The excretory process in this case is dependent on nonionized or lipid molecules, which may readily pass through biological membranes. Among the more common sites for this type of drug excretion are the salivary glands, the sweat glands, and the lungs. Although these organs do indeed have a drug excretory function, it is a small one. For example, approximately 90% of a 10-ounce dose of ethyl alcohol is metabolized by the liver and excreted in the urine. Of the remaining 10%, 2% will be excreted by the lungs, salivary and sweat glands, and the remainder will be excreted in the feces.

Drug Disappearance: A Clinical Example

The elimination of drugs from the body is primarily determined by the nature of the drug itself, its route of administration, and the efficiency of absorptive, metabolic, and excretory processes of the organism. The time required for the removal of a drug from the body, as a function of these factors, may be described by a drug disappearance curve. At this juncture, it seems appropriate to provide a clinical example of drug disappearance for a group of psychoactive compounds. The barbiturates provide an excellent framework for this discussion. The barbiturate drugs may be distinguished on the basis of their overall duration of action. When approached in this manner, three relatively distinct subclasses of barbiturates can be seen. There are the ultra-short-acting barbiturates, which are effective for up to 3 hours; the short- to intermediate-acting barbiturates, which may be effective up to about 6 hours, and the long-acting barbiturates, which exert their effects in excess of 6 hours.

Each of these subclasses of barbiturates is chemically distinct, and is processed by the body in quite a different way from the others. The ultra-short-acting barbiturate, thiopental, for example, is highly lipid soluble and, therefore, following administration it will be rapidly deposited in the fat tissue (and the nervous system). The selective deposition of thiopental in fat prevents it from being optimally distributed throughout the body (but it does have a high affinity for nervous tissue). Rather, thiopental is released from fat reservoirs as plasma levels of the drug decline and is thereafter degraded by the liver and excreted in the bile (and thus prevented from having extended effects). The short- to intermediate-acting barbiturate pentobarbital is less lipid soluble than thiopental and is not as rapidly deposited in fat tissue (or the nervous system). It is, however, degraded by the liver and excreted by the kidneys in a water-soluble form; yet because pentobarbital is present in the circulatory system in an active form for a longer period of time than thiopental, it will exert its behavioral effects for a longer duration. Lastly, the long-acting barbiturate phenobarbital is one of the least lipid-soluble barbiturates in general use. Its small degree of lipid solubility allows it to remain unmetabolized and bound to plasma proteins that act as a storage depot for the drug as it circulates in the blood. Since it passes into the tissue only with the greatest of difficulty, it will remain unmetabolized for very long periods of time and thus may remain in an active form longer than its more lipid-soluble relatives. Eventually, however, these relatively long-acting drugs too will be filtered by the kidneys and excreted in the urine still in active form.

THE MECHANISM OF DRUG ACTION

The issue of drug action may be viewed on several levels. On a phenomenological level, one may speak of altering perception, cognitive ability, or motivational state in the human subject. The manner in which these subjective states, as reported by the individual, are modified, may be described as the action of the drug. So too, one may study the behavior of laboratory animals or of human subjects subsequent to drug administration. Here, the action of a drug may be described objectively in terms of behavior under specific imposed conditions. On yet another level, the biological effects of drugs on physiological processes may be viewed as the action of the drug. All in all, each of these explanations provides a basis for understanding the impact of drugs on the psychological processes of the organism.

The cellular level of drug effects provides still another format by which the action of drugs can be assessed. In this regard, the most direct effect of a drug molecule on the biological activity of an organism is thought to result from physiochemical alterations in certain target organs and their component cells. These alterations in cell physiology can occur when drug molecules come in contact with specialized subcellular structures called receptors. Drug-receptor contact may occur by way of common chemical bonding and must be strong enough to resist disruptive processes. On the other hand, a strong combination of the drug with a receptor must be reversible; otherwise, prolonged contact could eventually result in cellular damage.

The determinations of the cellular effects of drugs are made by observing changes in cell activity. However, it must be made clear that, although certain physical changes in cells may be observed following drug administration, quite often it is not possible to conclude that a known alteration is the direct action of the drug. Indeed, some other biochemical or physical event may be the direct result of drug action; and this effect may then indirectly affect other physiological systems. By way of example, the drug digitalis (a heart stimulant) may have a direct effect on contractile proteins in cardiac muscle; it may compete or bond with the enzyme acetylcholinesterase, which normally functions to speed up the heart; or it may act directly on phorphoric acid synthesis, thus altering the energy production by cell muscles. Whatever the case may be, it is obvious that to espouse one distinct action of any drug is to presume a great deal, and thus such conclusions about drug action should be made with extreme caution.

FACTORS THAT MODIFY DRUG ACTION

Whichever level of analysis is employed in the study of drug action, one must take into account a number of factors that may modify the action and clinical effects of drugs. These factors include both quantitative and qualitative variations in the recipient organisms which may be of physiological or experiential origin.

Physiological Considerations

Age. Children are quite often more sensitive to drugs than are adults. Hormones, and particularly sex hormones, should be administered to children only with extreme caution. The possibility of inducing unwanted developmental side effects with sex hormones is particularly germane to cases involving very young children whose sexual anatomy may be markedly modified during early developmental periods (see Chapter 12).

In a similar fashion, the metabolic and excretory processes of infants are, in many cases, not fully developed; therefore, even small amounts of certain drugs may remain in the child's body for an extended duration and may, therefore, reach toxic levels. In addition, many drugs that will not normally enter the nervous system of adults may pass into the brains of infants. This may occur because of the immaturity of the infant brain itself as it relates to a functional blood-brain barrier. Some drugs may therefore have psychoactive effects on children that are not usually noted with adults (drugs may even have opposite effects in children and adults).

Elderly individuals may also respond to some drugs in an abnormal manner. Here, however, the basis of these abnormal variations most often results from a slowing up of metabolic and excretory functions. The higher probability of pathology in older persons also tends to make the effects of drugs unpredictable. Individuals with a history of pulmonary disease, for example, may be more sensitive to the respiratory depressive effects of many anesthetics or narcotics than are normal individuals.

Sex. Females are more sensitive than males to the effects of some drugs. The principal reason for this difference is due to smaller body size and the relatively higher amount of fat deposition in the female. However, since body size and amount of fat deposition are largely determined by individual hormonal events specific to females, the drug sensitivity seen in females may be related to endocrine physiology as well.

Tolerance. The frequent administration of certain drugs, whether in the treatment of disease states or in instances of "recreational" drug use often results in a phenomenon called *drug tolerance*. Tolerance is observed whenever a drug dosage must be increased to maintain a given drug effect. Tolerance develops to many psychoactive drugs, but foremost among these are the opiates, barbiturates, CNS depressants, the xanthenes (caffeine), and certain CNS stimulants such as the amphetamines. As tolerance occurs, cross tolerance also develops to related drugs, especially those which act at the same receptor sites. The effects of these related drugs will then be less than anticipated. In these cases the dosage of the drug must be elevated to achieve the desired effect.

Species differences. It is a common practice to test for the efficacy and possible harmful effects of drugs on laboratory animals prior to their distribution for human testing. This procedure is based on the assumption that there are enough similarities in physiological processes among lower mammals and humans to make accurate assessments of the effects of new drugs. There are, however, numerous examples of species variation in drug effects. The thalidomide episode, which saw thousands of malformed babies born to women taking this drug during pregnancy, illustrates a dramatic example of species differences in drug effects. Laboratory tests in several animal species were conducted prior to commercial use of thalidomide with no adverse effects uncovered from chronic administration. Only after its commercial distribution and the subsequent tragic events did it become apparent that the laboratory animals tested for chronic thalidomide toxicity were insensitive to its adverse teratogenic (causing malformations in a developing embryo) effects. It is unfortunate that even now we cannot be certain that similar instances will not recur.

Experiential Factors: Milieu

Many of the effects of psychoactive drugs are subject to influence by environmental factors present at the time of drug administration. The mental attitude, or "set," of an individual may vary widely and create quite unexpected results. The barbiturates, for example, may improve psychomotor performance under one set of circumstances, yet impair such activity under another set of conditions. This may be done by simply giving two kinds of instructions to the subject or by altering environmental contingencies. To a large extent, therefore, individuals will tend to behave in the way they expect a drug will affect them. This phenomenon, referred to as the *placebo effect*, is common to both clinical medicine and basic or applied research.

SUMMARY

The purpose of this chapter has been to provide a basic foundation of useful principles from the field of pharmacology. These principles are essential prerequisites to the study of psychopharmacology since this science utilizes many of the techniques and concepts of pharmacology in the study of psychoactive drugs. The overall effects of psychoactive drugs are to bring about changes in mood or behavior. The ways in which these alterations are accomplished, however, involve a complex interaction of pharmacological, physiological, and psychological factors. No one factor is prepotent in this regard, but each serves to contribute to the overall effectiveness that a drug will possess. In the pages to come, you will encounter many new and provocative concepts derived from psychopharmacological research. In this endeavor, the principles outlined here will serve as a foundation upon which a critical analysis of the material can be made.

2
BIOCHEMICAL
NEUROPHARMACOLOGY

Robert A. Levitt and Patrick D. Brophy

INTRODUCTION

The behavior of an organism is directly the result of events that occur in the nervous system. It follows, therefore, that a drug that influences behavior must do so by directly or indirectly altering nervous system processes. These nervous system processes that are the substrate for the behavioral effects of psychoactive drugs are generally of two types, nerve conduction and synaptic transmission.

Conduction

The first type of process (nerve conduction) involves the conduction of a nerve impulse from the receiving end of the neuron, the dendrites and cell body, to the output end, or axon, of the neuron. Drugs such as the general depressants (ethyl alcohol, barbiturates, general anesthetics) may alter, or more specifically depress, impulse conduction down the neuron and thereby exert profound physiological and behavioral effects. The depression of impulse conduction by the depressants may be achieved by changing the permeability of the cell membrane, or by interfering with cellular metabolic processes which provide energy for the conduction of neural impulses.

Transmission

A second means by which drugs may directly alter neural activity is by an influence on the transmission of neural impulses across the gap (synapse) that separates neurons. Various chemical substances called *synaptic transmitters* are released into the synapse and there act to transmit neural signals from one neuron to another. There are several suspected chemical substances that function as synaptic transmitters in the nervous system. Many drugs are capable of altering synaptic transmission by changing the status of one or more of these chemical transmission systems. This type of selective action on transmission can be contrasted with the previously mentioned action on impulse conduction within the neuron which is usually a general and diffuse effect on all neurons with which the drug comes into contact.

Indirect Actions

Although it is true that many psychoactive drugs directly affect the integrity of impulse conduction along neurons or transmission across synapses, nervous system processes may also be modified indirectly. Drugs that directly influence endocrine organs, for example, may initiate a sequence of hormonal events which ultimately affect the nervous system. These indirect effects may have mood altering or behavioral consequences for an organism. The important point, however, is that peripheral systems are reciprocally related to nervous system processes and if altered pharmacologically may indirectly influence behavior. The largest number of important and interesting indirect behavioral effects are via the endocrine system, and these will be considered in Chapters 11 and 12.

IMPULSE CONDUCTION DOWN THE NEURON

The structure of primary importance in a consideration of impulse conduction is the membrane of the neuron. This is a thin structure that separates the inside of a neuron or intracellular space which is filled with a fluid called *cytoplasm*, from the extracellular space containing extracellular fluid. The neuronal membrane may be considered to be a continuous barrier containing pores. If the neuron membrane had large pores, it would be equally permeable to all substances. However, this is not the case. There are only small pores along the membrane, and thus, only relatively small molecules may pass or diffuse through it. Therefore, the membrane is selectively permeable (a semipermeable membrane) because it lets some molecules pass through easily while slowing or stopping the passage of other, larger molecules. For example, water may freely pass through the membrane, but most organic molecules, which are relatively large, are unable to pass through the semipermeable membrane; and, since they are manufactured within the neuron, they are confined to the intracellular space.

Electrical Properties

Many molecules found in the intracellular or extracellular space are electrically charged, or ionized, and are thus called *ions*. Ions are characterized by positive or negative charges, which give them electrical properties that cause the ions to interact with each other in specific ways. Ions with like charges repel each other, whereas ions with unlike charges attract. Thus, two positive ions or two negative ions repel each other, whereas a positive and a negative ion attract each other. This phenomenon will to a large extent determine the concentration of ions on each side of the neuronal membrane.

Diffusion

A second process that influences the concentration of ions on each side of the neuronal membrane is diffusion. This term simply refers to the tendency of an ion to move from a region in which it is present in high concentration to an adjacent region in which it is present in lower concentration.

Active Transport

In addition to these passive mechanisms of diffusion and the electrical attraction and repulsion of molecules, there is also an active mechanism regulating the concentration of ions on the two sides of the neuronal membrane. This active transport mechanism (called the *sodium pump*) removes excess sodium ions that leak into the cytoplasm while the neuron is at rest (although sodium does tend to remain outside the neuron since it is a relatively large ion when it is in solution in water).

The Membrane Potential

There are four major ionic constituents of the neuronal cytoplasm and extracellular fluid. These are large negatively charged organic ions (OI^-), which are manufactured inside the cell, and also three inorganic ions which are brought into the body in ingested food and water. These inorganic ions are chloride (CI^-), which is also negatively charged, and sodium (Na^+), and potassium (K^+) both of which are positively charged.

Figure 2.1 illustrates in a simplified diagram the compromise that is reached between diffusion and electrical charge effects in establishing an equilibrium state across the nerve cell membrane. The sodium pump is also involved since it expels any sodium ions that manage to pass through the membrane into the cell. The negatively charged organic ions have been ignored for the purpose of simplicity. In Figure 2.1a the salts are placed into one side (extracellular space). Figure 2.1b illustrates equilibrium with only diffusion acting, while Figure 2.1c illustrates equilibrium with only electrical forces operative (note that in both figures the sodium ions are not able to penetrate the cytoplasm). In Figure 2.1d we see the compromise that is reached, at equilibrium, between the diffusional and electrical forces. With the addition of the large, intracellularly manufac- tured, negatively charged, organic ions, the intracellular fluid compartment becomes approximately 70 millivolts (mv) negative relative to the ionic charges in the extracellular space. Because of this polarity (−70 mv) across the membrane, the resting neuron is said to be *polarized*.

When an excitatory stimulus is applied to the receptive surface of the neuron, the membrane pores are thought to enlarge and the sodium pump to be rendered temporarily inoperative. The removal of calcium ions from the pores may be involved in both processes. During a brief period immediately following this

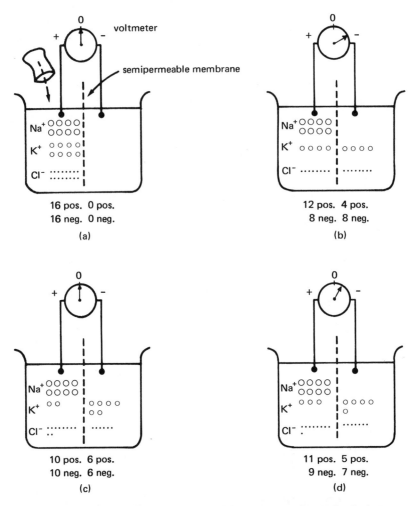

FIGURE 2.1. Simplified diagram of equilibrium or compromise tendencies between diffusion and electrical attraction/repulsion. (a) Salts dumped in one side. (b) If diffusion were the only force acting: potential (voltage) difference very large. (c) If electrical forces could override all other considerations: concentration differences very large. (d) A compromise between the two: potential smaller than in (b), concentration differences smaller than in (c). (Reprinted by permission from *A Primer of Physiological Psychology* by Robert L. Isaacson, Robert J. Douglas, Joel F. Lubar, and Leonard W. Schmaltz, [Harper & Row, 1971].)

excitatory stimulation, sodium ions rapidly pass through the semipermeable membrane and flood into the neuron until the intracellular fluid becomes about 30 mv positive (+30 mv) with respect to the extracellular space. Actually, the process is somewhat more complicated than this, but our explanation will suffice.

Graded Potentials

Chemical synaptic transmitter agents may tend to excite (depolarize) or inhibit (hyperpolarize) the receptive portion of a neuron on the dendrites and cell body. The excitatory inputs cause an excitatory postsynaptic potential (EPSP). The EPSP is a slight depolarization of the postsynaptic membrane which is not sufficient in and of itself to trigger the nerve impulse. The EPSP of the postsynaptic neuron does not enter the axon but is propagated throughout the dendrites and cell body in a decremental manner; that is, the amount of the depolarization is smaller at greater distances from the stimulus (synaptic input). If enough depolarizing stimuli are applied to the dendrites and cell body, resulting in a summation of several EPSPs, the potential difference across the membrane drops to about −60 mv at the beginning of the axon (axon hillock; where the axon leaves the soma), and an all-or-none nondecremental spike potential is generated (+30 mv). This all-or-none potential is initiated at the axon hillock and travels down the length of the axon.

While some synaptic transmitters trigger an excitatory EPSP, other synaptic transmitters may inhibit or hyperpolarize the receptive surface of the postsynaptic neuron (also in a decremental manner). The inhibitory transmitters cause an increased intracellular negativity (inhibitory postsynaptic potential, IPSP), probably by selectively allowing chloride ions to leak into or potassium ions to move out of the neuron. Figure 2.2a illustrates the summation of EPSPs and IPSPs and also shows the generation of a spike potential. If the spike potential is initiated at the axon hillock, it is then propagated down the axon, without decrement, until it reaches the end of the axon.

Summation

Spatial and temporal summation (Figure 2.2b), involving both EPSPs and IPSPs, have a role in bringing the potential difference at the axon hillock down to the threshold for the spike potential, or, in inhibiting the spike potential. In spatial summation, there is a summation of the excitatory or inhibitory activity of two or more inputs on different portions of the cell body and dendrites that together succeed in reaching threshold and triggering the spike potential, or in inhibiting the spike potential. In temporal summation, there is summation of two or more inputs arriving over the same input neuron close enough in time to add together and trigger, or to inhibit, a spike potential. If a spike potential is triggered, then following "the spike" the neuron undergoes an afterpotential period during which the neuron recovers from the impulse passage.

Synapse

Specific organelles, called *vesicles*, which have become differentiated for a secretory function can be identified in the axonal endings in the region of the synapse (Bloom, 1970). These axonal endings are usually called the *presynaptic* surface. When the spike potential reaches these presynaptic vesicles, the release

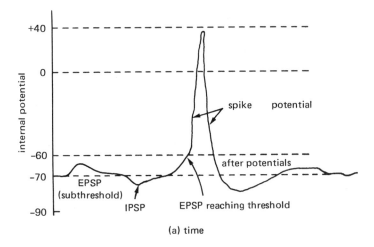

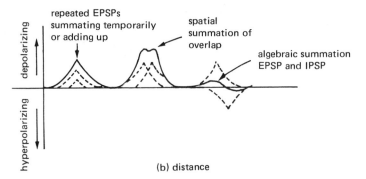

FIGURE 2.2. (a) Potential changes over time in the graded and spike potentials. (b) Spatial and temporal summation of the graded potentials. concentration differences smaller than in (c). (Reprinted by permission from *A Primer of Physiological Psychology* by Robert L. Isaacson, Robert J. Douglas, Joel F. Lubar, and Leonard W. Schmaltz, [Harper & Row, 1971].)

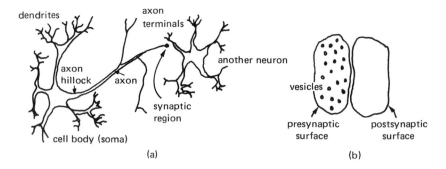

FIGURE 2.3. (a) Two neurons. (b) A synapse.

of a synaptic transmitter substance is greatly increased. The transmitter diffuses across the synaptic gap and may facilitate or inhibit the firing of the postsynaptic neuron. The parts of the cell body and dendrites on the opposite side of the synapse may be referred to as the *postsynaptic* surface (Ochs, 1965). At the synapse the spike potential is chemically transmitted across the gap (Figure 2.3; De Robertis, 1967).

THE DEVELOPMENT OF THE TRANSMITTER CONCEPT

It was initially thought that neurons were connected at the synapse and that this region was bridged by ionic and electrical events similar to those responsible for impulse conduction within the neuron. However, with the development of finer microscopic techniques a small gap was revealed between the presynaptic and postsynaptic membrane surfaces. It seemed unlikely that an electric current, which is what the spike potential is, could bridge this synaptic gap. Furthermore, there were a number of characteristics of nerve impulse transmission across the synaptic gap that were inconsistent with the electrical theory and suggested that the gap was bridged instead by a chemical mediator. These characteristics include the findings that synaptic transmission is subject to fatigue, electrical conduction is not; synaptic transmission is selectively sensitive to drugs, electrical conduction is not (although some drugs block conduction because of metabolic consequences); there is a brief delay in impulse transmission across the synapse, no such delay occurs in electrical conduction; synaptic transmission is unidirectional, electrical conduction is bidirectional; synaptic transmission exhibits temporal summation, electrical conduction does not; and, finally, synaptic transmission briefly outlasts the period of stimulation, while electrical conduction does not.

These discrepant phenomena led to the abandonment of the theory of electrical transmission across the synaptic gap. This earlier theory has now been replaced by the universally accepted theory of impulse transmission across the synaptic gap by means of chemical substances (McLennan, 1970; Ochs, 1965). The presynaptic neuron is now known to release a chemical substance that diffuses across the synaptic gap to combine with receptors on the surface membrane of the postsynaptic neuron. The interaction of the synaptic transmitter chemical with the postsynaptic receptor may be of an excitatory or depolarizing nature, or of an inhibitory or hyperpolarizing nature.

The synaptic transmitter chemicals are usually referred to simply as *neurotransmitters*, or *neurohumors*. Small packets or "quanta" of neurotransmitter (each quanta is presumed to include the contents of an individual vesicle) appear to be continually released by the presynaptic neurons, since small potentials can be recorded from the postsynaptic membrane surface even in the absence of the firing of spike potentials by the presynaptic neurons. The existence of these small potentials suggests that the firing of a spike potential does not initiate a new process, but instead greatly increases one that is already occurring—the continual release of small quantities of a neurotransmitter (Katz, 1971). The release rate of these transmitters then, determines the rate of impulse transmission between neurons (Bittner & Kennedy, 1970; Kuno, 1971; Rodahl & Issekutz, 1966), and ultimately, the behavior of the organism.

Early Evidence for Chemical Transmission

The concept of chemical synaptic transmission originally developed out of experiments that demonstrated that stimulation of the adrenal medulla and stimulation of the sympathetic nervous system had similar effects (Elliot, 1905). In these studies it was noted that the adrenal hormone, epinephrine (adrenaline), caused effects similar to those following stimulation of the sympathetic nervous system. This led to the suggestion that the sympathetic nerves acted through the liberation of the same compound that was produced by the adrenal glands. The sympathetic substance did not cause effects identical to those of adrenal epinephrine and is now known to be, instead, a slightly different compound, norepinephrine (noradrenaline).

The concept of chemical transmission was confirmed by Otto Loewi in 1920. Loewi knew that stimulation of the vagus nerve, which innervates the heart, would slow the beat of an isolated heart. Using this knowledge, Loewi took the fluid in which the heart of a frog had been bathed during stimulation of the vagus nerve, and bathed a second frog heart in it. The fluid now slowed the beat of this heart. This suggested that the vagus nerve had released a heart decelerating substance into the fluid. Loewi called this substance, which we now refer to as *acetylcholine* (ACh), "Vagusstoff." A second experiment showed that a heart accelerating substance was released from stimulation of the sympathetic nerves to the heart. Loewi referred to this substance, which we now call *norepinephrine* (NE), as "Acceleransstoff" (Friedman, 1971; Loewi, 1960).

Dale (1934, 1954) then proposed a biochemical classification of nerves as either adrenergic (releasing noradrenaline) or cholinergic (releasing acetylcholine) to indicate the chemical responsible for transmission across their synapses. This pharmacological classification of nerves formed the basis of Dale's principle of the "biochemical specificity of nerves." According to this principle, which is still accepted, each individual neuron manufactures only one transmitter, which is released at each of its terminals.

Criteria for Synaptic Transmitters

During the past 50 years a number of chemicals have been advanced as possible neurotransmitters. Each chemical is evaluated in terms of at least six criteria. These criteria act as guides and if a suspected (putative) transmitter meets most, or all, of them, it seems likely that the substance is a neurotransmitter (McLennan, 1970). These criteria are:

1. The substance must occur in neurons whose action it purportedly transmits.

2. Neurons must have enzymatic means of synthesizing the substance.

3. There must be a means by which the substance is inactivated.

4. Application of the substance to postsynaptic membranes must mimic stimulation of the presynaptic neuron.

5. During stimulation of the presynaptic neuron, the substance should be detectable in extracellular fluid near the synapse.

6. Pharmacological agents which alter the neuron's firing rate should similarly alter the effect on neuronal firing of the artificially applied putative transmitter.

Throughout the discussion of the putative transmitters in this and subsequent chapters, we will continually evaluate these substances in terms of the criteria just listed.

SYNAPTIC TRANSMISSION IN THE PERIPHERAL NERVOUS SYSTEM

The peripheral nervous system (PNS) consists of the neurons that connect the central nervous system (CNS), the brain and spinal cord, with the rest of the body. The structure of the PNS is readily understandable. It consists, in the human, of 43 pairs of nerves. There are 12 pairs of cranial nerves connecting the brain with the rest of the body, and 31 pairs of spinal nerves connecting the spinal cord with the body. Each of these nerves is a bundle containing a large number (hundreds or even thousands) of individual neuron fibers (axons).

Somatic and Autonomic Nervous Systems (SNS and ANS)

We can divide the PNS in two different ways. One is anatomical, into cranial or spinal nerves. The other is functional, into the somatic nervous system, which innervates the skeletal or voluntary muscles, and also provides the sensory information from most of the sense organs; and the ANS, which innervates the visceral structures. In the peripheral somatic nervous system, the spinal and cranial nerves carrying sensory information into the CNS from the receptors, and motor information from the CNS to skeletal muscles, consist of only one neuron with its long fiber process. There is no PNS synapse between the receptors and the CNS. However, there is a synapse between the motor nerve and the skeletal muscle. This particular synapse is called the *neuromuscular junction* and ACh is known to be the chemical synaptic transmitter substance at this site (Figure 2.4).

Certain cranial and spinal nerves contain parts of the autonomic nervous system in which there are two neurons between the CNS and the structure innervated. The ANS is relatively nonvoluntary and innervates the smooth muscles, cardiac muscle, and glands of the visceral structures. The viscera are the basic machinery of the body and consist of such structures as the heart and blood vessels, kidneys and bladder, stomach and intestines, lungs, pancreas, exocrine glands (ducted: for salivation, lacrimation and such) and endocrine glands (ductless: gonads, pituitary, thyroid).

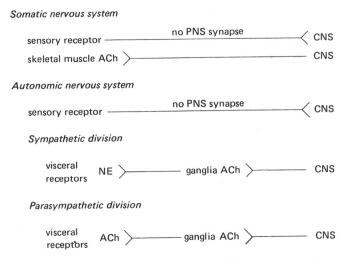

FIGURE 2.4. Synaptic transmitters in the peripheral nervous system.

The ANS is primarily a motor system consisting of the nerves to these visceral structures. The two neurons making up the ANS innervation of visceral structures connect (synapse) in ganglia (collections of cell bodies and synapses). These ganglia may be located either adjacent to the spinal cord (but outside of the vertebral column) or close to the organ to be innervated in the body or head region. The first neuron connecting the CNS to the ganglion is called the *preganglionic* neuron, and the second neuron beginning at the ganglion and going to the visceral organ is called the *postganglionic* neuron. This two-neuron pathway includes two synaptic connections. One of these is the synapse in the ganglion between the preganglionic axon fiber and the postganglionic neuron, and the other is the synapse between the postganglionic axon fiber and the effector muscle or gland.

There are two functional divisions of the ANS, the sympathetic and the parasympathetic. In general, these two divisions have opposite functions, but it must be made clear that the sympathetic and parasympathetic divisions are not constantly pulling the organism in two different directions. The two divisions are not in opposition, but each complements the actions of the other. The sympathetic division consists of some of the spinal cord fibers in the chest and upper abdominal regions and is primarily involved in the body's reactions to stress and emergency situations (fight or flight). The synaptic transmitter at the ganglia is acetylcholine while the transmitter secreted onto the effector organs by most sympathetic postganglionic neurons is norepinephrine.

The parasympathetic division consists of some of the fibers of several cranial nerves (III, VII, IX, X, XI) and some of the spinal nerve fibers in the lower abdominal region. This division of the ANS is primarily concerned with facilitating the performance of the body's housekeeping or maintenance activities (digestion, urination). The synaptic transmitter at both synapses in the parasympathetic division is acetylcholine. In the sympathetic division, many of the preganglionic neurons end in a chain of ganglia adjacent to the vertebral column. This feature allows extensive intercommunication between portions of the sympathetic division. In contrast, the ganglia in the parasympathetic division tend to be located close to the effector organs and are not connected into a chain (and thus parasympathetic actions are less well integrated than are sympathetic).

In summary, ACh is the synaptic transmitter in the peripheral nervous system at the neuromuscular junction, the synaptic site connecting somatic motor nerves with skeletal muscles; all autonomic ganglia (both sympathetic and parasympathetic); and at the neuroeffector junctions, the connections of the postganglionic neurons with smooth muscles, heart muscle, and glands, of the parasympathetic division. NE is the synaptic transmitter at the neuroeffector junctions between the sympathetic postganglionic neurons and the autonomic effector organs (Triggle, 1965; see Figure 2.4).

SYNAPTIC TRANSMISSION IN THE CENTRAL NERVOUS SYSTEM

In this section we discuss the major putative transmitters, including the biochemical pathway through which each transmitter is manufactured, the distribution of each transmitter in the CNS, and the way in which each transmitter is removed from the synapse and metabolized. The major putative CNS transmitters are acetylcholine (ACh), norepinephrine (NE), dopamine (D) and 5-hydroxytryptamine (5HT, also called *serotonin*). The CNS activity of other less well established putative transmitters will also be discussed. These include gamma-aminobutyric acid (GABA), the prostaglandins, histamine, other amino acids, and certain "brain specific" substances.

Acetylcholine

ACh, which was first synthesized in 1857, has been suspected of being a neurotransmitter since the 1920s. Although it has been studied for a longer period of time than any of the other putative transmitters, the evidence on its role in neural communication is still incomplete. One of the major technical problems that has yet to be overcome is the development of accurate and reliable chemical assay procedures (Cooper, Bloom, & Roth, 1974, Ch. 4). Bioassay preparations such as the dorsal muscle of the leech and the guinea pig ileum (which contract when ACh is applied to them) are presently the most sensitive and specific means of determining ACh, but are often unreliable. The recent wave of information on catecholamines, for which sensitive chemical assays have recently been developed, may soon be followed by information on ACh once similar procedures are perfected.

Synthesis. The first step in the biosynthesis of ACh involves the transport of choline, which is both an amine and an alcohol, into the neuron. This process requires sodium. Once inside the neuron, the choline combines with acetyl-coenzyme A (acetyl-CoA), a product of oxidation in the mitochondria, to form ACh. This reaction is catalyzed by an enzyme called *choline acetyltransferase*, with the availability of choline as the major factor controlling the rate of synthesis (Figure 2.5).

Once formed, ACh is stored in the synaptic vesicles until released. The rate of ACh synthesis is regulated by a feedback mechanism; therefore, synthesis varies directly with the rate of the release. This phenomenon is called *end product inhibition*. The end product, in this case ACh, inhibits the activity of an earlier enzyme in the synthetic pathway (choline acetyltransferase). Therefore, as ACh level is increased, its further synthesis is retarded.

As increased amounts of transmitter are used at the synapse, increased amounts are synthesized. This phenomenon, which also occurs with the other putative transmitters, suggests that turnover rate, as opposed to overall tissue levels, is a more appropriate measure of transmitter activity (Costa & Neff, 1970; Macon, Sokoloff, & Glowinski, 1971). Commonly used techniques to estimate turnover rate include the radioactive labeling of precursors or of the transmitter itself, and the subsequent measurement of the rate of decline of tissue radioactivity, or of the radioactivity of a perfusate gathered from the tissue. Another method involves the inhibition of synthesis and the subsequent measurement of the rate of decline of tissue levels of ACh.

Distribution. ACh is found in highest concentrations in the peripheral nervous system in somatic motor fibers, autonomic ganglia, and in

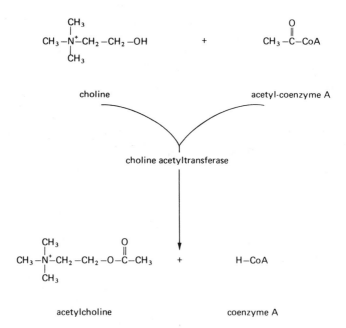

FIGURE 2.5. Synthesis of acetylcholine.

parasympathetic postganglionic fibers. Centrally, ACh is found throughout the brain and spinal cord (Figure 2.6a). It is rather difficult to measure CNS levels of ACh, since it decomposes very rapidly during the currently used assay procedures. However, indirect evidence for the activity of ACh may be obtained by measuring local concentrations of choline acetyltransferase. The highest activity of this enzyme is found in the caudate nucleus, basal ganglia, retina, and anterior (ventral) spinal roots (Cooper et al., 1974, Ch. 4; Koelle, 1955). The posterior (dorsal) spinal roots and cerebellum show only trace amounts of this enzyme, indicating a low level of ACh activity. The inference in these studies is that levels of this enzyme are correlated with levels of ACh.

Release and inactivation. The inward movement of calcium across the neuronal membrane is a critical step in the release of ACh (Rubin, 1970; Simpson, 1968). It may be that calcium molecules have a role in regulating the diameter of the "membrane pores." The arrival of a spike potential at the presynaptic vesicles causes the cell membrane to become highly permeable to calcium, which then rushes in and promotes the release of the transmitter. The spike potential may in some manner cause calcium to be released from the pores. This process of transmitter release is often referred to as *exocytosis.* Calcium appears essential to the process of release in all candidate transmitters studied thus far. After the release of ACh, the calcium is re-bound by the membrane with a subsequent decrease in membrane permeability to this ion.

The release of ACh is quantal, i.e., the amount released is not continually graded, but occurs as a multiple of a basic number or "quantum" of molecules. The quanta (perhaps the amount of ACh contained in a single vesicle) act on the postsynaptic membrane in an as yet unknown way to change the membrane's permeability to ions. This change in membrane ionic permeability initiates a spike potential if the membrane is depolarized by the ionic fluxes, or renders the membrane temporarily inexcitable if the membrane is hyperpolarized. The former effect is excitatory and the latter is inhibitory. Paradoxically, application of ACh to single neurons in the CNS has produced both effects (Bloom, Oliver, & Salmoiraghi, 1963). This suggests, of course, that ACh may serve as either an excitatory transmitter or an inhibitory transmitter in different anatomical regions and functional systems.

Released ACh diffuses across the synapse to act on the postsynaptic (receptor) membrane. Cholinergic receptors are thought to be located in or on the postsynaptic membrane but to date have not been isolated. One suggestion currently being given serious consideration is that the ACh receptor on the postsynaptic membrane consists of acetylcholinesterase and is also involved in the splitting up (deactivation) of the ACh molecule.

ACh is inactivated by being hydrolyzed by cholinesterase. The cholinesterase reacts with the ACh to break it down into choline and acetic acid. At least part of the liberated choline then passes back into the presynaptic nerve, a process called *reuptake,* for reuse in the synthesis of ACh. It is not clear how many cholinesterases (enzymes capable of hydrolyzing ACh) exist in vivo, as these

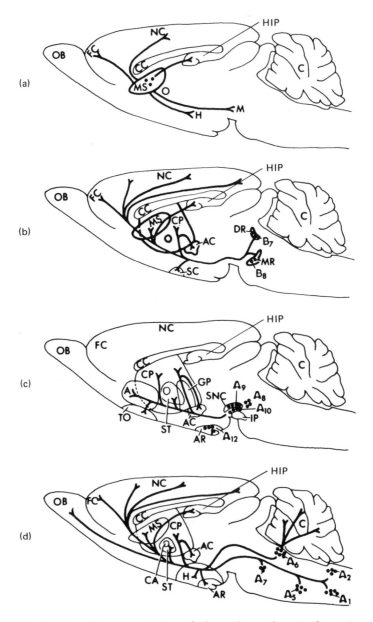

FIGURE 2.6. Schematic representation of the major pathways of putative synaptic transmitters in brain. Black dots represent the location of cell bodies and solid lines the pathways. Cell bodies are numbered according to Dahlstrom and Fuxe (1964), the letter A indicating catecholamine and the letter B serotonin cell bodies. (Reprinted by permission from J. A. Harvey, Discussion: Use of the ablation method in the pharmacological analysis of thirst. In A. N. Epstein, H. D. Kissileff, and E. Stellar [Eds.], *The Neuropsychology of Thirst,* p. 298. Copyright © 1973 by V. H. Winston and Sons.)

FIGURE 2.6a. Cholinergic pathways (Lewis & Shute, 1967; Shute & Lewis, 1967. The dorsal and ventral tegmental pathways have not been verified and so are not shown in the figure.): (1) Dorsal tegmental pathway. From cells located in nucleus cuniformis to tectum and thalamus. (2) Ventral tegmental pathway. From cells located in ventral tegmental area and substantia nigra to subthalamus, hypothalamus, and basal forebrain areas. (3) Septal projections. From cells in medial septal nuclei to the hippocampus, and from cells within the septal area (origin not certain) to cerebral cortex, hypothalamus, and mesencephalon.

FIGURE 2.6b. Serotonergic pathways: Forebrain pathway. From cells located in the dorsal and median raphe nuclei (B_7 and B_8) via the ventral tegmentum and medial forebrain bundle and innervating: suprachiasmatic nucleus and entire telencephalon including septum, caudate-putamen, amygdala, hippocampus, cingulate cortex, and entire neocortex.

FIGURE 2.6c. Dopaminergic pathways:(1) Nigrostriatal bundle. From cells located in the pars compacta of the substantia nigra (A_9) and in ventral tegmentum (A_8) via the ventral tegmentum, medial forebrain bundle, internal capsule, and globus pallidus to the caudate-putamen, and amygdala. (2) Mesolimbic pathway. From cells located dorsal to the interpeduncular nucleus (A_{10}) via the ventral tegmentum and medial forebrain bundle to the accumbens nucleus, interstitial nucleus of the stria terminalis, dorsal part, and olfactory tubercle. (3) Tuberoinfundibular pathway. From cells in arcuate nucleus (A_{12}) to the external layer of the median eminence.

FIGURE 2.6d. Noradrenergic pathways: (1) Dorsal pathway. From cells located primarily in locus coeruleus (A_6) via ventral tegmentum and medial forebrain bundle and innervating; cerebellum, geniculate bodies, thalamic nuclei, hypothalamus (sparse), and entire telencephalon including septum, caudate-putamen, amygdala, hyppocampus, cingulate cortex, and entire neocortex. (2) Ventral pathway. From cells located primarily in medulla oblongata and pons (cell groups A_1, A_2, A_5, A_7) via the ventral tegmentum and medial forebrain bundle and innnervating: the brainstem, especially hypothalamic structures such as dorsomedial, periventricular, paraventricular, supraoptic, arcuate and preoptic nuclei, as well as the area ventral to the fornix and median eminence.

Abbreviations used in text figure: A, accumbens nucleus; AC, central amygdaloid nucleus; AR, arcuate nucleus; C, cerebellum; CA, anterior commissure; CC, corpus callosum; CP, caudate-putamen; DR, dorsal raphe nucleus; FC, frontal cortex; GP globus pallidus; H, hypothalamus; HIP, hippocampus; IP, interpeduncular nucleus; M, mesencephalon; MR, median raphe nucleus; MS medial septal nucleus; NC, neocortex; OB, olfactory bulb; SC, suprachiasmatic nucleus; SNC, substantia nigra, pars compacta; ST, interstitial nucleus of the stria terminalis; TO, olfactory tubercle.

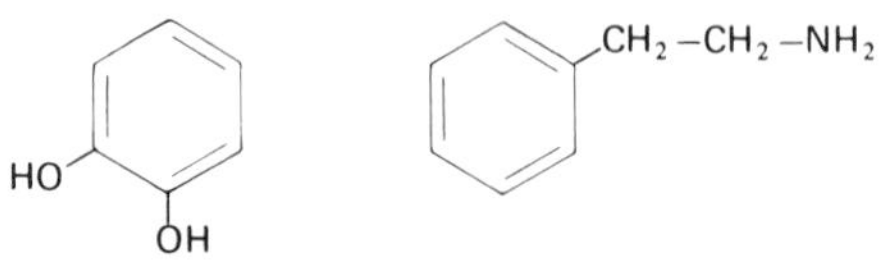

FIGURE 2.7. Structural basis of catecholamines.

esterases will hydrolyze not only ACh but other similar chemicals. However, two general types of cholinesterase are usually specified; acetylcholinesterase (AChE) and butyrocholinesterase (also called pseudocholinesterase) (ChE). The former is found primarily in nervous tissue and the latter in nonneural tissue. Because of the widespread distribution of cholinesterase in the body, and the relative nonspecificity of cholinesterase activity, simple tissue levels of AChE or ChE have been poor indicators of a functional ACh "system" (Cooper et al., 1974, Ch. 4; Koelle, 1963).

Catecholamines

The structural basis of the catecholamines (CAs) is a catechol nucleus (a 6-carbon benzene ring with two adjacent hydroxyl groups attached to it). The catecholamines then have an ethylamine group (CH_2-CH_2-NH_2) attached to the catechol nucleus (the parent compound for the CAs, containing a benzene ring and ethylamine group, but lacking the adjacent hydroxyl groups on the ring, is called phenylethylamine; Figure 2.7). The catecholamines of most interest to psychopharmacologists are the two neurotransmitter candidates, norepinephrine (NE) and dopamine (D) and the adrenal medullary hormone, epinephrine (E) (Axelrod, 1971; von Euler, 1971).

Synthesis. In mammals, tyrosine, the amino acid precursor of the CAs, can be derived from another amino acid, phenylalanine. Phenylalanine is normally ingested as a constituent of dietary protein and then metabolized in the liver by the enzyme, phenylalanine hydroxylase, to form tyrosine (McGeer, 1971). Since tyrosine itself is usually abundant in the diet, phenylalanine is not required for normal CA functioning and tyrosine is considered the amino acid from which the catecholamines are synthesized. The first step in the CA synthetic pathway is the hydroxylation of tyrosine to dihydroxyphenylalanine (dopa) by the enzyme tyrosine hydroxylase. This reaction occurs within the neuron and is the rate-limiting (slowest) step in the biosynthesis of catecholamines. Drugs which inhibit tyrosine hydroxylase also effectively reduce tissue levels of catecholamines. Tyrosine hydroxylase, in contrast to the other enzymes involved in CA biosynthesis, shows a high degree of substrate specificity (Axelrod, 1971). This means that it acts only on tyrosine and not on other similar amines. Although phenylalanine hydroxylase and tyrosine hydroxylase are functionally similar in that each adds a single hydroxyl group to the benzene ring; they appear to be two distinct enzymes, as both are necessary to convert phenylalanine to dopa.

The next enzyme involved in CA biosynthesis is dihydroxyphenylalanine decarboxylase (dopa decarboxylase) which converts dopa to dopamine (D). This enzyme is also referred to as *aromatic amino acid decarboxylase* (Cooper et al., 1974, Ch. 5) since it is relatively nonspecific with respect to the aromatic amino acids (amino acids containing a ring structure) it will decarboxylate (remove the carboxyl, COOH, group). It will also remove the carboxyl group from histidine, tyrosine, tryptophan, phenylalanine, and 5-hydroxytryptophan. Aromatic amino acid decarboxylase is found in a high concentration in many structures of the body and may also have important roles outside the nervous system.

Dopamine may then be converted to NE by the enzyme dopamine-β-hydroxylase (also called dopamine-β-oxidase). This enzyme is localized in the synaptic vesicles and does not show a high degree of substrate specificity in that it will oxidize almost any phenylethylamine to its corresponding phenylethanolamine (Molinoff, Weinshilboum, & Axelrod, 1971). Aromatic amino acid decarboxylase and dopamine-β-hydroxylase are about 100 to 1,000 times more active enzymatically than is tyrosine hydroxylase.

In the adrenal medulla, NE is *N*-methylated (a methyl, CH_3, group is added to the N, nitrogen, ion) to epinephrine by phenylethanolamine-*N*-methyl-transferase (PNMT). This enzyme is largely restricted to the adrenal medulla, although it is also found to have a low level of activity in some brain sites (White, Handler, & Smith, 1968, Chs. 4–5). Figure 2.8 depicts this biosynthetic pathway for the catecholamines.

In general, the degree of adrenergic activity in the PNS or CNS does not change the endogenous levels of NE. The reason for this is thought to be the existence of a homeostatic mechanism that maintains a constant transmitter level in adrenergic nerve endings, regardless of the level of activity (Costa & Neff, 1970). Apparently this homeostatic feedback is accomplished by means of end product inhibition, so that a high level of NE feeds back to inhibit tyrosine hydroxylase activity and a low NE level, due to adrenergic activity, releases the enzyme from this inhibition (Weiner, 1970). This mechanism of end product inhibition by which the final chemical in a synthetic pathway can act on an early enzyme in the pathway to inhibit further manufacture, is an efficient means of maintaining optimal levels of transmitters and other substances and is found for many biochemical systems.

Distribution. Norepinephrine was identified as the transmitter substance in postganglionic sympathetic nerves by von Euler in 1946. Vogt then showed in 1954 that brain NE was concentrated in the hypothalamus. Dopamine was identified in the brain in 1957 and was found to have a distribution different from that of NE. This differential distribution suggests that D is not simply present as a precursor of NE, but may also function as a transmitter itself in some systems (Hornykiewicz, 1966). The concentration of E is relatively low in mammalian brain, being about 10% of the NE content. However, certain brain areas such as the olfactory bulb contain substantial amounts of

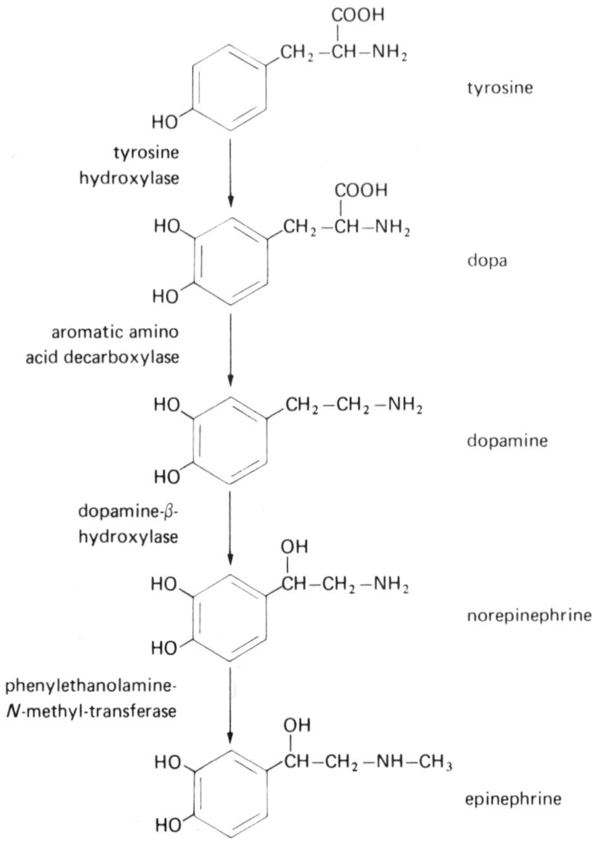

FIGURE 2.8. Primary pathway in the formation of catecholamines.

phenylethanolamine-*N*-methyl-transferase and are capable of synthesizing E, suggesting that E might have some transmitter role in the neural mediation of olfaction.

The distribution of the CAs has recently been analyzed in detail using a histochemical fluorescence technique (Fuxe, Hokfelt, & Ungerstedt, 1970a, 1770b; Hillarp, Fuxe, and Dahlström, 1966; Ungerstedt, 1971b). This method is based on the discovery that the amines can be converted into strongly fluorescent compounds if exposed to formaldehyde gas in the presence of protein (Falck, Hillarp, Thieme, & Torp, 1962). Using this technique, nerve cell bodies that contain concentrations of catecholamines have been located in the brainstem. These nerve cell bodies give rise to fibers which divide into fine terminal branches when they reach the brain area to be innervated. The fluorescence in the terminals is concentrated on small enlargements of the terminal branches. These enlargements contain extremely small amounts of amines, but because of the small size of the enlargements, enormous concentrations are reached. Almost the entire amine content of the brain is present in these enlargements. The amines appear to be present in granules or vesicles within these enlargements and the evidence suggests that these amine-containing vesicles are produced in the cell bodies and transported down to the terminals via the axons (Bloom, 1970). It is necessary to differentiate the D nerve terminals from the NE nerve terminals by the use of a number of pharmacological tests because the fluorescent compounds formed from D and NE are similar in color and appearance (Bjorkland, Ehinger, & Falck, 1968). The CNS distributions of D and NE are illustrated in Figures 2.6c and 2.6d.

The dopaminergic neuron systems consist of pathways ascending from cell bodies in the brainstem, primarily the substantia nigra (a nuclear group involved in motor coordination), to certain forebrain structures. Some of these fibers ascend as a part of the fiber system called the *medial forebrain bundle* (MFB) to terminate either in the forebrain or on the capillaries of the pituitary portal system. The D system terminating in the pituitary portal system participates in the regulation of gonadotropin secretion (see Chapters 11 and 12). Another ascending system that passes above the MFB is called the *nigrostriatal bundle* and innervates the basal ganglia, terminating in the caudate nucleus and putamen (Ungerstedt, 1971b). This neuron system containing D, with cell bodies in the substantia nigra and terminals in the basal ganglia, has been implicated in the control of motor coordination (Ungerstedt & Arbuthnott, 1970). Patients suffering from Parkinsonism, a disease characterized by defects in coordination (rigidity and tremors), have been found upon autopsy to have abnormally low concentrations of D in these brain structures (see Chapter 3).

The NE-containing cell bodies are found primarily in the lateral part of the reticular formation of the pons and medulla. Some noradrenergic nerve fibers descend from this region in the anterior and lateral fiber bundles of the spinal cord to innervate the gray matter of the ventral horn. These fibers have some role in the control of movement. There are also two ascending systems. One travels in the medial forebrain bundle to innervate the hypothalamus and other related limbic system structures. This fiber system appears to be the major substrate for self-stimulation reward and defective functioning may precipitate mental disorders (see Chapter 3). The other ascending system begins in the locus coeruleus of the brainstem reticular formation and travels above the medial forebrain bundle to innervate the hippocampus and cerebral cortex. This fiber system has been implicated in the control of sleep (Jouvet, 1969).

Storage and release. Most of the NE present in the brain is located in specialized cellular structures sometimes called *granules* (or vesicles). These vesicles also contain the enzyme, dopamine-β-hydroxylase. They appear to bind and store NE and serve as a depot for the transmitter, thus protecting it from enzymatic destruction. NE is probably formed from D within these vesicles, which are believed to be formed in the neuron cell bodies and transported to the nerve terminals by axoplasmic flow (Dahlstrom, 1970; Dahlstrom & Haggendal, 1966).

Much of our knowledge of the mechanism of CA release comes from the study of the adrenal medulla. It has not been possible to determine the mechanism of transmitter release in the CNS because of its relative inaccessibility and complexity. In the adrenal medulla, it is believed that the ACh secreted by sympathetic preganglionic neurons combines with receptors on the membranes of the CA-containing cells and produces a change in membrane protein conformation. This may then alter the membrane permeability to calcium ions,

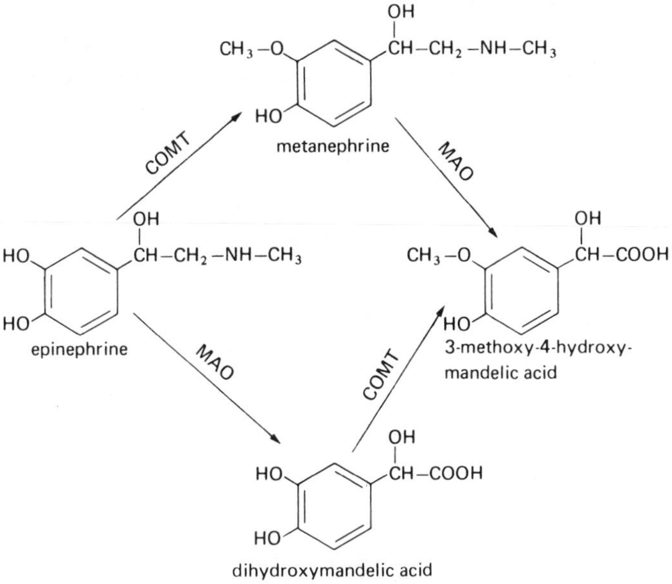

FIGURE 2.9. Metabolic degradation of the catecholamines.

which move inward. The inward flow of calcium is then believed to be the stimulus causing CA mobilization and secretion (Simpson, 1968).

Inactivation. The actions of CAs at the postsynaptic receptors are believed to be terminated by several mechanisms (Glowinski & Baldessarini, 1966). The decreased concentration of the amine in the synaptic cleft may be the result of (1) diffusion away from the receptor area, (2) enzymatic destruction, or (3) active uptake (usually called *reuptake*) into the presynaptic nerve terminal.

The enzymatic destruction of the catecholamines is carried out by two enzymes, monoamine oxidase (MAO) and catechol-*O*-methyltransferase (COMT) (Figure 2.9). MAO is located both intraneuronally and extraneuronally (Goridis & Neff, 1971); whereas COMT is located primarily extraneuronally. COMT converts norepinephrine and dopamine to their inactive 3-methoxy derivatives, normetanephrine and methoxytyramine. In the adrenal medulla COMT also converts epinephrine to metanephrine. Although extraneuronal MAO may deaminate the catecholamines or their O-methyl derivatives, this enzyme is not believed to play an important role in terminating the actions of the catecholamines in the synaptic cleft. MAO is believed primarily to destroy catecholamines that leak out of the storage vesicles but remain in the intracellular fluid. COMT is the primary destruction mechanism for extra-neuronal catecholamines (Axelrod, 1971; Glowinski & Baldessarini, 1966).

However, it is thought that the primary mechanism for removing synaptically excreted catecholamines is not by metabolic degradation, but rather by their reuptake back into the presynaptic terminal for reutilization. The processes of

CA reuptake should be further differentiated (Anden, Carlsson, & Haggendal, 1969). There are two separate uptake processes in catecholamine-containing neurons. One, located in the neuronal membrane, actively transports catecholamines and certain other amines into the neuron. The other uptake system is located in the membrane of the synaptic vesicles and transports intraneuronal (but extravesicular) catecholamines into the vesicles. This method of terminating the postsynaptic actions of the CAs is analogous to the uptake of choline by cholinergic neurons. Both reuptake processes provide a means of conserving and "recycling" bodily biochemical resources.

5-Hydroxytryptamine (5HT, Serotonin)

5HT is widely distributed in the tissues of both vertebrates and invertebrates. It was initially studied because of its role as a vasoconstrictor substance found in the blood plasma (hence its name *sero*tonin from *ser*um) and because of its high concentration in the intestinal mucosa. Approximately 98% of the body's 5HT is found in the gastrointestinal tract and in the blood platelets. The remaining 1% or 2% of endogenous 5HT is found in the CNS and most of this is located in the pineal gland which actually is peripheral to the blood-brain barrier (Cooper et al., 1974, Ch. 7). It appears, however, that the small amount of 5HT found in the CNS is synthesized there since 5HT does not readily penetrate the blood-brain barrier. Although many experiments on the behavioral role of 5HT have been undertaken, and this agent has been the subject of much speculation, its functional role remains unclear (Brodie & Reid, 1968; Moore, 1971). Behavioral roles for 5HT will be discussed in several of the subsequent chapters.

Synthesis. The first step in the synthesis of 5HT involves the active uptake of tryptophan, into the neuron. Tryptophan is an amino acid obtained from dietary protein. The structural basis of tryptophan is a complex organic double ring called an *indole*, containing one nitrogen atom (White, Handler, & Smith, 1968). The tryptophan is then hydroxylated to 5-hydroxytryptophan (5HTP) by the enzyme, tryptophan hydroxylase. This is the rate-limiting step in the synthesis of 5HT (Koe, 1971). The 5HTP is then decarboxylated to 5HT by aromatic amino acid decarboxylase, the same enzyme that decarboxylates dopa in the catecholamine pathway (Figure 2.10).

In the pineal gland, 5HT is further metabolized to melatonin in a two-step reaction. First, the 5HT is converted by 5HT-*N*-acetylase to *N*-acetylserotonin. Then an enzyme called 5-hydroxyindole-*O*-methyl-transferase converts this intermediate to melatonin. These two converting enzymes and also melatonin are only found in the pineal gland, which also contains about 50 times as much 5HT as that found in whole brain (on a per-gram-of-tissue basis). Melatonin is a skin-lightening agent; its production is partially controlled by the light cycle, and it appears to have a role in sexual physiology and behavior (Axelrod, 1974; Wurtman, Axelrod, & Phillips, 1963).

Distribution. 5HT can be identified in tissues by the same histochemical fluorescence technique used for the catecholamines. 5HT-containing cell bodies

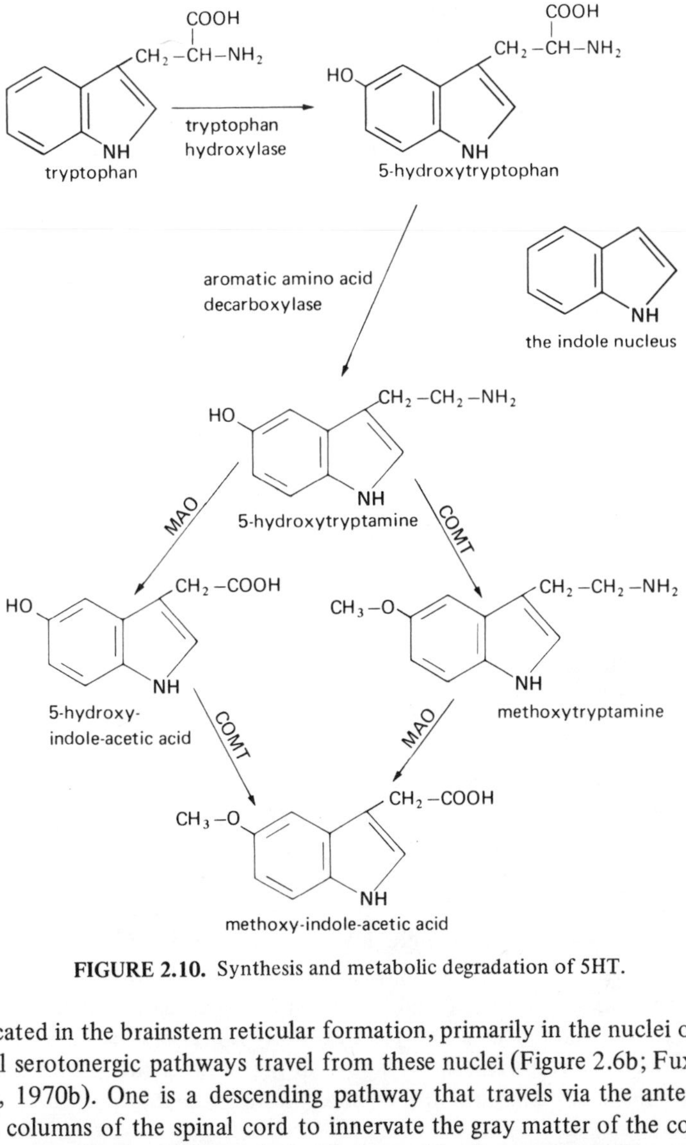

FIGURE 2.10. Synthesis and metabolic degradation of 5HT.

are located in the brainstem reticular formation, primarily in the nuclei of raphe. Several serotonergic pathways travel from these nuclei (Figure 2.6b; Fuxe et al., 1970a, 1970b). One is a descending pathway that travels via the anterior and lateral columns of the spinal cord to innervate the gray matter of the cord. This system probably has some role in the control of movement. The ascending serotonergic pathways travel through the lateral hypothalamic area in the medial forebrain bundle (in close proximity to the ascending noradrenergic pathway) to innervate the basal ganglia and cerebral cortex. One role of the ascending systems may be to participate with an ascending noradrenergic pathway in the control of sleep (Jouvet, 1969).

Inactivation. In the brain, 5HT is oxidatively deaminated by MAO (which appears to be identical to the MAO that deactivates the catecholamines) to form

5-hydroxyindoleacetic acid (5HIAA) (Meek & Fuxe, 1971). COMT may also be involved in 5HT metabolism (Figure 2.10). The concentration of 5HT appears to be under feedback control (end product inhibition) as is the case with the other transmitters (Macon et al., 1971). Central 5HT turnover can be inferred from measurement of 5HIAA in cerebrospinal fluid.

Gamma-Aminobutyric Acid (GABA)

The mammalian brain contains nearly eight times as much amino acids as blood plasma, and nearly one-seventh of this is GABA. GABA is localized exclusively in the CNS and the retina of the eye (which is morphologically an extension of the brain (Cooper et al., 1974, Ch. 8). It appears unlikely that GABA leaves the brain intact since no other physiological tissue contains more than a trace of this amino acid. Although conclusive proof of the role this compound plays in the mammalian CNS is lacking, much evidence supports the hypothesis that GABA is an inhibitory transmitter (Iverson, 1970).

Synthesis. GABA is formed by the decarboxylation of the amino acid, glutamic acid. This reaction is catalyzed by glutamic acid decarboxylase (GAD). This appears to be the only pathway for GABA formation in brain and this enzyme is found only in the CNS of mammals (with a distribution paralleling that of GABA; see Figure 2.11).

Distribution. In vertebrates the highest levels of GABA are found in the substantia nigra, globus pallidus, hypothalamus, and the superior and inferior colliculi of the midbrain. In the cerebral cortex and cerebellum, GABA is found primarily in areas involved in inhibitory synaptic functions (the outer layers of the cerebral cortex and the Purkinje cells of the cerebellum) (Fahn & Cote, 1968). Application of GABA to these areas mimics the hyperpolarizing potential changes found after naturally elicited inhibitory-postsynaptic potentials.

Further metabolism of GABA. There seems to be no mechanism for the rapid destruction of GABA, nor has a rapid reuptake mechanism been demonstrated. GABA is intimately involved in the oxidative metabolism of carbohydrates in the CNS by means of the "GABA shunt" involving its production from glutamic acid and its metabolism to succinic semialdehyde and then to succinic acid (which enters the tricarboxylic acid or Krebs cycle).

GABA as a neurotransmitter. There is strong evidence that GABA functions as a transmitter at inhibitory nerve endings to crustacean muscle fibers and

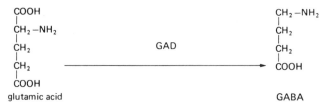

FIGURE 2.11. Decarboxylation of glutamic acid to GABA.

stretch receptors (Cooper et al., 1974, Ch. 8; Kravitz, 1967; Roberts & Kuriyama, 1968). This invertebrate neurotransmitter role may be considered indirect evidence for neurotransmitter function in the mammalian nervous system. However, it is especially difficult to conclude a mammalian neurotransmitter role for GABA and the other amino acids since they also have general metabolic roles. Although there is good evidence for the production and storage of GABA in the mammalian CNS (DeFeudis et al., 1970), and GABA possesses inhibitory pharmacological activity when applied to the CNS, an association with specific inhibitory pathways has yet to be demonstrated.

Other Endogenous Compounds
with Neuropharmacological Activity

A number of other endogenous substances that are found in the CNS possess neuropharmacological activity and may function as synaptic transmitters or as modulators of synaptic activity (Cooper et al., 1974, Chs. 8 & 9).

Glycine. This amino acid may function as an inhibitory transmitter in the mammalian spinal cord (Aprison & Werman, 1968). It is found there, especially in gray matter, in high concentrations. Found in association with inhibitory interneurons, glycine hyperpolarizes motor neurons to the same level as normal postsynaptic inhibition. Furthermore, strychnine, a drug which blocks the action of glycine, also blocks postsynaptic inhibition.

Histamine. This substance is found in certain mammalian CNS locations (especially the hypothalamus and pituitary gland), peripheral nerves, and sensory receptors, as well as throughout the body. Histamine is formed in the brain from the amino acid, histidine, by the action of an enzyme called histidine decarboxylase (Cooper et al., 1974, Ch. 9; Douglas, 1970). Histamine has wide distribution in body tissue and is involved in the body's defense reaction to foreign substances. Its metabolism in the brain is influenced by centrally active drugs such as reserpine and chlorpromazine, and the chemical may function in the CNS as a modulator of neural firing. Recently, injection of histamine into the lateral hypothalamus of rats has been found to inhibit electrical self-stimulation (Cohn, Ball, & Hirsch, 1973; also see Chapter 3 in this book), suggesting perhaps a modulatory role in the neural substrate of reward.

Other amino acids. Both glutamic and aspartic acids are found in the CNS in significant quantities and have excitant properties when pharmacologically applied (Johnson & Aprison, 1970). However, these amino acids demonstrate a rather nonselective ability to activate neural discharges and do not show an asymmetric distribution, suggesting a general role in synaptic transmission.

Prostaglandins. These lipids were first isolated from human seminal plasma and sheep seminal vesicles. Their release in peripheral tissues appears related to neural activity and they may have a neuromodulator role (Cooper et al., 1974, Ch. 9). Several different prostaglandins have now been isolated from the

CNS and they have been found to be widely distributed. They are released by electrical brain stimulation and a number of psychoactive drugs and cause changes in transmitter activity when applied to brain. Catatonia and somnolence have been produced by perfusing prostaglandins into the ventricles of the cat. These agents are being investigated on a number of fronts (analgesia, contraception, temperature regulation) and appear to have an important role in cellular metabolism.

Adenosine 3', 5'-monophosphate (cyclic AMP). Sutherland recently received the Nobel prize for his work demonstrating the role of cyclic AMP in cellular functioning. It appears to be the mediator of a variety of hormone actions at the cellular level, such as epinephrine-stimulated glycogenolysis in skeletal muscle (the production of glucose from glycogen), the secretion of insulin, lipolysis in fat cells (the production of glucose from fat), and the release of thyroid-stimulating hormone.

Of all mammalian tissues, brain has the highest levels of adenylate cyclase, the enzyme that catalyzes the synthesis of cyclic AMP from adenosine triphosphate (ATP), and also of phosphodiesterase, the enzyme that inactivates cyclic AMP. The formation and degradation of cyclic AMP in the nervous system, furthermore, have been shown to be regulated by the same factors that affect impulse transmission by neurons.

The application on NE, 5HT, or histamine in vitro to brain slices alters neuronal firing by combining with certain receptors on the neurons, apparently then stimulating the activity of adenylate cyclase. Cyclic AMP release appears to be an intermediate step between activation of receptors on the neuron and the firing of the cell, for the synapses of noradrenergic neurons from the locus coeruleus onto the Purkinje cells of the cerebellum, for dopaminergic synapses in the basal ganglia, and for certain dopaminergic interneuron synapses in ANS sympathetic ganglia. It may be that cyclic AMP is an intermediate between receptor binding and cell response for many or all of the neurotransmitter systems in the nervous system (Glessa et al., 1970; Marx, 1972; Sutherland, 1972). However, see Lake and Jordan (1974) for contrary evidence.

Brain-specific substances. A number of investigators are attempting to isolate and identify substances found only in the CNS. Such substances may be found to have a unique role in brain function. Several have been isolated and are currently under study (Cooper et al., 1974, Ch. 9).

Substance P is a polypeptide, isolated from brain, whose physiological function is obscure. Pharmacologically, it has been shown to have smooth muscle contraction and vasodilator properties. Although Substance P has a localized distribution in brain tissue, it has not been conclusively shown to have any significant effect when administered to the CNS.

Ergothioneine is a substance that has been found in cerebellar extracts and optic nerve and that increases cerebellar electrical activity when injected into the cerebral circulation.

PSYCHOACTIVE DRUGS AND SYNAPTIC TRANSMISSION

There are numerous ways in which a drug can alter synaptic transmission. Some of these mechanisms of drug action have already been mentioned. The specific effects of drugs on cholinergic, catecholaminergic, and serotonergic systems, warrant a detailed treatment in order to understand how psychoactive drugs influence these major biochemical systems of the CNS.

Mechanisms of Drug Action

Most psychoactive drugs achieve their effects by some alteration of synaptic transmission (Koelle, 1971). Alterations in neural firing can result when a drug modifies the synthesis, storage, release, reuptake, or degradation of the synaptic transmitter. Furthermore, drugs can influence neural firing by altering impulse conduction within the neuron by affecting membrane ionic permeabilities or cellular metabolism. Other drugs may mimic the actions of the transmitter at the postsynaptic receptor sites or combine with the receptors, without actually triggering the neural impulse. These last drugs are called competitive inhibitors.

One can readily see from the previous sections of this chapter that the events involved in neural conduction and synaptic transmission are indeed quite complex. Many different substances must interact in a precise sequence and to a particular degree to assure normal neural functioning. Psychoactive drugs can facilitate or inhibit neural conduction and synaptic transmission by acting on any or all of the participants in a particular reaction. Furthermore, the original substance may undergo several subsequent reactions in a sequence so that an effect early in the sequence, or pathway, may be greatly magnified later in the sequence. By modifying the rate at which each reaction proceeds and then observing the organism's behavior we are able to infer what function the intermediates play in behavior (Cooper et al., 1974).

Drugs and Cholinergic Transmission

Receptor types. In the PNS, ACh is the synaptic transmitter at all autonomic ganglia (both sympathetic and parasympathetic), at the neuroeffector junctions of the postganglionic parasympathetic fibers, and at the neuromuscular junction between the somatic nervous system motor neurons and skeletal muscle (Triggle, 1965; also see the section entitled "Synaptic Transmission in the Peripheral Nervous System," earlier in this chapter, and Figure 2.4).

These three PNS sites differ from each other, however, with regard to their interactions with acetylcholine substitutes and antagonists. One drug, muscarine, mimics ACh at smooth muscle, cardiac muscle, and glands (neuroeffector junctions), without affecting ganglionic transmission or skeletal muscles; while a second drug, nicotine, selectively stimulates autonomic ganglia and also skeletal muscles. Therefore, a muscarinic cholinergic drug affects the parasympathetic neuroeffector junction, whereas a nicotinic cholinergic drug affects autonomic ganglia and the neuromuscular junction (skeletal muscle).

Another class of drugs selectively blocks cholinergic synapses by competitive inhibition; for example, the cholinergic postganglionic neuroeffector junction is blocked by atropine or scopolamine, the neuromuscular junction is blocked by curare, and autonomic ganglia may be blocked by the drug, hexamethonium (Goth, 1974, Chs. 9-11; Innes & Nickerson, 1970b; Koelle, 1970a, 1970b, 1970c, 1970d; Volle, 1966; Volle & Koelle, 1970). The existence of these drugs, which selectively stimulate or inhibit only at certain of the cholinergic synapses, suggests that there are structural and functional differences at these sites; all cholinergic synapses are not alike (Schechter & Rosencrans, 1971). Since as far as is known, all presynaptic neurons produce an identical ACh, it seems likely that the major differences have to do with properties of the receptors located on the postsynaptic membrane (Koelle, 1970b).

Cholinergic facilitators. A variety of drugs increases cholinergic activity both in the PNS and the CNS. Muscarine and nicotine will each mimic ACh at some, but not all, CNS cholinergic sites. This finding suggests that CNS cholinergic sites may also be distinguishable as muscarinic and nicotinic. Pilocarpine is an alkaloid (a chemical found in plants, as are muscarine and nicotine) which mimics the stimulant actions of ACh on postsynaptic receptors. Pilocarpine differs in action, however, from muscarine and nicotine in that it is effective at both muscarinic and nicotinic sites in the PNS and CNS. A number of drugs, called *choline esters*, have very similar chemical structures to ACh, and mimic this chemical transmitter, to some extent, at all of its sites of activity. Unlike the alkaloids, these choline esters, of which carbachol is an example, are not found in nature, but are synthesized (Koelle, 1970d).

Several drugs increase central and peripheral cholinergic activity by combining with AChE, thus inhibiting the enzymatic destruction of ACh. Two types of such cholinesterase inhibitors are usually recognized. One type is called *reversible inhibitors*. The bond between these agents (physostigmine and neostigmine are examples) and the AChE is temporary, thus the AChE is eventually released and again available for ACh metabolism. The other type of cholinesterase inhibitor is irreversible. Since these agents (diisopropyl fluorophosphate [DFP] is an example) do not unbind from the AChE, their action is prolonged; new AChE must be synthesized in order for ACh to be metabolized. It is interesting to point out that both of these groups of cholinesterase inhibitors can be considered as competitive blockers of ACh. However, due to some unknown property, they compete with ACh for AChE rather than for the postsynaptic receptor sites. These agents increase cholinergic activity by competing with ACh for AChE, while the receptor blocking agents decrease cholinergic activity by competing with ACh for the postsynaptic receptor sites.

Cholinergic inhibitors. There are a variety of ways in which both PNS and CNS cholinergic transmission can be blocked. The receptor blocking agents, such as atropine, curare, and hexamethonium, are also each effective at some CNS

TABLE 2.1

Drugs and the Cholinergic Synapse

Site or function	Increase cholinergic activity	Decrease cholinergic activity
Neuroeffector junctions	Muscarine	Atropine Scopolamine
Autonomic ganglia	Nicotine	Hexamethonium
Neuromuscular junctions	Nicotine	Curare
ACh mimickers	Pilocarpine Carbachol	
Cholinesterase inhibitors	Physostigmine Neostigmine DFP	
Choline transport inhibitor		Hemicholinium
ACh release inhibitor		Botulin toxin

sites, again suggesting an organization of CNS cholinergic receptor types along similar lines to the PNS receptor types. Hemicholinium is a drug that inhibits the transport of choline into the nerve terminal, thus inhibiting the manufacture of ACh. The release of ACh from the presynaptic endings is blocked by botulin toxin. This toxin consists of proteins liberated by the microorganism *Clostridium botulinum*. These proteins are among the deadliest poisons known and have been responsible for numerous deaths due to "food poisoning." Some of the drugs that alter cholinergic transmission and their mechanisms of action are listed in Table 2.1. The cholinergic drugs and their physiological and behavioral actions will be discussed in detail in Chapter 4.

Drugs and Catecholamine Transmission

The postganglionic PNS sympathetic fibers secrete NE. An exception to this rule is the sympathetic postganglionic fibers to the sweat glands and certain facial blood vessels that are involved in blushing. These postganglionic sympathetic fibers anomalously secrete ACh. Another unusual case is the sympathetic innervation of the adrenal medulla. The sympathetic neurons synapsing on the secretory cells of this gland are preganglionic, and, therefore, secrete ACh. The adrenal medulla, then, which is analogous to sympathetic postganglionic fibers, secretes E as well as smaller amounts of NE (see Chapter 11 of this book and also Triggle, 1965).

Receptor types. Many adrenergic receptors in both the PNS and the CNS may be classified into two different types as either alpha receptors or beta receptors (Ahlquist, 1948). This classification system is based on experiments showing that adrenergic stimulants and blockers are most effective only at certain adrenergic receptor sites (Fitzgerald, 1969; Nickerson, 1970). For example, NE is a potent alpha stimulant, isoproterenol is a beta stimulant, and E is effective at both types of receptor sites (Innes & Nickerson, 1970a).

Receptor blocking agents (competitive inhibitors) tend to be much more effective at one of the two receptor sites. Phentolamine and phenoxybenzamine, for example, are potent alpha blockers, while propranolol is a potent beta blocker (Fitzgerald, 1969; Nickerson, 1970). As with the cholinergic system, these selective drug effects suggest that there are structural and functional differences between the postsynaptic receptors at alpha and beta sites. This subject, and the nature of these alpha- and beta-receptor functions, will be discussed in Chapter 3.

Adrenergic stimulants. Many drugs act by enhancing or mimicking the activity of catecholamines (Baldessarini & Kopin, 1967; Glowinski & Baldessarini, 1966; Snyder, 1970; Sulser & Sanders-Bush, 1971). Drugs can mimic CA effects either by combining with the receptors (direct-acting amines: NE, E, D, isoproterenol) or by releasing CAs from presynaptic nerve terminals (indirect-acting amines: tyramine, amphetamine) (Carr & Moore, 1969; Glowinski & Baldessarini, 1966; Innes & Nickerson, 1970a).

COMT inhibitors. Although the enzyme COMT is thought to be the major extraneuronal metabolizer of catecholamines, inhibition of COMT (for example, with pyrogallol) does not increase the effectiveness of sympathetic nerve stimulation or catecholaminergic drugs. In some cases the effect of dopa in humans has been potentiated by a COMT inhibitor (Ericsson, 1971). However, in general, deactivation of the CAs by COMT seems less important than deactivation by MAO or presynaptic reuptake. Therefore, investigators wishing to prolong CA activity usually attempt to accomplish this end by means of inhibitors of MAO or presynaptic reuptake.

Antidepressants: MAO inhibitors and tricyclics. MAO is located both within the neuron and extracellularly, but is believed to control primarily the intraneuronal concentration of amines. The brain content of NE, D, and also 5HT increases when MAO is inhibited by drugs (iproniazid, nialamide). These MAO inhibitors frequently induce signs of CNS stimulation and elevated mood, and also potentiate the actions of exogenous NE and D, or their precursors, on peripheral sympathetic effector organs (Hendley & Snyder, 1968; Jarvik, 1970).

The tricyclic antidepressants (imipramine) are a group of drugs that, like the MAO inhibitors, produce CNS stimulation and elevated mood (Kety, 1959, 1966). In moderate doses these agents have little effect on the normal behavior of animals or humans. However, they exhibit antidepressant properties when administered to sedated animals or to emotionally depressed humans. The mechanism of action of these compounds is believed to be related to a slowing down of the reuptake of NE by the presynaptic nerve terminals, thereby allowing a more prolonged activation of postsynaptic receptors (Jarvik, 1970). The local anesthetic, cocaine, also has central excitatory properties which may result from slowing the reuptake of NE by presynaptic nerve terminals.

Synthesis inhibitors: False transmitters. Since dopamine-β-hydroxylase contains copper ions, its activity may be inhibited by compounds that themselves bind to copper, such as disulfiram (Cooper et al., 1974, Ch. 6). This drug inhibits the conversion of D to NE and produces a reduction in brain NE together with a concomitant increase in brain D.

Inhibitors of tyrosine hydroxylase, the rate-limiting step in CA synthesis, disrupt the synthesis of dopa, D, NE, and E (Kopin, 1968). Alphamethyl-paratyrosine (AMPT) or 3-iodotyrosine, analogues of tyrosine, inhibit this enzyme in vitro and reduce CA tissue stores in vivo. These agents (AMPT and 3-iodotyrosine) disrupt CA functioning because of the formation of false transmitters (Kopin, 1968). The last two enzymes in the biosynthesis of NE are relatively nonspecific and will metabolize many abnormal or exogenous amino acids. These abnormal compounds may then be treated qualitatively the same as the physiological transmitters and this may lead to the storage and release of abnormal compounds from dopaminergic and noradrenergic nerve terminals (Sjoerdsma, 1971). Compounds that are synthesized and stored in place of endogenous catecholamines and subsequently released by nerve stimulation are, therefore, referred to as *false transmitters*. These false transmitters are generally less active than the normal transmitter (at the postsynaptic receptor sites) and may even, by their presence, damage the presynaptic storage vesicles (Groppetti & Costa, 1969: Moore, 1971).

Administration of 6-hydroxydopamine causes an acute degeneration of noradrenergic and dopaminergic nerve terminals in the peripheral and central nervous systems (Laverty & Taylor, 1970; Malmfors & Sachs, 1968; Ungerstedt, 1971a), resulting in sedation and depression when administered to the CNS of animals. This drug is taken up into the nerve terminals, then acts as a false transmitter, and is also toxic, destroying these terminals by causing an acute degeneration (Malmfors & Thoenen, 1971). This drug, 6-hydroxydopamine, has assumed considerable prominence in behavioral research on CA functioning, and its use is discussed in detail in the next chapter.

Release inhibitors. Another way of blocking CA activity is by preventing the release of NE from the terminals of sympathetic neurons. Several drugs, including bretylium (Abbs & Robertson, 1970) and guanethidine (Abbs, 1966), have this action (Boura & Green, 1965).

Vesicular reuptake inhibitors. Metabolic destruction by MAO and COMT is probably not the primary mechanism by which the actions of catecholamines are terminated. Transport back into the presynaptic nerve terminals, and then also into the vesicles, seems to be the primary mechanism for removing catecholamines from the synaptic cleft. It is of major interest that stores of catecholamines can be depleted by a number of drugs that can block vesicular reuptake (Glowinski, 1970; Glowinski & Baldessarini, 1966; Jarvik, 1970). These drugs tend to produce sedation and depression when given to animals or humans. Reserpine depletes tissue stores of catecholamines (NE and D) for 2 weeks or more following a single injection (Giachetti & Shore, 1970). Other compounds have a shorter duration of action. A single injection of tetrabenazine reduces the brain catecholamine content for 1 to 3 days. These compounds do not act at the neuronal membrane to block uptake of CA into the neuron, but instead, they disrupt the transport of intraneuronal CAs into their storage vesicles. Thus, intraneuronal CA is not protected from MAO and is subjected to oxidative deamination. Following administration of reserpine or reserpinelike compounds, CAs are slowly depleted from the brain and peripheral tissues. These CAs are lost from neurons as inactive, deaminated products (deactivated by MAO). Pretreatment with MAO inhibitors may partially prevent this reserpine-induced depletion of CA stores. Reserpine also blocks the uptake of 5HT by the serotonergic storage vesicles (Jarvik, 1970; Koelle, 1970b; Moore, 1971).

Some of the drugs that alter noradrenergic transmission and their mechanisms of action are listed in Table 2.2. The physiological and behavioral roles of CA systems, and the physiological and behavioral actions of the drugs that alter CA activity, will be the subject of many of the chapters to come.

Drugs and Serotonergic Transmission

Receptors for 5HT have been classified into two types, just as have the adrenergic and cholinergic receptors. The M or nervous type is antagonized by morphine or atropine and potentiated by AChE inhibitors, but is unaffected by LSD (Cooper et al., 1974, Ch. 7). The D or muscular type, is antagonized by LSD and related compounds (but not affected by AChE inhibitors).

Reserpine and LSD both have the indole nucleus in common with 5HT. Furthermore, reserpine depletes brain stores of 5HT just as it depletes the catecholamines. These findings led to the question of whether reserpine-induced sedation could be attributed primarily to either CA or 5HT depletion. It was then discovered that AMPT, which is metabolized to form a false transmitter for the CAs, also produces behavioral sedation and a reserpine-type depression. However, parachlorophenylalanine (PCPA), an analogous false transmitter precursor for 5HT, does not produce sedation (Koe & Weissman, 1968; Volicer, 1969). PCPA blocks the synthesis of 5HTP from tryptophan by competing with tryptophan for the enzyme, tryptophan hydroxylase (Bloom & Giarman, 1968). In addition, the finding that PCPA-treated rats that already are devoid of 5HT (but do not exhibit sedation), do then exhibit sedation following reserpine treatment, leads to the conclusion that the sedative effect of reserpine is the result of CA depletion (Bloom & Giarman, 1968).

A possible role for 5HT in the hallucinogenic properties of LSD has been reponsible for much of the interest in 5HT. The finding that LSD interfered with

TABLE 2.2

Drugs and the Noradrenergic Synapse

Site or function	Increase noradrenergic activity	Decrease noradrenergic activity
Alpha receptors	Norepinephrine Epinephrine	Phentolamine Phenoxybenzamine
Beta receptors	Isoproterenol Epinephrine	Propranolol
Indirect-acting amines	Amphetamine Tyramine	
COMT inhibitor	Pyrogallol	
MAO inhibitors	Iproniazid Nialamide	
Presynaptic reuptake inhibitors	Imipramine Cocaine	
Synthesis inhibitors		Disulfiram AMPT 3-Iodotyrosine
Presynaptic terminal degeneration		6-Hydroxydopamine
Release inhibitors		Bretylium Guanethidine
Vesicular reuptake inhibitors		Reserpine Tetrabenazine

the action of 5HT on smooth muscle preparations led to the proposal that an inhibition of brain 5HT by LSD might be the hallucinogenic mechanism. However, since other 5HT blocking agents produce few behavioral effects, this relationship is unclear (Douglas, 1970; Jarvik, 1970). It has even been found that very low concentrations of LSD, rather than blocking 5HT action, could potentiate it.

Many of the drugs that affect CA metabolism also affect 5HT in a similar manner (Meek & Fuxe, 1971). Cocaine and imipramine block the presynaptic reuptake of the CAs and likewise block the reuptake of 5HT. Reserpine and

TABLE 2.3

Drugs and the Serotonergic Synapse

Site or function	Increase serotonergic activity	Decrease serotonergic activity
Nervous-type receptors	AChE inhibitors	Morphine Atropine
Muscular-type receptors		LSD
Presynaptic reuptake inhibitors	Imipramine Cocaine	
MAO inhibitors	Iproniazid Nialamide	
Vesicular reuptake inhibitors		Reserpine Tetrabenazine
Synthesis inhibitor		PCPA

tetrabenazine both deplete tissue stores of the catecholamines and likewise deplete tissue stores of 5HT. The MAO inhibitors increase the available amounts of both the catecholamines and 5HT (Gyermek, 1961). Table 2.3 lists some of the drugs which affect the serotonergic system and their mechanisms of action. Notice the similarities between Tables 2.2 and 2.3.

Drugs and the Other Putative Transmitters

As yet, no specific relationship between the psychoactive drugs and GABA has been established. However, strychnine and picrotoxin, which are behavioral stimulants and convulsants (Chapter 8), block synaptic transmission at inhibitory synapses, and thus, may be inhibiting the action of GABA. Since GABA does not penetrate the blood-brain barrier, it has not been possible to increase its CNS concentration by peripheral administration (Curtis & Watkins, 1965).

Research on drug effects on the other putative transmitters, such as glycine, the prostaglandins, and Substance P is just beginning, and no relationships are yet firmly established.

CONCLUSIONS

The purpose of this chapter has been to provide an introduction to the biochemistry of neuronal activity. The biochemical processes involved in the conduction of the neural impulse down the neuron and transmission across the synapse appear to be the substrates for the behavioral effects on many drugs with psychoactive properties. The reader should now have a general understanding of these neurobiochemical systems. The types of biochemical alterations that drugs can produce have been reviewed with particular emphasis on the cholinergic, catecholaminergic, and serotonergic synaptic transmitter systems. These are complex biochemical systems, but the unraveling of their functioning provides a firm basis for unlocking the "mysteries of the mind." In the chapters ahead we will see that behavioral and physiological studies of these systems, employing drugs as a major tool, are leading to important advances in our understanding of rewards and punishments (Chapters 3 and 4), mental disorders (Chapters 3-6, 8, and 9), pain (Chapter 7), and learning and memory (Chapter 10). Effective pharmacotherapy for a variety of behavioral disorders is also rapidly advancing (Chapters 3-9).

3
ADRENERGIC DRUGS

Robert A. Levitt and Daniel J. Lonowski

INTRODUCTION

With this chapter we begin a comprehensive survey of psychoactive drugs. Viewed from a biological standpoint, psychoactive drugs can be seen to cause profound modifications of the ongoing biochemical and physiological processes of mammalian organisms. The manner in which these physical changes in biological functioning are expressed, however, may be more overtly described in terms of alterations in perceptual, motor, or behavioral phenomena.

The effects of psychoactive drugs are to a large degree dependent on the history and present physiological and environmental status of the organism. Yet, these qualifying factors act more as modulators of the highly specific biological actions characteristic of any psychoactive drug under study. The influence of psychoactive agents on natural or endogenous biochemical processes, therefore, provides a rational basis for studying these chemical compounds.

The adrenergic drugs compose the first group of psychoactive compounds to be considered. These drugs are designated as adrenergic because of their intimate relationship with the sympathetic division of the autonomic nervous system. In this system the adrenergic transmitter norepinephrine (NE) is released from sympathetic postganglionic neurons and also from the adrenal medulla (hence the name *adren*ergic). In contrast, the parasympathetic division of the peripheral nervous system secretes acetylcholine (ACh), the cholinergic transmitter (the subject of Chapter 4).

Biological Homeostasis and Behavior

In the autonomic nervous system, the adrenergic sympathetic and the cholinergic parasympathetic divisions have complementary actions. These actions are generally directed toward the maintenance of biological homeostasis. The term *homeostasis* refers to the maintenance of an optimal level of biological functioning for the survival of the organism. The interaction of the sympathetic and the parasympathetic nervous systems in response to environmental or physiological states exerts corrective changes to maintain a relative biological balance for the organism.

Although physiological events are commonly regarded as operating in the pursuit of biological homeostasis, it is important to recognize that behavioral processes are as much an integral part of homeostatic management as are physiological processes. One might even consider that the traditional dichotomy drawn between physiological and behavioral processes is more definitional than factual. These processes, therefore, should be conceived of as different ways of explaining a single underlying biochemical phenomenon. The events referred to as physiological, biochemical, and behavioral should all be considered as reflections of biological homeostatic demands placed on the organism. These processes are in turn controlled by the organism's needs or motivational state, by the organism's past history and experiences, and by present environmental factors.

In order to illustrate this point, consider an organism deprived of food. In response to food deprivation a series of biological homeostatic processes are activated. These involve autonomic and hormonal changes that help conserve energy and facilitate the conversion of body food stores to usable energy. Furthermore, reflexive or learned food-seeking behavior patterns are activated; or in the absence of food or when food-seeking is prevented, these behavior patterns are deactivated in order to reduce exertion and conserve energy.

Similarly, in hot environments blood flow is channelled to the body surfaces to increase heat removal, and water is conserved as a result of urine retention. An organism will typically show behavior directed towards locating a cooler environment such as a body of water or the shade of a rock or tree. These illustrations are merely two in a multitude of possible examples which show that behavioral processes are as much a reflection of biological homeostatic demands as are biochemical and physiological ones.

Peripheral vs Central Actions

Much of our terminology and knowledge concerning the actions of adrenergic and cholinergic drugs are derived from studies of the sympathetic and parasympathetic nervous systems. In contrast, research into the roles of NE and ACh in the central nervous system (CNS) is more recent and our knowledge of

CNS physiology is more primitive and speculative. Since NE and ACh have been shown to be neurotransmitters in the peripheral nervous system, it is a tempting and a logical extension of this information to propose a similar function for these substances in the CNS. However, study of the central actions of these agents is fraught with difficulty, and a conclusive demonstration of their action in the CNS has not been achieved as yet. Thus, generalizations that adrenergic and cholinergic systems have complementary actions in the CNS, or in the regulation of behavioral processes, should at this point be approached very carefully. This situation is, of course, quite disconcerting to the psychopharmacologist, since it is these CNS actions of the various chemical agents that are of most interest to us. At any rate, such attempts are being made and progress in this area has been achieved.

Endogenous Adrenergic Chemicals

Three related adrenergic compounds are found in mammalian organisms. These substances are dopamine (D), norepinephrine (NE), and epinephrine (E). Each of these chemicals is distributed throughout the body and found to varying degrees in the peripheral and central nervous systems. D and NE are synaptic transmitters, while E is the main hormone of the adrenal medulla.

Three Integrating Concepts

The actions of D, NE, and E in the regulation of homeostasis are complex. However, there appear to be three somewhat distinct phenomena which conceptually can provide an understanding of the overall functions of these adrenergic compounds. The first of these phenomena relates to the role of NE released by the peripheral sympathetic nervous system and of E from the adrenal medulla in reactions to stress and to the press of environmental demands and needs. Several characteristic physiological responses are subserved by these components of the peripheral sympathetic nervous system.

The second phenomenon is related to the effects of centrally produced NE. Brain NE appears to facilitate many physiological and behavioral processes under the control of the CNS. In response to increased levels of brain NE, an organism becomes aroused or alerted, exhibits more activity, and typically shows an augmentation of learning and performance. These behavioral changes are, of course, consistent with the sympathetic function of reacting to stress and emergency demands. Moreover, we will attempt to show that NE acts as a synaptic transmitter in a specialized brain system that underlies the reinforcement of behavior. The arousal, activity, and learning effects may, therefore, reflect the positive reinforcement or "stamping in" role of brain NE. Any deficits in such a system could conceivably result in misdirected behavior patterns (non–goal-directed) and inappropriate behavior in response to reinforcement. Disorders of brain NE have in fact been recently linked to serious mental diseases such as schizophrenia, mania, and depression.

A third and final aspect of adrenergic processes relates to the role of brain D in the mediation of motor functions and certain forms of sensorimotor integration. A deficit of brain dopaminergic systems has been shown to be related to the motor disorder, Parkinson's disease.

To summarize, the three conceptual systems to be employed are the peripheral sympathetic system (NE and E), a CNS reinforcement system (NE), and a CNS motor control system (D). Alterations in any of these systems will influence the status of the organism and set into play a series of modified patterns of behavior. The scope of this chapter, therefore, will be to examine the various drugs which affect the levels of E, NE, and D in therapeutic or experimental situations, and to examine the physiological and behavioral effects of such alterations of endogenous systems.

BIOCHEMICAL CONSIDERATIONS

We will now discuss several matters pertaining to the biochemistry of the actions of adrenergic drugs. These include the ways in which adrenergic drugs are chemically designated, optical isomerism, direct vs indirect mechanisms of action for adrenergic stimulants, and the alpha- and beta-receptor designations.

Chemical Pharmacology

Dopamine, norepinephrine, and epinephrine are biologically active chemicals that are normally found in the body. These three chemicals are commonly referred to as the *catecholamines* (CAs). This term is derived from the fact that D, NE, and E share a basic structure called *catechol* consisting of a benzene ring with two adjacent hydroxyl groups (OH) attached to it (Figure 3.1). The *amine* in catecholamine refers to the fact that each chemical contains nitrogen (N). The biologically active catecholamines are derived from the basic phenylethylamine structure, also shown in Figure 3.1.

Synthetic drugs that have actions on these CA systems, whether facilitative or inhibitory, tend to have considerable chemical similarity to the endogenous chemicals. Small structural differences between drugs, as well as the small structural differences between the endogenous D, NE, and E, have quite significant effects on the actions of the drug or chemical.

Optical isomers. The endogenous chemicals, NE and E, and also many of the adrenergic drugs, may each be found in two different forms which, essentially, are mirror images of each other. That is, a particular chemical, for example NE, may exist in nature in two different states which are mirror images. Both forms of the NE, in this example, would share the chemical structure shown in Figure 3.1; yet, if examined more closely it would be found that the two versions of the compound interact with light in different ways. In general terms, one version would have the property of rotating polarized light waves in a clockwise direction and would be referred to as the *dextro* form of the compound, while the other version would rotate light counterclockwise and be called the *levo*

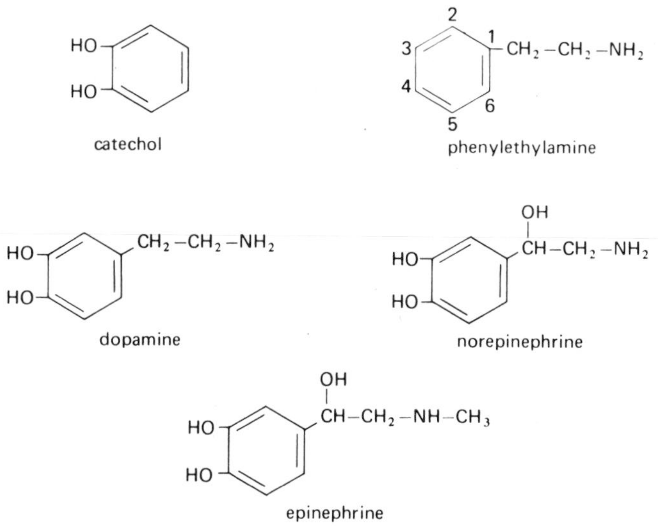

FIGURE 3.1. Catechol, phenylethylamine, and the endogenous CAs.

form of the compound. The slightly different spatial relationship of the structural parts, for instance as in NE, is shown below:

$$\overset{\displaystyle OH}{\overset{|}{-CH-CH_2-NH_2}} \qquad vs \qquad \underset{\displaystyle OH}{\underset{|}{-CH-CH_2-NH_2}}$$

When two chemicals share the same structural formula but exist as mirror images with respect to the direction in which they rotate polarized light, they are said to be *optical isomers* of each other. The endogenous biologically active catecholamines, NE and E, rotate polarized light counterclockwise and are the levo (*l*) isomers of these compounds. The dextro (*d*) isomers are not endogenous, and are without biological activity. Quite often *d* and *l* isomers are combined for pharmacological purposes. When this is done, the compound is called a *racemic mixture*. D does not have two optical forms, since it does not possess the assymetry found with NE and E (Figure 3.1).

Direct vs Indirect Mechanisms of Action

The three endogenous CAs, dopamine, norepinephrine, and epinephrine, achieve their physiological and behavioral effects by directly combining with and stimulating receptors on neurons or effector organs. When naturally produced in the body or when administered to an organism in pharmacological doses, these compounds are said to exert their effects by a *direct action* on receptor sites.

The adrenergic stimulants which are not endogenous to the body may achieve their effects by a similar direct action on receptors. However, they may also achieve their adrenergic-stimulating action by a second mechanism, referred to as an *indirect action*. This indirect adrenergic-stimulating action results from the drug being taken up into the transmitter-containing vesicles of the presynaptic ending, and there replacing the endogenous transmitter while causing its expulsion from the vesicle. The adrenergic activation then results from the expelled endogenous transmitter combining with the receptors (Carr & Moore, 1969; Weissman, Koe, & Tenen, 1966). An indirect-acting adrenergic stimulant would have less of an effect if it were administered to an organism whose own CAs had been depleted in some manner; however, a direct-acting stimulant would still be effective under these conditions. It is possible for a particular adrenergic stimulant to act by both direct and indirect mechanisms. The relative contribution of direct and indirect actions may depend on drug dose, the species of animal, and the particular physiological or behavioral response under study.

Alpha and Beta Receptors

An important consideration, in a discussion of the mechanism of action of adrenergic stimulant or inhibitory drugs, is the concept of alpha- and beta-receptor sites. This concept developed from research findings that particular adrenergic drugs were differentially capable of achieving certain physiological responses (Ahlquist, 1948). These data showed that the various adrenergic receptor sites are not equally responsive to all adrenergic drugs. It appeared necessary, therefore, to postulate two different receptor types, now called *alpha receptors* and *beta receptors,* to account for most of the physiological patterns observed. Certain adrenergic compounds, however, may facilitate both alpha and beta actions; while other adrenergic stimulants are excitatory only at alpha or beta sites (Table 3.1). Certain of these alpha or beta actions are listed in Table 3.2.

It is important to realize that two different receptors have not actually been isolated or identified. This concept is simply based on the different actions of adrenergic drugs in different systems. In fact, alpha and beta receptors may

TABLE 3.1

Mechanisms of Action of the Major Sympathetic Stimulants

Mechanism	Stimulant	
	Direct	Indirect
Activates both alpha and beta receptors	Epinephrine	Amphetamine and methamphetamine[a]
Activates alpha receptors	Norepinephrine	
Activates beta receptors	Isoproterenol	

[a]These may also have certain other effects.

TABLE 3.2

Receptors Mediating Various Adrenergic Drug Effects

Effector organ	Receptor	Response
Heart	Beta	Increased rate and force of beat
Blood vessels		
To skin and viscera	Alpha	Contraction
To skeletal muscles	Alpha	Contraction
To skeletal muscles	Beta	Relaxation
Gastrointestinal smooth muscle		
To stomach	Beta	Decreased motility
To intestine	Beta	Decreased motility
To intestine	Alpha	Decreased motility
Gastrointestinal sphincters	Alpha	Constriction
Urinary bladder and kidney smooth muscle	Alpha	Relaxation
Urinary bladder sphincters	Alpha	Constriction
Lungs (bronchial tubes)	Beta	Dilation
Pupil of the eye	Alpha	Dilation
Metabolic	?	Increased glucose availability
CNS	?	Alerting, rewarding, improved learning and performance

actually be a somewhat different structure on various cells, or they may reflect different sensitivities of cells to these chemicals. Furthermore, it would be incorrect to think of one of these "receptor sites" as being excitatory and the other inhibitory. This is not the case. Instead, alpha and beta agonists simply produce qualitatively different actions in the organism. The designation as alpha or beta simply refers to the ease with which drugs influence one or the other of the conceptual receptor sites. These designations do not specifically denote the response that is then produced by the particular adrenergic system.

ADRENERGIC STIMULANTS

Adrenergic stimulants produce behavioral arousal or activation. The sites of action for particular effects of adrenergic stimulants may be peripheral or central, and may involve direct or indirect mechanisms. This section will include a consideration of several adrenergic compounds, emphasizing their physiological actions and therapeutic uses. Some of the more common adrenergic stimulants and their modes of action on peripheral receptors are shown in Table 3.1.

Epinephrine, Norepinephrine,
and Autonomic Arousal

During exercise or times of stress the sympathetic division of the autonomic nervous system is activated. The primary CNS structure organizing and controlling the autonomic nervous system is the hypothalamus. The hypothalamic regulation of autonomic functioning is, in turn, under the influence of a variety of mechanisms, including other brain structures, sensory input, blood-borne hormones, nutrients, toxins, and cognitive processes reflective of past experience and learning.

The increased sympathetic nervous system activity is carried to the body viscera over spinal motor nerves that leave the spinal cord at the level of the upper and lower back. These nerves innervate visceral structures such as the glands, kidneys, bladder, liver, stomach, intestines, heart, and blood vessels. Many of these structures also receive complementary input from the cholinergic parasympathetic division of the ANS (see Chapter 4).

The sympathetic autonomic activation is accomplished by two mechanisms, release of norepinephrine onto the receptive surfaces by the sympathetic neurons, and release of epinephrine (and smaller amounts of norepinephrine) into the bloodstream by the adrenal medulla. During autonomic arousal, the sympathetic nervous system neuronally stimulates the cells of the adrenal medulla, which then secrete E (and also some NE). These hormones, released into the circulatory system, are carried in the blood to the various adrenergic receptor sites (see Chapter 11). Since E is effective in activating both alpha and beta receptors, while NE is effective primarily at alpha sites, activation of the adrenal medulla produces both alpha and beta effects, whereas sympathetic activation (without adrenal medullary activity) achieves only alpha-receptor effects. Table 3.2 illustrates the types of receptors found on various visceral organs. The particular response of each respective peripheral system is thus a reflection of differential sensitivities to circulating levels of NE and E.

Cardiovascular system. Adrenal medullary E is both an alpha- and beta-receptor stimulant. Its action is to constrict blood vessels and generally to produce a rise in blood pressure. However, not all blood vessels are constricted by E. For example, the blood vessels to the skin and visceral structures contain only alpha receptors and E will reduce blood flow to the skin and viscera by constricting the diameter of these blood vessels. However, the blood vessels innervating skeletal muscles contain both alpha and beta receptors. Here, the beta receptors have a lower threshold, and are, thus, more sensitive to E. Therefore, E, by beta receptor action, will dilate the blood vessels innervating the skeletal muscles. This blood redistribution is an important part of the homeostatic mechanisms for dealing with stress and emergency situations. Adrenal medullary E also increases the rate and force of the heart by a beta receptor stimulating action. In general, the rise in blood pressure produced by E is due to its effects on cardiac output. Thus, although a redistribution of blood is accomplished via constriction and dilation of blood vessels, this effect does not in itself alter blood pressure.

NE, in contrast to E, is primarily an alpha-receptor stimulant. NE, released by the nervous system, increases blood pressure by constricting the blood vessels to the skin and viscera. NE has little effect on blood flow to the skeletal muscles (perhaps a slight decrease) or on the cardiac output. Thus, what emerges is that E increases blood pressure mainly by increasing cardiac output, while NE increases blood pressure mainly by constricting blood vessels to the skin and viscera.

Excretory systems. The smooth muscles of the stomach contain beta receptors, while the smooth muscles of the intestines contain both alpha and beta receptors. Since E affects alpha and beta receptors, its release will precipitate a relaxation and decreased motility of both the stomach and intestines. NE, on the other hand, will only affect the alpha receptors of the intestines, causing decreased motility. The sphincters of the gastrointestinal system are constricted by the alpha-agonist action of E or NE. The smooth muscles of the kidneys and bladder are relaxed, leading to an inhibition of urine formation, whereas the bladder sphincter is contracted, inhibiting urine flow. These various actions are consistent with the reorganization of bodily processes produced by sympathetic arousal, emphasizing skeletal muscle responding and CNS activation, and temporarily damping down bodily maintenance activities.

Bronchial muscle. E dilates the smooth muscle lining the bronchial tubes which lead to the lungs. Since this is a beta-receptor-mediated action, it is not achieved by NE. This action of E and of certain beta-agonist drugs is used in the treatment of asthma and certain other respiratory diseases.

Carbohydrate metabolism. Both E and NE increase the conversion of stored carbohydrates, fats, and proteins to glucose, the main source of energy for the body. Blood levels of glucose and cellular glucose metabolism are, therefore, increased by either substance. However, the receptors responsible for these actions are not specifiable as either alpha or beta.

Summary. Adrenal medullary E and sympathetic NE are extremely important bodily mechanisms for maintaining biological homeostasis, and for reacting to stress and emergency situations. By their joint effects on the heart, blood vessels, visceral structures, carbohydrate metabolism, and the CNS, they produce a redistribution of the body's resources from maintenance activities to a facilitation in the status of skeletal muscle and brain functions.

These agents (E and NE) are little used in clinical medicine. E is employed as a heart stimulant and in the treatment of asthma or other allergic conditions (directly into the heart or by systemic injection during emergencies). Many of their derivatives, however, receive a great deal of medical use.

Dopamine and Levodopa

Dopamine is an endogenous CA that is the immediate precursor to NE in the synthetic pathway. D has been found in both the CNS and the PNS, and there is now strong evidence that it is a synaptic transmitter in the CNS, as well as in interneurons in PNS autonomic ganglia. Many of the drugs that facilitate or inhibit the action of NE and E have similar effects on D systems. However, the CNS dopaminergic receptors have not been shown to conform to any classification system, such as the alpha- and beta-receptor concepts for NE and E.

At certain sites in the CNS, the CA synthesis is not carried through to NE, but instead stops at D. It appears, therefore, that at these sites, dopamine-β-hydroxylase, the enzyme that converts D to NE, is either absent or deficient. One CNS pathway known to be dopaminergic has its cell bodies in the substantia nigra of the midbrain, and its synaptic terminals in the basal ganglia (caudate nucleus, putamen, globus pallidus) of the forebrain (see Chapter 2).

This nigrostriatal pathway appears to have a role in involuntary bodily movements (coordination, posture). A defect in the functioning of this pathway has now been implicated in the etiology of Parkinson's disease. This name is applied to a motor system disorder, characterized by tremors, rigidity of the muscles, and a loss of the reflexes that usually function to maintain posture. Parkinson's disease usually begins in late middle age, and is chronic and progressive. Although the cause of the Parkinsonian symptoms and the deficiency of D is not known, the disease has been associated with a history of brain inflammation (encephalitis). The symptoms may also occur in persons undergoing prolonged treatment with the tranquilizers used to treat schizophrenia (Chapter 5), although in this case the motor symptoms usually subside when the tranquilizer is withdrawn. Trauma to the brain, a brain tumor in the basal ganglia region, and carbon monoxide poisoning, are other possible causes of Parkinsonian symptoms.

The lesions found in Parkinsonism are usually in the substantia nigra, globus pallidus, or both. Recent bioassay studies of the brains of deceased Parkinsonian patients have confirmed cellular damage, a deficiency of dopamine, and of aromatic amino acid decarboxylase, the enzyme that converts dopa to dopamine (Chapter 2) (Lloyd & Hornykiewicz, 1970). Symptoms resembling those of Parkinsonism can be produced in experimental animals by brain lesions or by the application of certain adrenergic blocking agents (see the section entitled "6-hydroxydopamine" later in this chapter) to this system.

There is some evidence that a cholinergic system in the basal ganglia normally opposes or complements the function of this D system. Until recently the most effective treatment for Parkinsonism used anticholinergic drugs (Chapter 4). Dopamine has been used to treat Parkinsonism, but is ineffective since it does not pass the blood-brain barrier. Currently the immediate precursor of D, dopa, is the most effective treatment for many cases of Parkinsonism. The drug used is actually levodopa, the levoisomer, which is the isomer endogenous to the CNS, and is considerably more active than the dextro isomer. Unlike D, levodopa (dihydroxyphenylalanine) does pass the blood-brain barrier, and presumably is then converted to D in the brain, where it can act in place of the deficient transmitter. This drug is effective to a variable degree in ameliorating the tremor, rigidity, incoordination, and lack of balance (Esplin, 1970; Hornykiewicz, 1966). However, abnormal involuntary movements are a serious side effect of the continuous high dosage therapy that is required (Cotzias et al., 1971; Goldstein et al., 1973).

Isoproterenol (Isuprel)

Isoproterenol is structurally similar to the other catecholamines, but is a synthetic drug and is not endogenous to the body. It is a direct-acting stimulant and is selectively effective at beta-receptor adrenergic sites (Figure 3.2 and Table 3.1). Isoproterenol is our most effective beta-stimulant, and its primary effects are, thus, to stimulate the heart, relax the bronchial tubes, dilate the blood vessels to skeletal muscles, and relax the gastrointestinal tract (Table 3.2). The levoisomer is about 50 times as active as the dextroisomer. This drug is the one of choice for the inhalation treatment of asthma.

Amphetamine and Methamphetamine

These two drugs are not catecholamines; they lack the catechol nucleus (the adjacent hydroxyl groups on the benzene ring). However, their structural formulas are similar to those of the CAs (Figure 3.2). The peripheral physiological, CNS, and behavioral actions of amphetamine and methamphetamine are quite similar. These drugs are indirect-acting adrenergic stimulants and, thus, are somewhat effective in activating both alpha- and beta-receptor functions. However, they both may also have, to some degree, a direct action, and also may inhibit the reuptake and enzymatic destruction of endogenous CAs by MAO. The ratio of direct to indirect action may vary with the particular drug, the dose, the species, and the system under study. One can see, therefore, that these agents have complex actions in humans and other species. There is, however, controversy surrounding this subject, and most investigators believe these agents primarily achieve their effects via an indirect stimulant action.

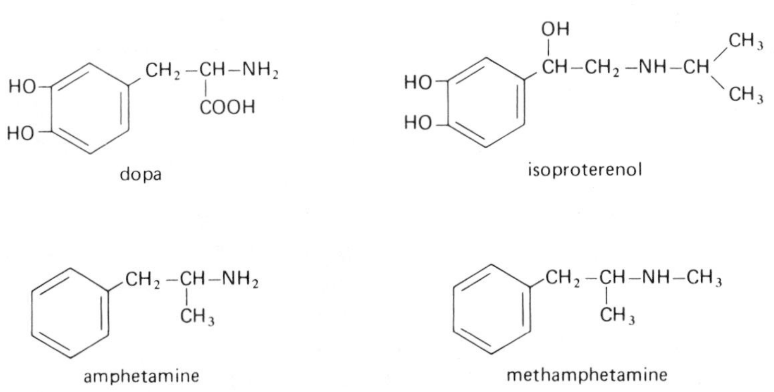

FIGURE 3.2. Some adrenergic stimulants.

The indirect action of the amphetamines is illustrated by the finding that they lower the level of brain NE in animals. The released NE is metabolized primarily by O-methylation by COMT, suggesting the release of active NE into the synaptic cleft (Baldessarini & Kopin, 1967; Carr & Moore, 1969; Glowinski & Axelrod, 1966). However, amphetamine still exerts certain of its CNS stimulatory effects after NE depletion by reserpine, suggesting a possible direct action. Amphetamine may also, under certain conditions, inhibit NE reuptake by the neuronal membrane and also by the storage vesicles (Snyder, 1970). Furthermore, the possibility that the amphetamines achieve their CNS effects by MAO inhibition has been suggested. However, the amphetamines are still effective in subjects whose brain MAO activity has been reduced by MAO inhibitors (Chapter 8). It has also been suggested that a false transmitter may be manufactured from the amphetamines and be responsible for some of their central effects (Baldessarini & Kopin, 1967; Groppetti & Costa, 1969; Innes & Nickerson, 1970a; Kopin, 1968; Weissman, Koe, & Tenen, 1966). These complex and varied possible mechanisms of action should not be so surprising to the student since the amphetamines share much of the chemical structure of the catecholamines. They may be capable in the appropriate circumstances of replacing or duplicating the actions of E and NE in a variety of respects.

The controversy surrounding the proposed actions of the amphetamines raises several possibilities. A direct-stimulating action would result from the amphetamines combining with and activating adrenergic receptors; an indirect action from the drugs being taken up by the neuronal and vesicular membrane into the vesicle, thus replacing some NE and forcing the NE out of the vesicle. If the amphetamines are taken up by the neuronal and vesicular membranes, they would be competing with NE at these sites, and thus, would inhibit NE reuptake. A similar competition between the amphetamines and NE for the destructive enzyme, MAO, would also not be surprising, and would inhibit the degradation and prolong the action of endogenous NE. Amphetamines do not compete for COMT, since they contain no hydroxyl groups on the benzene ring (for methylation). It also appears likely that the amphetamines interact with the serotonergic system (Chapter 2), at least by a direct-stimulating action on these receptors (Bradley, 1968; Brodie & Shore, 1957; Carlsson, 1969; Shore, 1962), further complicating the picture.

Amphetamine (Benzedrine, the racemic mixture consisting of both the levo- and dextro-rotating molecules) is a powerful adrenergic stimulant in both the peripheral and central nervous systems. The dextroisomer (dextroamphetamine, Dexedrine) is three to four times as potent as the levoisomer with respect to CNS stimulation. Since the amphetamines are not solely dependent on a direct mimetic action, dextro-isomerism does not limit their activity. Methamphetamine (Desoxyn, Methedrine) produces somewhat stronger CNS effects than dextro- or levo-amphetamine, and has become quite popular for self-administration as an alerting and euphoric agent. "On the street" it is commonly referred to as "speed." All three of these agents are effective when taken orally, in contrast to NE and E, which are rapidly metabolized in the gastrointestinal tract (and also do not pass the blood-brain barrier).

Other Adrenergic Stimulants

There are a large number of other adrenergic stimulant drugs which need not be discussed since their actions are very similar to those drugs we have included. For information on the pharmacology and use of these other agents, consult Goth (1974) or Innes and Nickerson (1970a). All of these agents have potent adrenergic stimulant actions, to varying degrees, in both the peripheral and central nervous systems. Many are used in clinical medicine for their vascular actions; they help to temporarily clear the nasal passages or eyes by local vasoconstrictor actions. Other major uses are as behavioral stimulants and alerting agents, and as appetite suppressants in the treatment of obesity. The CNS and behavioral effects of the various adrenergic stimulants will be discussed later in this chapter.

ADRENERGIC INHIBITORS

In this section the peripheral physiological actions and the therapeutic uses of the adrenergic blocking agents will be considered. These drugs inhibit responses to adrenergic nerve stimulation and to adrenergic drugs by competitive blockade of the receptors on the postsynaptic neurons or effector cells. This class of blocking agents is very selective and the blockade action of each drug is primarily on either alpha- or beta-receptor actions (Goth, 1974; Nickerson, 1970). We will also explore a drug which has recently achieved dominance in studies of adrenergic functions. This agent, 6-hydroxydopamine, selectively destroys adrenergic nerve terminals and, in a sense, also blocks adrenergic activity.

Alpha-Adrenergic Blocking Agents

These agents include phenoxybenzamine (Dibenzyline), dibenamine, phentolamine (Regitine), tolazoline (Priscoline), and the alkaloids of ergot. With the exception of the ergot alkaloids, which will be discussed separately below, the pharmacology of these drugs is very similar. The structural formulas for phenoxybenzamine and phentolamine, which are the drugs predominantly used in behavioral research, are shown in Figure 3.3.

An interesting effect achieved by these agents is known as "epinephrine reversal." Injection of E usually produces a characteristic rise in blood pressure, which is the result of an interaction between its alpha-receptor vasoconstrictor properties, its beta-receptor vasodilator properties and its beta-receptor cardiac stimulant action. These alpha-blocking agents reverse the usual pressor effect of E, and produce a depressor effect, by selectively blocking the alpha receptors mediating vasoconstriction.

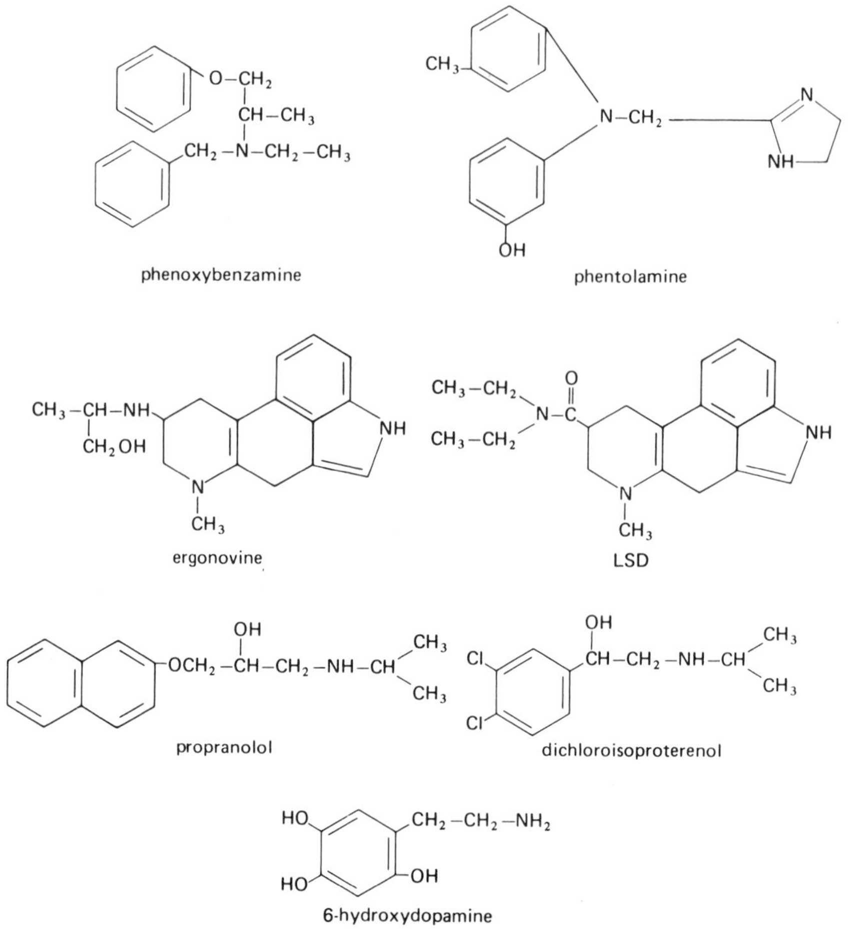

phenoxybenzamine

phentolamine

ergonovine

LSD

propranolol

dichloroisoproterenol

6-hydroxydopamine

FIGURE 3.3. Some adrenergic inhibitors (and LSD).

One use of these agents is in the diagnosis of a rare form of hypertension called *pheochromocytoma*. In this disease the hypertension results from an E- and/or NE-secreting tumor of the adrenal medulla. When the hypertension is caused by such a tumor, an injection of one of the alpha-adrenergic blocking agents will produce a striking immediate fall in blood pressure. Alpha-adrenergic blockers are also used in clinical medicine in the treatment of certain peripheral vascular diseases in which the circulation is impaired due to peripheral blood vessel constriction.

The ergot alkaloids. Ergot is a naturally occurring substance found in a fungus (*Claviceps purpurea*) that infects rye and other edible grains. This fungus is highly toxic and was responsible for widespread outbreaks of poisoning in medieval Europe (from ingesting infected bread). Unlike the other alpha-adrenergic blocking agents, ergot is a potent vasoconstrictor, and produces gangrene of the extremities, and abortion due to uterine gangrene. This vasoconstrictor action is independent of ergot's effect on adrenergic receptors. The vasoconstriction is due to a direct constrictor action on the smooth muscles that circle the blood vessels. Thus, this action bypasses the adrenergic receptors. Paradoxically, however, ergot will still reverse the vasoconstrictor actions of alpha-adrenergic stimulants, and will also block the other alpha-adrenergic effects listed in Table 3.2.

Three of the alkaloids of ergot (ergotamine, ergotoxine, and ergonovine) have been isolated and their chemical structure identified. It is worth pointing out that they share their basic chemical structure with LSD (see ergonovine and LSD in Figure 3.3). Although the ergot alkaloids have not been found to produce LSD-like hallucinatory side effects in clinical use, convulsions, insomnia, and various disturbances of "consciousness and thinking" do occur in ergotism (ergot poisoning, usually from ingesting infected bread; also called St. Anthony's fire), suggesting either some hallucinogenic action for the ergot alkaloids, or their conversion to LSD (or some other related substance; see Chapter 9 for more details).

The alkaloids of ergot are currently used in clinical medicine, not for their adrenergic inhibiting actions, but for their vasoconstrictor action. They are used following birth to reduce uterine bleeding. They are also used in the treatment of migraine headaches, which appear to be caused by dilation of certain blood vessels surrounding the brain (Brazeau, 1970).

Beta-Receptor Blocking Agents

The beta-receptor antagonists can be considered as derivatives of isoproterenol, since they share its basic chemical structure. These compounds selectively compete for the beta-receptor sites. The common beta-adrenergic blockers, propranolol (Inderal), dichloroisoproterenol (DCI), pronethalol (Nethalid, Alderlin) and sotalol, have a common pharmacology. Propranolol and dichloroisoproterenol (Figure 3.3) are the drugs primarily used in CNS and behavioral research. Although they are not in general clinical use, these agents have been investigated for the treatment of certain conditions characterized by a rapid or irregular heartbeat. Two major dangers inherent in their use are heart failure and asthma, resulting from blockade of the adrenergic beta-receptor cardiac-excitatory and bronchial relaxant actions.

6-Hydroxydopamine (6OHDA)

This drug (Figure 3.3) has recently been shown to produce a chemical sympathectomy (Tranzer & Thoenen, 1968). It is now known to be selectively toxic to sympathetic neurons in the peripheral nervous system, and to noradrenergic and dopaminergic neurons in the CNS as well (Malmfors & Thoenen, 1971). It is toxic both to cell bodies and processes, but is most highly destructive to the presynaptic vesicles. The 6OHDA is selectively taken up into the vesicle by the reuptake processes normally operating for NE and D. It is, however, highly toxic to the vesicle and consequently causes an immediate depletion of the endogenous transmitter, and a permanent destruction of the presynaptic ending; at low doses recovery may take place. Now 6OHDA has become one of the brain researcher's most potent tools for the investigation of adrenergic processes.

ADRENERGIC MECHANISMS:
THE CNS AND BEHAVIOR

Investigations of the regulation of biological processes in the peripheral nervous system have, in the last 15 years, been extended to an analysis of endogenous catecholamines in the CNS. With this trend, substantial insight has been gained into the nature of adrenergic systems. Much of this research has been directed at anatomical and biochemical identification of adrenergic systems in the CNS, as well as to the effects of drugs on these systems, and on behavior. It now appears that an integration of the physiological, pharmacological, and behavioral information can be accomplished.

We will attempt to show that several seemingly unrelated behavioral phenomena are related to two basic systems in the CNS: a noradrenergic reinforcement system and a dopaminergic motor system. In this endeavor, the CNS actions of adrenergic drugs will be discussed under the following headings: reinforcement processes, instrumental responding, and arousal, as they relate to the noradrenergic system; and motor functions as they relate to the dopaminergic system. We will also describe the interplay of these two systems in the mediation of ingestive behaviors (feeding and drinking). Finally we will attempt to show how several severe mental disorders (schizophrenia, mania, and depression) may best be understood as reflections of pathology of the noradrenergic and dopaminergic systems. Thus these conditions will be referred to as brain disorders.

Reinforcement Processes

The goal of this section is to show that rewarding effects can be produced by electrical stimulation of the brain. Furthermore, this behavioral phenomenon will be shown to be subserved by a noradrenergic system involving the medial forebrain bundle.

It is generally agreed that behavior is maintained by its consequences for the organism. This generality appears to apply to innate or reflex responses as well as to learned behaviors. If the consequences of behavior are experienced as pleasurable or rewarding, an organism is likely to repeat the behavior under similar circumstances. Under these conditions an organism's behavior is said to be under the control of reinforcement contingencies. Common reinforcers are food, water, and physical contact, as well as learned or acquired reinforcers like money, compliments, and school grades. In a similar sense, reinforcement may be represented by an organism breaking contact with painful or threatening stimuli such as extreme temperature or predators. In either case, the reinforcement serves to strengthen behavior that has potential survival value for the organism. Thus, these adaptive behaviors help to maintain biological homeostasis.

Behavior, however, is not controlled solely by its positive consequences. There appears to exist a complementary phenomenon which we will refer to as *aversion*. This process directs behavior along similar adaptive lines but differs qualitatively from reinforcement. The consequences of aversive stimuli are that on future occasions an organism will be less likely to engage in the same behavior; the behavior is inhibited. Importantly, it does not appear that this regulatory process is subserved by the noradrenergic system. Rather, data seem to suggest that a cholinergic system forms the basis of aversive processes (see the next chapter).

Brain stimulation as reinforcer. In the early 1950s it was discovered that a brief pulse of electricity delivered to the brains of rats could serve as a potent reinforcer or punishment. Whether the brain stimulation was reinforcing or punishing depended primarily on the location of the electrode in the brain and the strength of the electrical stimulation that was delivered. These positive and negative consequences of electrical brain-stimulation (*EBS*) have been found in all species of animals that have been tested, including humans. Organisms will perform any of a variety of responses in order to turn on or turn off electrical stimulation of the brain. Responses used have included lever-pressing, maze-running, crossing-over to the other side of a shuttle box, and pole-climbing. The most common response that is used in studies of the reinforcement consequences of brain stimulation is a lever press. Since an organism has direct control of the response and is able to self-administer the EBS, the lever-pressing response in these situations is generally referred to as self-stimulation (SS).

Self-stimulation can be obtained using electrical stimulation at a variety of brain locations. Although there is some discrepancy in the findings as to the location of SS sites in different species, there also is a great deal of consistency in the results. The phenomenon appears to have its focus in the brainstem, hypothalamus, and limbic system. Noradrenergic systems have been identified that travel from the brainstem, including the locus coeruleus and other sites, through the lateral regions of the hypothalamus to terminate in many limbic system structures, including the hypothalamus, septal area, amygdala, hippocampus, parts of the thalamus, and cerebral cortex.

Dopaminergic and serotonergic neuron fibers, also, have been found to ascend from the brainstem in the lateral region of the hypothalamus on the way to innervate limbic system structures, the basal ganglia, and the cerebral cortex. The dopaminergic pathway is usually called the *nigrostriatal bundle,* while the NE and 5HT pathways are collectively called the *medial forebrain bundle* (MFB) (Olds, 1962; Olds & Olds, 1964; Stein, 1964, 1969).

Certain other regions of the brain appear to mediate aversive effects. Electrical stimulation of these areas will support escape or avoidance behavior. The focus of these aversive effects seems to be the periventricular system (PVS), a group of neuron fibers which travels from the midbrain to the thalamus, with subsequent extensions into the hypothalamus, basal ganglia, limbic system, and cerebral cortex. There is some evidence that this PVS mechanism is cholinergic in nature (Stein, 1964). The anatomical distributions of the MFB and PVS systems are shown for a primitive mammalian brain in Figure 3.4. The MFB and PVS appear to be capable of interacting by distributing fibers to a number of common sites along their paths.

MEDIAL FOREBRAIN BUNDLE
(REWARD)

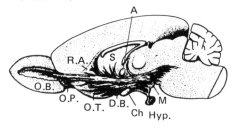

PERIVENTRICULAR SYSTEM
(PUNISHMENT)

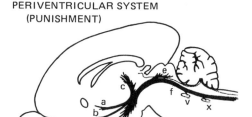

FIGURE 3.4. (*Top*) diagram representing medial forebrain bundle—presumed substrate of reward mechanism—in a generalized and primitive mammalian brain.

(*Bottom*) diagram representing periventricular system of fibers—presumed substrate of punishment mechanism.

Abbreviations: A, anterior commissure; D.B., nucleus of the diagonal band; M, mammillary body; S, septum; b, anterior hypothalamus; c, thalamus; d, posterior hypothalamus; e, tectum. (After Le Gros Clark, Beattie, Riddoch, & Dott, 1938.)

A great deal of interest in the reinforcement systems of the brain has resulted from the notion that biochemical or structural defects in these systems may be the basis of a variety of human mental disorders, which we could now perhaps speak of as brain disorders (Bishop, Elder, & Heath, 1964; Olds, 1962; Olds & Olds, 1964; Stein, 1967). However, this material will be discussed in the last section of this chapter, which deals with brain disorders. In the rest of this section on reinforcement we will review and evaluate the data suggesting that ascending noradrenergic MFB neurons function as the CNS basis for behavior maintained by its rewarding consequences.

Norepinephrine, the MFB, and reinforcement. Several lines of evidence provide strong support for the statement that an MFB neuronal system, in which NE is the synaptic transmitter, functions as the biological basis of reinforcement in mammalian species (including the human). This evidence includes the following findings: NE is found in MFB neurons; synthesizing and inactivating enzymes for NE are found in the MFB; application of NE to the MFB mimics the effects of activating the MFB via presynaptic neurons; electrical stimulation of the MFB results in an increase in recoverable NE and its metabolites in synaptic regions; and drugs that increase or decrease the action of NE also have a similar stimulant or depressant action on the MFB neurons. Furthermore, each treatment that facilitates or inhibits the action of these noradrenergic MFB neurons has an analogous facilitative or inhibitory action on self-stimulation reward and on the reinforcement consequences of natural rewards.

Identification, synthesis, and degradation: Using the histochemical fluorescent technique discussed in Chapter 2, a noradrenergic pathway having its cell bodies in the brainstem has been found to then travel through the lateral hypothalamus in the MFB to the limbic system and cerebral cortex (Fuxe, 1965; Hillarp, Fuxe, & Dahlström, 1966). This pathway has also already been reviewed in this chapter. Using another technique, NE-containing synaptic vesicles have been isolated in homogenates of hypothalamic tissue (Glowinski & Iverson, 1966b). Furthermore, unilateral hypothalamic lesions interrupting the MFB produce a reduction in NE levels at limbic system sites anterior and ipsilateral (on the same side of the brain) to the lesion, but not posterior and contralateral (on the opposite side of the brain) (Heller & Moore, 1968; Heller, Seiden, & Moore, 1966.) Therefore, these studies lead to the conclusion that NE is found in MFB neurons.

Synthesizing and deactivating enzyme systems and a reuptake mechanism for NE have also each been demonstrated in the MFB region. For instance, if radioactively tagged dopa is injected into the lateral ventricle of the rat, radioactive NE can then be recovered from the MFB region (Coyle & Axelrod, 1971; Glowinski & Axelrod, 1966). In vitro studies have also shown that electrical stimulation of isolated hypothalamic tissue leads to the release of NE (Baldessarini & Kopin, 1967). Both COMT and MAO, and also an NE reuptake mechanism that incorporates radioactive NE into MFB neurons, have been demonstrated (Glowinski & Iverson, 1966a).

Neural firing changes: Studies employing a microelectrophoretic technique for injecting small amounts of NE into the extracellular space of one or a few MFB neurons have shown that these neurons respond to NE by a change in their firing rate. With this technique, multibarreled hollow glass microelectrodes are used to deliver a minute quantity of chemical to the region of a neuron, whose firing rate can also be recorded with the same electrode. The firing rate of particular MFB nerve cells may be augmented or decreased by NE. Adrenergic blocking agents characteristically have opposite effects to NE (Salmoiraghi, 1966; Salmoiraghi & Bloom, 1964).

Reinforcement and NE release: An extremely important study by Stein and Wise (1969; Stein, 1969) provides perhaps the most cogent evidence for NE being a synaptic transmitter in an MFB reinforcement system. This is an elegant and complex experiment and thus will be reviewed in some detail. The subjects were rats, each receiving three separate implants (see Figure 3.5). A cannula in the lateral ventricle was used to inject radioactively tagged NE. An electrode placed posteriorly in the MFB was used to deliver electrical stimulation to the brain (EBS). The third implant was a concentric push-pull cannula aimed at the MFB either in the anterior hypothalamus or the amygdala. This push-pull cannula was used to recover material from the brain. With the push-pull cannula a fluid similar in constitution to extracellular fluid was continually perfused under low pressure in very small amounts through the inner cannula into the brain substance. The fluid was then immediately and continually retrieved from the brain by slight suction through the outer cannula.

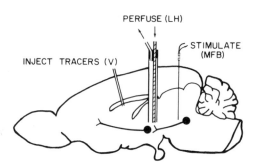

FIGURE 3.5. Diagram of perfusion experiment showing relative locations of stimulating electrode in the medial forebrain bundle (MFB), perfusion cannula in lateral hypothalamus (LH), and needle for injection of radioisotopes in lateral ventricle (V) on an outline of rat brain. (From L. Stein and C. D. Wise, Release of norepinephrine from hypothalamus and amygdala by rewarding medial forebrain bundle stimulation and amphetamine. *Journal of Comparative and Physiological Psychology,* 1969, **67**, 189–198. Copyright 1969 by the American Psychological Association. Reprinted by permission.)

The animals were first tested behaviorally for the reinforcing consequences of the EBS delivered through the posterior MFB electrode. Sites were classified as reinforcing (the rat self-stimulated), punishing (the rat avoided pressing the lever), or neutral (the rat depressed the lever at a low rate). On the next test, radioactively labeled NE was injected into the lateral ventricle and EBS was automatically delivered to the rat via the posterior MFB electrode. The amount of labeled NE and its metabolites recovered by the push-pull cannula in the anterior hypothalamus or amygdala was then measured. The experimenters found that delivering reinforcing EBS to the posterior MFB increased the amount of NE and its metabolites recovered from the push-pull cannula, whereas delivering punishing EBS decreased the amount of NE and its metabolites recovered. These changes occurred both for cannulae in the anterior hypothalamus and the amygdala. Delivering neutral EBS to the posterior MFB did not alter the amount of radioactively labeled NE and its metabolites recovered from the two anterior sites, when compared to control periods during which no electrical stimulation was delivered. These data provide strong evidence that reinforcing consequences of MFB stimulation are correlated with the incorporation of exogenous NE into MFB neurons and its subsequent release into the synaptic cleft.

Pharmacological manipulations: A variety of pharmacological studies are also consistent with the MFB noradrenergic reinforcement system hypothesis. NE itself has been found to enhance SS rates when administered intraventricularly (Wise & Stein, 1969). Amphetamine also increases noradrenergic activity and has been found to enhance the effect of rewarding EBS; following amphetamine administration, SS rates increase, while electrical current threshold for SS decreases (Stein, 1964; Stein & Wise, 1970). MAO inhibitors also increase noradrenergic activity and have been found to increase SS rate when systemically injected in rats (Poschel & Ninteman, 1964).

Reserpine depletes NE stores and decreases SS rate for MFB brain stimulation in the rat. However, if animals are pretreated with an MAO inhibitor before reserpine treatment, brain NE stores are much less depleted by reserpine, and SS rate is only slightly reduced. Alpha-methylparatyrosine (AMPT), a precursor for a false transmitter for NE, also reduces brain NE levels and SS rate in animals. Chlorpromazine (a phenothiazine tranquilizer) blocks the reuptake of NE (and dopamine), leading to an NE depletion, and reduces SS rate, while increasing the threshold for SS in animals (Poschel & Ninteman, 1963, 1964, 1966; Stein, 1964; Stein & Wise, 1970).

It is thought that the antischizophrenic tranquilizers (especially the phenothiazines and the butyrophenones; see Chapter 5) are primarily active in blocking the reuptake of dopamine (rather than NE). This reuptake selectivity has been integrated into a current biochemical theory of schizophrenia (see the section entitled "Brain Disorders" later in this chapter) that suggests D is secreted in the brain of schizophrenic patients at sites in the reinforcement system where NE is secreted in the brains of "normal" individuals (Hökfelt, Ljungdahl, Fuxe, & Johansson, 1974).

These pharmacological manipulations of the reinforcement system, by their consistency, provide considerable evidence for NE as a transmitter in an ascending MFB reinforcement system. Those drugs which enhance noradrenergic activity, also facilitate SS, whereas drugs that inhibit noradrenergic activity inhibit SS. It should also be pointed out that those drugs that enhance NE and SS tend to produce pleasurable and euphoric effects, whereas drugs that depress NE and SS tend to have sedating and depressive effects. These data suggest that the reward system may be involved in abnormal euphoria or depression and that pharmacological manipulation of this system may be a way of treating certain disordered behavioral states (see the section entitled "Brain Disorders" later in this chapter).

Instrumental Responding

There has been a great deal of research on the effects of adrenergic drugs on instrumental responding. For the most part these experiments have employed the peripheral injection of adrenergic stimulants or blocking agents. The endogenous adrenergic chemicals, NE and E, seem to have little effect on instrumental responding when systemically injected, probably because they do not readily pass the blood-brain barrier, and therefore do not directly affect brain functions. The adrenergic-stimulating drugs that do pass the blood-brain barrier (the amphetamines) for the most part have a facilitative action on instrumental responding, whether the behavior is maintained by its aversive or its appetitive consequences. In contrast, systemic injections of adrenergic antagonists (which also pass the blood-brain barrier) primarily have an inhibitory action on instrumental responding.

We propose that the facilitation or inhibition of instrumental responding by adrenergic stimulants and antagonists is via a direct action on the noradrenergic reinforcement mechanism which directs behavior along adaptive lines. The purpose of the next sections is to build a case for the noradrenergic reinforcement system as the basis of the actions of adrenergic drugs on aversively controlled and appetitive behaviors. Thus, the noradrenergic reinforcement system would not only be the basis of self-stimulation reward and drug effects on SS, but would also be the basis of natural rewards and of the actions of adrenergic drugs on learned behavior controlled by reinforcement contingencies.

Aversively controlled behavior—peripheral NE and E. It has been suggested that conditioned autonomic responses are mediated by the adrenal medulla and have an important role in the learning and performance of behavior maintained by aversive stimulation (Mowrer, 1947; Wynn & Solomon, 1955). This hypothesis would seem to predict that E injections would facilitate, and removal of the adrenal medulla would inhibit, the acquisition or performance of avoidance responses. This is not the case. Surgical removal of the adrenal medulla (the source of much of the endogenous catecholamines) has little effect on avoidance behavior (Moyer & Bunnell, 1959). E or NE administration also has little effect on avoidance behavior. However, since endogenous adrenal medullary E (or NE) and peripherally administered E or NE do not enter the brain in any appreciable amount, these findings are not informative as to the role of CNS noradrenergic system in instrumental responding.

Although NE or E does not facilitate avoidance behavior when systemically administered, they may under certain conditions enhance the fear reaction of animals to novel stimuli (Moyer & Bunnell, 1958; Stewart & Brookshire, 1967, 1968). This enhancement of fear reactions would appear to result from a facilitation of sympathetic nervous system arousal. Such fear reactions as vocalization, jumping, crouching, defecating, and urinating are increased by NE or E administration in mildly aversive situations (Grossman & Sclafani, 1971; Singer, 1963).

Amphetamines: Although the catecholamines (NE and E) appear to have little effect in avoidance situations, numerous studies show that the amphetamines (which readily pass the blood-brain barrier), when administered in low to moderate doses, will facilitate the learning or performance of instrumental avoidance responses. This finding has been supported by studies in the rat employing a variety of test situations, such as: Sidman avoidance (the animal is punished unless it presses a lever at least once every 20 seconds) (Carlton, 1961a, 1961b; Verhave, 1958); discriminated lever-pressing (Hearst & Whalen, 1963); shuttle box avoidance (Cardo, 1959); pole-jumping avoidance (Lynch, Aceto, & Thomas, 1960); and in escape-responding situations where the noxious stimulation is presented without warning and cannot be avoided (in such situations amphetamine decreases the latency of escape responses) (Keleman & Bovet, 1961; Mize & Isaac, 1962). Although one early investigator found passive avoidance responses to be impaired (Cardo, 1959), most other studies find passive avoidance to be improved by low doses of amphetamine (Geller & Seifter, 1960; Teitelbaum & Derks, 1958).

Two types of explanations have been provided for the facilitation of avoidance responding by amphetamines. One is via an action on learning processes per se, while the other is via an alteration of emotional reactivity. The learning interpretation has generally received only partial support since only a small number of studies have found the facilitation of avoidance behavior to persist after amphetamine injection (Kulkarni, 1968). The temporary action of amphetamine, in this case, would suggest a performance rather than a learning effect. Most authors seem to favor an explanation of the facilitative action of the amphetamines on avoidance responding based on an increase in "emotional reactivity", or on a suppression of freezing behavior (Hearst & Whalen, 1963; also see Chapter 11 in this book). We believe that the facilitation of CNS reinforcement processes provides the best explanation of these facilitative drug effects, and is also consistent with these other explanations.

Several experiments provide data consistent with the notion that the facilitation of avoidance responding by the amphetamines is due to their actions on endogenous CNS catecholamine functioning. In cats, amphetamine reversed a reserpine-induced inhibition of avoidance behavior, whereas pretreatment with

AMPT (an NE depleter) blocked this action of amphetamine (Hanson, 1967). Further support is provided by Grossman's finding (1964a) in the rat that direct microinjection of NE into the septal region of the brain facilitated avoidance performance, while microinjection of an adrenergic blocking agent had an opposite action.

Appetitive behavior. For the most part, systemic administration of NE or E has been found to suppress instrumental behavior directed at obtaining food or water (the studies have employed a variety of doses, species, and reinforcement schedules) (Breggin, 1965; Wentink, 1938; Wurtman, Frank, Morse, & Dews, 1959). Therefore, the peripheral administration of the CAs would seem to have a general inhibitory effect on appetitive responding. Since systemic injections of NE and E have also been shown to suppress food and water intake in a simple consummatory response situation (an anorexic action), it may be that this action could account for the suppression in instrumental responding for rewards. However, the blood-brain barrier constraint suggests that the suppression of appetitive behavior by peripherally administered NE and E is a consequence of peripheral sympathetic arousal, rather than effects related to the CNS.

Amphetamines: The involvement of adrenergic processes in instrumental behavior has best been established with the use of amphetamines, which do pass the blood-brain barrier. Under certain conditions, peripherally injected amphetamine has been shown to facilitate instrumental repsonses directed at obtaining food or water. Dews (1958) found a response facilitation by amphetamine in rats maintained on fixed interval (FI) and fixed ratio (FR) schedules designed to generate relatively low response rates. This response enhancement was obtained at low dosage levels, whereas higher doses depressed conditioned behavior. A similar finding has been reported by McMillan (1969).

On the other hand, there are a number of studies which suggest a disruptive effect of amphetamine on appetitive behavior. Low doses of amphetamine will increase responding on reinforcement schedules designed to generate extremely low response rates (differential reinforcement of low rates, DRL), and will decrease responding on schedules that generate very high response rates (Dews & Morse, 1961; Grossman & Sclafani, 1971; Kelleher & Morse, 1968). Either of these disruptive effects leads to a reduction of food or water rewards.

It does not appear that the anorexic action of amphetamine can account for this disruption of appetitive behavior since facilitation of this behavior has also been reported. Rather, the effect of amphetamine administration on appetitive conditioning seems to be schedule dependent. Clark and Steele (1966) have demonstrated this by using multiple chained schedules designed to maintain both low and high response rates during different segments of an individual experimental session. Under these conditions a single dose of amphetamine clearly increased low rate responding and decreased high rate responding.

One possible explanation for the amphetamine disruption of conditioned behavior on schedules generating low or high response rates may be related to yet another action of this drug. Amphetamines produce a heightened state of arousal. Such a state could lead to attentional shifts or competing responses antagonistic to the conditioned response. The introduction of competing responses (without amphetamines) does disrupt behavior maintained on DRL schedules (Laties, Weiss, Clark, & Reynolds, 1965). Similarly, amphetamines have been reported to increase "irrelevant" and otherwise antagonistic responses in the runway apparatus (Carlson, Doyle, & Bidder, 1965).

It thus appears that with schedules of reinforcement that require an organism to develop complex mediating or timing behaviors to receive rewards, amphetamines have a disruptive effect. Yet, amphetamine does facilitate instrumental behavior when less stringent schedules are employed. It is proposed that under these conditions amphetamines are acting to enhance the reinforcement value of the total environmental complex, including stimulus and response components. This potentiation of reinforcement is the result of amphetamine activation of noradrenergic reinforcement processes which have been shown to be markedly influenced by this drug. By so doing, response increments are produced.

It is further suggested that an identical condition is created for animals maintained on more stringent reinforcement schedules. However, on DRL schedules a facilitation of reinforcement processes makes suppression of responding more difficult, leading to disruptions of the conditioned response. Likewise, on variable interval (VI) schedules which generate high response rates, an amphetamine potentiation of reinforcement processes tends to overstimulate the organism, and thus behavioral decrements ensue.

Consistent behavioral-biochemical correlations. The facilitation of instrumental responding by adrenergic stimulants is proposed to occur through an enhancement of the MFB noradrenergic reinforcement system. Several very interesting recent studies serve to support this explanation. First, water-deprived rats performing a lever-pressing response for water reinforcement, exhibited an increase in NE metabolism in the brain (Lewy & Seiden, 1972). Therefore, reinforced instrumental responding was accompanied by enhanced noradrenergic functioning. Secondly, bilateral lesions of the noradrenergic nucleus locus coeruleus of the brainstem led to a decrease in NE levels along the entire ascending noradrenergic system. Such lesions impaired the learning of a running response by rats for a food reward in a simple runway (Anlezark, Crow, & Greenway, 1973). These authors also interpreted the learning deficit as we have, as a result of an interference with reinforcement processes. A third experiment in mice has shown that a drug that inhibits dopamine-β-hydroxylase, the enzyme that converts D to NE, depresses passive avoidance learning. This drug, diethyldithiocarbamate, decreased brain NE biosynthesis and also depressed the passive avoidance behavior (Randt, Quartermain, Goldstein, & Anagnoste, 1971). Fourth, reserpine and AMPT, drugs that decrease brain CA functioning, also cause a temporary failure to perform a well learned conditioned avoidance response (Seiden & Peterson, 1968). Each of these enhancement or depressant effects of manipulating noradrenergic mechanisms could result from an action on a reinforcement system.

Arousal

In general, one of the CNS actions of the adrenergic stimulants can be described as arousing or alerting. The organism is also more active than normal, and is more susceptible to emotion provoking stimuli. These actions are quite dose-dependent, and are replaced at high doses by a toxic depression. Experimenters have looked at this arousal action in a variety of ways; we will attempt to show a common basis, and furthermore, will relate the arousal action to our unifying reinforcement hypothesis.

Arousal action. If the amphetamines are administered orally or by systemic injection, an alerting or arousal effect is achieved. This may be seen in animals or humans as increased behavioral arousal, sleeplessness, increased motor activity, an improvement in problem solving and physical performance (swimming, running, solving math problems or word association tests, for example, especially with prolonged testing—fatigue and boredom are counteracted) and a more alert (desynchronized) EEG (Bradley & Elkes, 1957; Cole, 1967; Rothballer, 1959; Schulte, Reif, Bacher, Lawrence, & Tainter, 1941; Searle & Brown, 1938a, 1938b; Tormey & Lasagna, 1960; Utena, 1966; Zieve, 1937). The amphetamines are effective in this regard when given orally or by peripheral injection, since they are not deactivated in the gastrointestinal tract, and since they also pass the blood-brain barrier.

The CAs are not effective as arousants following systemic administration, but low to moderate doses of E, and especially NE, are arousing in animals and humans if injected into the cerebral ventricles or directly into the substance of the brain (Feldberg, 1963; Grossman, 1968; Hernández-Peón & Chávez-Ibarra, 1963; MacPhail & Miller, 1968; Marley, 1966; Marley & Key, 1963; Rothballer, 1956, 1957, 1959; Spooner & Winters, 1965; Yamaguchi et al., 1963, 1964). There is some indication that the brainstem reticular formation is the seat of these arousal or alerting actions (Bradley & Elkes, 1957).

Emotions. Several investigators have found that adrenergic agonists facilitate emotional reactivity or affective behavior in humans or other species. There have even been studies purporting to differentiate the involvement of NE and E with respect to the autonomic arousal seen in humans in states of anger and fear (Ax, 1953; Brady, 1967; Funkenstein, 1955; Funkenstein, Greenblatt, & Solomon, 1952; Hernández-Peón & Chávez-Ibarra, 1963; MacPhail & Miller, 1968; Schildkraut & Kety, 1967; Von Euler, 1964). The preponderance of data, however, is inconsistent with this notion of an adrenergic involvement in the type or kind of emotion that is displayed or "felt." This subject is dealt with in detail in Chapter 11 of this book and, therefore, the evidence will not now be reviewed. However, we might summarize our conclusions with the statement that peripheral adrenergic mechanisms have a nondifferentiated arousal or alerting function; and since arousal is a prerequisite to emotionality, the level of emotionality will correlate with adrenergic activity. In contrast, the type or kind of emotional experience, and the expression of the emotion, seem more dependent on past experiences and present environment (cognitive and perceptual processes). We, therefore, conclude that the involvement of adrenergic processes in emotions is simply an expression of their nonspecific arousal function. We will point out below our suggestion that the arousal occurs because the reinforcement system is facilitated by adrenergic stimulants, and thus animals and humans find the external stimuli in their environment more rewarding than they normally do.

Medical uses. The amphetamines have been used for their arousal action to counteract fatigue and depression. Administration of the amphetamines to humans tends to promote wakefulness, cause some elevation of mood (euphoria), decrease feelings of fatigue, and may improve learning or athletic performance. These effects are especially seen in sleepy or fatigued individuals. Amphetamines are thus prescribed for a variety of individuals and conditions which are not actually medical problems. These effects are quite dose dependent; at high doses an intoxication incompatible with optimal functioning sets in. Prolonged use is almost invariably followed by mental depression and fatigue (Weiss & Laties, 1962).

The amphetamines find therapeutic use in the treatment of depressive states. They also have been administered to children with certain behavioral problems— the so-called *hyperkinetic syndrome.* The amphetamines are also used for their stimulant action to relieve the hangover and depression following alcohol abuse and for counteracting the depression from poisoning with depressant drugs such as the barbiturates. Narcolepsy, a disease of unknown etiology, characterized by an inability to stay awake, has also been successfully treated with the amphetamines.

Self-administration. The amphetamines are used for self-administration to achieve arousal and also to achieve euphoria (in animal research studies amphetamine self-administration can also be produced). Physicians also prescribe the amphetamines for their arousal effect in patients who must or wish to work longer hours, or who simply like the way they feel under amphetamine. In occupations such as space flight, naval sonar operation, and military war activity the amphetamines are commonly used to maintain alertness. Since psychotic reactions accompanied by hallucinations and delusions may occur with high doses or prolonged use, this sort of use is not without its price. Also, since stress lowers the lethal dose of the amphetamines, a normally effective dose may be fatal when taken during acute stress (Chance, 1946; Höhn & Lasagna, 1960; Moore, 1963).

Conclusions. The CNS effects of the adrenergic system considered in this section can be interpreted as the result of increased arousal. In humans and in animals we presume this effect is perceived as reinforcing. We wish to suggest that the increased arousal and euphoria have a common basis in the noradrenergic reinforcement system. As such, the arousal, alertness, and increased locomotor activity may be regarded as the consequences of increased noradrenergic, functioning, which results in the organism being more intensely reinforced by environmental stimuli. Thus, the organism is more aroused, more attendant to stimuli, more active, and more euphoric, due to a facilitation of the MFB noradrenergic reinforcement system.

Motor Functions

We have already discussed the role of dopamine as a synaptic transmitter in a nigrostriatal motor system, and the involvement of this system in Parkinsonism. Unilateral damage (only one side of the brain) to this system, for instance, by a substantia nigral brain lesion or by injection of 60HDA into the substantia nigra, causes an asymmetry of movements in animals. This asymmetry is characterized by an asymmetrical posture, or under certain conditions by a vigorous continual body rotation toward the lesion (Ungerstedt, 1971c).

Certain recent studies now suggest that alterations of the dopaminergic system may also have more complex behavioral consequences. For instance, d-amphetamine is about 10 times more effective than l-amphetamine in activating brain norepinephrine (for example, by inhibiting reuptake), while these two drugs are equally effective in inhibiting reuptake of dopamine by the basal ganglia. In behavioral studies, d-amphetamine is also 10 times as potent as l-amphetamine in enhancing locomotor activity in rats (an arousal effect), but only twice as potent in eliciting a compulsive gnawing syndrome. These findings suggest a predominantly dopaminergic basis for the compulsive gnawing, which does not seem related to ingestive behavior, since animals will readily gnaw at the sides and floor of their metal cage. Presumably, if only D were involved, the dextro- and levoisomers would have been equally effective. Therefore, NE may also have some limited influence on this syndrome (Taylor & Snyder, 1970).

Even more provocative is the report by Ungerstedt (1971c) that bilateral (both sides of the brain) destruction of the dopaminergic pathway in the substantia nigra or along its route to the basal ganglia produces in rats a syndrome identical to the starvation syndrome produced by lateral hypothalamic lesions. In this syndrome there is an initial 1-to-2-day period of hyperactivity, followed by a marked reduction in movements, and death within about 5 days if the animals are not tube fed. With tube feedings the animals resume spontaneous eating within about 3 to 4 weeks. The critical involvement of the dopaminergic pathway in the lateral hypothalamic syndrome is further suggested by the finding that bilateral 60HDA destruction of the noradrenergic system does not produce this starvation syndrome. These findings have also been confirmed in part by Zigmond and Stricker (1972), who found the aphagia produced in rats by intraventricular 60HDA to be based on D, rather than NE, depletion. In another recent study, bilateral electrolytic lesions of the noradrenergic locus coeruleus, which produced learning deficits in rats (see the section entitled "Instrumental Responding" earlier in this chapter), did not affect body weight (Anlezark, Crow, & Greenway, 1973).

Ingestive Behavior

There are three phenomena pointing to a relationship between adrenergic systems and ingestive behavior. The first of these is the anorexic effect of systemically administered alpha-adrenergic agonists. Second is the increase in feeding that results from intracerebral administration of alpha-adrenergic stimulants in the rat. Third is the drinking that is produced by beta-adrenergic stimulants.

Amphetamine-induced anorexia. The peripheral administration of amphetamine may be used as an appetite depressant and as a means for reducing food intake in animals and humans. Unfortunately, certain undesirable side effects, such as tolerance, appear with chronic administration. Tolerance to the anorexic action of amphetamine develops relatively quickly and increased dosages are usually required to maintain the effect (Seaton, Rose, & Duncan, 1964; Tormey & Lasagna, 1960).

Amphetamines have a variety of peripheral physiological effects. These include a mobilization of free fatty acids (Santi & Guiliana, 1964); an increase in general metabolism (Kundstadter, 1940); a rise in oxygen consumption (Tainter, 1944); and a reduction in gastric motility (Ritvo, 1936). However, amphetamines continue to depress base levels of food intake in the absence of chemical changes in the blood circulation (Nathanson, 1937) and following denervation of peripheral nerves controlling gastrointestinal motility (Harris, Ivy, & Searle, 1947). Thus, the production of amphetamine-induced anorexia does not appear to be entirely dependent on changes in peripheral physiological processes. Instead, it has been suggested that amphetamine affects CNS processes directly and that this action is responsible for the anorexia.

Although it is generally agreed that amphetamine leads to anorexia by some effect on the CNS, the nature of this involvement is not completely understood. There is, however, rather compelling evidence that hypothalamic activity is markedly altered following amphetamine administration. Since the hypothalamus is intimately related to the regulation of consummatory behavior, it is suspected that pharmacological alterations of neural activity at this locus can markedly affect food intake.

At present there are two major theories which attempt to explain the mechanism of action for amphetamine-induced anorexia: the ventromedial-hypothalamic mimicking hypothesis; and the lateral-hypothalamic blocking hypothesis (Cole, 1973). These hypotheses are the culmination of a large body of literature linking the ventromedial (VMN) and lateral hypothalamic (LHA) nuclei to the control of consummatory behavior and are based on observations of the results of stimulation and destruction of these nuclear groups.

VMN-mimicking hypothesis: Electrical stimulation of the VMN leads to a reduction of food intake (Anand & Dua, 1955), whereas destruction of this nucleus produces a syndrome characterized by excessive food intake and obesity (Hetherington & Ranson, 1942). The VMN syndrome consists of a dynamic phase, during which time an animal eats excessively, and a static phase, at which time food intake drops off, but the added weight gain is maintained. The VMN, therefore, may function normally to limit the amount of food consumption needed by an organism to maintain a specified body weight. As such it may function as a satiety mechanism which keeps food intake and body weight within homeostatic limits.

Intravenous injections of amphetamine markedly alter VMN activity. Brobeck, Larsson, and Reyes (1956) found that amphetamine inhibited neural activity in most of the hypothalamus, with the exception of the VMN, which showed an increase in activity. These data were taken as evidence that amphetamine activates the VMN satiety mechanism and pharmacologically mimics processes involved in natural food satiation. These data also suggest that the VMN, when activated, may lead to an inhibition of other hypothalamic regions possibly involved in the regulation of food intake. Other data from single cell recording in the VMN supports the conclusion that amphetamine increases neural activity in this site (Krebs, Bindra, & Campbell, 1969).

The tenability of the VMN-mimicking hypothesis is somewhat weakened when one considers the effects of amphetamine on VMN-lesioned animals. A reduction or elimination of anorexia would be expected in such animals, since a functional VMN satiety mechanism is no longer present; in fact, an attenuation of amphetamine anorexia has been reported in VNM-lesioned animals (Sharp, Nielson, & Porter, 1962). Yet, it has also been reported that anorexia can still be obtained in VMN-lesioned subjects (Reynolds, 1959).

Reynolds' findings have raised doubts concerning the credibility of the VMN-mimicking hypothesis. But despite these conflicting data, there may be reason to suspect that a persistence of amphetamine-induced anorexia in VMN-lesioned animals is the result of denervation supersensitivity in the remaining VMN adrenergically sensitive neurons not destroyed by lesioning (Margules, 1969, 1970).

LHA-blocking hypothesis: At about the same time that the VMN was being implicated in the regulation of consummatory behavior, Brügger (1943) reported that electrical stimulation of the LHA in cats would elicit eating. Since then, there have been a number of studies demonstrating feeding elicited by LHA stimulation (Delgado & Anand, 1953; Devor et al., 1970; Miller, 1957, 1960; Smith, 1961). Destruction of the LHA creates a syndrome marked by an absence of feeding and drinking, a rapid decline in body weight, and death within several days (Anand & Brobeck, 1951). These deficits in consummatory behavior following damage to the LHA strongly implicate the LHA as a critical region operative in the initiation and regulation of food intake.

Booth (1968) has shown that direct injections of amphetamine in the LHA depress feeding in rats. A similar depressant effect has been obtained by direct application of procaine to the LHA (Epstein, 1960). These data, taken together, suggest that amphetamine directly reduces or blocks neural activity in the LHA and consequently leads to a reduction of feeding behavior. Consistent with the above conclusion are findings that amphetamine also decreases the amplitude of LHA electrical activity (Reiter, 1970), and raises the threshold for electrically elicited feeding in the LHA (Miller, 1960). In addition, amphetamine does not induce anorexia in recovered LHA-lesioned animals (Carlisle, 1964).

Conclusions: At the present state of our knowledge, neither of the theories just discussed can be rejected. Rather, the evidence suggests that the VMN and LHA both are in some way associated with the reduction of feeding following amphetamine administration. The specificity of this relationship, however, has recently been questioned.

Ahlskog and Hoebel (1973) have identified an ascending noradrenergic fiber system, which they propose functions as a satiety mechanism and acts as a substrate for amphetamine-induced anorexia. This system originates from cell groups in the reticular formation of the medulla oblongata and pons (locus coeruleus) and ascends ventrally to enter the medial forebrain bundle. Ahlskog and Hoebel showed that electrolytic or chemical destruction of this ventral noradrenergic bundle induces excessive eating. Furthermore, amphetamine was without anorexic action in ventral bundle–lesioned animals. These data seriously question the major theories of amphetamine-induced anorexia.

Feeding. It is rather paradoxical to find that central injection of norepinephrine, epinephrine, or their precursor, dopamine, into the lateral hypothalamic area results in the elicitation of food consumption in the rat (but not in the cat, monkey, or rabbit) (Feldberg & Sherwood, 1954; Grossman, 1962; Miller, 1965; Myers & Sharpe, 1968). Usually, 4 to 5 grams of food will be consumed during a 30-minute test. It has been shown that the "motivation" for food is truly increased, since animals will perform instrumental tasks in order to obtain access to food during these tests (Grossman, 1962). When food consumption is elicited due to the injection of catecholamines, there is usually an accompanying decrease in water consumption, a depression of locomotor activity, and an increase in blood sugar level (Grossman, 1962; Miller, 1965). The increased food intake has also been noted in rats to follow NE injection into other limbic system sites (Booth, 1967a; Coury, 1967). It is interesting to note, however, that application of epinephrine or norepinephrine into the amygdala increases the food consumption of deprived rats, but has no such effect in sated animals (Grossman, 1964b).

The basis for the opposite action of alpha-adrenergic stimulants following systemic and central administration is not understood. The same drug, for instance NE, will produce anorexia in the rat following systemic administration, but will increase feeding following central injection. Since the feeding augmentation has only been found in the rat, this phenomenon, in any event, would seem to be rather limited. However, a variety of explanations are available. One problem is that we cannot yet choose between them or integrate them into a unitary model. Since it has recently been shown that the same dose of NE that facilitates feeding in the rat during the lighted day inhibits feeding during the dark night, a circadian rhythm would seem to be indicated in the control of feeding behavior, and the feeding phenomenon would appear to be even more limited (Margules, Lewis, Dragovich, & Margules, 1972).

Endogenous hypothalamic NE levels are higher in the dark and lower in the light, and rats feed primarily in the dark, perhaps as a function of the raised NE levels. Therefore, it may be that in the dark, the cerebrally injected NE raises the noradrenergic activity above levels optimal for feeding, whereas during the light, injected NE raises noradrenergic activity to levels optimal for feeding (Margules et al., 1972).

Lesions of the lateral hypothalamic area produce starvation in rats, concomitant with a large reduction in endogenous levels of both NE and D. However, as discussed above, Ungerstedt (1971c) has shown that the lateral hypothalamic syndrome may very well result from damage to the dopaminergic pathway. In contrast, other authors (Berger, Wise, & Stein, 1971, 1973) have found intraventricular NE administration to facilitate recovery from the effects of bilateral lateral hypothalamic damage. These authors have suggested that the recovery is due to the reestablishment of a functioning noradrenergic reinforcement system. Consistent with this hypothesis is the finding that deficits in a variety of biological drives (that lead to feeding, drinking, copulation, pain avoidance) follow lateral hypothalamic lesions (Glickman & Schiff, 1967; Valenstein, 1966). Thus, these various deficits may result from partial destruction of a generalized reinforcement mechanism underlying all the species typical biological drive-type behaviors.

We might point out at this time that D (as well as NE) will elicit feeding in the light following application to the rat lateral hypothalamus. It may be that the adrenergic elicitation of feeding is completely or partially a dopaminergic, rather than a noradrenergic, action. In any event, it is not possible at this time to definitely specify the basis of the feeding following adrenergic stimulation and the starvation following lateral hypothalamic lesions. However, some combination or interaction of effects on the dopaminergic motor control system and the noradrenergic reinforcement system would seem to be responsible for both findings.

Drinking. Injection of the beta-adrenergic agonist, isoproterenol, will elicit water ingestion in the rat (and also other species) (Lehr, Mallow, & Krukowski, 1967). This result occurs following systemic injection, and also following direct injection into the brain. However, water ingestion following isoproterenol injection is eliminated by removing the kidneys (Houpt & Epstein, 1971). Since it has also been shown that beta-adrenergic stimulation causes renin release from the kidneys, and that renin is then converted to the potent dipsogen, angiotensin, it appears that the dipsogenic action of isoproterenol (even when injected directly into the brain) results from the action of angiotensin (see Chapters 4 and 11 in this book).

Brain Disorders

There are two classes of brain disorder in which the catecholamines have been etiologically implicated. The first class is the Parkinsonian-type motor disorder. A dopaminergic deficit seems to be causally related to this type of dysfunction. The other class of disorders has been referred to traditionally as the mental disorders. Our position is that mental (behavioral) disorders are the sole result of either learning or physiological dysfunction, or some combination of the two.

The two major classes of psychoses (the most profound and seriously incapacitating behavioral disorders) are schizophrenia and manic-depressive psychosis. There is now good evidence that a defect in the functioning of the noradrenergic reinforcement system is correlated with these disorders and probably related to their etiology. In schizophrenia an aberration of the thought processes and of the individual's pleasure resources seem to predominate. In manic-depressive psychosis an aberration of affective behavior and arousal seems to predominate. We will discuss the various lines of evidence suggesting the involvement of catecholamines in these processes. These include pharmacological studies, investigations of CA metabolites, and studies of brain function in schizophrenic and manic-depressive individuals.

The catecholamine hypothesis of affective disorders postulates that endogenous depression is due to a functional deficiency of brain catecholamines, and that mania is due to a contrasting overactivity. The catecholamine hypothesis of schizophrenia suggests that some abnormal product of NE or E metabolism existing in the brain is responsible for the primary symptoms of this disease. It has further been suggested that an enzymatic defect, perhaps genetically based, may be activated or potentiated by certain life situations and thus lead to this type of disorder (Kety, 1959; Mandell & Spooner, 1968; Schildkraut, 1965; Schildkraut & Kety, (1967). Much of the evidence for the catecholamine hypotheses of mental disorders is indirect and is partially based on the action of three groups of drugs: (1) reserpine and drugs related to reserpine, (2) amphetamine and the MAO inhibitors, and (3) the tricyclic antidepressants (Table 3.3) (Brady; 1967; Snyder, 1970; Stein, 1967).

Drug effects. The hypothesis that some forms of mania and depression are associated with a disturbance of brain norepinephrine function is based on the following arguments: (1) A drug-induced deficiency of brain catecholamines in animals is usually associated with sedation and inertia, whereas high levels of catecholamines are associated with overactivity and arousal. (2) Prolonged administration of reserpine, known to deplete brain catecholamines in animals, is likely to precipitate a severe depression, even suicide, in human beings. Depression has also been described as a side effect of treatment with alpha-methyldopa, a precursor of a false CA transmitter (alpha-methyldopamine), and thus an agent which specifically depletes brain norepinephrine stores, and with propranolol, a highly active blocking agent of beta-adrenergic receptors. The inference made from these studies is that depression is correlated with a depletion and a functional deactivation of brain NE. (3) Severe stress of a mental or physical nature often acts as a trigger for the onset of endogenous depression. Such stresses have been shown to reduce catecholamine levels in the animal brain. (4) MAO inhibitors and imipraminelike drugs are the most effective antidepressant agents (Chapter 8). Both types of drugs are antagonists or reserpine and potentiators of norepinephrine. (5) Electroconvulsive shock therapy, which

TABLE 3.3

Summary of Pharmacological Observations Compatible with Catecholamine Hypothesis of Affective Disorders

Drug	Effects on mood (humans)	Effects on behavior (animals)	Effects on catecholamines in brain (animals)
Reserpine	Sedation Depression (in some patients)	Sedation	Depletion (intracellular deamination and inactivation)
Tetrabenazine	Sedation Depression (in some patients)	Sedation	Depletion (intracellular deamination and inactivation)
Amphetamine	Stimulation	Stimulation Excitement	Releases norepinephrine (onto receptors) Inhibits cellular uptake (and inactivation) of norepinephrine
Monoamine oxidase inhibitors	Antidepressant	Excitement Prevents and reverses reserpine-induced sedation	Increases levels
Imipramine	Antidepressant	Prevents reserpine-induced sedation Potentiation of amphetamine effects	Inhibits cellular uptake (and inactivation) of norepinephrine–? potentiates action of norepinephrine (as in periphery)
Lithium salts	Treatment of mania		? Increases intracellular deamination of norepinephrine–? decreases norepinephrine available at receptors
AMPT	Sedation (transient) with hypomania upon withdrawal	Sedation (in some studies)	Inhibits synthesis

Note. Reprinted by permission from J. J. Schildkraut and S. S. Kety, Biogenic amines and emotion. *Science*, 1967, **156**, 21–30. Copyright 1967 by the American Association for the Advancement of Science.

is still used in the treatment of depression, is known to stimulate the sympathetic nervous system and produce a massive discharge of catecholamines (Welch, Hendley, & Turek, 1974). (6) Amphetamine, though no longer used as antidepressant because of its side effects, has marked euphoric and alerting effects. This action of amphetamine is complex; it is due partially to the release of NE, combined with a blockade of the neuronal reuptake of NE at presynaptic sites (Kety, 1959; Schildkraut & Kety, 1967; Stein, 1967; Stein & Wise, 1970).

The amphetamines and related drugs (methylphenidate) can also mimic the symptoms of schizophrenia. Large doses (500–1,000 mg per day) taken for a week or so produce a syndrome virtually identical to an acute attack of schizophrenia. This result has been found both in individuals self-administering amphetamines and in normal individuals taking amphetamines as part of an experiment. In very small doses amphetamines also exacerbate the symptoms of schizophrenic patients. In this case it appears that the schizophrenic symptoms are truly worsened, rather than the impositon of a "different" amphetamine psychosis on top of the schizophrenia. Another finding suggesting a similarity between this amphetamine-induced schizophrenia and natural schizophrenia is that the phenothiazines and butyrophenones, which are the most effective medications in natural schizophrenia, are also the best antidotes for amphetamine-induced schizophrenia or for the amphetamine-induced intensification of natural schizophrenia. It, therefore, appears that it is the "psychosis" produced by the amphetamines that is our best "model" for acute schizophrenia (Snyder, Banerjee, Yamamura, & Greenberg, 1974).

A unique metabolite. A number of supposedly unique metabolites of CAs have been discovered and studied in the blood or urine of schizophrenic patients. Such agents as adrenochrome, adrenolutin, ceruloplasma, and taraxein, first implicated as possible agents responsible for psychotic symptoms, are now considered with much more skepticism. In carefully controlled studies these agents are clearly not specifically identifiable with schizophrenia. For example, a protein extract (an alpha-2-globulin) obtained from the blood of schizophrenic patients has been found when injected into rats to impair rope-climbing skill and to alter the behavior of primates (monkeys). However, similar extracts from stressed surgical patients are equally as effective (Kety, 1959). Thus, although this particular protein may be elevated in the blood of many schizophrenics, it has not been proven that this compound, or any of its biochemical or behavioral effects, are directly related to the etiology of schizophrenia. Urinary analyses of particular chemical metabolites have also failed to provide any direct evidence for the role played by catecholamines in abnormal affective states (Kety, 1959). It is perhaps germane, however, to point out that patients exhibiting the cyclic form of the manic-depressive disorder have high excretion rates of CA metabolites associated with the manic phase and low rates associated with the depressive phase (Kety, 1959).

Recently, investigators have begun examining biogenic amine metabolites in the cerebrospinal fluid (CSF) of psychotic patients. In one such study, the concentration of a norepinephrine metabolite (3-methoxy-4-hydroxyphenylgly-col) was lower in the CSF of depressed patients than in normal or manic patients (which did not differ from each other). However, others have found this metabolite to be elevated in manics, and normal in depressives (Post, Gordon, Goodwin, & Bunney, 1973; Wilk et al., 1972). In yet another study, the serotonin metabolite, 5-hydroxy-indoleacetic acid, has been found reduced in the CSF of both manic and depressed patients (Mendels, Frazer, Fitzgerald, Ramsey, & Stokes, 1972). Whether any of these alterations in CSF levels of biogenic amine metabolites are etiologically related to the psychoses, however, remains unclear.

Brain function: A proposed genetic biochemical defect in schizophrenia. An early clue to the involvement of the brain's reinforcement system in psychotic disorders was provided by studies of electrical brain stimulation in humans. Heath (1964) found EBS to the septal region to be both reinforcing and sexually exciting in nonpsychotic humans; whereas, in another study, it was found that schizophrenic humans would not self-stimulate (Bishop, Elder, & Heath, 1964), suggesting that a reinforcement system dysfunction may underly this disease.

Recently, Stein (1971) and Stein and Wise (1971) have proposed that a genetic abnormality in the MFB noradrenergic reinforcement system, may be the basic mechanism responsible for the disordered behavior of schizophrenia. It is suggested that as a consequence of a genetic defect which leads to a deficiency of dopamine-β-hydroxylase (the enzyme that converts dopamine to norepineph-rine in the presynaptic terminal), much of the dopamine present in the presynaptic region is not converted into NE. It is thought that the unconverted dopamine is then oxygenated in the synaptic gap (or in the presynaptic terminal) to 6-hydroxydopamine. The dopamine and 6-hydroxydopamine may then fail to effectively activate the postsynaptic membrane as norepinephrine would have, and the 6-hydroxydopamine, to which some of the dopamine is metabolized, is taken up by the presynaptic membrane where it damages or destroys the membrane.

There is evidence that the injection of 6-hydroxydopamine causes a prolonged depletion of brain catecholamines and degeneration of noradrenergic nerve terminals (Tranzer & Thoenen, 1968). Also, 6-hydroxydopamine has been shown to induce degeneration of peripheral sympathetic nerve terminals. When injected intraventricularly in rats, 6-hydroxydopamine has caused a prolonged depletion of brain catecholamines, a decrease in self-stimulation bar-press rates, a decrease in ingestive behavior, and a catatoniclike stupor. Furthermore, compounds similar to 6-hydroxydopamine have been found to have hallucino-genic activity in humans.

A recent study in primates (macaques) may also be interpreted as supporting the psychopathology-reinforcement system hypothesis (Redmond, Hinrichs, Maas, & Kling, 1973). Intraventricular injection of 6-hydroxydopamine signifi-cantly disturbed the social behavior of treated animals in a free-ranging colony. The treated monkeys had "blank affectless faces," and exhibited decreases in social grooming, self-grooming, threats, attacks, and total social initiatives. The authors suggested that "damage to a 'reward-punishment system' . . . might be inferred from the decreased engagement in reinforced or rewarded behaviors . . . and from the failure of some animals to avoid punishment."

Wise and Stein (1973) have recently obtained further evidence consistent with their overall model of the cause of schizophrenia. They have shown that the levels of dopamine-β-hydroxylase in the brainstem, hypothalamus, and amygdala of schizophrenics are significantly lower than the amounts of this enzyme found in the same regions of nonschizophrenic brains. These data, obtained from autopsy material, can be expected to open up a new area of research. A great deal of provocative and important information on the biochemistry of psychopathology should be obtainable by biochemically analyzing autopsy brains.

Chlorpromazine (CPZ) and related drugs (Chapter 5) have been the drugs of choice in the treatment of schizophrenia. CPZ is an inhibitor of CA reuptake, especially that of dopamine, and antagonizes the CA-depleting action of 6-hydroxydopamine, and the reduction of self-stimulation produced by 6-hydroxydopamine. The basic model, shown in Figure 3.6, is that CPZ is effective in the treatment of schizophrenia because it protects the reward system of the schizophrenic by blocking the uptake of endogenously formed 6-hydroxydopamine into the noradrenergic nerve ending. The reduced efficacy of CPZ in so-called "burnt out" chronic schizophrenics may be a result of irreversible damage to the noradrenergic reward terminals from 6-hydroxydopamine.

Stein and Wise have further suggested that there are two ascending noradrenergic systems and that damage to a dorsal pathway that ascends to the cerebral cortex may produce thought disorders characteristic of schizophrenia, while damage to a ventral pathway innervating hypothalamic and limbic system structures may yield affective disorders such as mania and depression. Even if this model is completely in error, as it may very well be, it is important as an example of the type of biological malfunction that could easily lead to severe psychopathology. One important aspect of this hypothesis is the increase in precision and credibility as compared to previous speculation. We can see a progression from the analysis of substances in urine and blood, to the analysis of CSF, to the analysis of anatomically localized brain enzyme systems involved in synaptic transmission.

This Stein and Wise hypothesis of a noradrenergic reinforcement system basis for schizophrenia has, not surprisingly, aroused considerable controversy (see Antelman, Lippa, Fisher, Bowers, Van Woert, Strauss, Carpenter, Stein, & Wise, 1972, for an exchange of letters on the subject). One important question appears to relate to the temporary behavioral deficits produced by 6OHDA in rats, despite a permanent depression of brain catecholamine levels. This relationship, however, can be related to the episodic nature of the early course of schizophrenia in many patients. One explanation for this phenomenon involves a process called *denervation supersensitivity*. When catecholamine levels are

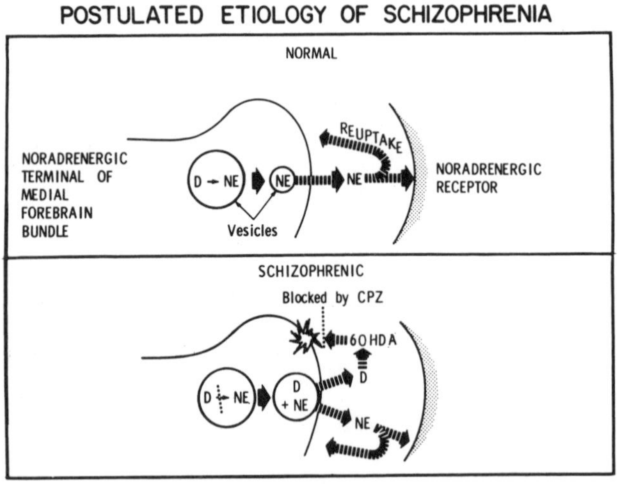

POSTULATED ETIOLOGY OF SCHIZOPHRENIA

FIGURE 3.6. Postulated etiology of schizophrenia–diagram of noradrenergic transmission in normal and schizophrenic brain based on the assumption that a pathological gene for schizophrenia causes reduced activity, or synthesis, of dopamine-β-hydroxylase. Normal: Virtually all dopamine (D) is converted to norepinephrine (NE) by dopamine-β-hydroxylase. Schizophrenic: Dopamine is only partially converted to norepinephrine. After release into synapse, some of the dopamine is autoxidized to 6-hydroxydopamine. When this toxic substance is taken up by the nerve terminals, it gradually destroys the vesicles and eventually the nerve endings. (Reprinted by permission from L. Stein and C. D. Wise, Possible etiology of schizophrenia: Progressive damage to the noradrenergic reward system by 6-hydroxydopamine. *Science*, 1971, **171**, 1032–1036. Copyright 1971 by the American Association for the Advancement of Science.)

depleted in the peripheral or central nervous system by damage to the CA neurons, the CA postsynaptic receptors become supersensitive to exogenously administered adrenergic agonists (and to whatever endogenous CAs remain). Several investigators have now reported experiments suggesting that the development of denervation supersensitivity does occur following depletion of CAs, and may account for the behavioral recovery of 6OHDA-treated rats, and for the episodic nature of schizophrenia (see the letter by Stein & Wise in Antelman et al., 1972; and also Glick, Greenstein, & Zimmerberg, 1972).

SUMMARY AND CONCLUSIONS

In this chapter we have reviewed the roles of adrenergic drugs and of the endogenous adrenergic systems both in the physiological functioning of mammalian organisms and in their behavior. A number of biochemical considerations are important to understanding the adrenergics. These include structure-activity relationships (that is, the relationship between the chemical structure of a compound and its physiological and behavioral actions), optical isomerism, direct vs indirect mechanisms of action, and the concepts of alpha and beta receptors.

The term *homeostasis* refers to the maintenance of an optimal level of biological functioning within specific normal limits. Although it is common to regard physiological processes as operating in the pursuit of biological homeostasis, we have also emphasized the importance of recognizing that behavioral events, too, are a part of homeostatis management.

The actions of D, NE, and E in the regulation of homeostasis are complex. However, there appear to be at least three somewhat distinct phenomena which conceptually provide an understanding of the physiological and behavioral functions of these adrenergic compounds. The first of these processes relates to the role of peripheral synaptically released NE and D and of adrenal medullary E in reactions to physical stress and to the press of environmental demands and needs. Several characteristic physiological responses and species-typical behaviors are subserved by these peripheral adrenergic mechanisms (usually referred to as *sympathetic arousal*).

The second phenomenon is related to the effects of centrally produced NE. Brain NE generally appears to facilitate physiological and behavioral processes under the control of the CNS. In response to increased levels of brain NE, an organism becomes aroused or alerted, exhibits more activity, and typically shows an augmentation of learning and performance. These behavioral changes are, of course, consistent with the homeostatic function of responding to stress and emergency demands.

Closely related to the arousing effect of brain NE is the concept of NE in the facilitation of reinforcement or reward processes. We have attempted to show that NE acts as a synaptic transmitter in a specialized brain system that underlies the reinforcement of behavior. The enhancement of arousal or alertness and of learned behavior may, therefore, reflect the reinforcement or "stamping in" role of brain NE. Any deficits in such a system could conceivably result in misdirected behavior patterns (non-goal-directed) and inappropriate behavior in response to reward contingencies. Deficits in brain NE have, in fact, been etiologically linked to the two most severe forms of mental disorders, schizophrenia and manic-depressive psychosis.

A third and final aspect of adrenergic processes relates to brain D in the mediation of motor functions and certain forms of sensorimotor integration. A deficit of brain dopaminergic systems has been shown to be related to the motor disorder, Parkinson's disease. Similarly, particular disorders of appetitive behavior (feeding) may follow damage to dopaminergic neurons.

The integrity of each of these adrenergic processes is dependent on optimal levels of D, NE, and E, respectively. Alterations in any one system may influence the physiological status of the organism and set into play a series of modified patterns of behavior. The intent of this chapter has been to examine the various adrenergic drugs which affect the levels of E, NE, and D in therapeutic or experimental situations and to examine the physiological and behavioral effects of such alterations of endogenous systems.

4
CHOLINERGIC DRUGS

Hugh E. Criswell and Robert A. Levitt

The cholinergic drugs, as with the adrenergics considered in the preceding chapter, profoundly act on the peripheral and central nervous systems. These actions result from either the stimulation or the inhibition of neuronal transmission at cholinergic junctions (those that utilize acetylcholine, ACh, as a transmitter). We have already learned in the chapter on biochemical neuro-pharmacology (Chapter 2) that ACh is a junctional transmitter at three distinguishable sites in the peripheral nervous system. These sites are (1) the synapses in the autonomic nervous system ganglia, both for the sympathetic and the parasympathetic divisions; (2) the synapselike junctions between the postganglionic fibers of the parasympathetic division and the autonomic effector organs (neuroeffector junctions); and (3) the synapselike junctions between the peripheral somatic nervous system motor fibers and the skeletal muscles (neuromuscular junctions). These last two junctions, which we have chosen to call *neuroeffector* and *neuromuscular*, are not actually synapses since they do not connect two neurons, but are synapselike in many of their properties. In fact, the neuromuscular junction has often been used as a model for the study of synaptic activity and much of our knowledge of synaptic events has been inferred from studies of the neuromuscular junction.

In this chapter we will first review the properties of ACh itself. We will then discuss the most important properties of the major drugs that facilitate or inhibit cholinergic transmission (these drugs and their modes of action were listed in Table 2.1). The last section of this chapter will be concerned with the behavioral roles of CNS cholinergic systems and with the effects of drugs on these CNS behavioral systems. The central integrating concept we will employ is that of a CNS cholinergic system as the neurological basis for the inhibition of behavior.

Evidence of this behavioral inhibition is seen in a variety of processes, including habituation, extinction, and the effects of aversive stimuli. Certain roles in homeostatic adjustments that do not fit into this behavioral inhibition concept will also be discussed. These homeostatic roles include fluid balance and aggressive behavior.

ACETYLCHOLINE

The steps in the biosynthesis of this neurotransmitter were detailed in Chapter 2 (Figure 2.5). The manufactured ACh is then stored in the vesicles of the presynaptic ending until the firing of a spike potential by the neuron causes its release. Following release into the synaptic cleft, the ACh diffuses across this space to the region of the postsynaptic neuron or effector. The effect of the ACh may be either excitatory or inhibitory depending upon the properties of the postsynaptic membrane. The ACh is then hydrolized by the enzyme acetylcholinesterase (AChE), thereby returning the postsynaptic membrane to its normal resting state.

Direct and Indirect Actions

Cholinergic drugs may act directly upon the postsynaptic ACh receptor (a direct action) or indirectly by altering the effective levels of endogenous ACh within the nervous system (an indirect action). Indirect-acting cholinergic drugs may alter the levels of ACh by acting at any point along the pathway of synthesis or destruction. Direct-acting cholinergic drugs have a sufficient resemblance to ACh to become bound to the postsynaptic membrane of a synaptic junction where ACh would normally function as the transmitter substance. Many of these substances not only bind to the ACh receptor but, once bound, cause an effect upon that receptor similar to that of ACh itself. These compounds mimic the effects of ACh and are, therefore, called *cholinomimetics* (or *cholinergic agonists*). Other substances, while similar enough to ACh that they will bind to the postsynaptic membrane, are not similar enough to produce the neurotransmitter effect of ACh at that site. These drugs, which passively occupy the ACh receptor site, prevent endogenous ACh from reaching that site and thereby block its action as a neurotransmitter. These substances are called *competitive receptor blocking agents* (*cholinergic antagonists* or *cholinolytics*).

Receptor Types

We have already pointed out that three distinct cholinergic receptors can be identified within the peripheral nervous system (see Chapter 2). These are the muscarinic receptors at the parasympathetic neuroeffector junctions, which are especially sensitive to stimulation by muscarine and blockade by atropinelike drugs; the nicotinic receptors of the autonomic ganglia, which are stimulated by nicotine and blocked by drugs such as hexamethonium; and the nicotinic receptors of the neuromuscular junctions, which are also stimulated by nicotine, but are sensitive to blockade by curarelike drugs rather than by hexamethonium. Thus, cholinergic junctions in the peripheral nervous system may be divided into three classes based upon their differing sensitivities to the various drugs that are agonistic or antagonistic to the action of ACh. These three categories are not entirely exclusive. Rather, the various drugs differ in their relative activities at these sites. Thus, ACh affects all three receptors, while muscarine acts on only one. Other drugs, such as nicotine, may have different potencies at the differing sites while having at least a minimal effect upon all three receptor types.

In comparing the peripheral cholinergic system with the adrenergic system, ACh can be seen as analogous to epinephrine, since ACh activates each of the types of cholinergic junctions (as epinephrine activates both alpha- and beta-adrenergic junctions). Another important point to be made again is that the evidence for ACh functioning as a CNS synaptic transmitter is not as strong as for its role in the peripheral nervous system. Furthermore, evidence of ACh synaptic activity in the CNS is primarily indirect and is partially inferred from its peripheral nervous system role.

Actions of ACh

ACh has many functions in the body, but it is of little therapeutic value as a drug, due to the rapid destruction of exogeneous ACh in the blood by cholinesterase. However, many of the drugs that mimic ACh, and which are not so rapidly destroyed, have potent and useful effects. We will, however, first describe the effects of endogenous ACh as a model for other cholinergic drugs.

ACh as a "universal transmitter"?   Since ACh stimulates synapses within the autonomic ganglia, it produces manifestations of both sympathetic and parasympathetic action. Within the parasympathetic nervous system, only one transmitter is released—ACh. Within the sympathetic nervous system, ACh is released by the first neuron in the two-neuron chain and this ACh then produces a spike potential in the second neuron. It is this second neuron which then releases NE at the neuroeffector junction. In fact, it appears that even here the NE release may be secondary to an initial ACh release. The drugs guanethidine and bretylium prevent the release of NE from the presynaptic terminal (see Table 2.2). When these drugs are administered at the sympathetic neuroeffector junction, stimulation of the sympathetic nervous system leads to parasympathetic rather than sympathetic effects (Guyton, 1971). This would be expected if small quantities of ACh were liberated from the sympathetic postganglionic neurons at the same time as larger quantities of NE were normally liberated. Blocking the release of NE would then allow the effects of the small amount of ACh released to be observed. This is consistent with a postulated intermediate event in synaptic transmission at adrenergic synapses; that is, it has been suggested that a spike potential causes the release of a small amount of ACh in autonomic fibers. This initial release of ACh then serves to activate the release of NE at the sympathetic neuroeffector junction or of more ACh at the parasympathetic neuroeffector junction (Koelle, 1962). The type of chemical which is released subsequent to the initial release of ACh then depends upon the type of neuron. This idea has been extended to cover CNS neurons as well; and ACh has been proposed as a "universal transmitter" that acts as an intermediate between the ionic spike potential events and the release of other transmitters. Since ACh appears to have a widespread distribution and also to be found intraneuronally throughout the neuron, it has further been suggested that ACh even has a role in triggering the spike potential itself (Burn & Rand, 1965; Nachmonsohn, 1970). These latter views are not now generally accepted, but could eventually prove to have some validity.

Cardiovascular system. The vascular system is extremely sensitive to the effects of administered ACh. Doses of ACh that are too small to produce effects upon the heart, skeletal muscle, or glands produce a drop in blood pressure due to the vasodilative effect of ACh. The actions of ACh upon the cardiac rhythm and conduction of impulses within the heart parallel almost exactly those produced by stimulation of the vagus nerve (cranial nerve X) which supplies the major parasympathetic innervation to the heart. These effects include slowing of the heartbeat and a decrease in impulse conduction (Volle, 1971a).

Smooth muscles. While ACh has a relaxing effect upon the smooth muscles lining the blood vessels, its effect upon the smooth muscles of most other organs is one of increased tone. Thus, ACh causes contraction of the smooth muscle cells of the bronchioles, uterus, ureters, bladder, stomach, small intestine, and colon.

Glands. The glands innervated (and activated) by cholinergic fibers include the adrenal medulla, and also the salivary, lacrimal (tear), and sweat glands, in addition to various secretory cells of the pancreas, bronchioles, and gastrointestinal mucosa (Guyton, 1971).

Sympathetic action. Most of the effects of ACh occur as a result of its direct action at the parasympathetic neuroeffector junction (muscarinic action). The nicotinic actions of ACh are usually masked by these more potent muscarinic effects. At high doses, however, the sympathetic division of the ANS is stimulated at the ganglia and many of the parasympathetic effects of the lower doses of ACh may be reversed. This is especially true if a muscarinic blocking agent, such as atropine, is given concomitantly with the ACh. If the muscarinic effects of ACh are blocked, it becomes a sympathomimetic rather than a parasympathomimetic drug (Koelle, 1970b; Volle, 1971a).

CNS. The CNS effects of high doses of ACh, or any of the drugs that stimulate cholinergic activity, are similar. They each will produce a disruption of the thought processes, characterized by confusion and delirium, and a generalized cortical excitation, which may lead to convulsions. In lesser doses, effects may be seen at subcortical sites. At high doses, a central respiratory arrest may be produced. This acts in concert with the peripheral paralysis of the respiratory musculature to produce death by asphyxiation.

OTHER CHOLINE ESTERS

These agents include methacholine, carbamylcholine (carbachol, Figure 4.1), and bethanechol, which are synthetic esters of choline similar in chemical structure to ACh. Muscarine (Figure 4.1), arecoline, and pilocarpine are naturally occurring choline esters found in plants that share many of the properties of ACh. Nicotine (Figure 4.1) is not a choline ester, but is a naturally occurring substance obtained from tobacco, which mimics certain of the effects of ACh.

Many of the choline esters have strong stimulant actions on muscarinic receptors and all are less sensitive to hydrolysis by cholinesterase than is ACh itself. The relative strength of their actions on the cardiovascular, gastrointestinal, and urinary tracts varies, as does the degree to which they also possess nicotinic actions. However, knowledge of these different patterns of action is not necessary for our purposes. Certain of these choline esters are used in clinical medicine to slow the heartbeat or to increase gastrointestinal or urinary activity when these functions are slowed by some pathological condition.

Muscarine

The most selective drug for action at the parasympathetic neuroeffector junction is muscarine. Muscarine is found in the mushroom *Amanita muscaria*

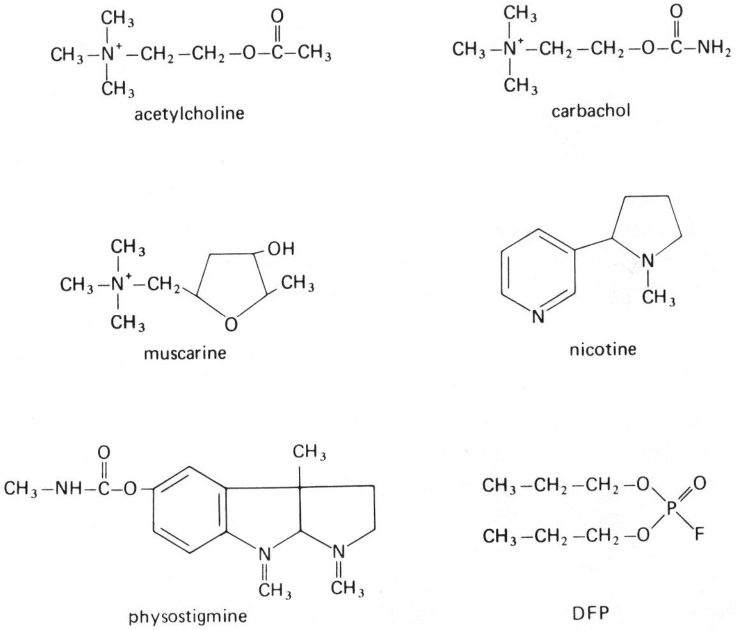

FIGURE 4.1. Representative cholinergic facilitators.

(fly agaric). The pharmacological properties of muscarine are due to its actions at the parasympathetic neuroeffector junction and are essentially identical to those of parasympathetic arousal. Either the administration of a muscarinic drug or the direct stimulation of the parasympathetic division of the ANS produces a syndrome of events which includes an increase in intestinal motility, an increase in the secretion of the glands supplying salivary and digestive fluids, and a relaxation of the sphincters of the bladder and intestine, with an accompanying constriction of the bladder musculature. These responses represent an integrated series of events which are consistent with the increase in vegetative function commonly associated with the arousal of the parasympathetic nervous system.

Muscarine also has an unexpected stimulant effect upon the sweat glands. The sweat glands are sympathetically innervated and would normally be expected to respond to NE rather than to a cholinergic drug. However, the muscarinic action of ACh upon the exocrine glands extends to the sweat glands as well, making this one of the few sympathetically mediated responses that results from a release of ACh rather than from NE at the sympathetic neuroeffector junction.

While ACh is rapidly destroyed by cholinesterase in the bloodstream, muscarine is relatively immune to such destruction. This results in a much higher potency for muscarine, which is about 100 times as effective as ACh for the production of parasympathetic arousal (Volle, 1971b).

Poisoning. As was previously noted, muscarine is present in some mushrooms. The poisoning which results from the ingestion of these mushrooms is due primarily to the extreme arousal of the parasympathetic neuroeffector junctions produced by muscarine. These symptoms develop rapidly (sometimes within minutes) following ingestion of the offending mushrooms (Koelle, 1970d). As we shall see, the muscarinic blocking agent, atropine, is an effective antidote for this type of mushroom poisoning.

Recreational use. Amanita muscaria grows wild in Europe and North America where it has been consumed for its hallucinatory effects. These effects are manifested as an initial depression of activity and as a dreamlike state during which "visions" may occur. The initial motor depression is followed by a period of excitement with sensory (primarily visual and auditory) distortions and hallucinations. These effects are probably not due to the muscarine present in *Amanita muscaria*, but to some combination of the many other pharmacologically active agents which are present. These include atropine, hyoscyamine, muscimol, ibotinic acid, muscazone, and possibly bufotenine. No one agent duplicates the effects of ingestion of the mushroom; the interaction of two or more of the pharmacologically active agents is probably responsible for the psychoactive effects of *Amanita muscaria* (Longo, 1972).

Pilocarpine and Arecoline

Pilocarpine is found in the leaves of *Pilocarpus jaberondi* and *Pilocarpus microphyllus*. When the leaves of these plants are chewed, they produce profuse salivation. Pilocarpine has a strong stimulant effect upon both the salivary and sweat glands. When injected in the human, pilocarpine can produce within a few hours as much as 3 liters of sweat and 350 milliliters of saliva (Koelle, 1970d). The muscarinic effects of pilocarpine are accompanied by additional activity at the ganglionic synapses which may result in an increase in blood pressure. The fact that pilocarpine lacks a quaternary nitrogen (a nitrogen attached to four other atoms) allows it to penetrate the blood-brain barrier more easily than other ACh-like drugs, and it has some central effects, which will be discussed later (Volle, 1971b).

Arecoline is found in the areca nut (betel nut). Betel, which consists of betel nuts and shells, the leaves from a pepper plant, and lime, has been chewed for centuries in the East Indies and is reputed to produce euphoria. Its peripheral effects are similar to those of pilocarpine (Koelle, 1970d; Volle, 1971b).

Nicotine

Nicotine is a naturally occurring chemical obtained from the tobacco plant. Tobacco was commonly smoked by the American Indians when it was discovered by European explorers in the 15th century. Nicotine has an extremely interesting history and the interested reader is referred to Brecher (1972). Nicotine penetrates the blood-brain barrier and has important central effects which will be discussed shortly. Its peripheral actions are due to its stimulant effects upon the autonomic ganglia, the adrenal medulla, and the neuromuscular junction. It is important to note that nicotine acts as a stimulant at these sites only when administered in very small doses.

Depolarization blockade. Nicotine is such an effective depolarizing agent at the postsynaptic membrane that at higher doses the membrane is depolarized and then maintained in the depolarized state for an extended period of time, thus blocking cholinergic transmission. The mechanism behind this effect is that neurons have an optimal setting of stimulus conditions that will yield a spike potential. If too little transmitter reaches the postsynaptic receptor, the EPSP will not be large or prolonged enough to generate a spike potential. Too much transmitter, on the other hand, leads to such an extended occupancy of the postsynaptic receptor sites that the neuron, once depolarized, cannot effectively repolarize to generate a second impulse. It is only when an optimal amount of transmitter (somewhere between these two extremes) reaches the postsynaptic membrane that neural transmission can occur (Koelle, 1970d; Volle, 1971b). The biphasic (stimulation followed by a blockade of transmission due to a maintained depolarization) action of many drugs at the nicotinic receptor complicates a description of the actions of the nicotinic drugs. The dose range between that producing excitation of the postsynaptic membrane and that producing a depolarizing blockade of the membrane is small for nicotine. Other nicotinic drugs do exist, however, which have a relatively large difference between the stimulation and blocking dosages (such as dimethylphenyl-piperazinium, DMPP).

Poisoning. The nicotinic drugs do not have therapeutic usefulness. They are, however, of great interest because of their widespread use by tobacco smokers and because of their occasional toxicological importance stemming from overindulgence in tobacco or accidental contamination from insecticides, many of which contain nicotine. The symptoms of nicotine poisoning will serve to describe both its stimulating and blocking actions at the nicotinic receptor.

At lethal drug levels there may be little symptomatic warning, as the action of nicotine is extremely rapid. A burning sensation in the mouth and stomach is followed by nausea, salivation, abdominal pain, vomiting, and diarrhea. A cold sweat, headache, dizziness, auditory and visual distortions, confusion, and weakness occur. Respiration is stimulated and blood pressure rises. The pupils are first constricted due to parasympathetic stimulation and then dilated due to the ensuing depolarizing blockade. The heart rate is first slowed by the parasympathetic stimulation from nicotine and then becomes rapid as the parasympathetic effects are blocked. The ensuing coma is accompanied by circulatory shock, convulsions, and respiratory paralysis, followed by death (Aviado, 1971). From the above description it can be seen that nicotine produces a combination of sympathetic and parasympathetic effects. This combination is due to the nonselective stimulation of all postganglionic neurons of the autonomic nervous system. Some of the sympathetic effects are also due to the release of epinephrine from the adrenal glands that results from ganglionic excitatory effects of nicotine upon the splanchnic nerve (Volle & Koelle, 1970).

Smoking. The average cigarette contains about 2% nicotine (20 to 30 mg) as compared to about 1% in the "denicotinized" preparations. A cigar may contain 10 times this amount. The acute lethal dose of nicotine is between 50 and 75 mg, but this level would be difficult to achieve from smoking, due to the slow absorption of nicotine via the inhalation route. A person actually absorbs only 2.5 to 3.5 mg of nicotine from a single cigarette. With this drug dose, the effects observed are comparable to those noted following a 1-mg dose injected intravenously (Volle & Koelle, 1970).

Many of the effects of cigarette smoking are unpredictable. This is due to a combination of factors including the ingredients other than nicotine that are in tobacco smoke (nearly 500 compounds other than nicotine have been isolated from tobacco smoke), the development of tolerance to nicotine upon continued intake, the biphasic action of nicotine, and the activity of nicotine at the autonomic ganglia of both sympathetic and parasympathetic divisions of the ANS, as well as a direct effect of nicotine at the neuromuscular junction. Some generalizations are, however, possible. The majority of persons respond to low levels of nicotine with a peripheral vasoconstriction which is often evidenced by cold hands. The peripheral vasoconstriction is usually accompanied by an increase in blood pressure. Some of the effects of smoking can be attributed to the release of E and NE from the adrenal gland.

Effects of chronic intake: Because of cigarette smoking, much interest has been generated in the effects of chronic nicotine intake. Typically, nicotine is ingested through smoking tobacco. The heat from the burning tobacco causes the nicotine to vaporize and about 10% of the available nicotine is inhaled; of this amount, 90% is absorbed into the bloodstream. As was previously pointed out, smoking results in the ingestion of many compounds other than nicotine and several of the effects of smoking may result from these other chemicals. In particular, the carcinogenic (cancer-producing) effects of tobacco smoke probably do not directly involve nicotine; research is currently underway to identify the carcinogenic agents in cigarette smoke and to attempt to produce a "cancerless" cigarette.

The other characteristics of chronic cigarette smoking may also be due to agents other than the nicotine in cigarettes. Cigarette smokers commonly complain of shortness of breath. This may be due to the fact that the carbon monoxide inhaled with the smoke combines with hemoglobin in the red blood cells to form carboxyhemoglobin. Approximately 10% of the body's hemoglobin may then be tied up in this way. Carboxyhemoglobin is a form of hemoglobin which does not permit oxygen binding; therefore the oxygen-carrying capability of the blood is decreased. All tobacco smoke contains carbon monoxide and, therefore, all tobacco products facilitate the production of carboxyhemoglobin. Cigarette smoke contains the least carbon monoxide (about 1%), pipe smoke about 2%, and cigar smoke about 6%. It may be this oxygen deprivation which causes the shortness of breath in the chronic smoker. The carbon monoxide may also be responsible for the smaller babies born to pregnant smokers. Not only are babies of pregnant smokers smaller, there is also an increase of from 200% to 300% in the number of premature babies and a significant increase in the incidence of stillborn children, or babies that die soon after birth (Brecher, 1972).

Many of the effects of cigarette smoking may be attributed to the effects of nicotine possibly interacting with other constituents of the smoke. Both nicotine and tobacco smoke have been shown to inhibit stomach contractions for about 1 hour and also to decrease the sensitivity of the taste buds. Perhaps this combination of effects is why people report a reduction of hunger after smoking cigarettes. Also, many report that they invariably gain weight when they cease smoking. Psychodynamic interpretations have suggested that smokers have a strong oral need and when cigarettes are no longer available, the smoker resorts to munching food. There may be other reasons. Food probably tastes better to a nonsmoker because the taste buds are no longer desensitized and he or she is aware of the stomach contractions which are associated with hunger. In addition to this, the metabolic rate decreases when a person stops smoking and there is a decrease in heart rate of about three beats per minute, as well as a 10% reduction in oxygen consumption. This would produce a situation where food is simply not being burned up as rapidly and instead is stored as fat (Aviado, 1971; Brecher, 1972; Volle & Koelle, 1970).

Addiction: While it is still possible to find persons who will claim that people who cannot quit smoking are simply weak and have no self control, more and more evidence is being accumulated which suggests that nicotine is an addicting drug. Much of this evidence is reviewed in Brecher (1972) who concludes that nicotine is most definitely an addicting drug, but one that has been "domesticated." Three requirements must be met before a drug is classified as addicitng. (1) Tolerance must develop to the pharmacological effects of the drug upon prolonged use. (2) Withdrawal symptoms must appear when the drug is discontinued following prolonged use. (3) There must be a strong tendency to continue the drug intake (craving) following prolonged use. All three of these qualifications have been met by nicotine.

The buildup of tolerance to nicotine is a part of folklore. Who has not heard of the novice smoker's experience with his first cigar? The novice smoker cannot usually tolerate the amount of nicotine present in a single cigarette, but after several years of smoking, may be able to smoke ten without experiencing the toxic symptoms of pallor, sweating, nausea, and vomiting.

Withdrawal from nicotine produces a whole constellation of symptoms in the chronic smoker. These include drowsiness, headache, digestive disorders, sweating, cramps, insomnia, and nervousness (Brecher, 1972). Yet, while narcotic or alcohol addiction has often been associated with antisocial behavior and a craving for the addicting substance, this has seldom been seen following chronic nicotine intake. Murder, robbery, mugging, bribery, extortion, etc., are not commonly associated with nicotine addiction. Why? It may be a case of availability rather than pharmacology. Heroin is not generally available and attempts to obtain it lead to socially unacceptable behavior. When heroin or methadone are made readily available to the addict in a "maintenance" program (see Chapter 7) the incidence of antisocial behavior associated with narcotic addiction declines markedly. In Germany during World War II, tobacco was rationed so that men were allowed only two packs per month and women were allowed only one pack per month. Studies have shown that with the unavailability of nicotine people stole, bartered, and black-marketed cigarettes— definitely antisocial behavior. Americans have lost sight of nicotine addiction and the dependence upon nicotine because of the constant availability of the drug. Rarely do we have to "walk a mile for a Camel." Clearly, more research into the mechanism of action of this potent drug is needed.

CHOLINESTERASE-INHIBITING AGENTS

The principal means by which ACh is removed from its sites of action is by hydrolysis by AChE. Inhibition of AChE allows the ACh to accumulate at the postsynaptic membrane. Thus, the responses of cholinergically innervated tissues are exaggerated and prolonged; we find increased skeletal muscle activity, increased glandular and smooth muscle activity, a decrease in heart rate (parasympathetic effects), and increased ganglionic transmission and CNS effects. All of these actions are seen following administration of the anticholinesterase agents (Koelle, 1970a; Volle, 1971a). There are two groups of anticholinesterases, the reversible and the irreversible inhibitors. In general, those agents possessing therapeutic value are reversible in action while the highly toxic drugs used in insecticides and chemical warfare act irreversibly.

Reversible Cholinesterase Inhibitors

AChE catalyzes the hydrolysis of ACh in the following way. When ACh and AChE come into contact, bonds are formed between the molecules, producing an ACh-AChE complex. The formation of this complex reduces the strength of the bond between the acidic and alcoholic components of the ACh and places this bond in a position where it can easily combine with a hydroxyl group (OH) to produce acetic acid, free choline, and a regenerated AChE molecule (Carrier, 1972; Triggle, 1971).

The reversible anticholinesterases (physostigmine, neostigmine, and edrophonium are examples) form a transient complex with the surface of the AChE molecule in much the same way as does ACh. The bonds formed by the anticholinesterase agents are stronger than those formed between ACh and AChE and the anti-AChE compounds act as competitive inhibitors for the active sites on the AChE molecule. The anti-AChE compounds thereby reduce the amount of AChE that is available for the hydrolysis of ACh and, therefore, increase the lifetime of ACh once it is released from the presynaptic terminal. The strength of the bond connecting the AChE and AChE inhibitor determines the period of action of the anti-AChE compound. Some compounds have a relatively short period of activity lasting about 1 to 2 hours, while others bind more strongly to AChE. The latter drugs deactivate the AChE molecule for 2 to 8 hours.

Small doses of an anti-AChE agent yield a predominantly muscarinic response, as would be expected from the predominantly muscarinic effects of ACh. Thus, vasodilation (and a consequent decrease in blood pressure), decreased heart rate, increased gastrointestinal activity, bronchial constriction and spasm, increased salivation and sweating, and pupillary constriction occur. At low doses, the effects upon the neuromuscular junction are minimal, but as the dosage is increased, muscle stimulation occurs, followed by paralysis due to a depolarizing block. The primary therapeutic use of the anti-AChE agents is in the treatment of myasthenia gravis. This is an interesting disorder of cholinergic transmission at the neuromuscular junction, and bears some discussion.

Myasthenia gravis. Myasthenia gravis is a disease which is characterized by weakness of the skeletal muscles. The weakness does not affect all muscles equally. Most often, the first signs are double vision (diplopia) which results from a weakening of the extraocular muscles. Another common form of the disease involves a gradual weakening of the muscles of the trunk and extremities, while a third form originates in the muscles involved in chewing and swallowing.

Once started, the disease gradually spreads to other muscles and the severity of the symptoms wax and wane. Myasthenia gravis is a disorder of cholinergic transmission at the neuromuscular junction and while its etiology is unknown, three hypotheses have been advanced: (1) The amount of ACh released presynaptically is less than normal. (2) A curarelike substance is synthesized by the affected individual. (3) The postsynaptic membrane is less sensitive to ACh than normal (Curtis et al., 1972). All three hypotheses have found some experimental support with the most recent information favoring the third hypothesis (Fambrough, Drachman, & Satymurty, 1973).

A logical corrolary to these hypotheses is that compounds which would increase the effectiveness of that ACh which is released at the neuromuscular junction should increase the strength of muscular contractions in persons suffering from myasthenia gravis. The anticholinesterase agents have just this effect and are, at present, the treatment of choice for myasthenia gravis. Their mechanism of action is as follows. As the effective amount of ACh reaching the postsynaptic terminal is decreased in myasthenia gravis (in some manner), AChE would normally deactivate this ACh before it reached the threshold for the production of a muscle endplate potential (this is the version of a neuron spike potential found at the neuromuscular junction). Inhibition of the destruction of ACh by an anti-AChE agent allows a buildup of endogenous ACh at the postsynaptic membrane where the increased amount of ACh is now able to initiate a muscle potential (Koelle, 1970a). It is important to remember that the neuromuscular junction responds to the nicotinic effects of ACh and that excess amounts of ACh may lead to a depolarization blockade of the neuromuscular junction. Indeed, the usual cause of death from anti-AChE poisoning is a paralysis of the respiratory muscles. For this reason, a most important consideration with these agents is the administration of a proper dosage. An overdose of the anti-AChE agent may lead to weakness by causing a depolarizing block at the neuromuscular junction, which is indistinguishable from that caused by myasthenia gravis itself. This task is further complicated by the ever-changing severity of the symptoms, which necessitates a constant adjustment of the dosage of the medication (Curtis et al., 1972).

The three reversible anti-AChE agents which have received the most extensive testing and which have been used in the treatment of myasthenia gravis are edrophonium (Tensilon), physostigmine (Eserine), and neostigmine. These three drugs differ in important ways. Edrophonium is, by far, the shortest acting. Physostigmine and neostigmine are both longer acting drugs, but their effects differ from each other in an important way. While physostigmine (Figure 4.1) is a tertiary amine (each nitrogen is connected to no more than three other atoms), and, therefore, penetrates the blood-brain barrier, neostigmine is a quaternary ammonium compound (a nitrogen connects to four atoms) and does not penetrate the blood-brain barrier in significant quantities. This difference makes neostigmine the superior drug for the treatment of myasthenia gravis where peripheral effects are desired and CNS effects would be detrimental (Meyers, Jawetz, & Goldfien, 1972). All three of these compounds also have some direct cholinergic activity at the neuromuscular junction and this action appears to be substantial, at least for edrophonium (Carrier, 1972).

Nonreversible Cholinesterase Inhibitors

The nonreversible anti-AChE agents are, for the most part, organophosphate compounds, which are the active ingredients in many insecticides. Because of their toxicity, these agents are of little therapeutic value. They have, however, found use chemical warfare agents and as insecticides. The toxicity of these compounds is of considerable importance due to the danger of accidental poisoning. The compound diisopropylfluorophosphate (DFP) (Figure 4.1) is typical of this class of anti-AChE agents.

DFP is a phosphoric acid ester which combines with AChE to form a phosphorus-enzyme complex. The signs of overdosage are due to the accumulation of ACh, with death due to a depression of respiration caused by central depression, paralysis of the diaphragm and intercostal muscles, bronchial spasm, and the accumulation of bronchial secretions. The DFP-AChE bond is very stable, and the duration of action of DFP ranges from several days to several weeks (the time it takes for new AChE to be manufactured) (Koelle, 1970a). Other anti-AChE agents include mipafox, sarin, parathion, malathion, and tepp, which were developed either as nerve gases or insecticides.

The severity of the side effects and the strong CNS effects of DFP, combined with its long duration of effect, make it unsuitable for most clinical applications. An exception is for the treatment of chronic glaucoma. The increased intraocular pressure of glaucoma may occasionally be reduced by the local application of DFP. The DFP produces a constriction of the iris which allows a freer flow of the ocular fluids and a resulting decrease in pressure. The local application of small amounts of DFP in this situation does not produce the previously mentioned side effects and the prolonged duration of the effect of DFP means that the patient need be treated only about once a week, rather than once a day as would be required if a reversible anti-AChE agent were employed (Koelle, 1970a).

Poisoning. Two forms of treatment are available for poisoning due to anti-AChE compounds. Atropine (or an atropinelike drug) antagonizes the muscarinic effects of these agents and thereby reduces bronchial secretions and the central respiratory depression. Atropine is ineffective at the neuromuscular junction, however, and the skeletal muscle paralysis of the anti-AChE agents is not counteracted. Artificial respiratory assistance may be required if paralysis of the respiratory muscles has occurred.

A second treatment involves the administration of an AChE reactivator such as pralidoxime (PAM) or diacetylmonoxime (DAM). These agents break the bond between AChE and the anti-AChE compound. However, they are slow acting and atropine should also be given (Koelle, 1970a).

CHOLINERGIC BLOCKING DRUGS

Up to this point, we have been primarily concerned with drugs which mimic the effects of ACh. Some of these drugs were also found to be capable of blocking the action of ACh. We will now turn our attention to a group of drugs whose primary function is the antagonism of cholinergic activity. These substances may produce their effects via a direct action upon the postsynaptic membrane, or by interfering with the synthesis or release of ACh from the presynaptic terminal (indirect action).

Agents which produce anticholinergic effects by a direct action upon the postsynaptic membrane of the cholinergic synapse fall into two categories, those which passively occupy the postsynaptic ACh receptor site, and thereby prevent endogenous ACh from producing an effect at that site (receptor blocking agents), and those which produce a prolonged ACh-like depolarization of the postsynaptic membrane (such as the previously discussed actions of nicotine).

As we have seen, the actions of ACh within the peripheral nervous system are threefold, at autonomic ganglia, at neuromuscular junctions, and at the postganglionic parasympathetic neuroeffector junctions. The cholinergic receptor blocking agents (competitive inhibitors) may also be conveniently divided into three groups of drugs, those blocking the action of ACh at the parasympathetic neuroeffector junction, those blocking the action of ACh at the autonomic ganglia, and those drugs causing a blockade of the neuromuscular junction.

Muscarinic Blocking Agents

Atropine and related drugs have the ability to selectively block the muscarinic effects of ACh. Drugs within this category are thus parasympatholytic. They act at the postsynaptic membrane of the parasympathetic neuroeffector junction to prevent the action of ACh upon smooth and cardiac muscle, and upon the glands. The ability of the antimuscarinic drugs to decrease the activity of smooth muscles and exocrine glands accounts for the extensive medical use of these drugs. The agents to be considered are atropine and scopolamine. They are similar enough in action to be discussed together.

Atropine (d, 1-hyoscyamine) (Figure 4.2) and scopolamine (hyoscine) are found together in the plants *Atropa belladonna* (deadly nightshade), *Datura stramonium* (Jamestown weed), and *Hyoscyamus niger* (henbane). The only structural difference between the two compounds is a single oxygen atom; both are tertiary amines and easily cross the blood-brain barrier. These drugs are collectively called the *belladonna alkaloids*. The term *belladonna* comes from the Italian and means "handsome woman" since the substance was used by the ladies of Venice to give them sparkling eyes (by dilating the pupils) (Cullumbine, 1971).

At therapeutic concentrations, atropine and scopolamine act as competitive inhibitors and their effects can, therefore, be reversed by high concentrations of ACh or other cholinergic drugs. Unless it is reversed by increased levels of ACh, the blockade of the postsynaptic cholinergic receptors may persist for 3 to 10 days. The specificity of these drugs for muscarinic receptors is so high that sensitivity to atropine is often used to define the muscarinic receptor (Carrier,

1972). An important point to remember is that a cholinergic blockade by a depolarizing blocking agent such as nicotine will be made worse by the application of a cholinomimetic compound, rather than being counteracted.

Effects on organ systems. Atropine and scopolamine prevent both heat- and emotion-induced sweating, and produce dryness of the mouth and respiratory passages. The reduction of respiratory system secretion makes these drugs useful in the preoperative preparation of patients where accumulation of fluid tends to block the respiratory tract and interfere with respiration during anesthesia. Atropine also inhibits the production of acid by the exocrine glands of the stomach and thereby reduces gastric acidity.

The smooth muscle stimulant actions of cholinergic drugs and of the parasympathetic nervous system are inhibited by atropine and scopolamine. This makes these drugs valuable as antispasmodic agents, to reduce the increased peristalsis which often accompanies emotional upset or ulcers. Atropine blocks the parasympathetic innervation of the iris and pupil with a resulting dilation of the iris and paralysis of the ability of the lens to accommodate (focus at varying distances). These effects occur with small quantities of atropine or scopolamine either locally (at the eye) or systemically (Guyton, 1971).

Toxicity. Although the fatal dose of either atropine or scopolamine is high, deaths have occurred (often from eating the deadly nightshade plant, thus the origin of this name). The toxic symptoms include dryness of the mouth and throat, dilated pupils, blurred vision, sensitivity to light, hot and dry skin, increased heart rate, and increased body temperature. The anti-AChE agent neostigmine counteracts many of these symptoms and is an antidote for atropine poisoning.

CNS. Atropine and scopolamine also have generalized effects within the CNS. Some of these effects are mediated by anticholinergic actions on the reticular activating system, while others may stem from direct cortical effects of these drugs. Scopolamine, in particular, produces drowsiness and sedation which is accompanied by amnesia for the period of the drug's action. The amnesic effects of scopolamine and the production of euphoria by this drug have led to its use combined with an analgesic to decrease the unpleasant aspects of childbirth. The combination of scopolamine and morphine produces in the mother a state termed *twilight sleep*. Atropine does not produce amnesia in this situation and has less of a sedative effect. Both of these drugs will produce convulsions in toxic doses. Scopolamine also has an inhibitory effect upon vestibular functions and is thus effective in the prevention of motion sickness (Cullumbine, 1971; Innes & Nickerson, 1970b).

Confusion, hallucinations, and delirium have been associated with the intake of high doses of the belladonna alkaloids and it is not presently known whether this is a result of a direct cortical action of these drugs or whether it represents a more generalized toxic reaction to the drugs. It should be remembered that many drugs produce a distortion of perception when given in toxic doses. This appears to result from a general disturbance of body chemistry.

Ganglionic Blocking Agents

These agents can be divided into quaternary compounds such as hexamethonium (Figure 4.2), which do not cross the blood-brain barrier and, therefore, have effects only upon the peripheral nervous system, and nonquaternary compounds, such as mecamylamine, which do cross the blood-brain barrier and cause central as well as peripheral effects. Hexamethonium was the forerunner of the compounds now used in the treatment of hypertension. Besides the lowered blood pressure, which is the clinically desirable effect of hexamethonium, other effects due to ganglionic blockade are also produced. Effects due to blockade of the sympathetic ganglia include vasodilation, hypotension, increased peripheral blood flow, and decreased venous return to the heart. Symptoms due to blockade of the parasympathetic ganglia include dilation of the pupil, inability to accommodate the lens, a fast heartbeat, and decreased gastrointestinal tone and motility. The use of ganglionic blocking drugs involves the risk of acute episodes of hypotension with blood pressure dropping to shock levels (Volle & Koelle, 1970). The nonquaternary compound mecamylamine has similar actions at the autonomic ganglia but due to its ease of entry into the CNS, its side effects include tremor, confusion, and hallucinations. The control of these side effects requires careful dosage adjustment (Volle & Koelle, 1970).

Neuromuscular Blocking Agents

The pharmacology of the neuromuscular blocking agents is of interest from several viewpoints. It is of practical concern because the neuromuscular blocking

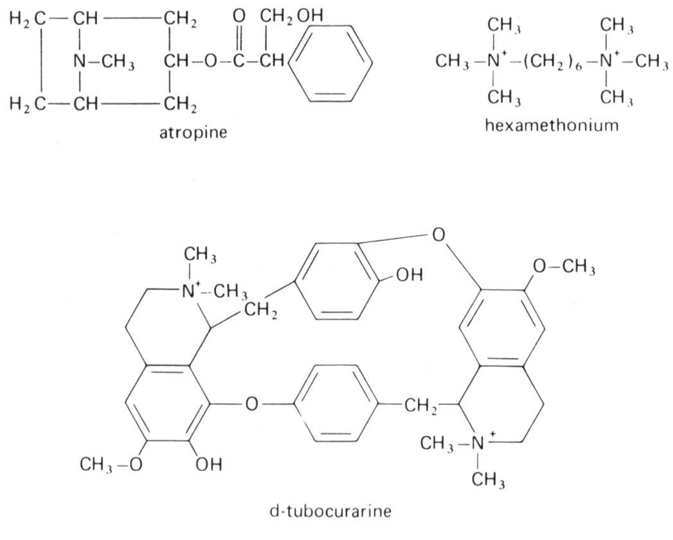

FIGURE 4.2. Representative cholinergic receptor blocking agents.

agents are used extensively in anesthesia to reduce the tone of the skeletal muscles and in psychiatric practice to reduce the intensity of the muscular contractions which accompany electroconvulsive therapy (Koelle, 1970c; Waud & Waud, 1971). From a more theoretical point of view, the area is of interest because the neuromuscular junction is the most accessible synapse for experimental work and serves as a model for intracellular impulse transmission and drug-receptor interactions (see Triggle, 1971). Finally, recent research has made use of neuromuscular blocking paralyzing drugs to study learning mediated by the autonomic nervous system.

The term *neuromuscular blocking agent* refers to those drugs which interfere with transmission from motor nerve endings to the membrane of the skeletal muscles. The members of this class form a part of a more general group of muscle relaxants which includes the depressant tranquilizers (for example, mephenesin and meprobamate) (see Chapter 5).

The most widely known of the neuromuscular blocking drugs is the South American Indian poison curare. Curare, or more accurately its active ingredient, d-tubocurarine (Figure 4.2), is a competitive inhibitor which selectively affects the neuromuscular junction. Intravenous administration of d-tubocurarine in humans causes muscle weakness and total flaccidity such that the muscles cannot be excited by nerve stimulation. The paralyses occur in a regular sequence eye and eyelid, face, neck and throat, trunk and extremities, and (last) the diaphragm. If artificial respiration is maintained during the time the diaphragm is inactive, no further drug effects are seen. Recovery of muscular function follows the reverse order of the paralysis (Carrier, 1972).

Besides its use in surgery and psychiatry, curare has been used in the psychological laboratory. Miller (1969) has reviewed a series of studies that have been conducted under his direction showing that voluntary control of the autonomic nervous system–mediated responses can be developed by simply rewarding a person or animal for producing a response such as lowered blood pressure, sweating, altered heart rate, dilated blood vessels, etc. These changes in autonomic function were originally thought to be independent of reinforcement contingencies and it was thought that they could be altered only by classical conditioning. To insure that these changes in autonomic responding were not simply secondary effects resulting from conditioning of the skeletal muscles (for example, an increase in heart rate might simply be a result of increased activity causing a greater load upon the heart), Miller curarized animals and demonstrated that the curarized animals could still control their autonomic functions. It was found that controlling the autonomic nervous system was even easier when the skeletal system was paralyzed by d-tubocurarine. This technique has not been extensively used in the human because paralysis by curare produces an extremely unpleasant emotional experience. Neuromuscular paralysis is unpleasant enough that it has been successfully used as an aversive stimulus for behavior control. Subjects have reported a feeling of suffocation and helplessness even when adequate ventilation was maintained and behaviors which are followed by the injection of a short-acting curarizing agent, such as succinylcholine, decrease in frequency (the drug acts as an aversive stimulus).

Indirect-acting Cholinergic Blocking Agents

Certain anticholinergic drugs act by decreasing the amount of ACh which is released from the presynaptic terminal. Hemicholinium (a synthesis inhibitor) acts by blocking the cellular uptake of choline. Following the administration of hemicholinium, the synthesis of ACh is prevented due to the resulting choline deficiency. Botulin toxin (a release inhibitor) acts by preventing the release of ACh from the presynaptic terminal. Botulin toxin is of toxicological interest as it is the responsible agent in botulism poisoning which commonly occurs following the ingestion of improperly handled home canned foods. Botulism occurs when insufficient heating of the canned food fails to kill the botulin bacteria which then act anaerobically to produce botulin toxin. This toxin is easily destroyed and properly heating the affected food before serving will destroy the toxin. This can be accomplished by boiling the food for 10 to 20 minutes. The symptoms of botulism poisoning are a direct result of its anticholinergic activity (Guyton, 1971).

CHOLINERGIC MECHANISMS: THE CNS AND BEHAVIOR

The survival of an organism is dependent upon the maintenance of a certain set of conditions which are often described in terms of biological homeostasis. Any major deviation from the homeostatic levels of food, water, mineral balance, body temperature, or any of several other biological variables, will result in the death of the organism. Within the organism's environment, we may conceive of three types of stimuli with which he may come into contact, and two types of behavior which are available. The types of stimuli are stimuli associated with biological benefit, stimuli associated with biological detriment, and neutral stimuli. The two behaviors which are available to an organism are approach toward a stimulus and avoidance of the stimulus. Clearly, only those organisms which have developed (through evolutionary processes) a system which leads to an approach response in the presence of biologically beneficial stimuli, and an avoidance response in the face of biologically detrimental stimuli, will survive to reproduce. Evolution would, therefore, favor the development of such a system (Glickman & Schiff, 1967).

In certain lower organisms, the responses to the environment appear to be highly specific and stereotyped. As we ascend the phylogenetic scale, however, responses become more variable and prior experience with the environment comes to play a major role in the determination of an organism's behavior. The mechanism whereby an organism maintains biological homeostasis can be considered to consist of three subsystems, an innate approach response to certain environmental stimuli, an innate avoidance response to other stimuli, and a mechanism whereby previously neutral stimuli may become included within one or the other of these groups of stimuli. The last process is termed *learning*.

In Chapter 3 we developed a model in which a system of adrenergic neurons, forming the medial forebrain bundle, subserved the function of reward or approach to certain stimuli. We now propose that a system of cholinergic neurons forming the periventricular system (see Figure 3.4 in Chapter 3) subserves the function of behavioral inhibition. The operation of this inhibitory system is seen in several behavioral phenomena, such as the effects of aversive stimuli, the suppression of incorrect responses, extinction, and habituation. We will also discuss the data suggesting a role for cholinergic mechanisms in species-specific behavior patterns such as water ingestion and aggression.

ACh and Aversive Stimuli

A cholinergic system, which includes the dorsal midbrain, the posterior and medial hypothalamus, and thalamic nuclei, has been implicated as the neural mechanism mediating the behavioral effects of aversive stimuli (stimuli which are unpleasant to the organism). This group of nuclei is termed the *periventricular system* (PVS) and stimulation of the PVS results in a suppression of responding, while a response contingent withholding of PVS stimulation results in an increase in the rate of responding (Stein, 1969). This implies that stimulation of the PVS is aversive. The PVS communicates with the limbic system circuit (Nauta, 1963) and many structures within this limbic circuit receive innervation from both the PVS and the MFB (Grossman, 1973).

Brain manipulations. An informative series of studies concerns the pharmacological manipulation of the medial hypothalamic portion of the PVS (Stein, 1969). When cannulae are inserted into this area for the purpose of injecting a drug, the damage to the brain that results from the introduction of the cannula has an effect upon behavior. Normally, if a rat is placed in a situation where a given behavior is followed by an electric shock, the animal ceases that behavior, thereby avoiding the shock. Often the animal is put into a box with a hole in one wall. If he goes through the hole into another box, he receives a shock. As he can avoid the shock by passively remaining in the original box, this technique is termed *passive avoidance learning*. The destruction of a brain area which mediates the effects of aversive stimuli would be expected to produce a deficit in passive avoidance. Penetration of the ventromedial nucleus of the hypothalamus (VMN) by a small cannula is sufficient to produce an increase in punished responses, sometimes termed a *passive avoidance deficit*. The decrease in the effectiveness of an aversive stimulus following injury to the VMN is consistent with its involvement in the PVS punishment circuit. If a cholinergic substance, such as carbachol or physostigmine, is injected into this area, the passive avoidance decrement is abolished and the aversive stimulus again becomes capable of inhibiting the responding of the organism. The microinjection of an anticholinergic substance (atropine) produces an even greater passive avoidance deficit. In other words, operations which interfere with cholinergic activity in the PVS (including either destruction of the neurons or a cholinergic blockade of the neurons) produce a deficit in passive avoidance behavior. When the cholinergic activity of the PVS is returned toward normal by agents which increase the effectiveness of the remaining cholinergic neurons, the passive avoidance deficit is counteracted. Taken together, these studies show that the suppression of behavior through punishment is mediated by the PVS, the mediation is based upon cholinergic transmission, and ACh acts as an excitatory transmitter within the PVS. The excitatory nature of the ACh activity within the PVS can be deduced from the similar effects of atropine, which reduces ACh activity, and lesions, which reduce neural activity.

Systemic drug injections. Further evidence for the involvement of ACh in the inhibition of behavior by punishment has been obtained from the systemic administration of drugs, such as atropine and scopolamine, which cross the blood-brain barrier easily and influence ACh-mediated neural activity in the brain.

Responses such as active avoidance in a shuttle box, where a rat must shuttle back and forth between two boxes, are difficult for a rat to learn. The shock which follows nonavoidance causes the animal to freeze (inhibits behavior), which results in further shocks. This is a common problem with learning situations which involve the use of an aversive stimulus. Quite often, the aversive stimulus will elicit behavior, such as freezing, which is incompatible with the response to be learned. In the situation described above, if the anticholinergic interferes with the inhibition of behavior that results from the aversive stimulus, it should improve the animal's performance in the active avoidance situation. Just that effect has been observed (Suits & Isaacson, 1968).

It is possible that the anticholinergic agent had a general effect upon learning and the animals which had been given an injection of atropine simply learned faster than the controls. If atropine or scopolamine improve learning, the improvement should also show up on passive avoidance. This does not occur; in fact, scopolamine has been found to interfere with the acquistion of a passive avoidance response. This is what we would expect if the scopolamine depresses the inhibitory effects of the aversive stimulus. Thus, anticholinergic drugs, by reducing freezing, facilitate the learning of a behavior which involves an active response to a stimulus signaling the presentation of an aversive stimulus and interfere with the learning of a behavior which involves the inhibition of responding (passive avoidance) to a stimulus signaling the presentation of an aversive stimulus.

Other Examples of Behavioral Inhibition

The behavioral effect of punishment is to suppress the punished behavior. The involvement of cholinergic neurons in the suppression of behavior, however, extends beyond their relation to punishment. Many other situations which do not involve the punishment of behavior also result in a suppression of that behavior.

The suppression of incorrect responses. When an organism learns to perform a certain behavior, such as turning to the left in a maze, it must, at the same time, suppress any tendency to turn to the right. Learning, therefore, is dependent upon the suppression of incorrect responses as well as upon the performance of the correct responses. Whitehouse (1964) has shown that scopolamine interferes with maze learning and that it results in an animal making more entries into the unrewarded alleys. This is consistent with a disinhibition of the unrewarded responses by the anticholinergic drug.

Extinction. Another example of the suppression of a behavior occurs when an organism has been trained to make a response, and, once a high level of responding is reached, the reinforcer is discontinued. Following the discontinuation of reinforcement, the organism decreases its rate of responding. This process of the extinction of a conditioned response can be viewed as a suppression of the previously rewarded behavior. If anticholinergic drugs disinhibit behavior, they would be expected to increase the number of responses that an animal will emit during extinction. Rats that have been given systemic injections of atropine will continue to emit a previously reinforced response during extinction long after nondrugged subjects stop responding (Carlton, 1969).

Habituation. Most animals have a tendency to explore a novel environment. This tendency is manifested in behaviors, such as increased locomotion upon being placed in a novel environment or performing an operant task which results in the presentation of a novel stimulus. Under normal conditions, these behaviors decrease in frequency as the stimuli lose their novelty. Anticholinergic drugs extend the period of time during which animals will show increased activity when they are placed in a novel environment (Carlton & Vogel, 1965) and during which they will press a lever to turn on a light in their cage (Carlton, 1969).

The above effects of the anticholinergic drugs are consistent with the hypothesis that a cholinergic system is involved in the inhibition of behavior and that the inhibited behavior is released by the anticholinergic drugs. Available evidence suggests that the cholinergic drugs in low doses have the opposite effect to the anticholinergics and actually increase the ability of an organism to suppress behavior. The neuroanatomical basis of these effects appears to be centered within the PVS.

ACh and Homeostatic Regulatory Behavior

Up to this point, we have concentrated upon the involvement of brain cholinergic pathways in the behavioral changes that result from learning. Cholinergic pathways are also implicated in the occurrence of certain stereotyped species-specific behaviors which may be unlearned responses to environmental and physiological cues. In particular, a great deal of research has centered around the homeostatic control of water and electrolyte balance. At least in the rat, this homeostatic mechanism involves a cholinergic neural circuit. Recently, a cholinergic neural mechanism has also been posited to underly mouse killing by rats. We will now examine the effects of cholinergic drugs on these behaviors.

Cholinergic drinking. In order to study the neural mechanisms underlying behavior, psychologists have often resorted to stimulating discrete areas of the brain and observing the changes in behavior that result from the stimulation. This technique has been particularly effective in the study of the areas of the brain which underly basic mechanisms such as food and water intake. Localized injection of microgram quantities of a chemical into the brain of an awake, behaving animal through a previously surgically implanted cannula (a technique called *chemical stimulation of the brain*) has provided some insight into brain-behavior relationships.

Water intake has been elicited by the stimulation of areas of the hypothalamus and other limbic system structures (Robinson, 1964). As water intake represents an easily measured index of homeostatic regulation, considerable data has been collected relating brain stimulation to drinking behavior, and some understanding of brain function has resulted from the study of drinking produced by brain stimulation. Not only have the areas of the brain that control the homeostatic regulation of water intake been localized, the chemical process underlying neural transmission within this system has been studied in some detail. The involvement of a cholinergic neural circuit in drinking is currently the subject of much research and debate.

The elicitation of drinking by cholinergic stimulation of the lateral hypothalamic area (LHA) of the rat (Grossman, 1960) was followed by a demonstration that drinking could also be cholinergically elicited from several sites within the limbic system. These sites ranged from the cingulate gyrus and septal region of the forebrain through the thalamus and hypothalamus to the midbrain (Fisher & Coury, 1962). The widespread distribution within the limbic system of sites from which drinking may be elicited by cholinergic stimulation and the ability of cholinergic blocking agents to interfere with the elicitation of drinking even when the two drugs are injected into separate sites within the limbic system has led some investigators to propose that a neural circuit, composed of several limbic system sites, underlies drinking behavior (Levitt, 1971; Levitt & Fisher, 1966, 1967; Miller, 1965).

Amygdala: Of the several brain sites involved in drinking behavior, three deserve special attention. Stimulation of the amygdala does not elicit drinking in a water-satiated rat. In a deprived rat, however, or in a rat from which drinking is elicited by the cholinergic stimulation of another site, cholinergic stimulation of the amygdala increases the amount of water drunk. This suggests that the amygdala may serve to modulate the drinking behavior that is elicited from other limbic system areas (Grossman, 1967).

LHA: Lesions of the LHA prevent the elicitation of drinking from other limbic system sites, but lesions of other limbic system sites do not prevent the elicitation of drinking by stimulation of the LHA (Stein & Levitt, 1971; Wolf & Miller, 1964). This suggests that a final common pathway for the production of drinking behavior may pass through the LHA.

Subfornical organ: Recently a new area has been implicated in drinking behavior. This is a small area, adjacent to the third ventricle just below the fornix, which is called the *subfornical organ* (SFO). Extremely small quantities of a cholinergic compound (a few nanograms) are capable of eliciting drinking when microinjected into the SFO. The extreme sensitivity of this site to cholinergic stimulation, coupled with its proximity to the third ventricle, has suggested to some investigators that all cholinergically elicited drinking may result from the diffusion of the chemicals into the ventricular system and their subsequent action upon the SFO (Simpson & Routtenberg, 1972, 1973). This interpretation has been called into question by studies showing that radioactively tagged compounds do not diffuse significantly from the site of their injection and that there is no correlation between the distance of a stimulation site from the ventricular system and either the latency to drink or the amount drunk following chemical stimulation (see Levitt, 1971, for an analysis of this question).

Cholinergic blockade: As was previously noted, atropine will block the drinking produced by carbachol microinjection, not only when the two agents are injected simultaneously into the same site, but also when carbachol is injected into one site and atropine into another site from which carbachol would elicit drinking. However, atropine blocks carbachol-induced drinking only when injected into a site from which carbachol itself elicits drinking. This suggests that the atropine may act by disrupting a part of the cholinergic drinking circuit, and that the disruption of any one part of the circuit by atropine prevents carbachol from activating the circuit from that site or from another site (Stein & Levitt, 1971). The interpretation of the action of atropine within the drinking circuit is complicated by the fact that while atropine will inhibit carbachol-induced drinking from certain sites within the limbic system, lesions of these same sites have no effect upon carbachol-induced drinking (Stein & Levitt, 1971). This type of data was cited by Routtenberg (1972) as evidence that the atropine was not acting at the site of injection, but was diffusing to the SFO, as was the carbachol from the other site. Thus, the atropine and carbachol were proposed to both act at the same site (the SFO), even when they were injected into separate sites.

Neural activity recording: However, recent evidence is not totally consistent with this idea. When carbachol is injected into sites from which drinking is elicited, it produces an increase in neural activity at that site (Buerger et al., 1973). This increase in neural activity which results from the microinjection of carbachol into a "drinking site" (a site from which drinking may be elicited), as well as the drinking itself, can be eliminated by the simultaneous microinjection of atropine into another drinking site (Snyder & Levitt, in press). So far, this phenomenon has not been adequately explained, but it would be difficult to explain in terms of the diffusion of both drugs into the ventricular system.

Muscarinic receptors: There is evidence that the drinking elicited by cholinergic stimulation results from muscarinic effects of the cholinergic compounds. Drinking can be elicited by the microinjection of ACh, carbachol, or muscarine (all of which have muscarinic effects), but not by nicotine. Furthermore, atropine but not d-tubocurarine or hexamethonium, will block the elicitation of drinking by carbachol (Levitt, 1969; Stein & Seifter, 1962).

Physostigmine: The above studies have been concerned with an activation of the cholinergic postsynaptic receptor by the direct-acting cholinergic drugs. The direct-acting cholinergic drugs may also act by stimulating fiber systems directly, rather than by an action upon the postsynaptic membrane; therefore, the microinjection of a direct-acting cholinergic compound into the LHA does not insure that it is acting at the synaptic junction. It may, instead, be acting upon fibers of passage (axons) traveling through the LHA.

Drinking can also be produced by the microinjection of physostigmine (an anti-AChE agent) into the LHA, but not into the fornix; while the direct-acting cholinergic drug, carbachol, will elicit drinking from both of these sites (Levitt & O'Hearn, 1972). Physostigmine increases the effective level of ACh at the postsynaptic junction by slowing its destruction by AChE. It is, therefore, effective in the LHA where the turnover rate of endogenous ACh is high and ineffective at the fornix, a fiber system with few synapses for the release of endogenous ACh. This study indicates that endogenous ACh can function to elicit drinking. Furthermore, had the physostigmine diffused from its injection site within the fornix, it would have been expected to reach a nuclear area where endogenous ACh would act to produce drinking. Therefore, it is likely that the physostigmine was confined to its fornix site of injection, rather than diffusing to the SFO or elsewhere.

Summary: Drinking may be elicited by cholinergic stimulation of sites which are widespread throughout the limbic system. Stimulation of a site which will normally elicit drinking may be rendered ineffective by anticholinergic blockade of another site which would also normally elicit drinking. Interestingly, while the atropine blockade of a drinking site renders the cholinergic stimulation of other sites ineffective, an electrolytic lesion of a drinking site does not block the elicitation of drinking from other sites. The exceptions to this rule are the LHA and the SFO, which appear to be major way stations in the cholinergic-drinking system. Finally, the postsynaptic membrane of the drinking system appears similar to that of the parasympathetic neuroeffector junction, as only muscarinic agents are effective in eliciting drinking from these brain sites, and only antimuscarinic agents in chemically blocking such elicited drinking.

The relation of cholinergic drinking to natural thirst. There is some question concerning the relationship between cholinergically elicited drinking and natural thirst. If the drinking elicited by microinjection of cholinergic drugs into the brain represents the cholinergic activation of the neural pathways which are involved in deprivation-induced drinking, the cholinergic blocking agents would be expected to interfere with deprivation-induced drinking. Atropine, administered either systemically or by brain microinjection, does produce a slight decrease in the water intake of deprived animals. The decrease is, however, much smaller than the decrease in carbachol-elicited water intake that is caused by atropine (Krikstone & Levitt, 1970). Thus, while the cholinergic drinking substrate may overlap that for deprivation-induced drinking, the overlap is not complete (Levitt, 1971).

Cholinergic drugs and aggression. It is possible to elicit aggressive behavior in many species through the electrical stimulation of certain subcortical brain structures. In the rat, electrical stimulation of the hypothalamus can elicit two different types of aggressive behavior (both of which can be directed toward mice). In affective attack the rat shows generalized arousal, learns to make an operant response to avoid the brain stimulation, and does not eat the mouse once it has been killed. In quiet biting attack, rats do not show arousal, do not attempt to escape the brain stimulation, and do eat the killed mice. The affective attack resembles the aggression which is caused by noxious stimulation (shock-elicited attack), while the quiet biting attack resembles the natural predatory response of rats toward mice (Moyer, 1968; Panksepp, 1971).

Mouse killing by rats is a stable phenomenon and rats can be divided into killers that will consistently kill a mouse which has been placed in their cages, but not a rat pup of the same size (Myer & White, 1965); and nonkillers, which will not kill a mouse placed in their cages, but may carry the mouse much as a female rat carries a pup (Lonowski, Levitt, & Larson, 1973). Early studies suggested that predatory aggression (quiet biting attack) might be cholinergically mediated. When carbachol was injected into the LHA of rats, it elicited mouse killing in rats which normally did not kill (Smith, King, & Hoebel, 1970). These authors also found that the microinjection of atropine into the LHA of killers inhibited their mouse killing. These studies have been called into question due to the extremely large doses of carbachol (100 μg) and atropine (50 μg) which were required to produce the effects (Bandler, 1969, 1970, 1971; Lonowski et al., 1973). More recent studies have suggested that stimulation of the LHA by large toxic doses of carbachol, which are known to produce convulsions, may cause an irritable aggression similar to affective attack, while more physiological doses of carbachol may actually decrease mouse killing by killer rats (Lonowski et al., 1973). This is currently an area of debate among psychologists and merits further research.

SUMMARY AND CONCLUSIONS

ACh is the chemical transmitter at three distinguishable sites in the peripheral nervous system: neuromuscular junctions, autonomic ganglia, and parasympathetic neuroeffector junctions. While ACh is effective at all three sites, certain drugs may primarily influence only one or two of these sites. These selective drug effects, such as the existence of drugs that are competitive receptor inhibitors at each site, suggest structural and functional differences between the postsynaptic receptors at the three sites. This organization of the cholinergic component of the peripheral nervous system also appears to provide a useful working model of the cholinergic component of the CNS. There is also some evidence that ACh may have a role in synaptic transmission and even in impulse conduction in adrenergic and other neurons, both in the peripheral nervous system and in the CNS.

There are a variety of drugs derived from plant sources or of synthetic origin that mimic or inhibit ACh at one or all of its sites of action. There are also drugs that facilitate cholinergic activity by combining with the enzyme, acetylcholinesterase, which normally deactivates endogenous ACh. Several especially important topics with respect to cholinergic physiology are the depolarizing, toxic, and addicting properties of nicotine; and the disease of the cholinergic neuromuscular junction called *myasthenia gravis*. In addition to prevalent recreational use of nicotine, both muscarine (fly agaric) and the antimuscarinic drugs (atropine) may have properties that lead to recreational and potentially abusive drug use. Neuromuscular blocking agents have important uses in surgery, and certain related depressant tranquilizers (meprobamate) may be effective because of the muscle relaxation they produce. Ganglionic blocking agents have effects due to the inhibiton of both parasympathetic and sympathetic actions. Several cholinergic chemicals, especially botulin toxin and the irreversible cholinesterase inhibitors, are of toxicological importance because of the danger of poisoning or because of their use in insecticides and chemical warfare agents.

The primary physiological effects of the cholinergic system can be seen in a facilitation of parasympathetic bodily homeostatic maintenance activities. The cholinergic system is also the basis of skeletal muscle voluntary movement because of its role at the neuromuscular junction. In the CNS, a cholinergic system appears to be the basis of behavioral inhibition (as a result of nonreward) in a variety of circumstances, such as the suppression of behavior by aversive stimuli (punishment), the suppression of incorrect responses in a reward situation, extinction, and habituation. This behavioral inhibition system should be conceived of as complementing (opposing?) and interacting with the behavioral facilitation (reward, pleasure) system presented in Chapter 3 as the MFB noradrenergic reward system. Cholinergic mechanisms in the brain also seem to have a role in such homeostatic survival activities as the control of water balance and aggression, just as the peripheral cholinergic system regulates homeostatic maintenance via the parasympathetic nervous system.

5
THE TRANQUILIZERS

Robert A. Levitt and Barry J. Krikstone

There is much confusion and controversy concerning the drugs we will discuss in this chapter. Some of this results from disagreement about the nature and causes of the behavioral pathologies themselves. Many view behavioral pathology from a psychoanalytic or dynamic orientation; others, the behavior therapists, from a learning process orientation; still others from a biological perspective.

It should already be clear that our orientation is biological. In Chapter 3 on adrenergic drugs we presented a model of the major psychoses (schizophrenia, depression, and mania), which emphasized the involvement of disordered biogenic amine functioning in these diseases. That is not to say that we believe an individual's experiences and environment are unimportant in the etiology and course of these disorders—quite the contrary. However, whether the etiology lies in "nature" or in "nurture," or, as is more likely, in some combination of the two, we believe that drugs which influence endogenous bioamines are one appropriate treatment modality.

The antischizophrenic tranquilizers (sometimes called *major* tranquilizers) comprise the first class of drugs we will discuss. These drugs are of use primarily in the treatment of schizophrenia. Lithium, a drug of use in the treatment of mania, will then be discussed. The depressant tranquilizers (sometimes called *minor* tranquilizers) are the last group of drugs in this chapter. These agents have much in common with the other depressants to be presented in the next chapter.

We believe that a simplistic overview of the behavioral disorders and their pharmacological treatment is required at this time to organize the information to be presented. Some of the research which is the basis of our approach was reviewed in the admittedly speculative section on brain disorders in Chapter 3. Schizophrenia can be viewed as resulting from some abnormal chemical substance (related to D and NE) selectively affecting brain function. We propose that the antischizophrenic tranquilizers have some effectiveness in this disorder because they ameliorate the effect of this substance on the brain, and thus to some extent "normalize" the aberrant behavior of the schizophrenic.

Continuing along this same line, mania and depression may be conceived as the result, respectively, of overactivity or underactivity in brain biogenic amine systems (probably primarily catecholaminic). Lithium may be effective in mania because it inhibits catecholamine functions. The depressant tranquilizers and the general depressants (the next chapter) may also be of some use in mania because of their sedating effects. The antidepressant drugs (Chapter 8) are of use in depression because they enhance the action of catecholamines. We believe the drugs we call the *depressant* tranquilizers are similar in their actions to the depressant drugs that we will discuss in the next chapter (for example, the barbiturates and alcohol). These various drugs have some effectiveness in the treatment of anxiety because they produce muscle relaxation or promote daytime sedation and (used in a higher dose) enable a tense and anxious individual to get to sleep in the evening.

THE ANTISCHIZOPHRENIC TRANQUILIZERS

The presenting symptoms generally agreed to result in a diagnosis of schizophrenia are restricted affect, poor insight, and disordered thoughts (incoherent speech; widespread, persecutory, bizarre, or nihilistic delusions) (see Table 5.1; Carpenter, Strauss, & Bartko, 1973). We have previously (Chapter 3) suggested that these behavioral symptoms result from damage to the noradrenergic reward system of the brain. The drugs that are effective as antischizophrenic agents normalize affect and ameliorate the delusions.

It has been estimated that over 250 million people have received at least one of these drugs (Crane, 1973). Over the years physicians have prescribed them for a variety of disorders, including schizophrenia, psychoticlike behavior associated with mental deficiency, paranoid states, senility, brain damage, mania, hyperactivity in children, narcotic addiction, and neurotic anxiety. However, only in the case of schizophrenia has the efficacy of these drugs been confirmed (Crane, 1973). The antischizophrenic drugs produce little, if any, dependency and are not addicting. There are, however, dangers associated with their use since the incidence of annoying and potentially dangerous side effects is high.

These drugs can be conveniently divided biochemically into three subgroups—the rauwolfia alkaloids, the phenothiazine derivatives, and the butyrophenones. The rauwolfia alkaloids and phenothiazines were responsible for the psychopharmacological revolution of the mid-1950s. Their effectiveness in the treatment of schizophrenia (especially in its early stages) was responsible for the dramatic reduction in the population of mental hospitals (from about 550,000 residents in government mental hospitals in 1955 to about 400,000 now (see Longo, 1972). The effectiveness of these drugs in correcting psychotic behavior

TABLE 5.1

Symptoms of Schizophrenia

Sign or symptom	Observation or question
Restricted affect	Blank, expressionless face. Very little or no emotion shown when delusion or normal material is discussed which would usually bring out emotion.
Poor insight	Overall rating of insight.
Poor rapport	Did the interviewer find it possible to establish good rapport with patient during interview?
Unreliable information	Was the information obtained in this interview credible or not?
Incoherent speech	Free and spontaneous flow of incoherent speech.
Thoughts aloud	Does patient feel thoughts are being broadcast, transmitted, so that everyone knows what he is thinking? Does he ever seem to hear his thoughts spoken aloud? (Almost as if someone standing nearby could hear them?)
Widespread delusions	How widespread are patient's delusions? How many areas in patient's life are interpreted delusionally?
Bizarre delusions	Are the delusions comprehensible?
Nihilistic delusions	Does patient feel that his body is decaying, rotting? Does he feel that some part of his body is missing, for example, head, brain, or arms? Does he ever have the feeling that he does not exist at all, that he is dead, dissolved?

Note. Reprinted by permission from W. T. Carpenter Jr., J. S. Strauss, and J. J. Bartko, Flexible system for the diagnosis of schizophrenia: Report from the WHO International pilot study of schizophrenia. *Science*, 1973, **182**, 1275–1277. Copyright 1973 by the American Association for the Advancement of Science.

was also the most significant factor responsible for the abandonment of frontal lobotomy as a psychotherapeutic approach (Valenstein, 1973).

The use of the rauwolfias in schizophrenia is no longer prevalent because of their side effects; however, a rauwolfia drug may still be tried after the other drug groups have failed to help a patient. The phenothiazines and the more recently introduced butyrophenones are now the drugs of choice, and they appear to be about equally effective. There are really no reliable objective criteria that permit us to make a choice between these last two groups of drugs.

Behavioral Effects

Each of these drug groups (rauwolfias, phenothiazines, butyrophenones) are sedating and cause slowing of the electroencephalogram (EEG) when first administered to schizophrenics, to normal humans, or to animals. In animal behavioral research the key feature of these drugs appears to be their ability to inhibit avoidance responding at doses too low to affect escape responding or reward conditioning. This means that the animal (for instance, a rat or cat) will not respond to a stimulus (a light or sound), that signals it must make a response to avoid a painful shock (this is called an *avoidance* response). The animal, however, still will make the appropriate response, called an *escape* response, once the shock itself is turned on. The animal also will perform a response while under the influence of the drug to obtain a reward such as food or water.

There is, however, a serious problem with considering the sedative and EEG-slowing actions in humans and animals or the avoidance inhibition in animals as related to antischizophrenic efficacy in human patients. These effects are only seen acutely, at the beginning of treatment; tolerance develops to them rather rapidly. In contrast, the normalizing action on the aberrant behavior of the schizophrenic patient is not seen for a few days, and may even not appear until the patient is tolerant to the sedative action. Moreover, tolerance does not develop to the antischizophrenic effects of these drugs in patients that are benefited. For this reason it is believed that the effectiveness of these drugs in schizophrenic patients is not dependent upon or related to their sedative, EEG slowing, or avoidance-inhibiting actions. When these agents are effective in normalizing the behavior of schizophrenics, they do so without sedating or depressing the patient's behavior or abilities (for instance, learning or task performance).

Is the Patient Cured?

These drugs may be of some use in chronic or "burnt out" schizophrenic patients, but their greatest efficacy is in the treatment of acute or recently developed cases. The drugs are usually considered as only a symptomatic treatment. But, in responsive patients, the effects can be dramatic (affect is normalized and the delusions cease) and it may be fair to consider the patient "cured" in the same sense that a patient with diabetes mellitus is cured by insulin. "While it is true that, in general, the drug acts mainly on the symptoms, the results obtained in certain cases, as for instance in early schizophrenia, are so dramatic, and the return to normal is so complete and long-lasting, that one may ask if there is only a symptomatic amelioration or also a basic modification of the psychotic process" (Longo, 1972, p. 10).

Large-scale investigations have proven that the antischizophrenic tranquilizers are more efficacious in schizophrenia than an inert substance (a placebo) or than the depressant sedatives. Using the ability of the patient to remain in the community as a criterion of drug effectiveness, 60% to 70% of acutely ill schizophrenic patients on no drugs are readmitted to a hospital within 1 year, while only 20% to 30% receiving antischizophrenic medication are readmitted. This difference between the drug-treated and nontreated patients in percentage not requiring hospitalization may become smaller over the years (Crane, 1973). Perhaps, as a better understanding of the biological etiology of this disease is achieved, more specific drugs and even greater pharmacological success will be possible.

The normalizing action of the antischizophrenic drugs may permit further benefit by rendering the patient more responsive to psychotherapy. However, in this particular behavioral disorder, schizophrenia, there is not conclusive evidence that any of the common psychotherapeutic approaches are beneficial.

Other Uses of the Antischizophrenic Drugs

Although these drugs have been tried for several other conditions, such as mania, hyperactivity in children, and neurotic anxiety, they are not specific for these disorders, and other drug groups are preferred. The limited degree of effectiveness that is found for the antischizophrenic drugs in these other disorders seems to be related to the short-lived sedating action. In patients with depression, the antischizophrenic drugs are actually contraindicated, since the depression is augmented by the sedating action of these drugs.

There is one other condition in which the antischizophrenic drugs are especially useful. They effectively control the "toxic psychoses" produced by the distorting drugs, such as LSD, mescaline, and psilocybin (see Chapter 9). For this use, chlorpromazine is most often employed, primarily because of the greater experience people have had with it. The selective effectiveness of these agents in the states induced by the distorting drugs suggests some relationship between the drug-induced states and schizophrenia itself.

Mechanism of Action

The antischizophrenic tranquilizers have in common an ability to increase the permeability of cellular and subcellular membranes. This results in a depletion of bioamines from storage sites and in an inability for their reuptake. To various degrees, and with some difference in pattern across drugs, these agents are, therefore, antiadrenergic, antidopaminergic, antiserotonergic, anticholinergic, and antihistaminergic. It was found first that reserpine depleted 5HT, leading to the suggestion that this action was responsible for its efficacy in schizophrenia (Brodie, 1959). Subsequently, it was found that reserpine also has similar effects on NE and D (Carlsson, 1960).

One curious and perhaps highly important finding is that all of the drugs with antischizophrenic activity also cause disorders of motor functioning. These disordered movements resemble those of Parkinson's disease, and suggest that the antischizophrenic and Parkinsonism effects may both result from a common mechanism—an inhibition of dopaminergic functioning. Attempts to develop antischizophrenic drugs without these disruptive side effects have failed and led to this idea. The problems of the motor and other side effects of these drugs will be discussed later.

In Chapter 3 we discussed the Stein and Wise (1971) hypothesis of the etiology of schizophrenia, which is supported by these motor effect findings. The antischizophrenic drugs such as the phenothiazines (for example, chlorpromazine, which Stein and Wise, 1971 used in their studies) may ameliorate schizophrenia by depleting the MFB noradrenergic reinforcement system of its aberrant D and 6-hydroxydopamine. At the same time, the Parkinsonismlike side effects would be an inevitable consequence of a concomitant depletion of D from the normally functioning dopaminergic nigrostriatal bundle (see Chapters 2 and 3).

Side Effects

The motor dysfunctions are produced by all of the effective antischizophrenic drugs. They are not seen, however, in all patients and are not equally prevalent with all drugs or drug groups. Yet, increasing the dosage of any of these drugs in any patient will bring them on. The Parkinsonian syndrome, if it is to appear, usually begins after 1 to 2 weeks of treatment. A perhaps related side effect found in some patients, usually those manifesting Parkinsonism, is called *akathisia*. This syndrome expresses itself in irresistible and uncontrollable impulses to engage in some motor activity, such as walking, hand rubbing, or hand cleaning (Longo, 1972).

Tardive dyskinesia. According to Crane (1973), permanent neurological disorders have become quite common in patients subjected to long-term therapy with the antischizophrenic drugs. The syndrome, called *tardive dyskinesia*, consists of "slow, rhythmical movements in the region of the mouth, with protrusion of the tongue, smacking of the lips, blowing of the cheeks, and side-to-side movements of the chin, as well as other bizarre muscular activity" (Crane, 1973, pp. 126–127). Not only the head, face, and mouth are involved; practically all parts of the body may exhibit motor disorders. This syndrome does not manifest itself until months or years after the initiation of drug therapy and may persist unchanged after medication is withdrawn. The syndrome is found primarily in those of advancing age and those who have taken antischizophrenic medication for several years, but has also been found in younger patients. Perhaps 5% of patients chronically taking these drugs develop the disorder. At the disorder's initial appearance, the drug should be withdrawn or the dosage reduced, or a different drug used, in an attempt to limit the syndrome.

The Rauwolfias

Rauwolfia serpentina, known as the snakeroot plant, has been used for thousands of years to treat snakebite wounds, epilepsy, and numerous other afflictions (including mental distresses). The first antipsychotic effects were reported in 1931 by Sen and Bose in an Indian medical journal. In 1952, Miller

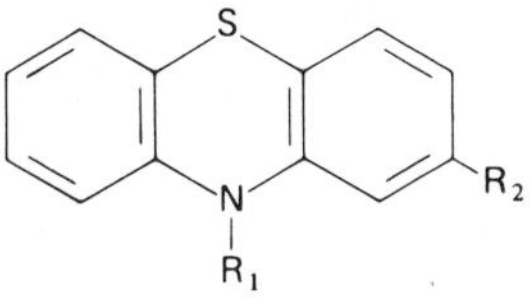

phenothiazine nucleus

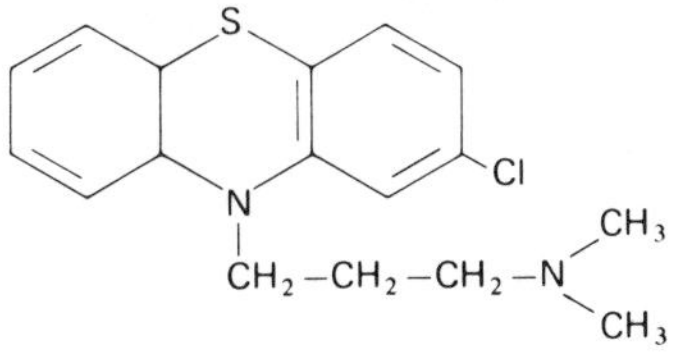

chlorpromazine

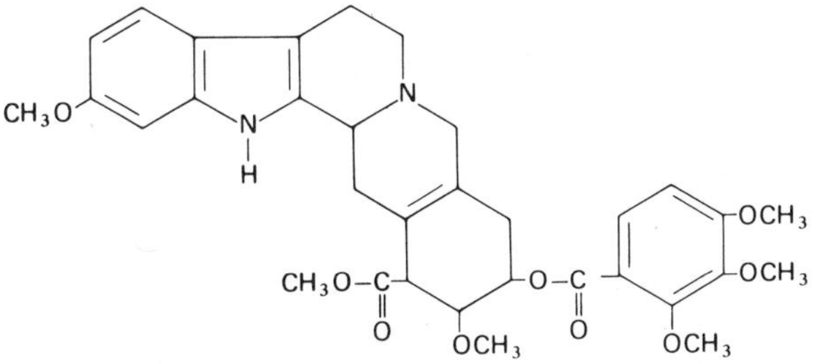

reserpine

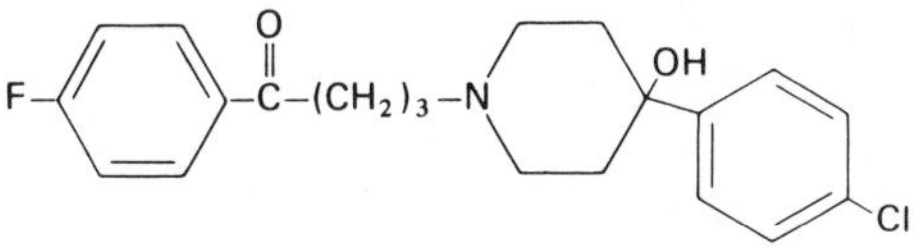

haloperidol

FIGURE 5.1. Representative antischizophrenic tranquilizers (and phenothiazine nucleus).

and his coworkers isolated reserpine (Figure 5.1), which accounts for approximately 50% of the activity of the entire *Rauwolfia serpentina* root. Reserpine was subsequently extracted from several other plants in the Rauwolfia genus, and in 1957 Woodward succeeded in synthesizing the chemical. The first report of the therapeutic effects of *Rauwolfia serpentina* in schizophrenic patients was presented in 1953 by Hakim.

Chemical structure. One group of chemicals obtained from rauwolfia contains an indole-ethylamine structure resembling that of serotonin and lysergic acid. Reserpine (Rauloydin, Raurine, Rau-sed, Reserpoid, Sandril, Serfin, Serpasil, Serpate) is the prototype of this chemical group which also includes the closely related psychoactive chemicals, deserpidine (Raudizin, Harmonyl), rescinnamine (Moderil), and syrosingopine (Singoserp).

Metabolism. The rauwolfia alkaloids have been termed "hit and run" drugs because of their rapid absorption, distribution, and excretion. In spite of these rapid changes, the rauwolfia drugs have a delayed onset of action and remain active for a considerable period of time. It may be that some unidentified metabolite of the alkaloids or a biochemical change produced by the rauwolfias persists long after the drug has been eliminated and is responsible for the behavioral effects. Studies of radioactively tagged rauwolfia alkaloids (see Ban, 1969) have indicated that the drugs are uniformly distributed throughout the body. Within 30 minutes of intravenous administration, the drug can be detected in most organs of the body. The drugs are not extensively stored in the organism, but instead are rapidly broken down and much of the drug is excreted very quickly. The main site of metabolic breakdown in humans is the liver, and about 50% of an oral dose of these drugs is excreted within 3 to 4 hours by the kidneys. In spite of this rapid excretion rate, the psychoactive properties of the rauwolfia drugs may last up to 5 days after a single dose and for several weeks after cessation of continuous drug treatment.

Biochemical effects.   Reserpine causes a depletion of bioamines (NE, 5HT) from the presynaptic storage vesicles. The depletion of NE seems to be responsible for the sedative effect of this drug since it is antagonized by dopa, an NE precursor; it can be duplicated by AMPT, the precursor of an NE false transmitter, but not by PCPA, the precursor of a 5HT false transmitter (see Chapter 2). The sedating action of reserpine, however, may not be directly related to its antischizophrenic action. Although there is agreement that bioamine depletion is responsible for many of the actions of reserpine, some consider an interaction with NE (Carlsson, 1960; Stein & Wise, 1971) and others with 5HT (Brodie, 1959) to be responsible for its efficacy in schizophrenia.

Neurophysiological effects.   The central effects of the rauwolfia drugs are varied. There is relatively little direct influence on the spinal cord or the lower medullary centers, but there is a dose-dependent effect on the reticular activating system. Low doses of reserpine produce an increased firing rate in the brainstem reticular formation and thalamic projection system. On the basis of these findings, it was suggested that the drug has a stimulating effect on the mesodiencephalic alerting systems. Large doses of the drug have opposite effects, i.e., an inhibition of neural firing rate.

Hypothalamic actions of the rauwolfia drugs have been noted in the posterior portion of the hypothalamus. The sedative effects and the lowering of blood pressure, heart rate, and body temperature produced by reserpine administration are very similar to the constellation of symptoms obtained by Hess (1954) upon stimulation of anterior hypothalamus, or the syndrome observed in patients with lesions in the posterior nuclei of the hypothalamus. This indirect evidence suggests that reserpine may inhibit the posterior nuclei of the hypothalamus, which exert partial control over the sympathetic outflow of the autonomic nervous system. "Sham rage" which consists of violent, poorly directed, stimulus-bound sympathetic responses in the decorticated animal is successfully controlled by reserpine.

Behavioral effects.   The psychoactive rauwolfia alkaloids induce a wide range of behavioral changes in humans and other species. This is strikingly demonstrated in wild animals. Monkeys can be handled easily following administration of this drug, even though they are not asleep and respond to stimuli of various kinds. The excitement in dogs or the playfulness seen in monkeys is soon depressed. At higher doses, the animals pass into a stage of quiescence, in which they pay little attention to their surroundings, have no interest in food, and sit motionless. Although these animals appear to be asleep, they are easily aroused by external stimulation. At certain dose levels the motor activity passes into a state called *catalepsy*, in which the animals may become fixed in unnatural postures.

In human studies a single dose of reserpine has been shown to lower the ability to make certain visual discriminations, disrupt paired associate learning, decrease tapping rate, and increase visual and auditory reaction time. Reserpine induces a state of quietness and calmness, and the patient usually exhibits decreased responsiveness to external stimuli, but responses to painful stimuli remain quite normal (see Ban, 1969).

Although reserpinized animals or humans remain awake, their response to depressant drugs such as barbiturates and alcohol is potentiated and the sleeping time following these hypnotics is prolonged. Reserpine gives no protection against the convulsions produced by electroshock or convulsant drugs (Chapter 8) and may even increase susceptibility to convulsions. Therefore, the depression produced by reserpine is far different from that produced by the barbiturates and other CNS depressants.

Escape responses do not seem to be inhibited, but avoidance responses are definitely impaired. Animals trained to avoid an electric footshock by pressing a lever, climbing a pole, or moving to another part of the cage do not perform the response to a warning signal, although they do when the shock is turned on.

Clinical use. The rauwolfia alkaloids have been administered to produce sedation in conditions ranging from snakebite to epilepsy. Today they are given alone or in combination with other drugs for hypertension (to reduce blood pressure and also to decrease anxiety). Less frequently they are used in vascular and allergic headaches and in the treatment of tachycardia (an abnormally fast heartbeat).

The rauwolfia alkaloids are no longer regularly used in the treatment of schizophrenia. They have been replaced by the phenothiazines and butyrophenones. This lack of use is primarily due to the disadvantageousness of the sedation and lowering of blood pressure also produced. Reserpine is sometimes administered to the violent schizophrenic patient and there is usually a decrease in violence or aggressive behavior and consequently less need for restraint (this use takes advantage of the sedative action). There also appears to be a remission of the hallucinations which plague the patient. Reserpine treatment is most effective in acute cases of schizophrenia and, as is also the case with the other drugs used in this disorder, with more chronic cases the efficacy of reserpine decreases.

Side effects. There are a variety of side effects associated with the clinical use of the rauwolfia drugs and they may be considered an extension of the normal pharmacological actions of the drugs. The rauwolfia drugs produce a sympathetic depression (or a parasympathetic dominance) which, if carried to a pathological extreme, may lead to slowing of the heart (bradycardia), excessive salivation, nausea, diarrhea, and nasal congestion. However, the most serious side effect of the rauwolfia drugs is the mental depression that may develop. In one experimental report (Quetsch, Achol, Litin, & Faucett, 1959) of effects in hypertensive patients receiving rauwolfia drugs, 26% were found to have become depressed, while only 5% depression was recorded for a control group. The depression produced by the rauwolfia compounds may be so great as to drive a patient to suicide, although intentional overdosing with the drug will not produce death.

Certain endocrinological side effects have also been reported. The rauwolfias have a blocking effect on the pituitary gonadotropins. Thus, the ovarian cycle is inhibited and fertility is depressed in females. In males, feminization and impairment of sexual function may also be found.

Summary.   The rauwolfia drugs reduce the blood pressure, calm or sedate the agitated subject, and have a normalizing action on the behavior of the schizophrenic. The use of the rauwolfia alkaloids in schizophrenia reached a peak in the 1950s and 1960s, but with the popularity of the phenothiazine and butyrophenone drugs the rauwolfias are no longer commonly used for this purpose. The disadvantages of the rauwolfias are their slow onset of action, and most importantly, a relatively high frequency of mental depression which may lead the patient to the edge of suicide. Because of these unwanted reactions, the use of the rauwolfia alkaloids has primarily been confined to those patients who are unable to take (or do not respond to) other antischizophrenic drugs.

The Phenothiazine Derivatives

The phenothiazines are today among the most widely used drugs in the treatment of behavioral disturbances. By far, the most used drug in this group of compounds is chlorpromazine (Thorazine). It has been estimated that, during the past decade, at least 50 million patients have received therapeutic doses of this drug, and over 10,000 research reports have been published covering almost all aspects of its metabolism, action, absorption, and most importantly, clinical usefulness (Jarvik, 1970). The other phenothiazine derivatives have not been prescribed as widely and there are relatively fewer articles published specifically dealing with the phenothiazine-derived tranquilizers other than chlorpromazine.

Although phenothiazine itself was synthesized in 1883, it was not until 1934 that it was first used in medicine (and as an insecticide). In the late 1930s a derivative of phenothiazine, promethazine, was found to have antihistaminic effects and, like many antihistamines, a sedative and calming effect. Attempts were made to treat motor agitation but, as with the other antihistaminic drugs, these proved unsuccessful (Guiraud & David, 1950). The drug was subsequently used to prolong sleeping time induced by barbiturate treatment, or as an adjunct with anesthetics to produce a more profound loss of sensation. In 1950,

Charpentier synthesized drug number 4560 RP, later called *chlorpromazine*. Two years later it was reported that this drug produced in animals a potentiation of anesthetic effects and "artificial hibernation," a state in which consciousness is maintained but an indifference to the surroundings develops (Laborit, Hugnenard, & Allusume, 1952).

The first report of the use of chlorpromazine in the treatment of behavioral disturbances was made by Delay and associates in 1952 (Delay & Deniker, 1952; Delay, Deniker & Harl, 1952). Subsequently, the drug was released in the United States and has since been widely used in the treatment of schizophrenia. In the mid-1950s, many psychiatrists were skeptical of the usefulness of the drug and thought it was no more effective than a placebo. They thought it would not long remain a reputable treatment for mental disorders. Yet today, after thousands of research investigations and millions of patients have been treated with the drug, it seems very likely that chlorpromazine will be used in one form or another for many years to come. Variations of the phenothiazine molecules have resulted in compounds that differ in potency and toxicity from clorpromazine, but the relative therapeutic superiority of one over the other has yet to be demonstrated clearly (the most popular phenothiazines are listed in Table 5.2). Even though several phenothiazine derivatives are used in clinical therapy, chlorpromazine has been subjected to the closest scientific scrutiny and given to the largest number of patients. Therefore, throughout this discussion we will be chlorpromazine as an example of the phenothiazine drugs.

Chemical structure. Phenothiazine has a three-ringed structure in which two benzene rings are attached by atoms of sulfur and nitrogen (see Figure 5.1). Molecular substitutions are most common at the carbon atom labeled R_2 and at the nitrogen atom R_1. Most of the effective phenothiazines have a halogen at R_2 (chloride or fluoride). All of the phenothiazines used in the treatment of

TABLE 5.2

Popular Phenothiazine-derived Antischizophrenic Drugs

Generic name	Trade name	Average oral dose (mg)[a]
Chlorpromazine	Thorazine	25–50
Promazine	Sparine	25–50
Triflupromazine	Vesprin	10–25
Fluphenazine	Prolixin, Permitil	.25–.50
Perphenazine	Trilifon	4–8
Prochlorperazine	Compazine	5–10
Trifluoperazine	Stelazine	2–10
Thioridazine	Mellaril	25–100
Acetophenazine	Tindal	20–120

[a] These doses are usually administered 3 to 4 times daily.

schizophrenia have a three-carbon sequence separating the ring structure from the nitrogen atom on the R_1 side chain.

Metabolism.   The phenothiazines are well absorbed from the gastrointestinal tract and from parenteral areas and follow similar routes of absorption, metabolism, and excretion. Chlorpromazine (CPZ), for example, is absorbed in 5 to 10 minutes after parenteral administration and in 30 to 60 minutes after it is taken by mouth. The phenothiazines are then rapidly distributed to all body tissues. Systematic studies (Gothelf & Karczmar, 1963) have shown that from 60% to 70% of an administered dose is rapidly removed from the circulation by the liver. Fifty percent of the daily dose is excreted in the urine, and another substantial portion is eliminated in the feces.

Neurophysiological effects.   Following phenothiazine administration, changes can be found throughout the CNS. Unfortunately, it is not yet possible to say which of these effects are related to therapeutic action and which are merely coincidental or indirect.

Cortex and EEG: Administration of therapeutic doses of CPZ produces an EEG in humans, characteristic of drowsiness and the early stages of sleep. Just as a patient develops a tolerance to the behavioral sedating effects of the drug, so too, tolerance develops to the EEG slowing effects. CPZ also increases the threshold in the cortex to peripheral sensory stimulation or spinal cord dorsal root electrical stimulation (Fink, 1959).

Hypothalamus: The effect of the phenothiazines on the hypothalamus is complex. A response which may be specific to the hypothalamus and which CPZ blocks is the "sham rage," which is seen in decorticated animals. This response is characterized by hyperactivity, hyperresponsiveness to stimuli, and outbursts of sympathetic activity. The rage is poorly oriented and persists only as long as the noxious stimulus is present. Such animals are very sensitive to the depressant effects of CPZ, which indicates that phenothiazine drugs may have an effect on the nuclei of the hypothalamus.

Limbic system: The effects of CPZ on the limbic system structures are still unclear. Doses of the drug which produce behavioral depressant effects usually have little no effect on the neural structures making up this system.

Basal ganglia: The actions of CPZ on the basal ganglia are of interest because this drug (as well as the other phenothiazines) is known to produce a Parkinsonian syndrome and the neurological structures comprising the basal ganglia have long been suspected of being involved in the etiology of Parkinson's disease. CPZ decreases spontaneous firing of single units in the caudate nucleus and the globus pallidus. This effect is similar to the neural activity seen at these structures in persons with Parkinson's disease.

Medulla: The actions of the phenothiazines on the medulla may be seen in the antiemetic (antivomiting) effect of these drugs. It has been shown that the sensitivity of a medullary vomiting mechanism is affected by the phenothiazine drugs. CPZ inhibits apomorphine-induced vomiting, and since apomorphine acts directly by stimulating the vomiting mechanism in the medulla, the phenothiazines may act by direct inhibition of this mechanism or by a competitive action with apomorphine for selective receptor sites (Jarvik, 1970).

Reticular formation: As we shall see in Chapter 6, the barbiturates produce a depression of the brainstem reticular formation response to peripheral stimuli. Responses to electrical stimulation of the brainstem reticular formation are also inhibited. The action of CPZ is more complex. Whereas the barbiturates produce a marked impairment of arousal, CPZ produces only a slight increase in the threshold of arousal to electrical stimulation of the brainstem. This shows that the effect of CPZ is not primarily to depress the ascending reticular activating system and, once stimuli get through to the brain, processing may continue as usual. EEG records do show, however, that chlorpromazine blocks auditory and other types of peripheral stimulation (Bradley, 1968). This seems to indicate that there may be a selective inhibitory effect on sensory collaterals impinging upon the reticular formation, but very little, if any, inhibition by CPZ within the brainstem reticular formation itself. Chlorpromazine blocks the peripheral stimulation, but if the stimulation can get to the brainstem, processing appears to go on uninhibited.

Autonomic nervous system: CPZ and the phenothiazine derivatives have important effects on both the sympathetic and parasympathetic segments of the autonomic nervous system. CPZ has strong adrenergic blocking effects as well as weaker peripheral cholinergic blocking effects. In the dog, CPZ inhibits the hypertension which is normally produced by epinephrine. Characteristic of this sympathetic blockade is the failure of the human patient to react to stressful situations. There is no increase in blood pressure and cardiac output fails to increase. Troublesome reactions to the phenothiazines which are mediated by the autonomic nervous system include dry mouth, nasal congestion, and, most importantly, hypotension.

Endocrine effects.   Since, as we have seen, CPZ has strong effects on the hypothalamus, and the hypothalamus is so intimately related to the pituitary gland, it would be expected that the drug would affect pituitary hormone production. In the female, CPZ has been shown to reduce urinary levels of gonadotropins leading to decreased blood levels of estrogens and progestins, to block ovulation and estrus cycles, and to produce infertility. In the male, CPZ produces a decrease in testicular weight. It also produces a retardation of growth which may be caused by an interference with somatotropin since this action is reversible upon somatotropin replacement therapy. CPZ also produces a decrease in the amount of ACTH released by the pituitary, leading to an inhibition of a rat's response to stress, and inhibits the release of oxytocin from the posterior lobe of the pituitary.

Behavioral effects.   These drugs have their effect by direct action on the central nervous system, but also affect almost every organ in the body. CPZ initially produces sedation, as was described in 1952 by Delay and Deniker, who labeled the drug effects as the "neuroleptic syndrome" characterized by psychomotor slowing, emotional quieting, and affective indifference:

> Sitting or lying, the patient is motionless in his bed, often pale and with eyelids lowered. He remains silent most of the time. If he is questioned, he answers slowly and deliberately in a monotonous indifferent voice; he expresses himself in few words and becomes silent. Without exception the response is fairly appropriate and adaptable, showing that the subject is capable of attention and of thought. But he rarely initiates a question and he does not express his anxieties, desires or preferences. He is usually aware of the improvement induced by the treatment but does not show euphoria. The apparent indifference or the slowing of responses to external stimuli, the diminution of initiative and of anxiety without a change in the state of waking and consciousness or of intellectual faculties constitute the psychological syndrome attributable to the drug. (As cited in Jarvik, 1970, p. 156)

Sedation: This sedative effect perhaps contributes to the antischizophrenic potency of CPZ, but it is not essential to it. Tolerance develops rather rapidly to the sedative effects, but not to the antischizophrenic effects of the drug. Also, several of the phenothiazines (for example, perphenazine) possess little sedative properties, but are very potent antischizophrenic agents.

Conditioned responses: The basic screening procedure for tranquilizer drugs has been to test the drug for its influence on escape responses (i.e., an unconditioned response) and conditioned avoidance responses (i.e., a conditioned response). It has been found (Cook & Weidley, 1957) that small doses of CPZ inhibit the performance of a conditioned avoidance response; the animals fail to respond by climbing a pole to an auditory cue that signals the onset of punishing shock. However, the drug does not inhibit the unconditioned escape responses once the shock is applied. In addition to CPZ, treatments with reserpine and morphine also produce an inhibition of the conditioned response at doses which do not debilitate the unconditioned escape responses. However, doses of barbital, pentobarbital, and meprobamate affect the conditioned as well as the unconditioned responses to about the same extent. In animals, CPZ not only blocks the performance of learned avoidance responses, but also suppresses the acquisition of new avoidance responses and accelerates the extinction of such responses (Rutledge & Doty, 1957; also see Jarvik, 1970).

Human performance: The phenothiazines also affect the more complex human learning tasks. CPZ reduces vigilance in human subjects performing continuous pursuit-rotor or tapping-speed tests (motor function tests that require the subject to follow a target). Yet, the drug produces relatively little impairment of digit-symbol substitution, a mathematical analogies test of intellectual functioning. Barbiturate sedatives have the opposite effects, in that greater impairment is seen in the digit-symbol test than in the pursuit-rotor or tapping-speed tasks. It has been suggested that drugs resembling CPZ impair sustained attention tasks because of their effects on the ascending reticular activating system.

Motor activity: In addition to the effects the phenothiazine drugs have on conditioned responses in animals and humans, we may also look at the effects these drugs have on general motor activity. The phenothiazines used in psychiatry have been shown to impair spontaneous motor behavior in each species of animal studied, including the human. In therapeutic doses, behavior may be slowed or inhibited, but rarely is it stopped. A consequence of this behavioral inhibition is that treated animals or humans may even do better than normals in tasks that require response inhibition. For example, animals receiving CPZ are apt to do better than controls with no drug treatment on passive avoidance tasks, which require an animal to inhibit a dominant response in order to be rewarded (Blough, 1958). Similarly, extinction of a learned response and habituation or adaptation to novel stimuli are hastened by treatment with CPZ. In high doses, cataleptic effects may be produced so that the bodies and limbs of animals may be molded into various postures and the animals remain immobile for long periods of time. It should be emphasized that a decrease in motor activity is characteristic of a wide variety of drugs acting on the CNS, including barbiturates, narcotic analgesics, meprobamate, and chlordiazepoxide, and hence a diminution in motor activity may not be used as a sole indicant of phenothiazine treatment.

Clinical use. CPZ and the related phenothiazines exert a quieting effect on excited or hyperactive psychotic patients; combativeness disappears and relaxation and cooperativeness become prominent. Increased communication and social interaction is usually seen. The improvement in behavior with phenothiazines involves not only reduction in anxiety and agitation, but also alleviation of a wide range of other schizophrenic symptoms, including thought disturbances, delusions, hallucinations, and deterioration in personal care. Not surprisingly, the efficacy of phenothiazines in the treatment of chronic schizophrenia, though still appreciable, is not as striking as it is with acute schizophrenia. This indicates the importance of early intervention with drug therapy in schizophrenia.

Side effects. There are several quite severe side effects associated with the use of phenothiazine tranquilizers. Sedation and drowsiness are prone to occur, but these effects are apparently unrelated to the antischizophrenic effect. Tolerance develops to the sedation effect of the drugs but not to the antischizophrenic effect. The potential for producing side effects involving nonvoluntary movements seems to be a concomitant of the antischizophrenic properties of phenothiazines. These effects are common, but sometimes can be managed by reduction of dosage, change of drug, or the use of an anti-Parkinsonian drug. Autonomic side effects, such as postural hypotension, dry mouth, constipation, and urinary retention, have also been reported. Again, a tolerance develops to these responses. Jaundice has been reported following prolonged phenothiazine therapy and convulsions have occurred in patients with a preexisting seizure disorder. The most serious of the side effects produced by phenothiazines, agranulocytosis (a deficiency in the number of white cells in the blood), has been seen mostly in association with CPZ. Such behavioral side effects as occasional paradoxical agitation, intensification of psychotic symptoms, delirium, or precipitation of depression have been observed on occasion. Menstrual irregularity, breast enlargement in men (due to testosterone inhibition), weight gain, and edema (fluid retention) may also occur.

In recent years attention has been drawn to three different syndromes occurring in chronically hospitalized patients receiving long-term phenothiazine treatment. The impact of these syndromes is to temper somewhat one's enthusiasm for prolonged maintenance drug treatment, especially at high doses. (1) The skin-eye syndrome involves a darkening of the skin due to diffused pigmentary depositions, and opacities of the anterior lens and posterior cornea. (2) An extrapyramidal syndrome of persistent, sometimes irreversible choreiform or ticlike movements, usually involving the mouth and face, and developing only after many months to years of phenothiazine treatment, has also been noted (and is called *tardive dyskinesia*). (3) Lastly, there appears to be a rare occurrence of sudden death associated with high phenothiazine dosage. Despite this imposing list of side effects, the phenothiazines as used in practice are a relatively safe class of drugs. They are not addicting. Dependence does not occur with their use. Craving for these drugs does not develop and no significant withdrawal syndrome follows discontinuation of the medication. Though they have been ingested frequently with suicidal intent, it seems almost impossible to kill oneself with this class of drugs.

The Butyrophenones

As so often occurs in pharmacology, useful properties of drugs are discovered accidentally. We saw that the phenothiazines were originally tested as antihistamines when their potent tranquilizing properties were uncovered. The butyrophenones were studied as potential analgesics because of a structural similarity to meperidine (Chapter 7) when their antischizophrenic properties were uncovered. These drugs were first introduced in therapy in Europe in 1958, and were initially marketed in the United States in 1967. They now appear to be an effective alternative to the phenothiazines. The two major drugs in this class that possess antischizophrenic effects are haloperidol and triperidol.

Chemical structure.   The chemical formula for haloperidol is shown in Figure 5.1. Triperidol differs from haloperidol in that the chlorine molecule is absent and is replaced by a CF_3 substitution (C = carbon, F = fluorine) on another part of the benzene ring.

Metabolism.   The absorption, distribution, and excretion of haloperidol has been widely studied in humans and lower animals. Studies have been completed both on normal subjects and on schizophrenic patients (Braun, Poos, & Soudyn, 1967; Johnson, Charalanupous, & Braun, 1967). Haloperidol is absorbed rapidly from the gastrointestinal tract in both animals and humans. Isotope studies have shown radioactively tagged drug present in the blood within the first hour after oral ingestion. Plasma concentrations in the blood reach a maximum about 2 to

6 hours after administration and remain at a high level for about 72 hours. After this period there is a slow decline in plasma haloperidol levels with significant amounts remaining in the circulation for weeks after the ingestion of even a small amount (Johnson et al., 1967).

Biochemical and neurophysiological effects. There is no single effect produced by the butyrophenones that may be labeled as the specific physiological or neurochemical event responsible for the calming properties of this class of drugs. The predominant neurochemical effects involve GABA and the brain amines. Janssen (1967) has suggested that the butyrophenones work by mimicking the action of gamma-aminobutyric acid and by blocking the action of glutamic acid. He has previously suggested that glutamic acid and GABA are in competition for the same neuronal site, and that glutamic acid, once bound to this site, excites the neuron via membrane depolarization, but GABA depresses cellular functioning and makes the receptor site unavailable to glutamic acid without altering the resting membrane potential. Most investigators, however, would instead attribute the clinical efficacy of the butyrophenones to their effects on the catecholaminergic system (especially dopamine).

Dopamine usually produces a fall in blood pressure, but this effect is counteracted by low doses of haloperidol and other butyrophenones, suggesting a dopamine-antagonist effect of the drug (Rossum & Janssen, 1967). Also, the butyrophenones prevent the increase of brain norepinephrine seen after the administration of tranylcypromine (see Chapter 2; Drease & DeMeyer, 1964). Like the phenothiazines, the butyrophenones have a potent antiemetic effect which probably is caused by a direct action on a central vomiting mechanism in the caudal medulla (Janssen & Niemegeers, 1961).

Other effects attributed to the butyrophenones include: (1) a depression of the reticular formation (Arrigo, Savoldi, & Tartara, 1962), (2) a stimulant effect on the supraoptic and paraventricular nuclei of the hypothalamus as seen through histological examination of brains of rabbits treated with triperidol, (3) a depression of activity in the telencephalic basal ganglia, (4) an increase in hippocampal seizure thresholds and reduction in duration of afterdischarges (Monti, Rance, & Killam, 1966), and (5) a slowing of the alpha wave activity seen in cortical EEG records (Muller & Warnes, 1964).

Behavioral effects. The antischizophrenic butyrophenones inhibit motor activity in animals tested in the open field situation, induce catalepsy (an abnormal condition of muscular rigidity and a loss of control over the muscles), and cause ptosis (drooping of the eyelids caused by muscular weakness) in rats. They depress food intake and reduce the mortality level of animals tested in stress (usually shock-producing) situations (Janssen, 1967). The butyrophenones have also been shown to depress conditioned avoidance responses at doses which do not produce any behavioral calming effects. Recently, investigators (Oberst & Crook, 1967) have reported an inhibition produced by haloperidol on a sustained physical exercise test. Dogs were trained to run a treadmill in a sequence consisting of 15 minutes of running followed by 2-minute rest periods. Untreated dogs could perform this task without difficulty but dogs given 12.5 mg/kg of haloperidol could not.

In humans, haloperidol produced a feeling of tiredness when tested in a double-blind experimental situation. It did not decrease the subject's ability to solve math problems but did cause the subject to constantly overestimate his success at the task. The butyrophenones when tested on a group of chronic schizophrenic patients tended to decrease performance on tasks involving visual perception and to increase performance on psychomotor and conceptual tasks (St. Jean, 1964).

Clinical use.   The butyrophenone drugs are primarily used in the treatment of schizophrenic patients. Carefully controlled studies have shown that these drugs are as effective in treating schizophrenia as are the more commonly prescribed phenothiazines.

The butyrophenones have also been used in the treatment of organic disorders. A particular usefulness of these drugs has been in the management of Gilles de la Tourette's disease, a syndrome characterized by involuntary tics and uncontrolled obscene outbursts.

Side effects.   Serious side effects are rare in normal therapeutic dose ranges but may be seen in elderly or debilitated patients or when high doses are administered. Gerle (1964) has collated data from 70 published studies including 6,500 patients and from 40 questionnaires covering an additional 6,000 patients. Side effects produced by high drug doses include insomnia, depression, delirium, and confusion. Neurological reactions may follow administration of haloperidol or triperidol. The most commonly seen are extrapyramidal signs such as a decrease or complete absence of reactivity to stimuli. These reactions are characterized by a lack of spontaneous movements, bent stance, a shuffling gait, and an expressionless face. Often it is accompanied by rigidity and tremor. Contractions or twitchings of the jaw, cheek, or fingers are also sometimes seen as side effects of treatment with a butyrophenone (tardive dyskinesia).

LITHIUM

Lithium is now the drug of choice in the treatment of mania. Lithium was first chemically isolated in 1818. It was not until 1949, however, that Cade reported the sedative action that high doses of lithium carbonate had on the guinea pig. About 2 hours after drug administration the guinea pigs became quiet and lethargic and did not respond to stimuli, although they remained conscious. He reasoned that the drug may also calm the manic and hyperexcitable subject. He administered the drug to patients suffering from manic disorders and found improvement. The first controlled clinical investigation of the therapeutic usefulness of lithium (Schou, 1954) concluded that in the treatment of mania the drug was better than placebos, superior to the phenothiazines, and "represents a very welcome addition to the therapeutic measures against a disease that is very resistant to most types of treatment or in which the improvement after treatment is frequently rather short-lived" (p. 258).

Chemistry. Lithium is a positively charged ion that is the lightest of the metals. It is usually found in the body only in very small amounts. Like its related metals, sodium and potassium, lithium salts are highly soluble in water.

Absorption and metabolism. Lithium is readily absorbed from the intestine when given orally. Peak plasma concentration is reached in 2 to 4 hours. Lithium penetrates the cerebrospinal fluid and peak concentrations are usually one-half of that seen in the plasma. Excretion is mainly through the kidneys and about half of a single dose of the compound is excreted in the first 24 hours. However, there appears to be a balance between sodium and lithium concentrations, for if sodium levels are low, the excretion rate of lithium is decreased, and severe side effects may result. For this reason lithium is not given to patients who are on a salt-free diet. Just as low sodium concentration causes increased amounts of lithium to be retained, so sodium administration facilitates the excretion rate of the lithium compounds.

Biochemical and neurophysiological effects. Lithium chloride was originally used as a sodium substitute but this was quickly halted when the toxicity of the ion was realized. Although the lithium ion is distributed throughout the body tissues, it appears that its prime effect is on the central nervous system. It has been suggested that the drug acts by increasing the uptake or decreasing the release of catecholamines. Yet, Corrodi, Fuxe, Hokfelt, and Schou (1967) reported lithium to produce no change in the content of norepinephrine in the brain. Turnover, though, does seem to be affected. For example, an inhibition of tyrosine hydroxylase, an enzyme critical to the normal production of norepinephrine, has been found. However, more recently lithium has been found to produce an acute increase in serotonin synthesis by nerve endings, followed by a compensatory decrease in serotonin synthesis (due to an initial increase, and then a delayed decrease in brain tryptophan hydroxylase activity). The latency of the clinical effectiveness of lithium in manic states is consistent with this finding (Knapp & Mandell, 1973). Lithium can also replace sodium ions in the extracellular fluid and severely impair neural conduction through interference with the transporting mechanisms of the sodium pump. The mechanism responsible for the efficacy is not yet established, but it seems most likely that catecholamines or serotonin are involved. An effect on sodium metabolism seems less likely to be crucial, but this possibility cannot be completely discounted.

Clinical use. As far as the therapeutic usefulness of the lithium salts, it appears that they exert a selective depressive effect on the manic patient. It has been estimated that 70% to 80% of manic patients treated with lithium can be expected to respond satisfactorily within 2 weeks. Johnson and Gershon (1968) have reported that 78% of the 28 patients they treated with 1.5 to 2.0 g per day of lithium showed marked improvement within 3 days.

The effect of lithium in mania cannot simply be attributed to sedation. The drug is more selective than that. First, doses that are effective in manic patients are not sedative to normal subjects. Secondly, lithium appears to be more specifically therapeutic. Lithium appears to normalize mood and ideation. Lithium has been ineffective in the treatment of psychoneurotic disorders or the schizophrenic psychoses. Sometimes lithium is employed as a prophylactic during the depressive or normal phases to prevent mood swings in the manic-depressive patient. However, commencing treatment during a depressive phase is contraindicated; the patient often gets worse. Yet, if treatment is begun before the depressive phase is entered, the lithium appears to be prophylactic.

Side effects. Side effects may be very serious with the use of lithium. Overdosage and sodium deficiency are regular occurrences and produce severe reactions. Usually patients feel fatigued and may complain of muscular weakness. Their speech may be slurred and there may be a slight tremor in the hands. Some side effects disappear with continued treatment, but excessive urination, thirst, and tremor may persist. In some patients, side effects have been more severe, including convulsions, coma, and death. Due to the extreme dangers of toxicity with the use of lithium, it is absolutely necessary to monitor plasma lithium levels at least once a week to prevent accidental poisoning, and some authorities insist upon twice weekly monitoring.

DEPRESSANT TRANQUILIZERS

Distinct from the psychoses (schizophrenia, mania, depression) are a large spectrum of psychological disturbances called the *neuroses*. We can characterize the neuroses as being milder behavioral disorders involving anxiety, tension, and mild depression. The antischizophrenic tranquilizers are not particularly useful in a therapy program for neurotic behavior. The depressants discussed in the next chapter can be effective in the neuroses because of their sedating effect. Two groups of depressant tranquilizers, the propanediols and the benzodiaze-pines, are also useful in the treatment of the neuroses. Psychotherapy, especially the behavioral and relational therapies, can also be shown to be ameliorative for the neuroses. A treatment program combining pharmacotherapy and psycho-therapy would appear most beneficial for dealing with neurotic behavior.

The depressant tranquilizers of this chapter and the depressants of the next chapter seem equally effective in the neuroses. Although there are those who favor one or another group of drugs, such distinctions cannot be objectively validated. The depressant tranquilizers are quite distinct from the anti-schizophrenia tranquilizers, but very similar to the other depressants. The key features of the depressant tranquilizers seem to be a sedative action, muscle relaxation, taming of aggressive behavior in animal studies, effects on conflict behavior in animal studies (see "Behavioral Effects," which follows), and an anticonvulsant action. The relaxation of voluntary muscles is especially suspected of being responsible for the ameliorative action in tense and anxious patients.

As with the depressants, but not the antischizophrenic tranquilizers, tolerance develops to the therapeutic effects of the depressant tranquilizers. Moreover, these drugs are addicting, especially when taken in higher doses. A dependence develops and a severe withdrawal syndrome resembling that for the other depressants can be observed. The abstinence syndrome may include tremors, motor incoordination, hallucinations, anxiety, and even convulsions. The finding of cross-tolerance between the depressant tranquilizers and the depressants further suggests similarities between these drug groups. One advantage of the depressant tranquilizers seems to be their greater safety due to higher lethal doses and a concomitant lower likelihood of accidentally or suicidally fatal overdosage.

The Propanediols

Mephenesin (Tolserol), a centrally acting muscle relaxant, was first synthesized in 1908. However, it was not until 1946 that the muscular relaxation properties of the drug were discovered. It was reported (Berger & Bradley, 1946) that small amounts of mephenesin produced tranquilization, muscular relaxation, and a sleeplike condition from which the subject could easily be aroused. However, mephenesin had one major drawback—it was only active for a short time, thus requiring large, continuous doses if therapeutic calming and relaxation were to be established. The rapid deactivation of the drug was due to the rapid oxidation of the hydroxyl groups on the molecule, and scientists tried to change the molecule so that the drug would be more resistant to enzymatic destruction. Over 1,200 compounds were tried and soon a product of esterification of the mephenesin molecule was found to produce a longer lasting reduction in anxiety and a mild tranquilizing effect. This drug was meprobamate (Miltown, Equanil). Meprobamate quickly grew in popularity, and within 2 years after its introduction in 1951 was widely prescribed as a daytime sedative agent. According to some, the widespread use of meprobamate was probably due to such factors as efficient drug advertising and a desire of the medical profession for a nonbarbiturate sedative, as well as the apparent effectiveness of meprobamate in relieving anxiety without producing excessive drowsiness.

Just as the precise nature of anxiety is unclear, so is the precise nature of meprobamate action unclear. The drowsiness and relief from tension that the drug produces is similar to that produced by the barbiturates or a double martini. Meprobamate is not similar to the phenothiazines, reserpine, or haloperidol, in that it is not effective in the schizophrenic patient, nor does it produce the extrapyramidal side effects or blockade of conditioned avoidance responses seen with the major tranquilizers.

Chemical structure. Mephenesin (Figure 5.2) is the basic compound in the chemical group known as the *propanediols*. Esterification of the mephenesin

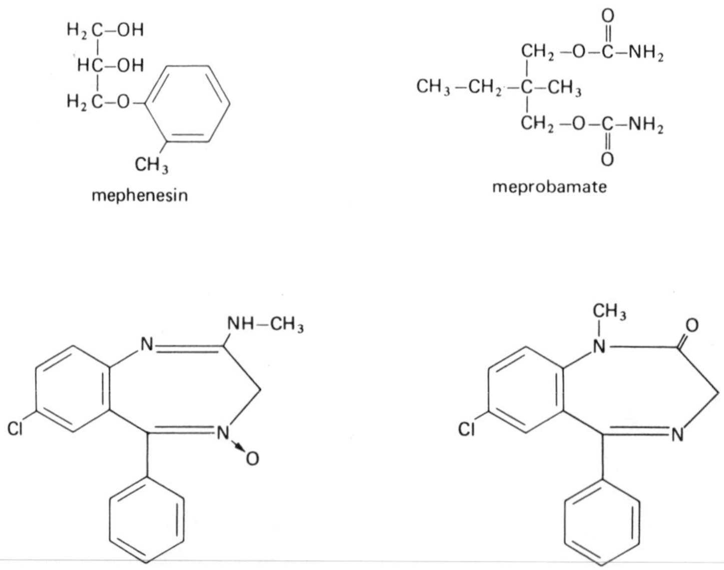

FIGURE 5.2.   Representative depressant tranquilizers.

molecule resulted in the compound commonly known as *meprobamate* (Figure 5.2). In a further search for a more potent and even less toxic propanediol than meprobamate, studies were directed toward modification of the meprobamate molecule. The major result was tybamate, a drug whose chemical structure is somewhat like that of meprobamate.

Metabolism.   Since meprobamate is the major drug of this class used in the treatment of neurotic behavior, discussion will be predominantly limited to it. Meprobamate is readily absorbed from the gastrointestinal tract and reaches peak plasma levels in 2 hours. A slow decline in plasma concentrations taking approximately 10 hours is then observed with a concomitant increase in body tissue concentrations. About 10% of the unchanged drug is excreted through the kidney in 24 hours. The remaining 90% is excreted in the urine in either the oxidized form or as the glucuronic acid metabolite.

Biochemical and neurophysiological effects.   Unlike the antischizophrenic tranquilizers, the propanediols do not suppress autonomic activities. Meprobamate and related drugs do not inhibit NE, D, 5HT, acetylcholine, or histamine (Berger, 1957).

Although no specific sites in the central nervous system have been identified as the critical locus of action of meprobamate, this drug does exert a blocking action on the interneurons of the spinal cord. This was first demonstrated in 1954 by Berger, who reported that the monosynaptic knee jerk reflex was uninhibited by meprobamate but that the multisynaptic crossed extensor and flexor reflexes were decreased or abolished. A similar effect has been produced by tybamate.

Numerous electroencephalographic changes have also been reported after meprobamate administration. For instance, early investigators (Hendley, 1954) have shown that low doses of the drug decrease the spontaneous electrical activity of the thalamic nuclei. Other scientists (Baird, Szekely, Wycis, & Spiegel, 1957) have observed slow wave activity in the basal ganglia (particularly the caudate nucleus) and the limbic structures in cats. These neurophysiological correlates may be secondary effects of the meprobamate, or they may reflect a primary neurophysiological substrate, which mediates the antianxiety effects. Continued research is needed in this area.

Behavioral effects. Unlike the antischizophrenics, the propanediols do not selectively inhibit avoidance responding. There are, however, two characteristic properties of the depressant tranquilizers (both the propanediols and the benzodiazepines). First, they tame the vicious behavior of aggressive animals. Naturally vicious animals such as monkeys are made placid, as are animals made vicious by isolation or brain lesions (for example, isolation of mice or septal region lesions in rats) (Hunt, 1957). With regard to this taming effect, the benzodiazepines are considerably more effective than the propanediols.

The second characteristic effect of the depressant tranquilizers on animal behavior is seen on tests of conflict. One test of this type, called *conditioned suppression*, demonstrates the property of an aversive (painful) stimulus to suppress ongoing behavior. In one application of this technique, a cat or rat that normally attacks a mouse is given a painful shock every time it does so. After a few trials it no longer attacks the mouse (the tendency to attack the mouse has been suppressed, hence the term *conditioned suppression*). An injection of meprobamate or a benzodiazepine will restore the suppressed attack response, despite the electric shock. In other procedures a food- or water-deprived animal (rat, cat, or other species) is shocked when it feeds or drinks. The ingestive behavior is suppressed by the shock. Again, administration of a depressant tranquilizer will restore the behavior that has been suppressed by shock.

In humans the usual therapeutic dose of 400 mg of meprobamate (generally taken four times a day) produces little, if any, impairment on psychological tests. However, this dose does decrease an electrodermal skin response (the galvanic skin response) to emotionally loaded verbal stimuli and impairs performance on a simple driving test (Loomis & West, 1958). In higher doses ranging up to 800 mg there is an increase in visual reaction times, an interference with motor coordination, and a depression of performance in learning tasks (Kornetsky, 1958). Other investigators (Paterson, 1963) have tested meprobamate in frustration-inducing situations and report that under the influence of the drug, the frustration threshold appears to be raised, thus allowing the subject to perform in stressful situations. In a study by Klerman, DiMascio, Havens, and Snell in 1960, meprobamate (400 and 800 mg) was compared to secobarbital (30 and 100 mg) and the antihistamine phenyltoloxamine (100 and 200 mg), and it was reported that meprobamate produced less sedation and calming than the barbiturate or the antihistamine.

Clinical use. In addition to their use as antianxiety agents, meprobamate and the propanediols are also administered for musculoskeletal disorders, like cerebral palsy and petit mal epilepsy. Of the related compounds, meputamate (Capla) has been used in the treatment of hypertension, carisoprodol (Rela, Soma) as an analgesic muscle relaxant, and ethinamate (Valmid) as a sedative-hypnotic drug.

Meprobamate is used primarily as an agent to relieve anxiety states. It is prescribed both as a daytime sedative and as a hypnotic in the treatment of insomnia. Meprobamate appears to be of some benefit to neurotic patients, increasing their ability to concentrate and lessening their distractability. Jarvik (1970) points out that the drug has become so popular since its introduction that it is widely prescribed, even if there is little chance of a therapeutic effect.

Side effects. In normal therapeutic doses, meprobamate and the related propanediols are safe and produce relatively rare incidences of serious side effects. The major areas of side effects may be viewed as neuropsychiatric, allergic, and compulsive use (which may lead to physical dependence).

One of the most frequent side effects is drowsiness. In isolated cases the drug has produced a state of euphoria, or a feeling of confusion, or panic. Both meprobamate and tybamate produce motor incoordination at high doses, and in some patients, at therapeutic doses, these drugs may still produce a motor incoordination and consequently interfere with driving skill.

The allergic reactions to the propanediols include fever, fainting, hypotension, anuria (inability to urinate), shock, and a respiratory depression which may lead to death. However, these serious side effects are extremely rare. Successful suicide attempts are also rare with these drugs, probably due to their low potency.

Compulsive use and physical dependence may definitely be seen with meprobamate. Withdrawal symptoms, seen after the abrupt discontinuation of high doses of meprobamate, include convulsions and coma. These may lead to death. The occurrence of meprobamate withdrawal symptoms is dependent on the dose of the drug used (Jarvik, 1970). Patients given a dose of 1.6 g per day for 4 months rarely exhibited the withdrawal symptoms; whereas in studies employing 3.2 g per day, a majority of the patients experienced symptoms including hallucinations, anxiety, and tremors. In a study employing 5.8 g per day, upon withdrawal the patients experienced tremors, insomnia, and gastrointestinal disturbances, and 10% of the patients had convulsions. It is usually recommended that doses of meprobamate not exceed 2.4 g per day to minimize the possibility of serious side effects.

Benzodiazepine Compounds

Three compounds which are derivatives of benzodiazepine are presently available to the physician, chlordiazepoxide (Librium), diazepam (Valium) and oxazepam (Serax). In the past 5 years chlordiazepoxide has probably been therapeutically administered as an anxiety-reducing drug more often than any other compound. However, the therapeutic efficacy of the drug is debated, and many hold that chlordiazepoxide is no more effective than the barbiturates in reducing anxiety.

Compounds of this type were initially prepared in 1933. Animal screening procedures indicated that chlordiazepoxide had muscle relaxant and anti-convulsant actions. Later it was reported (Randall, Schallek, Heise, Kieth, & Bagdon, 1960) that the drug had a "taming" effect on wild animals. These properties led to the drug's use in the treatment of anxiety, alcoholism, and psychoneurotic and psychosomatic disorders.

Chemical structure. The benzodiazepines were derived from compounds known as 3, 1, 4-benzodiazepines, which had no psychiatric use. In the 1950s Sternbach, Randall, and Gustafson (1964) studied the reaction of one of these chemicals and found a crystallized compound, 1, 4-benzodiazepine, more commonly known as *chlordiazepoxide* (see Figure 5.2). Diazepam (Figure 5.2), the second benzodiazepine derivative to be experimentally studied, has more potent pharmacological activity than the parent compound. Otherwise, its chemical and physical properties closely resemble those of chlordiazepoxide. Oxazepam is the third psychoactive benzodiazepine to be considered here.

Metabolism. The benzodiazepine drugs are rapidly absorbed from the gastrointestinal tract and from parenteral sites; however, peak plasma levels are not reached for several hours (4 to 8 hours). The major paths of benzodiazepine metabolism are demethylation, hydroxylation, and conjugation. These drugs are excreted slowly in the urine.

Biochemical and neurophysiological effects. Recent data (Wise et al., 1972) have been interpreted to suggest that the benzodiazepines reduce anxiety by reducing the turnover of serotonin in the brain. Turnover of norepinephrine, serotonin and other biogenic amines in the brain are all reduced by the benzodiazepines and also the barbiturates. In this study, one of the benzo-diazepines (oxazepam) was shown to increase punished responses in a conflict test (a supposed result of anxiety reduction), but also to decrease the rate of appetitive (nonpunished responses) in rats. A decrease in nonpunished responses is taken as an indication of depressant activity. Since selective serotonin antagonists (such as methylsergide and PCPA) have been found to selectively increase punished responses in the conflict test, while adrenergic antagonists do not, the authors conclude that the anxiety-reducing properties of the benzo-diazepines are due to serotonin blockade.

Early studies of the brain effects of the benzodiazepines (Schallek & Kuehn, 1965) led investigators to think that limbic system structures were depressed before reticular functions, thus providing the neurological substrate for reduced anxiety while maintaining a state of alertness. More recently, however, neural changes have been identified from the most caudal nuclei of the medulla to the most rostral cortical tissues. The benzodiazepines also have an inhibitory action on spinal reflexes, which may be countered by strychnine. The sensitivity of the reticular formation to chlordiazepoxide is low. However, high doses block EEG arousal produced by electrical stimulation of the brainstem reticular formation. Diencephalic influences of these drugs are mainly inhibitory. The benzo-diazepines have a depressive effect on the areas of the hypothalamus which regulate much of the sympathetic output. The drugs also decrease thalamic firing.

Like meprobamate and the barbiturates, chlordiazepoxide decreases the duration of electrical afterdischarges in the limbic system, including the septal region, the amygdala, and the hippocampus. The drug has also been shown to calm the hyperirritability seen in rats after bilateral septal region lesions. Some scientists believe that the anxiety-reducing effectiveness of the drugs is due to depression in these limbic system structures.

Behavioral effects. Chlordiazepoxide induces a variety of behavioral changes in animals and humans. Some of these can be easily observed, but others require sensitive behavioral measurement techniques to be assessed. Using the checklist designed by Norton (1957) for the monkey, it has been reported that chlordiazepoxide is more effective in reducing aggression than pentobarbital, meprobamate, or chlorpromazine. The behavioral effects were described as "decreasing defensive and aggressive hostility and increasing sociability" (from Norton, 1957, as cited by Ban, 1969, p. 330). It is difficult, however, to compare drugs on these behavioral tasks because the dose ranges are so varied. The benzodiazepines, as we discussed earlier for the propanediols, release behavior that has been suppressed by punishment (Ban, 1969).

An anticonvulsant action is also seen with the benzodiazepine drugs. It is greater than that of meprobamate and, as with the taming effect just discussed, it is produced at a dose below that which produces sedation or motor incoordination. Both chlordiazepoxide and diazepam block convulsions induced by strychnine, pentylenetetrazol, and electroshock. In studies on humans, diazepam was seen to produce drowsiness, slurring of speech, motor incoordina-tion, slowness of thinking, apathy, and impairment of memory functions as doses were increased from 15 mg to 40 mg per day for a month (DiMascio & Barrett, 1965).

Clinical use. Chlordiazepoxide, diazepam, and oxazepam have been used in the treatment of anxiety for their sedating and calming properties for the past two decades. They have also been used in the treatment of alcoholism, and diazepam has been used in certain types of epilepsy. The therapeutic effectiveness of the benzodiazepines in the treatment of neurotic disorders is convincing. The compounds have been used successfully in the treatment of nonspecific anxiety states and of phobic conditions. Ban (1969) lists a total of 31 researchers who have investigated and confirmed the therapeutic effectiveness of chlordiazepoxide and related benzodiazepines.

The use of chlordiazepoxide and diazepam has become popular for alcoholism, particularly for the symptoms of alcoholic withdrawal or the hyperexcitability and combativeness that occur during alcoholic intoxication. The drugs have also been used during postwithdrawal treatment to relieve anxiety and tension. Diazepam is frequently used as an adjunctive agent in the treatment of epileptic patients. Under the influence of diazepam the abnormal EEG is shifted toward the normal and seizure activity is reduced.

Side effects. There are several side effects which may occur with benzodiazepine treatment. Driving an automobile or any task requiring motor coordination and a sustained attention span are not recommended. Behavioral side effects may range from a slight reduction of spontaneous activity to toxic confusional states. The most frequent effects seen are somnolence and sleep disturbances.

A physical dependence develops with chlordiazepoxide as with the depressants (for example, the barbiturates) and meprobamate. In one study (Hollister, Motzenbecker, & Degan, 1961) 10 of 11 patients receiving 300 to 600 mg per day for several months experienced withdrawal symptoms when switched to a placebo. It should be noted, however, that these doses are approximately 10 times the normal therapeutic doses. Symptoms following withdrawal included agitation, insomnia, loss of appetite, and in two patients, convulsions.

Poisoning and successful suicide attempts are rare with these drugs. In a study (Zbinden, Bagdon, Keith, Phillips, & Randall, 1961) reviewing 22 attempts at suicide in patients who ingested from 0.2 to 2.25 g of chlordiazepoxide at one time, all patients were arousable. However, the patients were sedated and drowsy and blood pressure, respiration, and pulse were depressed. Larger doses of the drugs, however, may produce poisoning and death.

SUMMARY AND CONCLUSIONS

It is best to consider the tranquilizers as including two completely separate groups of drugs. The "antischizophrenic" tranquilizers (the phenothiazines, rauwolfia alkaloids and butyrophenones) are most effective in the treatment of the psychotic patient suffering from some form of schizophrenia. There appears to be a very strong predisposing genetic factor in this disease and a biochemical dysfunction seems to be involved; although, there may certainly be an interaction with the patient's experience and environment in determining the particular symptomology. All of the different subcategories of schizophrenia share a common set of symptoms which include deranged thought processes and inappropriate affective responding. Those symptoms, termed *primary* by Bleuler (1950), may represent the basic genetic-biochemical deficiency; whereas the secondary symptoms, which may include the more bizarre behaviors like hallucinations, delusions, and catatonic stupor, may be the result of an interaction between the biochemical dysfunction and the specific environmental stresses with which the patient has difficulty coping. The finding that the manic phase of manic-depressive psychosis is particularly amenable to drug therapy with lithium suggests, perhaps, some anatomical or biochemical distinction between the psychoses. The data point to some biochemical dysfunction of brain amine systems involved in reinforcement/motivational processes as the triggering abnormality (Rado, 1964; also see Chapter 3).

Psychotherapy should not be completely denigrated as a treatment of the psychoses. However, although drug treatments have been shown in carefully controlled studies to produce significant benefits, psychotherapy has not. The remission rate for the psychoses (schizophrenia, mania, and psychotic depression) when treated by psychotherapy has been shown to be no greater than that for untreated cases.

The "depressant tranquilizers," but not the antischizophrenic tranquilizers, seem to have some degree of effectiveness in the treatment of neurotic behaviors, which are primarily characterized by irrational anxiety. The neuroses are also treatable by psychotherapy. Both of these treatments, the depressant tranquilizers and psychotherapy, have been shown in controlled studies to be somewhat effective; some combination of pharmacotherapy and psychotherapy would seem to be the optimum treatment. However, the depressant tranquilizers have not been found to be more effective than treatment simply with a depressant sedative (next chapter). Although the neuroses appear to be experiential or learning disorders, we would not be surprised by the eventual isolation of an organic predisposing factor.

Clearly our present drugs for the treatment of both the psychoses and the neuroses are rather nonselective and provide primarily symptomatic relief. As the genetic and biochemical bases of both the psychoses and neuroses are discovered (and we believe they will be), we are confident that more specific medical "cures" will be developed. Surely, one of the most powerful of these medical treatments will be drugs with selective effects on the causative biochemical lesion.

6

THE DEPRESSANTS

Richard E. Wilcox and Robert A. Levitt

In this chapter we take up several groups of drugs which have in common their ability to depress neural activity. These drugs include the general anesthetics, ethanol (alcohol), the barbiturate sedatives, the nonbarbiturate sedatives, and the anticonvulsant agents.

With respect to depression, we could generate a continuum, starting with mild sedation and continuing through a comatose condition. In sedation the patient exhibits decreased movement and sensory responsiveness, but is awake; in hypnosis the patient is in a drug-induced sleep, but can be aroused; in anesthesia the depression is sufficiently deep to permit surgery without bringing the patient to consciousness; during a coma cardiovascular and respiratory collapse are imminent due to reduced neurological control of the visceral structures.

Theoretically, each class of depressants could be used to generate the stages of depression listed above, if the proper dose and route of administration were employed. Thus, the general anesthetics, ethanol, the barbiturate sedatives, and the nonbarbiturate sedatives may each be used as sedatives, hypnotics, or general anesthetics. As an example of the different levels of depression achievable with these agents, Figure 6.1 compares the sedative, hypnotic, anesthetic, and lethal doses in dogs for three of the barbiturates. Such factors as dose, route of administration, time until onset of the depression, and duration of the depression are important in determining whether mild sedation or deep anesthesia is produced. Continuing this point, the anticonvulsant drugs consist of sedatives which will produce mild daytime sedation at a low dose with a prolonged duration of action. With some of these drugs, sufficient depression is achieved to inhibit convulsive seizures without depressing the patient so much that daytime functioning is greatly impaired.

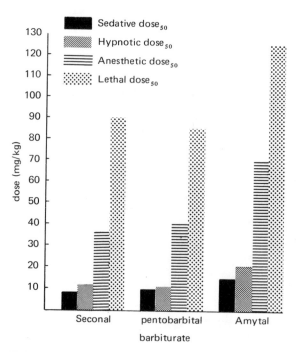

FIGURE 6.1. Activity of three barbiturates in dogs. A comparison of three barbiturates with regard to sedative, hypnotic, anesthetic, and lethal doses. Note that SD_{50} is approximately one fourth of AD_{50}, HD_{50} is about one third of AD_{50}, and AD_{50} is about one half of LD_{50}. (After Chen, 1954.)

All of the depressant drug classes produce at low doses a paradoxical excitatory effect on behavior. This excitatory and euphoric phase is the result of a disinhibition by depressing cortical functions before those of lower brain regions. It is this excitatory euphoric phase at low doses that is responsible for much of the nonclinical (recreational) use of these drugs. As the dose of each of these drugs is increased, the excitement is replaced by a progressively deepening depression of behavior and of neural activity.

The emphasis of this chapter will be somewhat different from that of the three previous chapters (Chapters 3-5). The adrenergic, cholinergic, and tranquilizer drugs have been widely used in basic studies of the mechanisms of brain function and of behavior. The general depressants have, in contrast, been less broadly employed in basic behavioral studies, but have been employed more widely to achieve behaviorally relevant therapeutic goals, and as agents of recreational use. Research with these agents has, therefore, primarily been directed toward furthering our understanding of their therapeutic effectiveness or to studying their nonclinical uses. For this reason the present chapter will concentrate on the physiological actions, therapeutic uses and side effects, and the problems of abuse (tolerance, physical dependence, and withdrawal) that arise with these agents.

GENERAL ANESTHETICS

Absence of sensation (which defines "anesthesia") is produced in addition to sleep and muscular relaxation by drugs such as ether. The term *anesthetic*, as used here, will be restricted to drugs producing a state of unconsciousness sufficiently complete to allow surgery to be performed (Adriani, 1968; Artusio & Puleo, 1963).

Ethanol, opium, and cannabis (hashish and marihuana) were the compounds used in the first attempts at anesthesia because of their shared property of inducing sleep. The safety margin between surgical anesthesia and death, however, is far too narrow to be adequately controlled for any of these drugs.

The introduction of the prototype anesthetic, ether, by William Morton is historically of note; the drama of the occasion qualifies it for repetition here.

Morton entered Harvard Medical School, consulting his chemistry teacher about the problem of anesthesia. He practiced on himself, the family dog, cats, hens and rats, successfully removing a tooth from a human patient under ether in 1846. He asked permission to test ether in an operation, the date set at October 16, 1846.

The operating room (ether dome) at the Massachusetts General Hospital remains as a memorial to this first public demonstration of surgical anesthesia. Skeptical spectators gathered in the gallery, attracted by news that a second-year medical student had developed a means for abolishing surgical pain. The patient was brought in while the surgeon waited in formal clothes (that is, a dress suit, surgical gown and gloves; even the bacterial origins of infection were unknown in that time). Everyone was ready and waiting, even the strong men to hold the patient down, but Morton did not appear. Fifteen minutes passed, and the impatient surgeon addressed the gallery, "As Dr. Morton has not arrived, I presume he is otherwise engaged." The audience smiled, the patient cringed, and the surgeon prepared to make his incision. Morton entered just then, his tardiness due to the necessity for completing an apparatus for ether administration. The surgeon stepped back (it is said) and, pointing to the man strapped to the operating table, said, "Well, sir, your patient is ready." Morton went quietly to work amidst a silent and unsympathetic audience. After a few minutes of ether inhalation, the patient was unconscious, whereupon Morton, looking to the surgeon, retorted, "Dr. Warren, *your* patient is ready!" The operation commenced: the patient, alive and breathing, gave not the slightest evidence of pain. The strong men were not needed. (Modified from Cohen & Dripps, 1970, pp. 43–44)

Stages of Anesthesia

The importance of controlling the depth of anesthesia has led to the adoption of a conventionalized scale for describing the stages of anesthetic action (Table 6.1). The effects involved in the stages of anesthesia define the major pharmacological actions of the depressants. This scale is equally useful in

TABLE 6.1

Stages of Anesthesia

Stage 1—Analgesia
 Plane 1—Normal memory and sensation
 Plane 2—Amnesia and partial analgesia
 Plane 3—Amnesia and analgesia

Stage 2—Excitement
 Begins with delirium, excitement (and possibly euphoria) and ends with loss of eyelid reflex; purposeless movements may occur and hyperreaction to stimuli present; pupils widely dilated; reflex vomiting may occur.

Stage 3—Surgical anesthesia
 Plane 1—Sleep
  Begins with loss of eyelid reflex and ends with eyes in resting position looking straight ahead; reflex swallowing present in light plane and maximum constriction of pupils present in deep plane; patient does not move and appears to be sleeping quietly.
 Plane 2—Sensory loss
  Begins when eyes come to rest and ends with onset of lower intercostal muscle paralysis; pupils begin to dilate and some skeletal muscle relaxation occurs; corneal reflex lost.
 Plane 3—Muscle tone loss
  Begins with onset of lower intercostal muscle paralysis and ends with complete intercostal muscle paralysis; marked skeletal muscle relaxation occurs, including beginning paralysis of diaphragm; pupils widely dilated, pupillary reflex to light lost, and lacrimation stops; laryngeal reflex becomes paralyzed.
 Plane 4—Intercostal paralysis
  Begins with onset of complete intercostal muscle paralysis and ends with complete diaphragmatic paralysis; corneal reflex lost and pupils maximally dilated; circulation depressed but still present.

Stage 4—Medullary paralysis
 Begins with complete respiratory paralysis which leads to complete circulatory failure.

Note. Reprinted by permission from A. Goth, *Medical Pharmacology* (7th ed.). Copyright 1974 by C. V. Mosby. (Also see Artusio, 1954.)

referring to the effects of all the depressant drugs and may serve as a reference for subsequent sections in which the properties of the other depressant drugs are considered.

 The alteration of CNS function by anesthetics follows a pattern characterized as a combination of ascending and descending depression that spares the medulla until large doses are used. This means that depression of the caudal sections of the spinal cord and of the neocortex occurs earliest. As dose is increased the depression spreads upward through the spinal cord and downward through diencephalic and midbrain functions until, eventually, actions on the medulla and the cervical (neck) spinal cord lead to vasomotor collapse and respiratory arrest. The stages of anesthesia are analgesia, excitement, surgical anesthesia, and medullary paralysis. As discussed in detail below, this overall pattern of depression, which applies to all depressant drugs, can be applied to several functions.

Behavior and state of consciousness. In Stage 1 (the analgesic stage) of anesthesia, the patient remains conscious and responsive, but, with depression of the neocortex and the beginnnings of disinhibition of lower telencephalic and diencephalic areas, euphoria and analgesia are experienced. In addition to the euphoria, the patient may experience a dreamlike state with disordered perceptions that are sometimes described as hallucinations. A variable degree of amnesia for the events of this stage occurs.

In Stage 2 (excitement) there is a more marked disinhibition, that is, neocortical influences are almost totally absent. The patient becomes excited, he may struggle and shout in a drunken, delirious manner, and lose consciousness.

Voluntary muscle responses. As the concentration of depressant in the body is increased, contraction of voluntary muscle is weakened and then abolished. The drug acts on the spinal cord and (in the case of the muscles innervated by cranial nerves) on the brainstem. Polysynaptic reflexes and tonic nerve impulse flow to muscle are reduced while monosynaptic reflexes persist. The patterns of respiration and eye movement (extraocular muscle activity) are of importance in describing the progressive depression of anesthesia.

Respiration is not altered during Stage 1 unless the agent used is a respiratory irritant (such as ether). In this case the rate may be increased and some irregularity in pattern may occur. During the stage of excitement there occurs a rapid, irregular, and rapidly changing pattern of respiration due to patient activity and exaggeration of respiratory reflexes. The entry into Stage 3 (surgical anesthesia) is marked by the onset of a regular pattern of respiration. Stage 3 is further divided into four planes.

In Planes 1 and 2, respiration continues to be full and regular (the border between these planes is marked by disappearance of eye movements). As depression deepens, those segments of the thoracic cord innervating the intercostal muscles are affected first. The diaphragm, which is innervated by the phrenic nerve from cervical segments is not paralyzed until later. Plane 3 is characterized by incomplete intercostal paralysis. Plane 4 begins when intercostal paralysis is complete. The purely abdominal (diaphragmatic) breathing is rapid and shallow. Accessory muscles of respiration are used. Because of medullary and cervical cord depression, no respiratory movements occur in Stage 4 (medullary paralysis).

When the extrinsic muscles of the eye are weakened, they no longer act in a coordinated way and the eyes rove (the eyeballs move slowly and not necessarily symmetrically). Movement is marked during Stage 2 and decreases progressively during Plane 1 of Stage 3. In Plane 2 or beyond, both eyes are fixed in the same position, either converging or diverging slightly.

Changes secondary to excitement and asphyxia. During the excitement stage of induction, sympathoadrenal discharge increases and the pupils dilate. Following excitement, and throughout Planes 1 and 2 of surgical anesthesia, the pupils return to their initial size (which may have been influenced by morphine or atropine used as preanesthetic medication). With the appearance of intercostal paralysis, sympathoadrenal stimulation (via carbon dioxide retention) leads once again to pupillary dilation.

During the period of excitement, pulse rate and blood pressure are both elevated just as the pupils are dilated. However, the progressive asphyxia (oxygen lack) accompanying deepening anesthesia leads to depression of medullary vasomotor centers. This results in an increased pulse rate, but also in a declining blood pressure. Respiration ceases before the heart stops and, if the patient can be artificially ventilated for a few breaths (to remove some of the anesthetic), the changes of Stage 4 are reversible.

Theories of Anesthesia

Theories of general anesthesia have been divided into those which account for the depression in terms of a blockade of axonal conduction (Seeman, 1972) and those which account for the phenomenon in terms of a disturbance in the mechanism of synaptic transmission (Nicoll, 1972; Richards, 1972; Streit, Akert, Sandrl, Livingston, & Moor, 1972). The same findings which hold true for anesthetics apply also to the other depressants.

Since general anesthetics block sensation at concentrations which do not block axonal conduction (Somjen, 1967), it is more likely that the depression is occurring at the synaptic site. Many investigations have demonstrated that general anesthetics depress excitatory postsynaptic potentials (EPSPs) (Richards, 1972; Chapter 2, this volume). Other researchers have shown that inhibitory postsynaptic potentials (IPSPs) are preserved under the same conditions (Larson & Major, 1970).

The synaptic mechanisms which have been proposed to account for general anesthesia include: (1) a decrease in the presynaptic release of excitatory transmitter; (2) an increase in the presynaptic release of inhibitory transmitter; (3) a decrease in the postsynaptic receptor sensitivity to excitatory transmitter; and (4) a stabilization of the postsynaptic membrane which inhibits action potential generation. Current evidence suggests that the action of general anesthetics and of the CNS depressants as a group is primarily postsynaptic in nature and involves a selective depression of EPSPs without changing IPSPs (Barker & Gainer, 1973). Briefly, in several crustacean and mollusc preparations of nerve cells, pentobarbital selectively and reversibly depressed both EPSPs and sodium-dependent postsynaptic responses to acetylcholine without affecting either IPSPs or chloride- and potassium-dependent depression of postsynaptic excitatory events. This same effect was also observed with chloroform (a general anesthetic), chloralose and urethane (nonbarbiturate sedative-hypnotic agents), diphenylhydantoin (an anticonvulsant), and ethanol (alcohol) as well as with a barbiturate (pentobarbital).

Metabolism

All drugs, both volatile and nonvolatile, are degraded in some degree by the body. When inhaled, the major portion of the volatile agents (ether, the halogenated hydrocarbons, and the gaseous agents) is eliminated unchanged from the lungs. Nonvolatile drugs (intravenous agents, such as thiopental) are totally or partly metabolized, primarily by the liver. (Adriani, 1962, 1970; Vandam, 1971b).

Following rapid absorption in the lungs, the volatile anesthetics enter the blood in a concentration proportional to that in the air of the lung alveoli. The consequence is that any desired depth of anesthesia may be attained by regulating the proportion of the vapors in the inhaled air. The relatively rich blood supply to the brain (15% of the total cardiac output for only 2% of the body mass) yields an equilibrium with the CNS anesthetic concentration following closely that of arterial blood (Vandam, 1971a). Whereas in acute intoxication with alcohol and the barbiturates artificial respiration does not help speed recovery, with the inhalational agents a substantial portion of the total dose may be removed quickly by this means (Wollman & Dripps, 1970).

Volatile Agents

The compounds within this group are either liquids (ether and the halogenated hydrocarbons) or gases (nitrous oxide, ethylene, and cyclopropane). These agents (when mixed with oxygen and inhaled at room temperature) reach a concentration in the arterial blood, CSF, and brain sufficient to depress the CNS to a level consistent with surgery. These agents are inert within the body (meaning that they are not metabolized; they have biological effects, and are not inert in that sense of the word) and are eliminated unchanged by exhalation.

Liquids. These highly soluble agents are potent in extremely low concentrations. High tissue solubility slows induction of anesthesia and permits a potentially dangerous situation to develop: increased depth of anesthesia over time. This is avoided in practice by initially administering a high concentration and then decreasing the amount of the agent until a safe, adequate level is reached.

The standard agent against which all new anesthetics are compared is ether. It is an irritating liquid which was for over a century the safest and most widely used agent capable of producing Stage 4 anesthesia (a complete anesthetic) (Price & Dripps, 1971b). Practically speaking, this last stage of anesthesia is not used clinically, since it is much too dangerous and because any procedure may be carried out in the third stage.

Ether may be administered by simple techniques, even by inexperienced personnel, making it of great value in primitive or emergency situations. It is safe because its irritant properties maintain (or even stimulate) respiration until the deeper planes of anesthesia; because there is a wide margin between the amount needed for anesthesia and that which results in medullary paralysis; and because it has no special toxic effects on the cardiovascular (or other) systems. Ether produces good muscle relaxation without the use of other drugs (for example, curare; see Chapter 4). Analgesia is so conspicuous that the patient may still be responsive to questions while some operations are performed.

Induction with ether is slow and unpleasant, but the use of other agents (thiopental sodium, a barbiturate) for induction overcomes this disadvantage. However, ether is explosive and recovery following its administration is prolonged. Its extreme gastrointestinal and respiratory irritation (more frequently accompanied by nausea and vomiting than is true for other agents) has resulted in a decline in its popularity.

Like ether, chloroform is analgesic in subanesthetic concentrations, but unlike ether, it produces serious cardiac depression. This halogenated hydrocarbon is more potent than ether and easily administered, but high initial concentrations may cause cardiac arrest by increasing parasympathetic (vagal) tone. This effect is avoided by premedication with a parasympathetic blocking agent (atropine) (see Chapter 4).

Deliberately produced in a search for a potent, nonexplosive anesthetic, halothane is a complete anesthetic and nonirritating, but poorly analgesic and toxic to the liver. It has become the most widely used inhalation agent because it is not explosive and only rarely causes serious adverse reactions. In combination with nitrous oxide (induces analgesia; see "Gases" below) and skeletal muscle relaxants, halothane is the current agent of choice (Deutsch & Vandam, 1971).

Gases. Like the volatile, liquid anesthetics, the anesthetic gases are well characterized by a few key attributes. Therefore, only the prototype agent, nitrous oxide, will be considered here.

Nitrogen narcosis (the "sleep of the deep" which often plagues divers) is related to the narcotic properties of nitrogen at high pressures. The effects in this case and in nitrous oxide anesthesia appear to result from decreased brain oxygen (hypoxia) due to a physical membrane-pore blockade of all cells in the body (Price & Dripps, 1971a). Since all cells depend on the presence of oxygen (which is kept out by the nitrous oxide) for their metabolism and since neural function is especially sensitive to lack of oxygen, it is no wonder that laughing gas (as nitrous oxide was popularly called in the 19th century) is an effective anesthetic. It is not a complete anesthetic, however, but will produce only analgesia and euphoria if administered at atmospheric pressure (hence the term, *laughing gas*). If higher than atmospheric concentrations are given (85% as opposed to 80%) the individual may progress to Stage 2 with a dreamy or fantasy state sometimes described as hallucinatory: giddiness, a pounding or ringing sensation in the head, and altered perceptions become manifest in addition to the analgesia and euphoria (Meyers et al., 1972).

Nitrous oxide is not toxic to any organ system and the adverse reactions which have occurred are due to administering it with inadequate oxygen. Therefore, it is administered under pressure with oxygen to yield a high degree of analgesia. Nitrous oxide's most important uses are as an induction agent and as a supplement to other drugs.

Nonvolatile Agents

These compounds must be sufficiently water soluble to be injected (usually intravenously) because they cannot be administered via the respiratory system. As a class these drugs block the reticular activating system and cause loss of consciousness. The patient responds by movement to painful stimuli, indicating that these drugs are not analgesic in safe dose levels. They must be administered in predetermined doses and, once administered, cannot be retrieved, but are deactivated in the liver and eliminated by the kidneys. This discussion will consider only thiopental, the current agent of choice (Whitehead & Virtue, 1971).

Barbiturates appear to act by depressing the spread of pain impulses to the cortex (Keats & Beecher, 1950). Tissue uptake depends on local blood flow and arterial concentrations of the drug; the brain receives 10% of a total thiopental dose within 40 seconds following intravenous injection (Price, H. L., Kovnak, Safer, Conner, & Price, M. L., 1960). The brain concentration diminishes to 50% of the peak value in 5 minutes and to 10% of the maximum within 30 minutes (consciousness returns) as areas of the body with a relatively poorer blood supply than the brain reach equilibrium.

Summary

What the general anesthetics may lack in obvious structural similarities they make up for by a common mechanism of action. There is no special distinction between general anesthetic agents and the sedative-hypnotics (other than duration of action due to differing routes of administration). As an example, note that thiopental (while normally used as an aid to induction of anesthesia) can by itself produce the full range of CNS depression from sedation through coma. Other barbiturates, such as secobarbital (Seconal), or ethanol (alcohol), if administered under the most carefully controlled conditions, may also yield all the stages of anesthesia discussed above in connection with ether.

A complete anesthetic induces coma, analgesia, and muscle relaxation. The prototype anesthetic, ether, does this by itself. More often the strengths of several agents (such as nitrous oxide and thiopental) are combined in producing balanced anesthesia. The almost immediate onset to action produced by inhalation of "laughing gas" provided the basis for the "instant drunk" which made this substance a popular entertainment device during the last century before its anesthetic effects were discovered. Other volatile anesthetics, such as ether, produce the same effect. This is a euphoric "rush" which parallels closely that produced by insufflating (inhaling or breathing into the nose) cocaine or amphetamine. This fact would make the volatile anesthetics choice agents for nonclinical use were it not for their extreme flammability and difficulty of administration. It is only the convenience in administering and obtaining other depressant drugs (plus the palatability of ethanol-containing beverages) that have made them more widely used to get "high."

ETHANOL

Ethanol (ethyl alcohol, "alcohol") is the most versatile of the depressant pharmacological agents. It is both a depressant and a food; it is a natural metabolite of certain chemical reactions in the body. Ethanol is highly soluble and diffusable in body tissues, thus, it can have an effect on every organ, tissue, and cell of the organism. These characteristics, together with its palatability, have been responsible for the unique and important place held by ethanol in the history of the human race. Most people refer to ethanol simply as alcohol. However, since we will discuss a second alcohol in this chapter (methyl alcohol, methanol), we will use the term *ethanol*.

Prolonged, excessive ethanol intake produces effects which result, somewhat paradoxically, from the beverage's nutritive value. Ethanol is a food and an efficient source of energy, but of little use otherwise. Particularly important is the fact that ethanol can be converted by the body to glucose and is thus a good source of calories, but contains no vitamins. An individual chronically ingesting large volumes of ethanol will have little appetite for other food, but will have ingested no proteins, minerals, or vitamins. Therefore, in chronic alcoholics certain of the toxic symptoms result from these deficiencies, rather than from the effects of the ethanol itself.

Source and Composition

Ethanol is the natural product of the action of yeast on the sugars present in fruits and vegetables. This process is referred to as *fermentation*. Under certain conditions fermentation occurs naturally, without human intervention. Early in the history of the human race, the pleasant effects of ingesting naturally fermented beverages were discovered, and humanity harnessed the fermentation process for its own use (Kissin & Beglister, 1971).

Types of ethanol-containing beverages include the products of fermentation (beer and wine), and distilled spirits (such as whiskey, vodka, gin). All exert their basic primary actions via the actual level of ethanol that they produce in the body (Forney & Harger, 1971). The main factors determining bodily ethanol concentration are the percentage of ethanol in the beverage and the amount of the beverage that is ingested. Beer and wine are fermented beverages containing between about 4% and 12% ethanol. To produce a higher concentration of ethanol the fermented fluid must be distilled. In distillation, the fluid is heated just to the boiling point of ethanol (which is lower than that of water). The ethanol is thus converted to a gas, which is carried by a system of tubes to a vat where it is cooled and converted back into a liquid. With this process, most of the water may be left behind, producing a distilled fluid containing as much as 95% ethanol. In order to produce 100% ethanol many distillations are required, increasing the cost of the process tremendously.

The ethanol content of beverages is usually designated by use of the term *proof*, rather than by percentage. This term *proof* (twice the percentage of ethanol by volume) originated from the Old English custom of testing the ethanol content of whiskey by moistening gun powder with the beverage and applying a flame to the mixture. Ignition resulted (with a presumed "poof!") when the combination contained slightly over 57% ethanol by volume (Ritchie, 1970a). Bonded straight bourbon and rye whiskies in the United States are 100-proof, while blended bourbon, rye, Scotch and Irish whiskies, and most gin and vodka are bottled at 80-, 86-, or 86.8-proof. The highest ethanol concentrations are found in the rums of Brazil, Jamaica, Puerto Rico, and British Guiana at 151-proof.

Metabolism

Because ethanol is a small, neutral, water-soluble molecule, it requires neither dissolution nor digestion, but is ready for absorption (by simple diffusion from the gastrointestinal tract) the moment it is ingested. Because the final distribution of the drug follows closely the water content of each tissue, the greatest concentration will remain in the blood so that it is the blood ethanol (also termed *blood alcohol*) level which provides the clearest indication of the total amount of ethanol in the body. Milk and other high protein foods, large fluid volumes, and nonethanolic components of ethanol-containing beverages may retard intestinal absorption enough so that a 6-hour period may be required for complete removal of the ethanol from the gastrointestinal tract (Forney & Harger, 1971; Ritchie, 1970a). Ethanol stimulates gastrointestinal activity, which helps to explain the gastric irritation induced by chronic consumption. The same fact may also indicate why individuals in some cultures may consume a glass or two of wine with meals throughout their lives and find that the ethanol benefits digestion.

Areas of the body which are highly vascularized, such as the brain, receive the largest initial ethanol concentration. The ethanol becomes partitioned more equitably as less vascular body areas, such as skeletal muscles, absorb the drug. This may explain the anecdotal observation of a person who becomes intoxicated on a single drink (by consuming a beer or martini at a gulp on an empty stomach, for example) and then sobers up quite suddenly an hour later (Muehlberger, 1958).

Almost 98% of the ethanol which enters the body is completely oxidized to carbon dioxide and water as a direct function of time. Since the liver is the chief site of ethanol breakdown, the amount of ethanol degraded per unit time is directly proportional to liver weight; that is, the rate of metabolism of ethanol is constant over time. In individuals with healthy livers, the rate of ethanol breakdown is proportional to lean (not fat) body weight. The heavier the individual's lean weight the greater the amount of ethanol which can be broken down per hour. An adult male of 150 lb would require 6 hours to metabolize 4 oz of whiskey or 1.25 quarts of beer, if his liver is intact. Any damage to this organ results in a much reduced capacity for drinking.

As the liver store of ethanol decreases, it is replaced by ethanol from the rest of the body. This yields a constant ratio of stored ethanol in the various tissues during the entire course of metabolism. Women tend to have more adipose tissue than men and, so, less lean body weight in which to store ethanol. Thus, following consumption of equal amounts of ethanol, a woman would have a higher blood level of the drug than would a man of equal weight. Also, when the blood ethanol level is increasing, it indicates that the metabolic capacity of the liver is being overwhelmed, forcing more and more of the drug to be partitioned within other systems of the body. When the blood ethanol level is declining, the capacity of the liver for metabolizing ethanol is not being exceeded. Thus, equal blood levels do not tell the entire story. Depending upon whether the level is rising or falling, quite different information is being provided about the body's metabolic capacity for the drug. An individual with a rising blood ethanol level is actually more "drunk" than he is later with a falling blood level of the ethanol, although the absolute levels are the same since more ethanol is contained in the body tissue in the first case.

There are three stages of ethanol metabolism (see Figure 6.2). They include: oxidation to acetaldehyde, the slowest (rate limiting) step in the elimination process; oxidation of acetaldehyde to acetic acid (normally an extremely rapid step); and then of the acetic acid to carbon dioxide and water (Jacobsen, 1952; Westerfeld, 1961). The rapid conversion of acetaldehyde to acetic acid is inhibited by disulfiram, which is an agent used to treat alcoholism. (See the section entitled "Disulfiram" later in this chapter.)

Effects on Organ Systems

An ounce or two of whiskey produces transient increases in blood pressure, pulse rate, and cardiac output. These effects may underlie the folk remedy of administering ethanol in the treatment of fainting. The peripheral blood vessel dilation (vasodilation) produced by the drug explains the flushed complexion and sensation of warmth experienced following the ingestion of moderate amounts. This vasodilation appears due to the action of acetaldehyde (Meyers, Jawetz, & Goldfien, 1972). Ethanol, which does *not* dilate the coronary arteries, has sometimes been prescribed in the treatment of cardiac pain due to coronary artery damage (angina pectoris) because of the mistaken belief that it does dilate the coronary arteries. Clinical trials with whiskey have shown that the relief of pain is due to the central effects of the ethanol, rather than to direct actions on the heart (Russek, Naegele, & Ragan, 1950). The increased urine output (diuresis) seen following the ingestion of ethanol-containing beverages is the result of a direct action to inhibit antidiuretic hormone release from the posterior pituitary gland (see Chapter 11).

In addition to the net water loss following ethanol ingestion, there is an increased excretion of catecholamines which appears due to the action of

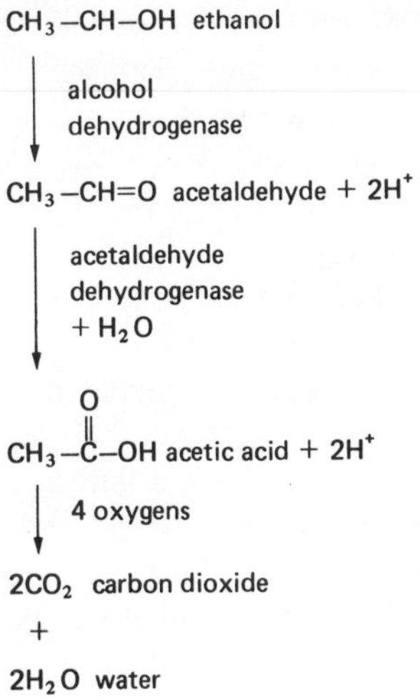

$CH_3-CH-OH$ ethanol

$\downarrow$ alcohol
dehydrogenase

$CH_3-CH=O$ acetaldehyde $+ 2H^+$

$\downarrow$ acetaldehyde
dehydrogenase
$+ H_2O$

$CH_3-\overset{\overset{O}{\|}}{C}-OH$ acetic acid $+ 2H^+$

$\downarrow$ 4 oxygens

$2CO_2$ carbon dioxide
$+$
$2H_2O$ water

FIGURE 6.2. The metabolism of ethanol.

ethanol's active metabolite, acetaldehyde. This increased CA release results in high blood levels of these compounds in response to ethanol, which is a similar situation to that seen following the activation of the sympathetic nervous system by stress. The dilated pupils, increased blood pressure, and increased blood sugar, which accompany the early stages of inebriation, result from this indirect sympathetic activation. In the later stages of intoxication, when the circulating epinephrine and norepinephrine have been excreted, the direct depressant effects of ethanol (lowered blood sugar and blood pressure) become apparent (Meyers et al., 1972).

The notion that ethanol has aphrodisiac properties is untrue. In their book *Human Sexual Response* (1966, p. 67), Masters and Johnson have this to say: "The syndrome of overindulgence has particular application to alcohol. While under its influence, many a male of any age has failed for the first time to achieve or maintain an erection. . . . Secondary impotence . . . has a higher incidence of direct association with excessive alcohol consumption than with any other single factor." That the effects of ethanol on sexual behavior are due to a loss of inhibition and not to increased coital capacity has been ably phrased in Macbeth (Act 2, Scene 3):

> *MacDuff*: What things does drink especially provoke?
> *Porter*: Lechery, sir, it provokes, and unprovokes; it provokes the desire, but takes away the performance.

Behavioral Effects

Ethanol acts as a stimulant only by releasing neocortical inhibitions on impulsive behavior. At all levels of the CNS, the principal pharmacologic action of ethanol is depression. Like the general anesthetics, ethanol is especially effective in depressing the reticular formation of the brainstem (Gray, 1971; Guyton, 1971). Mardones (1963) cites a classic report on the effects of graded doses of ethanol on performance. For simple tests of reaction time, dyna-mometer grip strength, reading, and memorizing, an initial improvement was observed (due, perhaps, to lowered distractibility) followed by performance decrements as dose was increased. Scores on tests of association, arithmetic calculation, and time estimation deteriorated at all dose levels used. The relation between concentration of ethanol in the blood and behavioral effect varies across individuals with such variables as tolerance, practice effects, and social pressures complicating the picture.

Impaired performance in real or simulated driving provides an index of drunkenness acceptable to the majority of researchers studying the effects of ethanol. A level of 100 mg ethanol per 100 ml blood which can be produced by consuming four whiskies in an hour is the basis for the legal definition of drunken driving in most states (Ray, 1972). Note that the level of drug referred to is 0.10% and not 100% (which is roughly 170 times a lethal dose; see Figure 6.3, which is from the April 22, 1974 issue of Time Magazine).

It is generally believed that memory for events occurring during ethanol ingestion is poor several hours later. It seems likely that this is true and one explanation may be the phenomenon of state-dependent learning (see Chapter 10). If true, then there is some probability that the memory could be recovered at a later time if additional ethanol were ingested. Rather weak dissociative effects have indeed been observed in several experiments which have utilized ethanol to produce a drug state in human subjects (Goodwin et al., 1969; Storm, Caird, & Korbin, 1967). In fact, of the drugs which acquire response control (state dependency) most rapidly, the depressants (including pentobarbital, phenobarbital, secobarbital, amobarbital, chloral hydrate, ethanol, and ether) are the most efficient (Overton, 1971).

Tolerance

Two kinds of tolerance following chronic alcohol consumption have been postulated: lowered blood alcohol levels at equal doses (metabolic tolerance); and decreased behavioral decrement at equal blood alcohol levels (tissue tolerance) (Mardones, 1963). For example, ethanol consumption initially increases electroshock seizure threshold in animals while suppressing the rapid eye movement (REM) phase of sleep in humans. Both return to normal levels with chronic consumption (Ban, 1969; Feinberg, 1969). This indicates that the body is able to adapt to a continual depression of neural activity by setting the baseline higher than normal. The higher baseline minus the depression due to the ethanol equals a level of activity nearly equal to that which preceded the period of ethanol administration.

Human subjects receiving constant daily doses of ethanol showed a continual decline in blood levels until a near zero level was reached on the tenth day of consumption (Ban, 1969). Thus, for a constant amount of ethanol entering the body, each day successively smaller portions of the total dose were partitioned to the blood (where the ethanol "awaited" its turn to be broken down by the

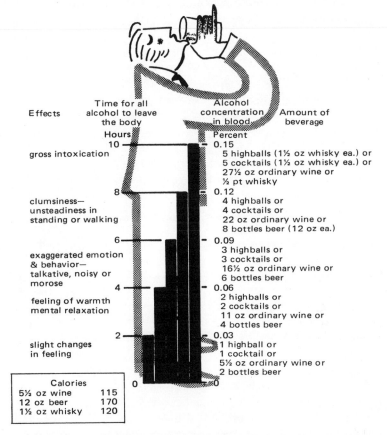

Effects	Time for all alcohol to leave the body Hours	Alcohol concentration in blood Percent	Amount of beverage
gross intoxication	10	0.15	5 highballs (1½ oz whisky ea.) or 5 cocktails (1½ oz whisky ea.) or 27½ oz ordinary wine or ½ pt whisky
clumsiness— unsteadiness in standing or walking	8	0.12	4 highballs or 4 cocktails or 22 oz ordinary wine or 8 bottles beer (12 oz ea.)
	6	0.09	3 highballs or 3 cocktails or 16½ oz ordinary wine or 6 bottles beer
exaggerated emotion & behavior— talkative, noisy or morose	4	0.06	2 highballs or 2 cocktails or 11 oz ordinary wine or 4 bottles beer
feeling of warmth mental relaxation			
slight changes in feeling	2	0.03	1 highball or 1 cocktail or 5½ oz ordinary wine or 2 bottles beer
	0	0	

Calories	
5½ oz wine	115
12 oz beer	170
1½ oz whisky	120

FIGURE 6.3. Alcohol levels in the blood—after drinks taken on an empty stomach by a 150-lb person. (Reprinted by permission from *Alcoholism, Time, The Weekly Newsmagazine*, April 22, 1974. Copyright 1974 by Time Inc.)

liver). This is because the liver became progressively more efficient in metabolizing the ethanol. Clearly, there is occurring here a process of compensation in the homeostatic mechanisms of these subjects. The "return to" equilibrium conditions now, however, does not indicate "normality." Ethanol ingestion is now as necessary for "normal" function as are protein, minerals, or vitamins. When the drug is withdrawn, the nervous system rebounds to a new, higher set point since the depressing effect of the ethanol is no longer present. REM levels, for example, show rather dramatic increases. This is important since REM periods are associated with dream activity. Alcoholics, and also barbiturate addicts, experience intense nightmares and hallucinations during drug withdrawal. These phenomena may be related to the intense REM activity and may function to drive the patient back to ethanol or barbiturates to relieve either the nightmares or the hallucinations or both.

Acute Intoxication

The signs of ethanol intoxication are so well known that an erroneous diagnosis of drunkenness is often made in patients who are suffering instead from the effects of barbiturates, paraldehyde (a nonbarbiturate sedative), stroke, fractured skull, or even schizophrenia. Breath odor is a notoriously unreliable guide.

The more rapid the consumption, the higher the peak blood ethanol concentration. Coma can be induced with ethanol by gulping a pint of 100-proof whiskey, while death could be induced by gulping two pints. Most acute ethanol deaths are due to the ingestion of a large additional amount of drug by a person who is already drunk (Forney & Harger, 1971).

As a sequel to ethanol ingestion the hangover is a common occurrence, more so than occurs after the use of short-acting sedative-hypnotic agents for two reasons. Firstly, ethanol is a slowly metabolized substance. Secondly, more doses of ethanol are ordinarily consumed than is the case with other depressant agents. Hangover is a state of drug withdrawal less completely developed than that seen with severe, chronic abuse. The symptoms of hangover include tremors fatigue, vertigo, throbbing headache, changing blood pressure, nausea and vomiting, acid blood pH (acidosis), and dehydration with persistent thirst (Meyers et al., 1972).

Treatment most logically begins during the period of ingestion (with restraint) but additional prophylactic measures may be carried out before retiring. Vomiting (emesis) may be induced with little difficulty to remove some of the absorbed alcohol. Fluids for dehydration, aspirin for headache, and sodium bicarbonate for the acidosis may also be administered.

Ethanol-associated Disturbances

The toxicity which develops following chronic ethanol abuse is due to two causes. First, there occurs in many alcoholics a nutritional deficit associated with the empty (that is, containing no protein, vitamins, or minerals) calories provided by alcoholic beverages. The chronic gastric irritation due to continued ethanol ingestion impairs the absorption of many nutrients (especially fats), adding further to the problem.

Second, no matter what the nutritional status of the individual, chronic ingestion of large amounts of ethanol exerts a direct toxic action on the body. The disease states which occur as a result of ethanol ingestion may loosely be divided into non-CNS and CNS disturbances. The non-CNS disturbances include: anemia, resulting from a deficiency of iron and certain B-complex vitamins (folic acid and cyanobalamin); pellagra, characterized by extensive dermatitis and inflammation of mucous membranes (due to deficiency of another B-complex vitamin, niacin); cardiac beriberi, heart failure from prolonged high output due to thiamine (another B-vitamin) deficiency; and cirrhosis of the liver. The CNS disturbances include: withdrawal (delirium tremens, DTs), dry beriberi, Wernicke's syndrome and Korsakoff's psychosis (Dreyfus, 1971).

Non-CNS disturbances. Only liver cirrhosis will be considered here. For a discussion of the other non-CNS disturbances the reader is referred to Dreyfus (1971). Liver cirrhosis is a disease characterized by inflammation and hardening of the liver tissue. There is some controversy as to whether this disorder is due solely to multiple nutritional deficits (protein, minerals, and vitamins) or whether there is some direct effect of ethanol (Dreyfus, 1971; Meyers et al., 1972). The weight of the evidence suggests that, while a nutritional deficit may complicate the picture by impairing the actions of a damaged liver, a direct toxic action of the ethanol may play the chief part.

Chronic alcoholics develop three major types of liver disease: fatty liver, alcoholic hepatitis, and cirrhosis (Gall & Mostof, 1973). While fatty liver is reversible when the ethanol is discontinued, alcoholic hepatitis (which may be the link between fatty liver and cirrhosis) appears not to be easily reversed. Inflammation and death of liver tissue are among the characteristic histologic features of the disorder. Both fatty liver and alcoholic hepatitis have been produced in baboons apparently as a direct result of ethanol toxicity. The diets of these animals contained excess proteins, vitamins, and minerals and pair-fed controls receiving the same diet with isocaloric substitution of sucrose for ethanol showed no degenerative changes upon microscopic examination of liver biopsy specimens. In contrast, the ethanol-fed animals showed marked changes (Rubin & Lieber, 1973). Since the weight of the animals at the time of sacrifice was not reported, it is possible that poor absorption of certain nutrients due to gastric irritation in the ethanol group may have been a factor. We shall see, however (below, "CNS disturbances"), that this appears not to be an important effect.

CNS disturbances. The various syndromes associated with CNS dysfunction due to ethanol are not separate entities. In an individual classified as having Korsakoff's syndrome, for example, some of the signs of Wernicke's disease will probably be present also. The disturbances discussed in this section all have the same basic etiology: ethanol.

Because of its rich vascularization, high degree of irritability, and a limited storage capacity for nutrients, CNS tissue is especially sensitive to complications subsequent to chronic ethanol intake. Brain damage and associated mental deterioration have been reported in alcoholic patients with no clinical history of malnutrition (Haug, 1968; Tumarkin, Wilson & Snyder, 1955). Thus, it is likely that ethanol exerts toxic effects on CNS function and learning despite adequate nutrition.

Animal behavior: Recent investigations using laboratory animals have supported this conclusion. By incorporating ethanol into liquid diets, it has been shown that mice (Freund, 1969; Walker & Zornetzer, in press) or rats (Hunter, Boast, Walker, & Zornetzer, in press) will consume substantial quantities of ethanol and subsequently develop withdrawal symptoms. The use of liquid diets as the sole source of calories and fluid provides for precise nutritional control. The calories provided by ethanol can be replaced in control diets by isocaloric quantities of sucrose. Further supplemental nutrients can be added to insure an excess of vitamins and minerals.

Using this technique, it has been shown that mice (Freund, 1970; Freund & Walker, 1971) or rats (Walker & Freund, 1971) consuming liquid diets for 3 to 7 months show impairment in shock avoidance learning when tested 2 to 18 weeks after ethanol was omitted from the diet. Further, rats tested for the acquisition of a differentially reinforced low response rate (DRL) following a period of prolonged consumption showed a similar deficit in acquisition (Freund, 1973; Walker & Freund, 1973). When compared with shock avoidance, the DRL is food-motivated rather than shock-motivated, requires response suppression rather than rapid response initiation, and acquisition is not contingent upon sensory processing of external stimuli. Thus, these are two quite distinct behavioral tasks. Since the animals in these studies showed an average weight gain, apparently their absorption of nutrients was adequate. These results suggest that prolonged ethanol consumption, despite adequate nutrition, results in impairment of the associative processes of learning.

Delirium tremens (DTs): In both alcoholic and nonalcoholic individuals an immediate sequel to about 2 weeks of excessive drinking is the delirium tremens which occur when the depressant effects of the ethanol are wearing off. Restlessness, tremor, copious sweating, insomnia, and headache present themselves as the initial part of the withdrawal syndrome. A second stage then ensues in which nightmares, hallucinations, delirium, and convulsions (in any combination) predominate. The agitated, muttering, anxious patient is constantly in motion: picking at his bedclothes (to remove fancied insects, snakes, or rodents); wandering around; or screaming. People, objects, even the date and time are unknown. The entire scope of the person's comprehension centers around the illusory, scurrying roaches and rats covering his body; around the all too real drenching sweat; high fever; and trip-hammering heart. After 3 to 5 days of this suffering, the patient falls into a sudden sleep, to awaken many hours later, DTs gone and amnesic for the entire episode (modified from Isbell, 1971).

The signs associated with withdrawal from ethanol are the opposite of those noted with drug administration: excitement versus depression. The reason may be due to a "tolerance" of the CNS to ethanol's depressant effects. The homeostatic reaction to the presence of ethanol within neural tissue over a prolonged period of time includes a shift in the set-point for baseline neural activity to a new, higher level. Since the presence of ethanol decreases neural activity, the shift in set-point would maintain the same relative equilibrium conditions in the presence of drug as in the predrug condition. If the ethanol is withdrawn suddenly, the set-point cannot be immediately lowered. The baseline of neural activity without drug is now much higher because the set-point is still high. This heightened CNS excitability without drug may correspond to the withdrawal syndrome (hallucinations, tremors, convulsions, etc.). The idea of an altered neural set-point may serve as a useful model upon which to hang many of the facts associated with depression, cross-tolerance, withdrawal, and so on, for any depressant drug.

Treatment of the DTs consists of fluids, salt (and other electrolytes), and vitamins. Carbohydrate solutions (dextrose in water) are often given but may actually precipitate or exaggerate the DTs if given without vitamins (since the metabolism of carbohydrates increases the demand for B vitamins). As is true for a hangover, the quickest way to terminate DTs is by administering ethanol. More commonly, long-acting sedative-hypnotic agents are administered (Meyers et al., 1972). Especially effective is the barbiturate hypnotic, phenobarbital, which illustrates the effect of *cross-tolerance*, which means that tolerance to one such depressant transfers to the other via mechanisms of action within the body which are similar enough to permit the transfer of effect (Forney & Hughs, 1968).

We have noted that at least some of the toxic effects of ethanol appear secondary to a nutritional deficit, especially of the water-soluble vitamins which cannot be stored in the body for any length of time. It is possible that a supplementation of alcoholic beverages with these (and other nutrients) would at least forestall some of the toxic consequences associated with chronic, heavy ethanol use.

Dry beriberi: Characterized by progressive muscle weakness and atrophy, dry beriberi (nutritional or alcoholic polyneuropathy) is the most common nutritional disease of the peripheral nervous system. An exaggeration followed by an abolition of the deep (tendon) reflexes suggests a progressive demyelination of peripheral nerves. Signs of irritation of ascending (sensory) and descending (motor) paths are also found (Grinker & Saks, 1966). Note that the term *dry beriberi* is usually used to refer to the peripheral nervous system consequences of B vitamin deficiencies in alcoholics, while cerebral beriberi refers to the brain disorders in these cases.

Cerebral beriberi—Korsakoff's and Wernicke's: Like dry beriberi, cerebral beriberi (which includes both Korsakoff's psychosis and Wernicke's disease) is a clinical syndrome associated with shortage of the water-soluble vitamins (especially thiamine). Either Korsakoff's psychosis, Wernicke's disease or both may constitute a third, more permanent stage of the ethanol withdrawal syndrome. Confusion, disorientation, and amnesia characterize the Korsakoff syndrome which is reminiscent of the cortical symptoms of DTs. The gradual loss of memory in chronic alcoholics can be permanent if the disease has progressed sufficiently; it appears to first involve more recent memories and may gradually progress further back in time. The Korsakoff syndrome proper is distinguished from simple withdrawal by the duration and intensity of symptoms which leads to another manifest feature of the psychosis: the tendency to fill in the memory gaps by supplying imaginary answers to questions (confabulation). Confabulation should not be considered a qualitatively distinct entity. It is a natural result of the individual's efforts to maintain his own esteem in the face of frightening amounts of confusion and memory loss (Merritt, 1967).

Wernicke's disease is manifested by a paralysis of sudden onset involving eye movements, by an inability to maintain balance when walking (ataxia), and by disturbances of consciousness (amnesia, disorientation with respect to time and place). Once again, this disorder, like dry beriberi and Korsakoff's syndrome, may be produced in complete abstainers who have the appropriate nutritional deficit. "Beriberi" is merely a generic term for a symptom pattern endemic to the orient, produced by a diet deficient in the B vitamins (for example, consisting primarily of polished rice). However, the direct toxic effects of ethanol almost certainly add further stress to an already damaged nervous system, just as was noted in the case of liver cirrhosis.

The pathology seen in the Wernicke-Korsakoff syndrome is quite constant. Lesions are found in the mammillary bodies, both fornices, near the third ventricle, and in the midbrain around the aqueduct of Sylvius. Thiamine administration can sometimes reverse many of the symptoms within a matter of hours (Merritt, 1967).

Probably the best way to conceptualize the CNS disorders in alcoholics is as a vitamin deficiency disease, complicated by the direct toxicity of ethanol. The term cerebral beriberi is used to characterize the entire disorder, while Wernicke's disease refers to the neurological consequences and Korsakoff's psychosis to the disorders of behavior and thought processes. The only reason for the use of three different terms is historical. They no longer seem necessary, but you should be aware of them since they are all still used.

Summary

Ethanol is completely miscible (soluble) in water; it is palatable in most common forms; it has caloric value. Nevertheless, ethanol is a typical short-acting central depressant. Its widespread use and availability make it reasonable to consider ethanol as the prototype depressant. Like the other agents considered in this chapter, ethanol has both central and general depressant actions (the central actions manifest themselves at lower dosages). Ethanol can be used as a general anesthetic capable of producing all four stages of anesthetic depression (although the safety margin between coma and death is very narrow). Because of the tendency for depressants to first inhibit polysynaptic and phylogenetically new pathways (such as neocortex) before other areas are affected, the individual inebriated with ethanol may initially be excited (Stage 2 anesthesia). This is a natural consequence of depressant action as higher brain areas are depressed and lower ones released from inhibitory control and, as we shall see, is a characteristic of all CNS depressants.

Disulfiram

Williams, in 1937, noted that workers exposed to tetramethylthiuram disulfide developed a hypersensitive reaction to ethanol. His suggestion that the drug be used in the treatment of alcoholism went unheeded. The ethyl analogue, disulfiram (tetraethylthiuram disulfide, Antabuse), had been used for some time in the rubber industry as a protection against oxidation. An ethanol hypersensitivity also occurred in workers exposed to disulfiram, but no published report appeared until two Danish physicians, who had themselves taken disulfiram in the course of research on its potential anthelmintic (an agent used to expel intestinal worms) usefulness, became ill at a cocktail party (Ritchie, 1970a).

The patient must agree to accept the drug daily with the understanding that ethanol ingestion will lead to a most unpleasant experience. At least 12 hours are required for the disulfiram effect to develop. The patient cannot ingest ethanol for 3 to 10 days after discontinuing the medication. After several days of drug administration (at first, 0.5 g, and later 0.25 g) a test dose of ethanol (1/2 oz of whiskey followed 30 minutes later, if necessary, by another 1/2 oz) will produce an unpleasant reaction within 20 minutes of ethanol administration. The reaction will then last up to 2 hours. The signs are hot, flushed face, then throbbing headache, respiratory difficulty, nausea, vomiting, profuse sweating, chest pain, blurred vision, dizziness, and weakness. The initial flush is replaced by pallor as the blood pressure falls, in some cases, all the way to levels found in shock (Ritchie, 1970a). Occasionally, the reaction has culminated in death (Kissin & Beglister, 1971). Even inhaled aftershave lotion (containing low levels of ethanol) has caused mild reactions (Meyers et al., 1972).

No obvious effects appear to be produced by the disulfiram itself. Instead, at least part of the effect is caused by the disulfiram preventing the conversion of acetaldehyde (ethanol's active metabolite) to acetic acid (in the breakdown of ethanol). When acetaldehyde is administered intravenously to human subjects not pretreated with disulfiram, several of the reactions noted above are induced.

We have noted earlier (Chapter 2) that the enzyme which catalyzes the conversion of dopamine to norepinephrine (dopamine-β-hydroxylase) contains copper ions. Disulfiram is one compound which is capable of binding to copper and so may inhibit the activity of the enzyme (Cooper et al., 1974). Since a defect in dopamine-β-hydroxylase (with concomitant oxidation of dopamine to 6-hydroxydopamine) is the basis for the Stein and Wise theory of schizophrenia (Chapter 3), it is at least possible that prolonged disulfiram treatment of chronic alcoholics might engender schizophrenic symptoms.

Methanol

This agent (wood alcohol, methyl alcohol, CH_3OH) is commonly encountered in duplicating machine fluid, in canned heat (Sterno), and as an industrial solvent. Methanol is often ingested mistakenly (or perhaps in desperation) by individuals desiring ethanol. For example, "squeeze" is Sterno placed inside a sock which is then wrung (squeezed) into a container. The liquid methanol so obtained is much more potent (and deadly) per volume than is ethanol since it is nearly pure methanol. All alcohols are capable of producing anesthesia and all are toxic. The toxicity generally increases with increasing molecular weight of the compound. The one exception to this linear trend is ethanol, which is less toxic than other members of the family.

Methanol is no different in regard to its depressant actions, but possesses additional toxic effects. The lethal dose of methanol is only 2 to 8 oz (Meyers et al., 1972). One cause of this low lethal dose is that methanol is metabolized to formic acid (a highly toxic derivative of the formaldehyde used in embalming).

While less active than ethanol as a central depressant, methanol produces a much more severe acidosis. Either the acidosis or the formic acid is the cause of the blindness (from optic nerve destruction) which frequently follows methanol ingestion. Following methanol ingestion the individual becomes intoxicated, as with ethanol. Between 6 and 36 hours later the headache, dizziness, nausea, acidosis, excitement, blindness, and coma or death appear. If the patient recovers at all, impaired vision is usually the minimal result (Cooper & Kini, 1962).

Treatment consists of combating the acidosis and retarding the production of formic acid. The former is accomplished via large amounts of sodium bicarbonate, the latter by administering ethanol. The reason is that simultaneously given alcohols compete with each other for the person's limited capability to metabolize alcohols. Because ethanol is metabolized preferentially over methanol, the conversion to formic acid is delayed. The ethanol should be given every 2 hours for about 4 days in order to be effective (Meyers et al., 1972).

THE BARBITURATES

Because of the development of the tranquilizers and antischizophrenic agents, this family of chemicals is currently used almost exclusively in the treatment of sleep disorders. The main therapeutic uses of the barbiturates are in the treatment of insomnia, anxiety, and epilepsy, and as short-acting anesthetics or as adjuncts to anesthesia (Sharpless, 1970a). The properties of this class of compounds are so similar that a discussion of a few prototypes covers the entire group. Indeed, of the 2,500 barbiturates which have been synthesized and the 50 agents marketed, about half a dozen compounds suffice for clinical needs. The choice among them is dependent on their onset and duration of action (Table 6.2; Sharpless, 1970a; Maynert, 1971b).

Neurologically equivalent doses of two drugs produce the same effects on neural tissue, such as equal amounts of EEG activation. Based on the duration of action of two such neurologically equal doses, the barbiturates are usually divided into long-acting (1 hour to onset, 6-to-10-hour duration; barbital and phenobarbital), intermediate-acting (1/2 hour to onset, 5-to-6-hour duration; butabarbital and amobarbital), short-acting (15 minutes to onset, 2-to-3-hour duration; pentobarbital and secobarbital), and ultra short-acting (when injected intravenously a 30-second latency to onset of anesthesia is common with a duration of anesthesia of 30 minutes; thiopental and hexobarbital).

TABLE 6.2
Selected Information on Some Common Barbiturates

Duration of action	Generic name	Trade name	Dose (oral) Sedative	Hypnotic	Selected chemical formulas*
Ultra-short acting	Thiopental	Pentothal	Used only as an anesthetic (intravenously)		(top structure)
Short-to-intermediate acting	Amobarbital Pentobarbital Secobarbital	Amytal Nembutal Seconal	.03 g Not used .05	.20 g .10 .20	(middle structure)
Long-acting	Phenobarbital Barbital	Luminal Veronal	.03 .05	.10 .30	(bottom structure)

*(Top) thiopental; (middle) pentobarbital; (bottom) phentobarbital.

Increasing the dose increases the duration of action. This is the case because the ability of the liver to metabolize the barbiturates is constant over time. This effect was already noted with the general anesthetics and with ethanol, and is the case for all depressants. In the usually recommended doses, phenobarbital is less effective in inducing sleep than is pentobarbital and the phenobarbital effect lasts no longer (Lasagna, 1956), because a much smaller dose of phenobarbital is usually prescribed than is the case for pentobarbital. Thus, the two drugs are normally not administered in equivalent doses.

Metabolism

Following absorption, the barbiturates are found in all tissues and fluids. The chief factors affecting barbiturate distribution and fate are lipid solubility and the ability to bind to plasma protein (Sharpless, 1970a). Thus, the more rapidly acting agents are highly lipid soluble and bind poorly (and so are rapidly degraded). Barbiturate depression is ended by physical redistribution, metabolic breakdown, and kidney excretion. All three methods reduce plasma concentrations of the drug. The reduced plasma concentration leads to a decreased concentration in cerebrospinal fluid and, in turn, in CNS sites of action.

Lipid solubility is the factor primarily determining which of the above methods is used in ending the CNS action. Long-acting agents are excreted in a largely unmetabolized form (65 % to 90% of a barbital dose) (Maynert, 1971b). In the case of an ultra-short-acting agent (such as thiopental used as an adjunct to anesthesia) a physical redistribution of the drug from brain to muscle occurs within 1/2 hour following injection. Even though the patient is likely to awaken at this time, the thiopental is still in his body. In fact only 0.3% of a dose goes unmetabolized with breakdown occurring at a rate of 10% to 15% per hour (Meyers et al., 1972). This slow breakdown explains the hangover characteristically experienced as an aftereffect of drug administration (Brodie, Mark, Popper, Lief, Bernstein & Rovenstein, 1950). Just as with ethanol, the barbiturates stimulate within the liver the mechanisms responsible for physical tolerance, the production of enzymes speeding up their metabolism (the process is called *enzyme induction*; Conney, 1967).

Mechanism and Sites of Action

The ascending reticular activating system, cerebral cortex, and limbic system are more sensitive than the rest of the nervous system to the barbiturates, as with all depressants. In clinical doses, it is the central depressant actions and not the general ones which are noted. The general depressant actions on peripheral nerves, on muscles, and on cell respiration do become manifest, however, in acute barbiturate poisoning.

Areas in the forebrain and brainstem, which appear to be significantly involved in the mediation of sleep, are depressed by the barbiturates. This neural depression is not, however, a requirement for behavioral depression. For example, the inhibitory areas of the medulla and basal ganglia appear to increase their overall firing in response to barbiturates. Thus, the behavioral effects seen following depressant administration are due to a new balance being established in the total firing pattern of the brain, not a decreased overall activity. Indeed, the brain in general seems to be quite active during times of behavioral quiescence whether artificially induced (via general anesthetics) or in sleep. There is no logical requirement that behavioral depressant drugs should depress all neural activity or that behavioral stimulants should increase it.

In fact, with depressants at least, it appears that they act by selectively inhibiting EPSPs and leaving IPSPs unaffected. This was noted earlier in the discussion of the general anesthetic agents. In the study cited, pentobarbital was one of the drugs which produced the EPSP decrement. It was noted also in that context that the so-called paradoxical excitation produced by depressant drugs is merely the result of a disinhibition of lower telencephalic and diencephalic areas of the brain from normal control, as the neocortex becomes depressed.

Chronic barbiturate intake results in smaller behavioral effects (tolerance, as with ethanol) and some return toward the original baseline of electrical activity. Increasing the dose to double or triple the clinically effective one at this time results in behavioral excitement (Stage 2 anesthesia; excitement phase). Once again, the setting in which the drug is taken and the expectations of the individual ingesting the drug play very important roles in the effects produced by any given dose. For example, as with ethanol, excitement is a common occurrence when the barbiturates are self-administered as "downers."

Physiological Effects

The inspiratory process is related primarily to the action of carbon dioxide on neurons within the respiratory control areas of the medulla, causing them to discharge. The termination of inspiration, resulting in expiration, occurs as a result of "feedback" of inhibitory influences to these neurons. This mechanism serves to keep the carbon dioxide concentration of arterial blood at a constant level in the presence of wide fluctuations in the oxygen concentration (Youmans, 1973). Because normal doses of the barbiturates do not alter carbon dioxide levels, barbiturate-induced sleep suppresses respiration in much the same way as does natural sleep. Respiratory stimulants appear to sensitize the medulla to carbon dioxide, so that, in the case of a barbiturate overdose, they may be of value in the treatment regime.

Clinical sedative or hypnotic doses of the barbiturates leave the circulation unaffected; anesthetic doses reduce blood pressure. Relative to the respiratory system, the circulation withstands barbiturate administration well. As in normal sleep, cerebral blood flow is slightly increased by barbiturates (Maynert, 1971b).

Even in barbiturate addicts, the liver appears not to be harmed by these compounds. As with ethanol, the rate of amino acid incorporation into liver microsomes and the rate of vitamin C usage and synthesis are increased by the barbiturates (Meyers et al., 1972). Thus, once again, these drugs lead to the development of tolerance to themselves by stimulating the processes responsible for their own metabolism.

Neural Effects

Among the various barbiturates as well as across the depressant drugs, differences in effect depend on dose, relative potency, and on the onset and duration of action. Modifications in the effects seen in a "standard" clinical situation may occur when route of administration, degree of CNS excitability, and previous drug experience are different than those of "normal" individuals. For example, when pentobarbital is injected into the gut (peritoneal cavity), rather than administered orally, the onset of the hypnotic effect is much more rapid because the absorption of the drug is also much more rapid. Also, an experienced user of ethanol will require larger initial sedative and hypnotic doses of phenobarbital, because of cross-tolerance, than will a complete abstainer. In fact, previous experience with any sedative-hypnotic agent, if that experience has resulted in some physical tolerance to the agent, will lead to a larger required dose of any barbiturate for sedation.

Sleep. Barbiturate-induced sleep in normal doses resembles normal sleep in most respects and does *not* reduce the amount of time spent in REM (Meyers et al., 1972). Therefore, in these doses the barbiturates do not result in REM rebound following their withdrawal. Further, these doses (such as 0.2 g pentobarbital at night) (Brecher, 1972) can be ingested over many months without the development of signs of physical dependence. However, larger doses do suppress REMs and do lead to signs of physical dependence. A similar effect was noted earlier in connection with ethanol.

Because REM periods are associated with increased activity of the cardio-vascular system as well as with greater CNS activity, cardiac patients are sometimes started on a treatment regime, which includes barbiturates at bedtime to decrease REM (Wikler, 1952). However, a dose of barbiturates sufficiently high to suppress REM sleep will induce physical dependence. If the agent is withdrawn gradually, REM sleep will increase; if it is withdrawn abruptly, convulsions are likely (which may be considered quite a complication in heart patients). Amphetamines (Chapter 3) share this REM-suppressing property with the barbiturates (Levitt, 1966, 1967), illustrating once more that neural and overt behavioral effects need not be correlated in any simple manner. Upon continued administration of the depressant, REM levels return to normal, as is also true for ethanol (Oswald, Berger, Jaramillo, Keddie, Olley, & Plunkett, 1963; Oswald & Priest, 1965). Since barbiturate withdrawal in chronic users of moderately large amounts of drug has been reported to precipitate a period of heightened REM and intense nightmare activity, individuals unaware of these natural consequences may continue taking the drug long after they had planned to stop (especially if they initially began taking the compound as an antianxiety agent).

Conditioning. To use an agent as a sedative is to use that compound to reduce anxiety (either anxiety with obvious cause, situational; or that with no apparent adequate stimulus, neurotic). The patient's conditioned responses to the drug must be given most careful consideration. For example, if a short-acting preparation is used, the effect appears quickly and decays rapidly, just as with ethanol. The patient soon associates the cyclic changes (3 to 4 times a day) with the medication. A situation is created with a high probability of nonclinical use via larger or more frequent doses. The long-acting, cumulative drugs (especially phenobarbital) will give constant blood levels of drug after a few days' administration (twice a day) and so are just as satisfactory for sedation. Since the cyclic changes are minimized the probability of nonclinical use is decreased (Meyers et al., 1972).

Hangover. Even a short-acting barbiturate taken before retiring may result in complaints of dizziness and weakness the following morning. This is exactly the same hangover as that seen with ethanol or in the recovery room following ether administration. Long-acting agents lead to a greater frequency of these signs, since a much more extended period is required for their metabolism. Subtle distortions of mood and impairment of judgment may persist for a full day following a 200-mg secobarbital (Seconal; intermediate-acting) dose. This indicates that as with ethanol, a person need not be rendered staggering drunk (the term referring to gait disturbances and uncontrolled eye movements) before he represents a danger to himself and others (McKenzie & Elliott, 1965). The combination of barbiturates and ethanol represents an especially dangerous situation. The multidose bottles of ethanol currently available and the ease with which multiple doses of a barbiturate (once obtained) may be ingested provide an easy opportunity for an individual to consume a lethal amount of depressant.

EEG effects. Because of the widespread use of the barbiturates in preventing seizures and in producing sedation, their EEG effects have been studied in detail in humans. The effects of gradual doses of barbiturates on the EEG are the same as those seen with proportionate doses of other depressants (such as general anesthetics and ethanol). Small doses are accompanied by increased fast activity and increased amplitude called *barbiturate activation*, not essentially different from the changes induced by normal sleep. Still-larger doses produce an EEG pattern characteristic of slow wave sleep. Anesthetic doses yield periods of complete EEG inactivity. At these dosage levels of the barbiturates both behavioral and EEG seizures are inhibited (Towman & Davis, 1949).

Pain. The barbiturates and ethanol differ from certain of the general anesthetics in that the general anesthetics decrease pain sensitivity in doses which do not appreciably affect the state of consciousness. In fact, small doses of the barbiturates may actually lower pain thresholds, while slightly larger doses may lead to excitement (from disinhibition).

Endocrine system. The barbiturates inhibit the secretion of corticotropin and the gonadotropic hormones by the anterior pituitary, while antidiuretic hormone secretion is increased (refer to Chapter 11 for a discussion of these compounds) when anesthetic doses are used (De Bodo & Prescott, 1945).

Tolerance and Addiction

Human subjects experiencing severe drowsiness with plasma phenobarbital concentrations of 5 μg per milliliter on Day 1 in a controlled study were unaware of any effects of the drug 12 days later at a plasma concentration five times as high (Butler, Mahaffee, & Waddell, 1954). Phenobarbital administration in rats increases the rate of hexobarbital metabolism sevenfold. Thus, tolerance to one member of the family transfers extensive tolerance to other members of the same family (cross-tolerance). This is used clinically in treating barbiturate withdrawal; it doesn't matter if the addict is going through withdrawal to pentobarbital, secobarbital, or even ethanol; phenobarbital administration can decrease the severity of the symptoms. Tolerance clearly has its limits. For example, many pentobarbital or secobarbital addicts achieve a maximal daily dose, which if exceeded by as little as 0.1 g results in coma. Laboratory animals made tolerant to the hypnotic actions of the barbiturates have a normal sensitivity to lethal doses. It is generally believed that humans do not differ from other animals in this respect (Maynert, 1971b).

Research on learning processes indicates that, other things being equal, the more immediate reinforcement is the more effective one (Kling & Schrier, 1971). Thus, the time to onset of action may be the primary reason why some depressants are more addicting (short- to intermediate-acting drugs, such as ethanol and secobarbital) than others (long-acting drugs, such as phenobarbital). Note that the longer a drug's duration of action, the longer its onset to action (refer to Chapter 1).

The barbiturates are becoming more commonly used nonclinically as preferred euphoric agents because of their ease of administration and all too great accessibility. They have been used as drugs for a "spree" and as substitutes for agents more expensive or difficult to obtain (ethanol, methamphetamine, and heroin).

Acute Toxicity

In large doses the barbiturates (and other depressant agents) produce deep, extended anesthesia, and depress respiration by a direct action on the medulla. If the medullary depression is severe, circulatory collapse is probable. The diagnosis in these instances must usually be made on circumstantial evidence (suicide note, phone call, or empty prescription container), since treatment (see next section) must be initiated before blood test results become available.

The lethal dose of a barbiturate depends to a large extent upon the interval between ingestion and treatment. If, for example, the individual is not discovered for several hours, 8 to 10 times the normal hypnotic dose (approximately 1 g) may be fatal. With prompt treatment, several times the lethal dose mentioned above may be consistent with survival. Generally, the quicker to onset of action of the drug, the lower the lethal plasma level: amobarbital levels one-half to one-third of phenobarbital levels are lethal.

Treatment. A group of Copenhagen physicians has developed a treatment program for acute intoxication with hypnotics. In 1949 the treatment of all cases of drug depression in the area was centralized in a single Copenhagen hospital. After the establishment of an intensive care unit and the introduction of a treatment program emphasizing maintenance of normal physiologic processes, the death rate in comparable groups of patients fell from 12% to 1% (Meyers et al., 1972; Setter, Maher, & Schreiner, 1966). The treatment of barbiturate intoxication (or ethanol overdose) consists of procedures which maintain life processes, while the liver metabolizes the drugs and the kidneys excrete both the drug and its metabolic products.

The most severe complication of acute depressant intoxication is shock: respiratory and circulatory collapse and irreversible kidney shutdown. Supportive therapy measures have occasionally been supplemented by central stimulants or by amphetamine. Since respiratory arrest is not a common cause of death in hospitalized patients (who have artificial airways established), the brief and weak actions of the convulsant stimulants when compared with the hazards (convulsions and postconvulsive depression) accompanying their use do not recommend them. Amphetamine is not a convulsive stimulant but an indirect-acting amine (causing norepinephrine release) so that it may be of some value in cases of depressant poisoning (Meyers et al., 1972; Myschetzky, 1961; Rubenstein, 1971).

Chronic Toxicity

Abrupt barbiturate withdrawal following chronic consumption of large quantities results in delirium and convulsions as intense as occur with any depressant drug. The delirium may consist of delusions, visual or auditory hallucinations, and disorientation with respect to time and place. In all respects the syndrome mirrors that seen following abrupt ethanol withdrawal. For example, among the several studies establishing the parallel between the barbiturates and ethanol, one small-scale experiment, conducted at the United States Public Health Service Hospital in Lexington, Kentucky, is of special interest because of the many details it provides.

> It was following withdrawal of barbiturate, however, that the parallel between that drug (pentobarbital, a short-acting barbiturate like ethanol in its onset to action) and alcohol was most impressively demonstrated. When an alcoholic who has been continuously drunk for days or weeks is abruptly deprived of his alcohol, he goes through a series of well-defined stages. . . . These five barbiturate addicts went through precisely this sequence of changes when their drug was withdrawn. . . . The similarity of the barbiturate withdrawal syndrome to alcoholic delirium tremens is striking. (Modified from Isbell, Altschule, Kornetsky, & Eisenman, 1950, p. 23, and Brecher, 1972, pp. 251–252.)

Therapeutic Uses

The range in barbiturate duration of action permits an extraordinary versatility in treatment. In individuals who haven't had much experience with depressant drugs (including ethanol), the recommended hypnotic dose of a short- or intermediate-acting agent will induce 6 or 7 hours of sleep, while a balanced sedative effect may be obtained by dividing the hypnotic dose of a long-acting agent into 3 or 4 equal portions to be taken during the day. Thus, the induction of sleep and the reduction of anxiety are the most common uses of these agents. Since depression and fatigue are common signs of anxiety, the barbiturates may combat these symptoms with the euphoria that they induce. Performance may be impaired while the subject believes (via the euphoria) that his performance has actually improved.

Because the barbiturates tend to reduce spontaneous activity in sedative doses, they may be used to advantage in situations were enforced bed rest is necessary. These agents previously found application in the control of marked (for example, maniacal) excitement but they are no longer used for this purpose since the needed amounts of the agents are massive (anesthetic doses).

The barbiturates also find extended use as anticonvulsants and as preanesthetic medication. The actions of other agents may often be advantageously modified by the barbiturates. For example, the excitement produced by dextroamphetamine may be decreased by the simultaneous administration of a barbiturate without reducing the stimulant-induced euphoria (Sharpless, 1970a). Indeed, since the barbiturates themselves induce a mood elevating effect, one might reasonably expect a drug interaction leading to a net summation of the euphoria. The barbiturates still maintain superiority over other agents in the treatment of acute convulsions such as occur from poisoning by stimulant drugs. During labor of childbirth, barbiturates are employed to render the patient sufficiently drowsy to sleep between pains and be amnesiac for the experience but, nevertheless, able to assist in the delivery ("twilight sleep") (Maynert, 1971b).

In the past, "douerschlaf" (prolonged sleep, often a week or more) via the barbiturates, was employed in the treatment of schizophrenia. The value of this treatment was never established. The use of barbiturates to provide greater suggestibility has seen these compounds applied to clinical psychotherapeutic programs and in criminal investigations. For the first use (narcoanalysis), the plan is to speed the development of rapport between the therapist and patient by relying on the sedative effects of the drugs; a drowsy patient is less likely to construct elaborate defenses for his actions. In criminal investigations, the misnomer "truth serum" has been applied to the drugs used. The probability of deceit does not decrease when barbiturates are used. It may, however, sometimes become easier for the authorities to trap the individual in a lie.

Due to a greater localization of speech than is the case with many other brain processes, hemispheric dominance becomes of vital concern when the neurosurgeon contemplates removal of part of the temporal lobe. When amobarbital is injected into the neck artery supplying one side of the head (carotid), hemispheric dominance is established on the injected side if speech disturbance and emotional depression result (Maynert, 1971b).

Summary

The barbiturates are used in the treatment of insomnia, anxiety, and epilepsy, and as short-acting anesthetic agents (especially as adjuncts to other drugs). They constitute a versatile class of drugs forming an alternative to ethanol in the clinical setting. The ease of administration of the barbiturates and the widely varying onsets to and duration of action of these drugs make them among the most useful agents available to the physician. Nevertheless, there is nothing special about them. The barbiturates comprise merely one group of CNS depressant; given under carefully controlled conditions they produce all the stages of anesthesia. In effect, the barbiturates are just a kind of solid ethanol.

NONBARBITURATE SEDATIVE–HYPNOTICS

The ability to produce a nonspecific, reversible depression of the CNS unites a number of compounds with otherwise diverse properties. This group of drugs includes the depressant tranquilizers (Chapter 5) and the agents discussed here. Although special claims have been made for most of these agents, generally their use is justified only when the barbiturates are contraindicated. This is because the properties of the barbiturates are better known and because they are less expensive. For the most part these nonbarbiturate sedative-hypnotic agents are closely related chemically to the barbiturates (methyprylon, glutethimide, thalidomide) or are alcohols or alcohol derivatives (chloral hydrate, paraldehyde, ethchlorvynol).

In classifying the sedatives in relation to their use, duration of action is the most important property (as is also true of the barbiturates). Just as with the barbiturates, the nonbarbiturate agents preferred for prolonged treatment of anxiety are long acting. For the induction of sleep, the short-acting nonbarbiturates are most useful (Table 6.3).

Short-acting Agents

The drugs considered here are chloral hydrate, paraldehyde, ethchlorvynol, and methyprylon. The prototype short-acting chemicals are pentobarbital and ethanol. The properties of the agents discussed here will be compared with those of the prototypes.

Chloral hydrate. Chloral hydrate was first introduced into medicine in 1869 when only ethanol, opium, and cannabis (hashish and marihuana) were available for hypnosis and sedation. Chloral hydrate is converted to an active derivative (trichloroethanol) in all tissues and to an inactive form in the liver. Like the barbiturates and ethanol, chloral hydrate provides the physical basis for

TABLE 6.3

Some Nonbarbiturate Sedative-Hypnotics

Length of action	Generic name	Trade name	Dose (oral)	
			Sedative	Hypnotic
Short-acting	Methyprylon	Noludar		
	Ethchlorvynol	Placidyl	0.1–0.2 g	0.5–1.0 g
	Chloral hydrate	Noctec	–	0.5–2.0 g
	Paraldehyde		–	3–8 ml
Intermediate-acting	Glutethimide	Doriden	.125–.25 g	.5 g
	Thalidomide		.025–.05 g	.1–.2 g
Long-acting	Bromide salts	Bromo Seltzer Miles Nervine	3–5 g	–

tolerance by increasing the drug metabolizing activity of liver microsomes (Sharpless, 1970b). The depressant effects are also similar. As with ethanol, the safety margin for chloral hydrate anesthesia is too narrow to permit clinical use. Like the barbiturates, little analgesic action is induced by chloral hydrate in hypnotic dosages. In contrast to ethanol and the barbiturates, chloral hydrate induces neither REM suppression when administered nor REM rebound when withdrawn (Kales, Malmstrom, Scharf, & Rubin, 1969).

The combination of chloral hydrate with ethanol ("knockout drops" or a "Mickey Finn") is the infamous mixture used prior to 1900 to render sailors unconscious to be shanghaied for the long trip to the Orient (Gessner & Cabana, 1967; Ray, 1972). The signs of acute intoxication are similar to those seen with ethanol.

Because of the rapid onset and short duration of action, a 1-g chloral hydrate dose is effective in individuals whose chief difficulty is falling asleep (but not remaining asleep), especially in the elderly and the very young. A major disadvantage of using chloral hydrate is that it is a gastric irritant. Repeated use leads to considerable stomach upset.

Paraldehyde, ethchlorvynol, and methyprylon. Paraldehyde was synthesized in 1824 and introduced clinically in 1882. Paraldehyde would probably be in wide use today because of its effectiveness as a CNS depressant with little respiratory depression and a wide safety margin, except for two characteristics. It has both a noxious taste and a disagreeable odor that permeates the user's breath. Thus, its use is usually restricted to hospital situations. In terms of potency, paraldehyde falls between ethanol and chloral hydrate. Habituation and addiction to paraldehyde are relatively uncommon because of the unpleasant taste and the disagreeable breath odor which it causes. When addiction does occur, it and the abstinence syndrome resemble those due to ethanol. The paraldehyde addict is often a former alcoholic who became acquainted with the drug when it was used in the DT therapy mentioned previously. Paraldehyde is indicated in individuals with renal disease since it is broken down to acetaldehyde which is then metabolized completely (to carbon dioxide and water), placing no added burden on the kidneys (Maynert, 1971a).

Ethchlorvynol, a substituted alcohol, is an effective hypnotic with both a short latency to onset (1/2 hour) and a short duration of action (3 hours) (Algeri, Katsas, & Zuango, 1962). As with the barbiturates, a therapeutic dose of ethchlorvynol may prove lethal in the presence of ethanol but, taken alone, 5 to 10 times the normal dose is more commonly required.

Methyprylon in hypnotic doses produces an effect virtually indistinguishable from that produced by 200 mg of secobarbital (Richels & Bass, 1963). Habituation, tolerance, addiction, and physical dependence have been reported. The abstinence syndrome is characteristic of the prototype depressants (Sharpless, 1970b).

Intermediate-acting Agents

The single compound to be considered here as a currently used drug is glutethimide. Meprobamate and diazepam are agents with similar properties which were discussed in Chapter 5. The prototype drug for this section is amobarbital. We shall also consider one agent no longer used clinically, thalidomide, to illustrate the necessity for study of all of the actions of any chemical before that chemical is allowed to be used clinically.

Glutethimide. The history of this agent is representative of that of many of the newer hypnotics. Upon its introduction, glutethimide was acclaimed as an effective "nonbarbiturate" hypnotic and sedative, free of a good many of the disadvantages of barbiturates and probably, in addition, lacking in ability to induce addiction. The drug gained instant, widespread acceptance, becoming within 2 years one of the most popular hypnotic agents in this country. It was, in 1955, the most widely prescribed nonbarbiturate sedative (cited by McBay & Katsas, 1957). Then cases of acute intoxication from glutethimide began to be reported in ever-increasing frequency. Also, unusual features of the poisoning made management difficult and may have been one reason for the fatalities reported. Furthermore, cases of glutethimide dependence, frank addiction, and a withdrawal syndrome of the type associated with withdrawal from barbiturates, led to a replacement of the initial optimism by caution. Glutethimide is now regarded as a typical central depressant having no special advantage over the barbiturates, as is true for most of the nonbarbiturate hypnotics. It is considered a satisfactory alternative to them, should one be needed (Sharpless, 1970b).

Thalidomide. This agent is structurally related to both glutethimide and methyprylon but, unlike them, is no longer available as a sedative-hypnotic. The discussion which follows of the abnormalities in fetal development (teratogenesis) induced by this agent should suggest caution in the application of all pharmacologic agents (both new ones and those in current use). All pharmaceuticals are toxic to some degree and, thus, all are at least potentially capable of inducing teratogenic effects in the newborn. Because drugs used clinically or in research have a multitude of effects within the organism, the example of thalidomide may inspire more careful research into drug properties so that both clinician and researcher may make their decisions for application of the chemicals based on a knowledge of the balance between desirable and undesirable properties of the compound in question (Mellin & Katzenstein, 1962).

Recorded instances exist of teratogenesis in both animals and humans as a result of exposure to weed-killing agents. In addition, abnormalities in human development caused by a German measles virus epidemic have been widely noted in the literature. Yet neither was sufficient to alert the medical community to the possibility that increasing use of insufficiently tested drugs by the public might one day result in tragedy. It required, instead, a major catastrophe to demonstrate that what had happened in other species could befall our own (Goldstein, Aronow, & Kalman, 1973).

In laboratory animals the largest possible oral dose of thalidomide which could be administered (5 g per kilogram of body weight) causes neither death nor even loss of the righting reflex. This is due to the relative insolubility of thalidomide in both lipids and water, which hinders its absorption. There is a marked decrease in motor activity, without an impairment of coordination. A most unusual finding was that 0.1 g of thalidomide produces hypnotic effects equal to the same amount of secobarbital (the barbiturate equivalent in terms of onset to and duration of action). Unlike the case with the barbiturate, however, individuals taking 140 times the normal hypnotic dose (14 g) in suicide attempts could be roused without the use of stimulants. This remarkable safety margin plus a low incidence of side effects led to availability without restriction (in some cases, without prescription) first in West Germany in 1958, then elsewhere. The stage was set for the tragedy to follow.

About 1960, scattered reports appeared of neurologic disturbance among patients receiving chronic treatment with thalidomide. The reports went unheeded. There was at this same time an increase in the number of infants born with flipperlike or absent limbs (phocomelia): no cases at all had been cited in the literature from 1949–1959; a single case was noted in 1959; three instances in 1960; and in 1961, 154 cases. Comparable increases occurred in countries other than West Germany; in fact increases in phocomelia spread throughout all countries where thalidomide was in use. By 1962, when the connection with thalidomide was verified 7,000 infants had been born with drug-induced malformations.

During a key period between Weeks 3 and 8 of gestation, even a few doses sufficed to produce the effect. Ingestion during gestational Days 21 and 22 resulted in a child with absence of the external ears and cranial nerve paralysis. Three to five days later the phocomelic effect was at its peak, with the development of flipperlike or absent limbs. The drug-sensitive period then tapered off around Day 36 and the resultant child suffered deformed internal organs and thumbs.

Long-acting Agents

The bromides will be considered here. Chlordiazepoxide and oxazepam are compounds with similar actions considered in Chapter 5. Phenobarbital may be considered prototypic.

Bromides. The ability of any bromide salt to depress the CNS was first utilized in 1857 in the treatment of epilepsy. Potassium bromide had been reported capable of diminishing sexual desires (anaphrodisiac quality). At that time some forms of epilepsy were regarded as consequences of masturbation or coitus interruptus. The drug was tried as a means of inhibiting this behavior and found successful in reducing epileptic attacks (if for the wrong reasons) (Sharpless, 1970b). In the latter half of the 19th century the bromides were employed on an enormous scale. More efficient and less toxic compounds have now supplanted them in therapy. Occasional use is still found for the bromides in the treatment of grand mal and focal epilepsy, but only if the plasma levels of bromide can be monitored and the patient kept under close observation.

Serious bromide intoxication still occurs because of the use of the chemical in headache remedies and "nerve tonics." For example, Bromo Seltzer contains 160 mg of potassium bromide per capful, and Miles Nervine, 620 mg per capful of triple bromides. These water-soluble salts all depend for their action on the bromide ion.

Bromide tends to be so highly irritating to the gastrointestinal tract that it is difficult to ingest and retain a toxic amount without vomiting. For this reason, the drug is useless as a hypnotic agent. Bromide is employed only for prolonged sedation or for the antiepileptic effects which are obtainable with sedative doses.

The absorption and distribution of bromide are similar to that for chloride: more than 24 hours are required for peak concentrations to be reached in cerebrospinal fluid, for example. In some species (cats) bromide enters the hypothalamus more readily than it does other brain regions (Maynert, 1971a). The ion is removed from brain and cerebrospinal fluid via active transport processes, while renal excretion is slightly less than, but otherwise similar to, that of chloride. Diuretic agents which increase chloride excretion also increase that of bromide.

Under conditions of a fixed daily dose, an average diet, and normal kidney function, the bromide ion accumulates for a month or more. At this time the daily rate of elimination equals the intake. Chronic intoxication (known as *bromism*) leads to alterations in nervous function so varied as to simulate almost every variety of neural pathology. This is because bromide and chloride compete with each other (being of like charge, and similar size) so that high bromide levels lead to low blood chloride. Low chloride levels in the cerebrospinal fluid are associated with such specific entities as inflammation of CNS tissue (for example, meningitis) (Bannister, 1969), but when the amount of a key biological anion is disturbed the following symptoms might also be anticipated. They include depression, fatigability, inability to concentrate, loss of memory, lack of appetite, and poor sleep, with confusion, disorientation, and even hallucinations in more severe cases. The physical symptoms variably encompass slurred speech, unsteady gait (ataxia), tremor, and decreased tendon reflexes. The patient may become comatose. When delirium, hallucinations, fear reactions, and mania result from excess bromide, the term *bromide psychosis* is often applied. This excitement is treated with other sedative-hypnotic agents (Brain & Walton, 1969); the bromide overdose itself is treated with chloride salts (Meyers et al., 1972).

Summary

The actions of the nonbarbiturate sedative-hypnotic agents mirror those of the other depressants so far considered: depression of the CNS from top (neocortex) down and bottom (spinal cord) up; anticonvulsant actions, but only in anesthetic doses; addicting actions leading to seizures following withdrawal of chronic, high doses. They have a selective action on the reticular activating system as do other depressants. Like them also, the nonbarbiturate sedative-hypnotics depress REM sleep (chloral hydrate being a notable exception). Cross-tolerance may occur with any of the agents so far discussed in the chapter; also, the depressant effects of any combination of these agents summate. All of the agents discussed depend on the same enzyme systems within the liver microsomes for their degradation. At any given moment the liver's metabolic capacity is constant as is the ability of the kidneys to excrete drug and decomposition products. As with the barbiturates, the nonbarbiturate sedative-hypnotics are used clinically in the treatment of anxiety (as well as in the induction of sleep). Like both the barbiturates and ethanol, these agents seem to find nonclinical use because of the disinhibition of lower telencephalic and diencephalic areas (following inhibition of neocortex) which they yield (engendering the euphoria characteristic of Stage 2 anesthesia). The chances for the disinhibition, euphoria, and an association between the time of medication and relief from anxiety are increased as the time to onset of action is decreased. Any depressant classified as short acting (and, hence, with a very brief onset to action) will have a maximum likelihood of being selected as a drug of "abuse."

EPILEPSY AND THE ANTICONVULSANT DRUGS

Epilepsy is a generic term for recurrent seizures of any origin. The periodicity of the attacks differentiate epilepsy from convulsions due to withdrawal from depressants. There are two types of epileptic seizures, classified according to point of origin, as local or generalized (Yahr, 1971). Generalized seizures are further divided into grand mal (a dramatic stiffening and jerking of the body with loss of consciousness for several minutes), petit mal (a momentary loss of consciousness camouflaged between normal actions), and myoclonic-akinetic (respectively, a sudden jerk or a sudden loss of muscle tonus throughout the body). Each type of epilepsy presents a unique EEG pattern which, like the behavioral seizure, is secondary to a more central causative process (Woodbury, 1969).

The Anticonvulsant Drugs

The main emphasis here is on compounds used in the treatment of epilepsy. The same chemicals effective as antiepileptics are also useful in controlling seizures due to other causes (for example, tumor inside the skull, mechanical trauma, or blood toxins). Because most patients who are treated for epileptic states receive more than one drug and because treatment is continuous for many years, the chronic toxicity of the anticonvulsant agents is of particular importance. Drugs with anticonvulsant activity include the long-acting barbiturates, diphenylhydantoin (and related drugs), trimethadione (and related drugs) and the succinimides.

Barbiturates. All of the sedative-hypnotic agents so far considered may be used to terminate an acute convulsive state. Large doses are required and for chronic administration only the long-acting depressants are satisfactory. Phenobarbital is the standard, but other long-acting drugs such as chlordiazepoxide are useful. Intermediate-acting compounds (such as meprobamate and diazepam) have been used, but their rapidly changing blood levels render them less suitable.

Phenobarbital is anticonvulsant in doses that are not normally sedative (100-200 mg daily). One point of view is that this is due to a specific anticonvulsant action of phenobarbital, while another position is that the usefulness of this drug derives from its sustained, constant level of CNS depression (Gunn, Gogerty, & Wolf, 1961).

The most common adverse reactions to the sedatives during antiepileptic treatment are related to sedation and disinhibition. These effects may be minimized by using combinations of anticonvulsant agents, each in doses smaller than those which yield disturbances.

Epileptic patients are unusually susceptible to the hyperexcitable state induced by a total withdrawal or a too rapid reduction in dose of an anticonvulsant drug. Because of its long duration of action, phenobarbital appears not to lead to addiction even when administered over long time periods. The anticonvulsant actions of this agent continue essentially unchanged without increases in the initial dose (Meyers et al., 1972). The overall intelligence and learning ability of epileptic children is probably not impaired by chronic treatment with the usual anticonvulsant doses of phenobarbital. This is because of the fact that tolerance to the sedative effects develops while the anticonvulsant usefulness is unimpaired (Wapner, Thurston, & Holowach, 1962); however, see the section that follows for a discussion of a secondary vitamin deficiency with behavioral concomitants.

Diphenylhydantoin (Dilantin). This agent was introduced in 1938 for the symptomatic treatment of epilepsy. In all species tested, the drug inhibits the spread of the seizure without depressing the discharging focus itself. Maximum blood levels of the compound are not reached until eight hours following oral administration. The metabolism is slow; the half-life of diphenylhydantoin in the plasma following discontinuance of long-term medication averages 22 hours (Arnold & Gerber, 1970). When the drug is given chronically, excretion matches absorption after 1 week's administration of a fixed dose.

If the usual daily dose of 400 to 700 mg diphenylhydantoin is substituted for phenobarbital, the barbiturate must be withdrawn gradually since diphenylhydantoin does not confer protection against barbiturate withdrawal seizures. This demonstrates that similarity of behavioral effect alone (the seizures due to barbiturate withdrawal are grand mal–like in appearance) carries no guarantee of identity of the underlying neural substrate. For treatment of grand mal epilepsy, symptomatic convulsions nonepileptic in nature, and for psychomotor attacks diphenylhydantoin (alone or in combination with phenobarbital) is the most adequate drug. Since petit mal attacks may be exacerbated by the drug, it is not used for treating this form of epilepsy or when the petit mal pattern is superimposed on that of grand mal in mixed epilepsy. Concurrent use of diphenylhydantoin and a barbiturate is advantageous because the differing side effects of the two drugs permit full doses of each and consequently, a relatively greater common anticonvulsive effect.

It has also been established that youthful epileptics who are treated for extended periods may undergo progressive mental deterioration that is independent of any preexisting brain damage. This is not a direct effect on associative processes but rather one associated with a nutritional deficiency of one of the water-soluble B-complex vitamins (folic acid). Prevention and treatment of the disorder are effectively carried out by administering a combination of folic acid and B_{12} in conjunction with the anticonvulsant medication (Meyers et al., 1972). All anticonvulsant agents tend to produce a folate deficiency; thus, the combination of diphenylhydantoin and phenobarbital is especially likely to cause the condition because each agent is taken at a full dose.

Trimethadione (Tridion). A new era in the treatment of epilepsy began in 1945 when the effects of trimethadione against petit mal were discovered. The compound is useful in reducing the number of petit mal attacks whether they are of the typical pattern or one of the variants with associated motor signs. Patients subject to these attacks have characteristic abnormal EEG patterns (diffuse, symmetric, and characterized by a 3-per-second spike-and-dome EEG pattern) more or less continuously rather than only during the clinical episode (as is usually the case in grand mal). Trimethadione may act by damping both inhibitory and excitatory activity in thalamic circuits, while the barbiturates may actually potentiate the inhibitory factors involved in petit mal discharges by their action to selectively depress EPSPs (Barker & Gainer, 1973; Morrell, Bradley, & Ptashne, 1959).

Ethosuximide (Zarontin) is another drug used for petit mal epilepsy, with properties similar to trimethadione (Glaser, 1971).

Summary

All of the agents classed as depressants are anticonvulsant and may be used acutely to terminate a convulsive state. Large doses are required for all but the long-acting agents: phenobarbital and chlordiazepoxide (Chapter 5) which are often effective in sedative dosages. An agent used to treat epilepsy should always be long acting, if possible, because the constancy of the induced depression appears as important as "special anticonvulsive effects" in the chemicals normally used. In general, all anticonvulsants appear to act by limiting seizure spread from the epileptic focus. They do this by means of the normal depressant action of inhibiting neural activity from neocortex downwards.

"HOW MANY WAYS CAN YOU GET DRUNK?"

One of the most dramatic rejoinders to this question was a study done by Dr. Harris Isbell and his associates (1950) to which we alluded earlier in our discussion of barbiturate withdrawal. The study compared acute and chronic barbiturate intoxication and withdrawal with that due to ethanol. Preliminary to the study, five prisoner volunteers serving sentences for narcotics violations were subjected to a battery of neurological and psychological tests. Then, in an isolated hospital research ward, the first phase of the study began. This was the administration of a large dose of pentobarbital. Both pentobarbital and ethanol are depressants with a short onset to action and a brief duration of activity within the body. The result was an intoxication which resembled to these researchers (who had been studying ethanol intoxication for years) that from ethanol in "almost all respects." The manifest psychological signs included a decrement in performance on the battery of psychological tests; the neurological signs (such as tremors and incoordination) were likewise indicative of individuals who were "dead drunk." The signs of the intoxication disappeared in about the same time that an equally large dose of ethanol would wear off (5 hours). The subjects slept poorly that night, as is common following an evening of ethanol ingestion and they complained of hangover (nervousness, tremulousness, loss of appetite, and headache) the following day.

The second phase of the experiment consisted of an attempt to reproduce by means of barbiturates all the behavioral signs seen in chronic alcoholism. For more than 3 months, doses of pentobarbital were given five times per day, from an initial "eye opener" before breakfast to a nightcap at 11 p.m. This method of administration was designed to duplicate the ingestion pattern seen with chronic alcoholics. Generally, the signs of intoxication were minimal early in the morning and increased throughout the day with their behavior and appearance indistinguishable from the skid row alcohol addict (Brecher, 1972).

The most impressive demonstration of the barbiturate-ethanol parallel occurred following withdrawal of the pentobarbital. The reader may benefit by referring back to the description of delirium tremens and then to the discussion of barbiturate withdrawal symptoms shown by the subjects in the Isbell experiment (as discussed earlier in the chapter). The barbiturate DTs were found to be just as serious as DTs due to ethanol withdrawal, because barbiturate DTs are indistinguishable from those produced by withdrawal from their liquid counterpart. The short-acting barbiturates (such as pentobarbital in this study) may be termed *solid alcohols* with some justification.

The similarity between depressants is highlighted by the phenomenon of cross-tolerance discussed earlier. Alcoholic DTs may be terminated by a dose of ethanol or by administration of a barbiturate (phenobarbital is usually given) or by administration of any other depressant. It is easier to give a pill than to administer ether but there is no logical reason why an anesthetic couldn't be used to end DTs. By the same token, an individual feeling the initial signs of withdrawal from secobarbital can stop the incipient full-blown reaction by taking a few drinks.

The parallel among depressants includes the anesthetics, as we have suggested. Ether was used for recreational purposes as early as the 18th century (Nagle, 1968). By the mid-1800s it had become the chief substitute for ethanol in Northern Ireland. This massive changeover from one drug to another occurred because the British government had placed a high tax on alcoholic beverages while the local constabularies at the same time cracked down on the sale and production of home-distilled Irish whiskey. Ether wasn't subject to a tax and was produced in London. It was no great problem, therefore, to ship huge amounts to Draperstown and other places in Ireland. The drug was preferred in some ways to the then-expensive whiskey since the drunk was almost instantaneous, it was cheap, it could be achieved several times a day without hangover, and if arrested for drunkenness "the offender would be sober by the time the police station was reached" (Nagle, 1968, p. 28). A surgeon visiting Draperstown in 1878 remarked that the main street smelled like his surgery (where ether was used as an anesthetic). Old ether "topers" could (by this surgeon's report) finish off a 3-oz wineglassful of ether at a single swig without even taking water for a chaser.

Let us return for a moment to the nonbarbiturate sedative-hypnotic agents chloral hydrate and paraldehyde. These depressants, like the rest, can produce drunkenness, addiction, and the full withdrawal syndrome (including DTs and convulsions) hardly distinguishable from those caused by ethanol and the barbiturates. It seems that there are as many ways to get drunk as there are CNS depressants available.

SUMMARY

All of the drugs considered in this chapter can produce the entire spectrum of CNS depression from Stage 1 through Stage 4 anesthesia. The chief differences among the depressants are due to their relative onsets to and durations of action. These, in turn, are functions of the dosage and route by which the drug is administered. If one has complete control over both the dosage and route parameters, he may produce at will identical syndromes of behavioral depression with any given pair of depressant drugs.

The behavioral consequences of taking a depressant result essentially from what is depressed and when. The initial depression is at the top and bottom of the CNS, the neocortex and caudal spinal cord, respectively. Thus, the individual becomes unsteady in gait before his hand coordination is much impaired; he may manifest an initial excitement (due to disinhibition of lower telencephalic and diencephalic brain areas) before he becomes drowsy as the ascending reticular activating system is affected.

While taken as antianxiety or sleep-inducing agents by most individuals, the depressants are effective anticonvulsants in high doses. The anticonvulsants also have sedative properties, which occasionally present some problems when their administration must be chronic. These primary effects of the depressants are due to the special sensitivity of neural tissue relative to other tissue to the actions of these drugs. We have seen that how long a drug remains in the body (a function of its lipid solubility, generally), and what tissue with which it is in contact, determine the drug's properties.

Chronic actions of the depressants are not basically different from the effects seen with acute administration. Any apparent differences are due to the development of tolerance by the body to the effects of the drug. Only where there is tolerance can there be a withdrawal syndrome. The fact that the withdrawal syndrome for any depressant reflects a heightened excitability of the CNS may be explained by the homeostatic set-point concept: behavior during withdrawal is the opposite of behavior under the drug because the nervous system compensates for a drug by changing its baseline level of activity so that the predrug levels of firing are maintained.

Finally, we have not meant to suggest that there are no differences among the depressants. Chemical compounds are as distinct as fingerprints; therein lies their utility for the student of pharmacology. For example, ethanol is more likely to lead to serious malnutrition and to gastrointestinal irritation than are the barbiturates, and perhaps also more likely to lead to neurological damage. It is far easier to self-administer a lethal handful of "downers" than it is to gulp down a quart of whiskey. Ether (which can be drunk like whiskey) leaves little hangover because it is excreted by the lungs (rapidly) rather than by the kidneys (over a period of hours). Yet it does seem reasonable at this point to conclude that the similarities of the depressant drugs far outweigh their differences, as far as the behaviorist is concerned. It matters not nearly so much whether one ingests chloral hydrate, halothane, glutethimide, secobarbital, or whiskey as how much is ingested and how it is ingested.

7
THE NARCOTIC ANALGESICS

Hugh E. Criswell and Robert A. Levitt

The narcotic analgesics are of major theoretical interest to the psychologist because of their significant behavioral actions. They are of major practical interest because of their high potential for abuse. The illicit use of narcotics has been a serious drug abuse problem in the United States since the early 20th century. This problem appears to have become even more severe in the 1960s and on into the present time. These drugs produce euphoria and a severe withdrawal syndrome in a tolerant individual (a regular user), and therefore have a high addiction liability. Attempts to find a successful means of treating narcotic addiction and returning the addict to a productive life have met with varying amounts of success, but all are considered controversial by some people. The criminal activities of many addicts, caused by the high cost of illicitly obtaining the drugs and the absence of a nominally priced licit supply, have resulted in a major crime problem. In this chapter we will touch on each of these subjects.

In spite of the problems detailed above, the narcotic analgesics are still one of the important pharmacological tools available to the physician. We can distinguish two general goals of medical treatment. The first is the prevention, cure, or amelioration of illness and disease. This may be accomplished in many ways: surgery, dietary alteration, and the use of drugs are just a few examples of medical treatments.

The narcotic drugs are employed by the physician for a different purpose, as an adjunct to the treatment of many kinds of illnesses and diseases. These are drugs that usually do not directly contribute to the amelioration or cure of the disease, but are, nonetheless, of striking clinical importance. These analgesics are used to treat the second most important clinical problem (after ameliorating, arresting, or curing the disease), that of pain and suffering. These drugs are so important because they combat the misery of the sickness and because they are useful in treating diseases of all the systems of the body.

Analgesics are defined as substances that reduce the sensation of pain without simultaneously reducing other sensations such as touch and pressure. This specific action on pain perception distinguishes the analgesics from the anesthetics, which block the perception of all incoming sensory information. Thus, when the dentist administers procaine (a local anesthetic) all sensory perceptions from the affected area are blocked. If a general anesthetic such as thiopental is used, unconsciousness results and no perception occurs. However, when an analgesic such as morphine is given, only the pain is supressed; other sense modalities such as touch, temperature, and proprioception remain.

Analgesics can be divided into two categories: (1) the *narcotic analgesics* like morphine, which are very powerful but produce dangerous side effects such as tolerance and addiction; and (2) the *anti-inflammatory, antipyretic analgesics* such as aspirin, which are weaker than the narcotics but do not usually produce such dangerous side effects. The narcotic analgesics reduce pain because of actions on the central nervous system. These agents are related to opium or are synthetic drugs that duplicate many of the effects of opium. It is the narcotic analgesics that produce profound behavioral effects and are subject to addiction and an acute withdrawal syndrome. The nonnarcotic analgesics, such as aspirin, appear to reduce pain, due to blocking actions on the sensory receptors. These agents have not been found to have major actions on the central nervous system nor to have behavioral manifestations in nontoxic doses. Therefore the nonnarcotic analgesics will not be discussed. This chapter will first discuss the mechanisms of pain perception and the problems involved in measuring pain and analgesia and will then discuss the narcotic analgesics. The many nonanalgesic effects of the narcotics will also be discussed as they relate to narcotic use and abuse.

PAIN

The perception of pain depends on reception of the painful stimulus by a nociceptor (pain receptor) and the transmission of the stimulus information to the brain. In the brain, the sensory information is analyzed and integrated with past experience and present context to result in the perceptual experience that we call pain. This perception is associated almost exclusively with damage or potential damage to tissue. Pain, thus, acts as a warning that damage to the organism is imminent. It is, therefore, not surprising from an evolutionary viewpoint that the perception of pain is unpleasant and that the escape or avoidance of pain is a potent reinforcer. An analgesic can reduce pain by acting at any point along the pathway from the pain receptor through the highest parts of the brain. Some understanding of the basic neurophysiology of pain will aid in understanding the effects of the narcotic analgesics.

Pain Reception

The type of sensory receptor responsible for the initiation of the neural activity perceived as pain is not known with certainty. Intense stimulation of each sensory system may be capable of producing the sensation of pain. One specific type of sensory receptor, the free nerve ending, however, is known to respond to painful stimulation. The free nerve ending is the only sense receptor found on the cornea of the eye and the sensitivity of the cornea to painful stimulation is well known to anyone who has worn contact lenses. These pain receptors are also sensitive to chemical stimulation and may be classified as chemoreceptors. Stimulation of free nerve endings by irritant chemicals such as bradykinin or histamine results in the perception of intense pain at the site of stimulation. These chemicals have been shown to be released by injured cells following tissue injury (Lim & Guzman, 1968). It is, therefore, probable that the production of pain may result from two different factors: (1) mechanical stimulation of the nerve endings themselves, and (2) chemical action of histamine and bradykinin (released by other injured cells at the site of stimulation) on the free nerve endings.

Pain Pathways

Fibers traveling from the pain receptors in the trunk and limbs enter at the rear of the spinal cord, while most fibers from pain receptors in the face, head, and neck enter the brainstem via one of the cranial nerves (Number V, the trigeminal nerve). The fibers then synapse on nuclei in the spinal cord or brainstem, respectively. Second order axons then leave these nuclei, cross over to the other side of the spinal cord or brainstem, and travel up to the thalamus in the lateral spinothalamic tract (for the trunk and limbs) or the tract of the trigeminal nerve (for the face, head, and neck). These second order fibers end in the thalamus. Third order fibers then travel from the thalamus to a part of the parietal lobe of the cerebral cortex. Note that pain information is traveling in the brain and spinal cord on the opposite side from which the pain originated. Because the fibers in this pain pathway are relatively small, conduction of pain impulses is quite slow. Under some conditions, painful stimulation may not be perceived for as long as 2 to 4 seconds after the stimulation. Such is the time required for neural impulses to travel through the small fibers from the heel to the brain (Collins, Nuylsen, & Shealy, 1966).

The simple three-neuron pathway just described represents the classical pain pathway. There is some question, however, as to the meaningfulness of this system with regard to the perception of pain, since many collaterals leave this system to project into the reticular formation and limbic system. In fact, so many fibers in the pain system fail to follow the classical three-neuron pathway that it has been suggested that the classical pathway is relatively unimportant for the perception of pain. At the least, the student should realize that the neurophysiological basis of pain is not well understood. Which neural pathways and structures are critically involved in the different aspects of pain perception and of pain-motivated behavior remain unclear. This, of course, makes the understanding of the mechanism of action of analgesic drugs very difficult. However, some progress seems to have been made and will be reviewed when we discuss "Morphine" later in this chapter.

The Perception of Pain

Pain perception is a complex process depending not only on the physical stimulation of the nociceptor, but also on the organism's past experience (memory) and present emotional and motivational state. Melzack and Wall (1965) have developed an interesting and useful conceptual organization of the pain system. Three primary dimensions have been attributed to pain. The first is the cognitive-evaluative aspect of pain. This is made possible by the modification of the neural information regarding a potential painful stimulus by such structures as the frontal cortex. The neural information is modified in light of the individual's past experience and present situation. Thus, the football player who is intent on a game may not notice the pain of a bone fracture. In this case, tactile and proprioceptive information arriving over rapidly conducting pathways may give rise to information which is fed back down to the pain pathway to inhibit this more slowly traveling information. This inhibition of incoming neural activity in the pain pathway may occur as early as the first synapse in the pain circuit and certainly before it reaches the higher brain centers.

A second aspect of pain is the motivational-affective component. The narcotic analgesics may act primarily on this aspect of pain. The person who has received a narcotic analgesic continues to feel the pain but "doesn't mind any more." Since similar results have been obtained by prefrontal lobotomy, the prefrontal area may be involved in this emotional aspect (the suffering) of pain.

The third aspect of pain is the sensory-discriminative component. This component is the raw information on which the perception of a painful stimulus is based. It is dependent on an intact spinal (or trigeminal) pain pathway which can deliver the raw data to the brain. Local anesthetics such as procaine act on this most basic aspect of pain by blocking the conduction of pain impulses before they reach the central nervous system.

The Problem of Measuring Pain

The fact that pain is a complex sensation consisting of cognitive, emotional, and sensory components presents a serious problem of measurement for the scientist. In science, a concept must be operationally defined before it can be investigated. Thus, the method of measurement is included in the definition. An example of an operational definition which could be used in the study of pain is: "A person will be said to have experienced pain if, when asked, 'Did that hurt?' he replies, 'Yes'." Pain is then measured by the person's verbal report of whether or not a given stimulus produced pain. This method seems reasonable, but, surprisingly, is not useful for the evaluation of many analgesics. If the pain threshold for electric shock is determined by this method and the person is then given an injection of morphine (one of the most potent analgesics), the experimenter will probably find that the pain threshold has not been changed by the analgesic. This is because the question asked, "Do you feel pain?", taps only the sensory-discriminative aspect of pain. In the middle of open heart surgery, where morphine is sometimes the only drug given, the patient is awake and if asked, "Does it hurt?" may nod, "Yes" (Jameson & Hasbrouck, 1971). The important fact is that the patient "doesn't mind" the fact that it hurts and is quite willing to go on with the surgery. Had the question been changed to "Do you mind the pain?", there would have been a large difference between the drugged and nondrugged states. It is, therefore, clear that the method of measurement can have a great effect on the determination of analgesic potency for a given drug.

It is necessary to screen large numbers of drugs for analgesic properties. Because it is neither ethical nor practical to test unknown drugs on humans, many methods have been devised for testing analgesic action on animals. A direct verbal report is, of course, not obtainable from the animal and the experience of pain must, therefore, be inferred from behavioral measures. Extreme caution must be exercised when making the generalization from animal behavior to human experience (which must also be measured in terms of observable behavior). Nonetheless, much information concerning the effectiveness of analgesics has been obtained from animal studies.

Methods for testing analgesic effects in animals. The commonly used methods for the evaluation of analgesic effectiveness of experimental drugs may be divided into two categories. First, there are direct methods, where a noxious stimulus is presented and the innate unlearned responses of the subject to that stimulus are recorded. Second, there are the indirect methods, in which the animal is trained to make a response that will allow it to escape or avoid the noxious stimulation, and the occurrence of these trained responses is recorded. The noxious stimulation may be provided by thermal, electrical, mechanical, or chemical stimuli. The responses measured may consist of any of the animal's innate responses to pain such as vocalization or reflex withdrawal of the stimulated limb. When training methods are used, two of the more commonly employed behavioral measures are lever-pressing and maze-running.

Thermal stimulation: When radiant heat is focused on the base of a rat's tail, pain can be produced (D'Amour & Smith, 1941). This remains one of the most popular methods of producing graded intensities of noxious stimulation for the evaluation of analgesics. An effective analgesic will increase the duration or intensity of heat necessary to produce vocalization by the animal. A modification of this procedure is called the *tail flick test* and involves measurement of the duration of stimulation by radiant energy to the rat's tail necessary for the elicitation of a reflex tail movement (Winter, 1965). A weakness of the radiant heat method of producing noxious stimulation is that repeated presentation of the painful stimulus sensitizes the receptors, resulting in increased responsiveness to the stimulus.

Electrical stimulation: The tail, the hind limb, or the tooth pulp can be electrically stimulated as a means of producing pain. Electrical stimulation of the tail produces several responses in the rat, any of which may be used as indication of pain perception. These include reflex movements of the hind legs, stimulus bound vocalization (vocalization which lasts only as long as the noxious stimulus is present) and vocalization which continues after the cessation of the stimulus. It is interesting to note that each of these measurements may result in a different evaluation of the potency of a suspected analgesic (Hoffmeister, 1968).

Mechanical stimulation: Winter (1965) cites several mechanical methods of pain production which have been used in the study of analgesics. These include tail-pinching, application of a metal clip to the toe, or inflaming an area such as a toe by the injection of a small amount of yeast followed by the application of pressure to the inflamed area. Several calibrated devices for the production of known amounts of pressure have also been designed. This method is subject to the same criticism as the use of radiant heat in that the stimulated area becomes sensitized and further stimulation will produce a stronger response.

Chemical stimulation: Pain may be elicited by direct chemical stimulation of the pain receptors by certain chemicals which may be released by damaged cells in response to injury. These chemicals include bradykinin, histamine, and prostaglandin. Injections of these substances produce an intense pain at the site of injection, which can be diminished by the mild analgesics such as aspirin. This type of pain is one of the few which will respond significantly to the mild analgesics that appear to act at the pain receptor rather than by exerting an effect upon the higher brain centers (Lim & Guzman, 1968).

The Straub test: If a method of testing analgesic effectiveness is to be valid, it need only predict the effectiveness of a given drug. The test itself may seem completely unrelated to pain perception. An excellent example of this type of test is the Straub test. In the Straub test, a mouse is injected with a suspected analgesic. Many analgesic drugs related to morphine will cause the animal's tail to become erect due to a constrictive action on the anal sphincter. An example of a positive Straub test is presented in Figure 7.1. Tail erection is not directly related to analgesia but most drugs which cause the Straub reaction are also powerful analgesics. This action on the anal sphincter is a property of the narcotic analgesics (which are constipating), but not the peripherally acting non-narcotic analgesics such as aspirin.

Operant techniques: These are attractive to investigators with a background in psychology because they closely resemble the behavioral responses seen in situations where pain is to be avoided or escaped. These techniques include avoidance conditioning where, by making a learned response, the animal can avoid a noxious stimulus (typically an electric shock) and escape conditioning where, by making a response during the presentation of the noxious stimulus, the animal can escape from that stimulus. There is an inherent weakness in the use of operant methods for the evaluation of analgesics. When a rat fails to press a lever in order to avoid the presentation of an electric shock, the reason may be

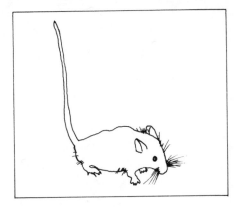

FIGURE 7.1. The Straub test as elicited by the injection of morphine in the mouse. Note the stiffening of the tail induced by contraction of the anal sphincter.

that analgesia has occurred and the stimulus has lost its aversiveness, or it may simply be due to weakness or lethargy due to toxic reactions to the drug. Some drugs interfere with memory (see Chapter 10), and a failure to escape or avoid a noxious stimulus may indicate that the animal no longer remembers the correct response. These problems severely limit the usefulness of operant techniques in the study of analgesic effectiveness (Winter, 1965).

The Testing of Analgesics in Humans

Once a possible analgesic has been found through animal testing and has been proven safe to animals, the drug is then tested on humans. Humans respond differently than other species to many drugs, and a good analgesic for rats might prove useless for humans. Two of the most important methodological problems involve the placebo effect and the use of the double-blind procedure.

The placebo effect. This is a psychological effect due to the subject's belief that he or she is going to be helped. This is extremely potent in the relief of pain. An injection of isotonic saline (a placebo) has been found to be 35% effective in reducing postoperative pain. This presumably is due to the cognitive aspect of the pain. In one aspect of his study, Beecher (1966) even failed to find a difference between the effects of morphine and a placebo on the relief of postoperative pain. If the patient can be made to think that the pain will decrease, it often does. Figure 7.2 shows the effect of morphine versus that of a placebo. For the first hour, there is little difference between the two conditions. This placebo effect must be taken into account in any attempted evaluation of an analgesic. To be truly effective, an analgesic must be more effective than a placebo.

The double-blind method. Most means of measuring pain in the human are subjective. Typically, a physician will ask the patient how the drug affected him.

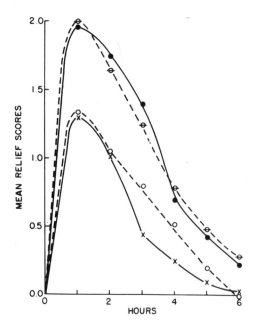

FIGURE 7.2. Time-effect curves for a saline pacebo (*X*), 10 mg of morphine sulfate (●), 25 mg of chlorpromazine (O), and a combination of 10 mg of morphine sulfate and 25 mg of chlorpromazine (⊖) in 34 patients with pain due to cancer. Pain relief (ordinate) is plotted against time in hours after drug administration (abscissa). The data represent the mean relief scores as determined by the patients' own ratings of pain intensity before and after the intramuscular administration of each medication. The drugs (61 doses each drug) were administered in a randomized order, and all 34 patients received all medications—27 of them receiving each medication twice. (Reprinted by permission from R. W. Houde, On assaying analgesics in man. In R. S. Knighton and P. R. Dumke, *Pain,* Copyright 1966 by Little, Brown.)

To obtain reliable results with a subjective test, the person scoring the test must not influence the results. As Rosenthal (1966) has shown, the only way to accomplish this end is to use the double-blind method. In this method, neither the scorer nor the subject knows the correct response. In cases where an analgesic drug is being tested, the physician must not know whether the patient is being given a placebo or an active drug. Also, the patient must not know whether he is being given a placebo or an active drug so that his statements about the pain will be unbiased.

When the above precautions are observed, it is almost impossible to show an effect of any of the analgesics on experimentally induced pain in the human (Beecher, 1966). Yet, the same drug that has no effect on pain produced by electrical stimulation in the laboratory will significantly reduce postoperative pain in the hospital. In the laboratory situation, the subject knows that he is going to receive a painful stimulus and he also knows that it can be stopped whenever he wants. This results in a different cognition from the person in the hospital who knows that he hurts but does not know how long the pain will last. A solution to the problem of evaluating the cognitive and emotional effects of an analgesic is to assess the analgesic in the clinical situation.

Summary

Although there is a considerable amount of experimental data on the neurology of pain, the relevance of these data for an understanding of the perception of pain and of pain-motivated behavior is not completely clear. Since the various techniques for evaluating analgesic potency show only a partial correlation, several should be used, as well as several different species of animals, in a screening program for analgesics. This animal screening is as important in bringing to light side effects and other contraindications as in establishing analgesic potency. The next step, laboratory tests in humans, can still be dangerous since human toxicity may not be predictable from animal studies. The final critical test, and really the only truly predictive one, is controlled clinical trials on the pain and suffering of human patients.

NARCOTIC ANALGESICS

The medical term *narcotic* refers to a group of drugs which has both sedative and analgesic properties. Until recently, this term was essentially restricted to the opiates (opium alkaloids which are derived from the dried juice of the unripe pod of the poppy, *Papaver somniferum,* and semi-synthetic derivatives of these alkaloids). The term is now also used to refer to certain synthetic drugs which share many of the properties of the opiates. Awareness of opium as a potent drug dates back to at least 4,000 B.C. Its use is clearly indicated in the Egyptian, Greek, and Roman cultures. Surprisingly, opium is still obtained by the methods used over 1,000 years ago. During the brief period between the time that the petals fall from the opium poppy and the time that the seed pod matures, opium is produced. Shallow cuts are made in the seed pods allowing the opium to escape. During the hours after the cuts are made in the pod, the opium seeps out and dries. The next day it is scraped off the pod as a latexlike substance. It is this sap from the opium poppy which is the base of the opiates such as morphine and codeine, and from which heroin is synthesized.

Opium has not always been known primarily as an analgesic. Galen (the Greek physician) stated that opium "resists poison and venomous bites, cures chronic headache, vertigo, deafness, epilepsy, apoplexy, dimness of sight, loss of voice, asthma, coughs of all kinds, spitting of blood, tightness of breath, colic, the iliac poison, jaundice, hardness of the spleen, stone urinary complaints, fevers, dropsies, leprosies, the troubles to which women are subject, melancholy, and all pestilences" (Scott, 1969, p. 111). Clearly, a drug of this potency deserves a place in history.

The modern spread of opium throughout the Western World may have begun with its use by Arabian physicians for the treatment of dysentery. Arabian traders then brought opium to China and the Orient as a cure for dysentery. The social use of opium by smoking became popular in the Orient only later in the 18th century. By the 18th century opium had also been introduced into Europe, but there the custom was opium eating rather than smoking. Many famous Europeans, including such literary greats as Elizabeth Barrett Browning, were addicted to a drug called *laudanum,* which is, according to one recipe, composed of one part each of opium, ipecac, and licorice to four parts each of potassium nitrate (saltpeter) and tartar. Thomas DeQuincy wrote of the visions seen under the influence of opium and the "Kubla Khan" was written by Coleridge upon awakening from an opium dream.

The development of the hypodermic syringe by Alexander Wood in 1853 ushered in the more serious problems resulting from the injection of opiates. Wood's wife holds the distinction of being the first person to die from a parenterally administered overdose of morphine (Cohen, 1970). Of possible interest to the student of psychology is the fact that Sigmund Freud, often cited as the founder of modern psychology, also died from an overdose of morphine, administered at his request when the pain of his facial cancer became too great (Schur, 1972).

In the early United States, opiate use advanced on two fronts. The Chinese workers, imported to build the rail lines connecting the east and west coast, brought with them the social custom of opium smoking. At the same time, a sudden upsurge in the use of patent medicines (most of which contained some form of opiate and a goodly amount of alcohol) brought drug addiction within reach of the common man. These patent medicines were advertised to bring relief from almost any ailment known to man. At one time in the late 1800s it was estimated that over 1% of the population of the United States was addicted to opiates, primarily from the intake of patent medicines.

Due to the ease of obtaining opiates during this period and their relatively low price, the problems of the opiate addict were similar to those of the alcoholic, and the severe social and legal problems attached to current narcotic use were not present. The Harrison Act in 1914 changed the situation of the opiate addict in the United States by making the nonprescription sale of opiates a criminal offense, thereby removing narcotic drugs from the open market. The opiate user was then forced to obtain his drugs by illegal means. This has led to the development of a modern drug problem with a government estimate of 250,000 heroin addicts in 1971, most of whom are young and from disadvantaged neighborhoods.

With the modern trend toward social acceptance of unusual lifestyles, more and more middle class youth are becoming addicted to opiates. The extent of the problem is suggested by the fact that more teenagers were killed in the city of New York during 1969 by heroin than by any other cause, including automobile accidents. In 1970, 1,154 deaths were attributed to drug addiction in New York City, with about 70% being a direct result of drug overdose while the other 30% resulted from drug related causes, such as hepatitis due to

THE NARCOTIC ANALGESICS 197

infected needles or impure drugs. For a more extensive review of the history of opiate use and the modern drug problem, see Ray (1972) or Brecher (1972).

The narcotic analgesics may be divided into three categories: (1) natural drugs, which include opium and the various alkaloids of opium such as morphine and codeine; (2) the semisynthetic drugs that are prepared by chemical synthesis from the natural drugs, the best example being heroin; (3) synthetic drugs which are prepared from a nonopiate base and some of which bear little chemical resemblance to the natural drugs. Examples of this class are meperidine and methadone.

Raw Opium

Raw opium contains several alkaloids, including some which are clinically useful as analgesics. The clinically useful alkaloids of opium are listed in Table 7.1. It can be seen that they may be divided into two classes based on their chemical structure. These two basic groups consist of the phenanthrenes and the benzylisoquinolines. The phenanthrenes, include morphine and codeine, which are known to be powerful analgesics, and thebaine, which is not an analgesic but produces convulsions in relatively low doses. The benzylisoquinoline derivative, papaverine, is a smooth muscle relaxant, while noscapine has found use as a cough suppressant. The chemical formulas for these alkaloids are shown in Figure 7.3.

Opium is available as a powder, or as gum opium, either of which contains 10% morphine as the primary active ingredient. Opium is also available as paregoric (camphorated opium tincture) or as laudanum. The main active ingredient in all of these preparations is morphine and the pharmacology of opium is essentially that of morphine.

Although many routes of administration are available for opium—smoking, snorting (using as snuff), parenteral, and oral—oral administration of opium is

TABLE 7.1

Alkaloids of Opium

Class	Natural alkaloid	Percentage in opium
Phenanthrene	Morphine	10.0
	Codeine	0.5
	Thebaine	0.2
Benzylquinoline	Papaverine	1.0
	Noscapine	6.0

Note. Reprinted by permission from J. H. Jaffe, Narcotic analgesics. In L. S. Goodman and A. Gilman (Eds.), *The Pharmacological Basis of Therapeutics* (4th ed.). Copyright 1970 by Macmillan Publishing Co.

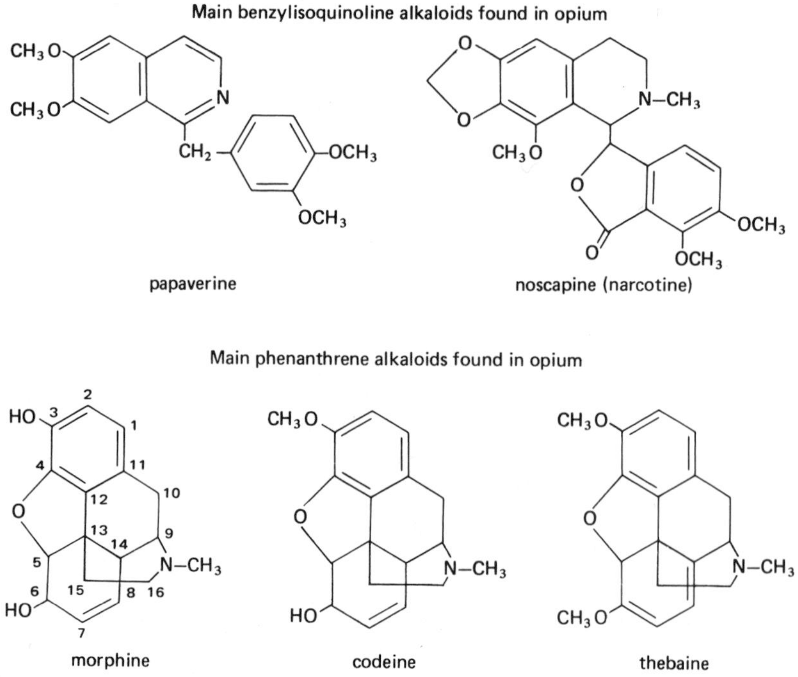

Main benzylisoquinoline alkaloids found in opium

papaverine

noscapine (narcotine)

Main phenanthrene alkaloids found in opium

morphine

codeine

thebaine

FIGURE 7.3.   The active opium alkaloids: Chemical structure.

the most common route (Jaffe, 1970b; Ray, 1972). These preparations of natural opium have previously found use for the relief of pain and in the treatment of intestinal overactivity. Although they are now little used as analgesics, paregoric is still used for infant colic and for diarrhea.

Morphine

Morphine is the primary alkaloid of opium and at the present time it is the most widely used analgesic for the relief of severe pain, a position which it has held from the time it was first isolated. The mechanism of action of this powerful drug, however, remains a mystery. This is due, in great part, to the large variety of effects produced by morphine. It is possible that the mechanism underlying the analgesic action of morphine may differ from the mechanism underlying the development of morphine dependence or that underlying the production of nausea. In spite of these complications, the mystery surrounding the analgesic action of morphine is decreasing. In this chapter we will review the available information concerning the locus and mechanism of the analgesic and other effects of morphine. Studies of metabolism, excretion, and brain uptake will be presented to assess the availability of morphine to the brain where its analgesic activity is thought to occur. Data concerning the areas of the brain involved in the analgesic and other effects of morphine will be presented and the interaction between morphine and certain putative neurotransmitters will be discussed.

Absorption. Morphine is usually administered parenterally and is approximately 30 times more potent by this route than when orally administered. For this reason, oral administration is not often practical. This is one major disadvantage of most of the narcotic analgesics. The level of morphine in the brain peaks between 30 minutes and 4 hours following an intraperitoneal injection. Following intravenous injection, morphine rarely requires more than 30 minutes to reach peak concentration (Clouet, 1971). It is generally recognized that the effects of morphine on pain perception are primarily of central origin. The entry of morphine into the brain is, therefore, a critical event. When morphine is administered either orally or parenterally, it must travel through the circulatory system to the brain and then pass from the blood into the brain. Many chemicals including morphine do not pass easily from blood to brain; a blood-brain barrier must be crossed before morphine can exert an effect on the brain. The mechanism underlying the blood-brain barrier to morphine is not well understood. It may simply be a passive barrier whereby the diffusion of morphine into the brain is hindered (Wang & Takemori, 1972), or it may involve the active transport of morphine both into and out of the brain (Loh, Shen & Way, 1971; Scrafani & Hug, 1968; Way, 1967). An important aspect of the blood-brain barrier to morphine is the fact that this barrier is not well developed in infants, and the dosage of morphine required for an infant is, therefore, lower than would be expected from studies on the adult. Heroin, which enters the brain more easily than morphine, does not show such an increased effectiveness in infants (Way, 1967; Way, W. L., Costle, & Way, E. L., 1965).

Metabolism and excretion. The metabolic breakdown of narcotic analgesics differs from drug to drug and from species to species. Nevertheless, the two most important routes are *N*-dealkylation and conjugation as glucuronides. Most of the metabolic breakdown occurs in the liver and care must be exercised when administering narcotic analgesics to patients with liver dysfunction. In the human, approximately 90% of the morphine can be accounted for by excretion through the kidneys as a glucuronide (Jaffe, 1970b).

The locus of action of morphine within the brain. Morphine may have some effect on pain at the level of the spinal cord. Inhibition of the reflex withdrawal of a painfully stimulated limb has been demonstrated in human patients with complete spinal cord transection above the level of the stimulation (Jaffe, 1970b). Nonetheless, the major effect of morphine on pain and suffering does not seem to occur at the spinal level. The inhibition of spinal reflexes is slight and occurs at relatively high doses. The major effect of morphine is thought to be on the integration of sensory information once it has reached the brain and minute quantities of morphine injected directly into the substance of the brain or into the ventricles have been shown to produce analgesia. This leaves little doubt that the primary analgesic effect of morphine is on the brain.

Three basic strategies have been followed in attempts to determine the locus of action of morphine in the brain. In order for a drug to influence the brain, it must first make physical contact with cells in the area to be affected. This involves binding of the drug to these cells and, therefore, involves an increase in the drug concentration as compared to areas where the drug is not effective. By measuring the concentration of morphine in various areas of the brain, the sites of morphine binding can be determined. A second common method of determining whether an area is involved in a given drug effect is to remove that brain area and look at the effect of this removal on drug activity. The third method involves the microinjection of small quantities of a drug into a circumscribed brain area. The drug can only directly affect primarily the area into which it was injected and any behavioral change resulting from microinjection would, therefore, be due to action at the site of injection.

The site of morphine binding. A commonly accepted mode for the action of psychoactive drugs involves the attachment, or binding of the drug to certain sites (called *receptor sites*) on a neuron. Only drugs with certain physical and chemical properties will become attached to a given receptor site. Once bound to its receptor, the drug then exerts its behavioral effect by causing a change in the excitability of the neuron to which it has become bound.

The binding of a narcotic drug to the receptor site is a necessary step in the production of a behavioral effect. Recent studies (Pert & Snyder, 1973) have shown that there is a site on the neuron which acts as a morphine receptor. Binding sites for morphine have been found on the neurons of many vertebrate brains, including mammals, birds, reptiles, amphibia, and fish. Morphine binding sites have not been observed in arthropods or platyhelminths (Pert, Pasternak, & Snyder, 1973). The binding of morphine to neural tissue occurs primarily at the synapse and most probably at the post-synaptic membrane. Thus, the attachment of morphine to this receptor site would influence synaptic transmission at that site (Pert, Snowman & Snyder, 1974).

Not all neurons contain morphine receptors and the direct effect of morphine is restricted to those neurons which do have a morphine receptor. By determining which areas of the brain contain neurons with morphine receptors, one can locate areas of potential analgesic activity. Brain structures found to be especially rich in morphine receptors include the basal ganglia and midbrain, while the cerebral cortex and cerebellum contain few such receptors. From these data, one might suspect that the basal ganglia and midbrain are areas where morphine has its greatest effect. Unfortunately, while the binding of a drug to its receptor site is necessary for the production of a change in the activity of a neuron, it is not necessarily sufficient. Furthermore, morphine produces many effects, only some of which are related to analgesia. Thus, while morphine binds most strongly in the basal ganglia, microinjections of morphine into this area do not produce analgesia. Microinjection of morphine into the midbrain, however, does produce analgesia (Tsou & Jang, 1964).

Studies attempting to determine the site of action of morphine by selective lesioning of the brain have for the most part been unsuccessful. One bright note is a study by Kerr and Pozuelo (1971), which showed that if rats were made physically dependent upon morphine by chronic morphine injections, lesions of the ventromedial hypothalamus or rostral septum resulted in a loss of their tolerance. These areas may, therefore, be involved in the development of morphine tolerance. This result raises the rather disturbing possibility of employing brain lesions as a treatment for opiate dependence in human addicts. It should be mentioned that there currently are neurosurgeons employing brain lesions in humans (psychosurgery) as a treatment for a variety of sociopathic behaviors (Holden, 1973).

Microinjection studies. Precise localization of the areas of the brain responsible for the various actions of morphine has been attempted using the method of chemical microinjection. Injection of morphine into the ventricles is 500 times as effective in the production of analgesia as is systemic injection of morphine (Tsou & Jang, 1964). Similar results have been found for the addictive properties of morphine (Herz, Teschemacher, Albus, & Zeiglgansberger, 1972). In rabbits made tolerant by continued systemic administration of morphine, microinjections of a morphine antagonist into the lateral or third ventricle produce mild withdrawal symptoms. In contrast, if the antagonist is injected into the fourth ventricle, severe withdrawal symptoms are produced, with death occurring in some animals. This suggests that the area around the fourth ventricle is strongly involved in the maintenance of tolerance to morphine (Herz et al., 1972).

Rather than injecting morphine into the ventricular system, several investigators have made injections directly into brain tissue. This latter method allows a more precise localization of the area affected by the microinjection. Tsou and Jang (1964) microinjected morphine into several sites in the rabbit brain and tested for analgesia as a result of these microinjections. They found that morphine was effective in producing analgesia when injected into the periventricular or periaqueductal gray of the midbrain, but was ineffective when injected into the posteromedial thalamus, the region of the lateral geniculate body, the midbrain reticular formation, tectum, hippocampus, caudate nucleus, or the septal region. This would suggest a rather well-localized analgesic effect of morphine which is confined to the periventricular and periaqueductal gray areas of the midbrain. Wei and others (1972) microinjected a narcotic antagonist into several areas of the brain in morphine-addicted rats. Microinjections into medial thalamus, periaqueductal gray, and periventricular gray precipitated withdrawal symptoms, while microinjections into the midbrain reticular system, hippocampus, or cerebral cortex produced no effect. The areas of overlap in these last two studies suggest that the production of analgesia and of physical dependence may involve overlapping structures.

It is also interesting that these areas directly overlap those from which analgesia may be produced by electrical stimulation. Several investigators

(Mayer, Wolfle, Akil, Carder, & Liebeskind, 1971; Reynolds, 1969) have described analgesia in the rat following electrical stimulation of the periventricular or periaqueductal gray. The similarity between morphine analgesia and analgesia produced by electrical stimulation of the central gray of the midbrain is further suggested by Akil and Mayer (1972) who found that both morphine analgesia and analgesia produced by electrical stimulation of the central gray were reduced by the serotonin synthesis inhibitor, parachlorophenylalanine.

Interestingly, while the areas where electrical and chemical stimulation by morphine will elicit analgesia overlap, the overlap is not complete. Electrical stimulation of the periventricular or periaqueductal gray of the rat produces a strong analgesic effect, while the microinjection of morphine into the same areas produces an extreme hypersensitivity to stimulation. Following the microinjection of morphine into these areas in the rat, the slightest noise is sufficient to produce a violent stereotyped jumping response, which is often accompanied by vocalization and which is so severe that rats occasionally die from convulsions produced when their heads strike the ceiling or walls of the experimental chamber (Jacquet & Lajtha, 1973). This anomalous effect of morphine microinjection does not appear to occur in the rabbit (as we have reported earlier). Tsou and Jang (1964) found analgesia when they microinjected morphine into the periventricular or periaqueductal gray of the rabbit. Thus, the microinjection of morphine into discreet brain sites does not necessarily mimic the effects of systemic morphine injections. This should not be surprising in light of the many differing effects of systemic morphine injections. It was suggested earlier that some of the effects of morphine administration could be separated chemically and this study by Jacquet and Lajtha shows that it is also possible to separate these effects neuroanatomically as well.

The small circumscribed area suggested responsible for the analgesic activity of morphine by these studies has not been confirmed by all investigators. In one study, morphine was found to be effective in producing analgesia when microinjected into several brain areas, including the anterior hypothalamus and preoptic area (Lotti, Lomax, & George, 1965). This discrepancy emphasizes the need for further investigation of the site of narcotic analgesic activity under better controlled conditions. Studies employing differing definitions of analgesia cannot be directly compared, as morphine microinjected into a given site may produce analgesia for only a limited area of the body. While a tail pinch might not reveal analgesia, a toe pinch might.

Biochemical correlates. Transmission of information between neurons in the mammalian nervous system is mediated by certain chemicals acting as synaptic transmitters. It has been known for some years (Miller, 1965) that a given brain locus may participate in several response systems and that these overlapping systems may retain their functional discreteness through the chemical specificity of synapses at the site of overlap.

Therefore, the microinjection of a drug, for instance morphine, into a given site may also produce several effects. Microinjections of morphine have produced changes in body temperature, catatonia, and both increases and decreases in behavioral motility, as well as analgesia and physical dependence (Herz & Teschemacher, 1971; Lotti et al., 1965). Several investigators have attempted to separate these effects neurochemically to determine which, if any, of the suspected neurotransmitters are involved in the analgesic action of morphine. These investigators have found interactions between morphine and the cholinergic, adrenergic, and serotonergic neurotransmitter systems.

If, indeed, the multitude of effects attributed to the action of morphine on the nervous system may be separated neurochemically, these effects might then be amenable to selective modification by the administration of a blocking agent which affects only the neurotransmitter system involved in the production of a specified effect. A large body of data has been collected concerning the interaction of morphine with the various putative neurotransmitter systems. Only a small portion of the available information will be reviewed here. The interested reader is referred to Clouet (1971) for a more detailed review of the neurochemical correlates of morphine administration.

The cholinergic system: Acetylcholine is almost certainly a neurotransmitter in the brain (see Chapter 2). There is some evidence that the analgesic effects of morphine are mediated, at least in part, by this system. Several cholinergic compounds including arecoline, oxotremorine, and RS–86 (Sandoz) have been shown to produce analgesia when injected peripherally. These drugs also produce analgesia when microinjected into certain sites in the brain. The cholinergic drug, carbachol, which is a quaternary ammonium compound and will not pass across the blood-brain barrier, does not produce analgesia when injected systemically. It does produce analgesia, however, when microinjected directly into the brain. This suggests that the analgesia produced by these cholinergic compounds is of central origin.

Even though the brain sites where microinjection of cholinergic compounds will produce analgesia overlap those sites where morphine microinjection will produce analgesia, the analgesic action of morphine does not appear to be due entirely to its activity on cholinergic neurons. This is shown by the fact that while the analgesia produced by the cholinergic substances is reversed by the systemic injection of the cholinergic blocking agent atropine, analgesia produced by morphine injection is not affected by atropine (Herz & Metys, 1968; Metys, Wagner, Metysova, & Herz, 1969). It may be that, although the morphine receptor is sensitive to cholinergic agonists, the receptor is not truly cholinergic, or at least does not conform to the peripheral nervous system model of cholinergic receptors (and thus is not blocked by a cholinergic receptor blocking agent).

The mechanism underlying the interaction between morphine and the cholinergic system is not clear, but morphine has been shown to affect several aspects of the entire cholinergic system, from the release of acetylcholine at the presynaptic junction through its destruction by hydrolysis. Morphine has been shown to inhibit the release of acetylcholine from preganglionic fibers and from whole brain preparations (Beleslin & Polak, 1965). Morphine has also been shown to be a competitive inhibitor of the postsynaptic acetylcholine binding system (Kuriyama, Roberts, & Vos, 1968) and has been shown to block the hydrolysis of acetylcholine by cholinesterase (Schaumann, 1959). Thus, morphine interferes with the release, binding, and hydrolysis of acetylcholine, suggesting a complex relationship between morphine and cholinergic neurons in the brain.

The catecholamine system: The analgesic and excitant effects of morphine have been shown to be intimately related to the catecholamine content of the brain. Injections of morphine cause the release of catecholamines from both the brain and the adrenal glands (Ray, Mukherj, & Ghosh, 1968). Drugs which alter the level of brain catecholamines have been shown to affect morphine-induced analgesia. The administration of reserpine, which causes an initial release of norepinephrine, followed by eventual depletion of the norepinephrine stores of the brain, has been shown to increase the analgesic effect of morphine if injected simultaneously with the morphine but to decrease or eliminate the analgesic effects of morphine if administered 24 hours prior to the morphine. Thus, the initial release of norepinephrine caused by reserpine injection was related to an increase in morphine-induced analgesia while the later depletion of norepinephrine stores was correlated with a decrease in morphine-induced analgesia. This implies that norepinephrine-containing neurons must be functional for morphine to produce analgesia.

The involvement of norepinephrine-containing neurons is further documented by the correlation between the amount of norepinephrine released in the brain by an injection of morphine and the level of analgesia resulting from that injection. When given equal doses of morphine, animals that show greater release of norepinephrine also show greater analgesia (Paalzow & Paalzow, 1971). Morphine administration appears to result in the increased release and eventual depletion of norepinephrine. This effect is blocked by the morphine antagonist, naloxone, which also blocks the analgesic action of morphine. Furthermore, the decrease in analgesia that accompanies the development of tolerance to morphine is paralleled by a decrease in the ability of morphine to liberate norepinephrine (Rethy, Smith, & Villarreal, 1971).

It would, therefore, seem that the release and subsequent depletion of norepinephrine stores in the brain by morphine are directly related to the analgesic effects of this alkaloid and its derivatives. Unfortunately, the use of agents like reserpine results in a decrease in brain levels of serotonin as well as of norepinephrine. The relative contributions of these two substances is, therefore, unclear. Attempts to alter the norepinephrine level without concurrently changing serotonin levels have met with rather mixed results. Both increases and decreases in the level of morphine analgesia have been found following pretreatment with alpha-methylparatyrosine (AMPT) or disulfiram, both of which deplete norepinephrine levels independently of serotonin levels (Major & Pleuvry, 1971). Recently, studies using 6-hydroxydopamine, which selectively destroys noradrenergic nerve endings and thereby reduces the concentration of norepinephrine in the brain, have demonstrated an effect of lowered norepinephrine content on morphine-induced analgesia. There is some question as to the direction of the effect, however, as Samanin and Bernasconi (1972) found an increase in morphine-induced analgesia following intraventricularly administered 6-hydroxydopamine, while Ayhan (1972) found a decrease in morphine-induced analgesia following a similar procedure. Clearly, more research is needed in this area, the only point agreed upon is that changes in adrenergic neurons are correlated with changes in the analgesic effectiveness of morphine.

Morphine is generally described as a sedating agent. Earlier in the chapter, however, it was stated that morphine acts as a behavioral excitant in some species. There is evidence that a similar excitant effect occurs in the human, but that it is masked by a stronger depressive effect. At the extremely high doses required for morphine anesthesia (as high as 600 to 800 mg) convulsive movements occur and a muscle relaxant must be used before surgery may be continued (Hasbrouck, 1970). There is also some evidence from animal studies that the excitant and depressive effects of morphine may be separated neurochemically. Following chronic administration of large doses of morphine, tolerance develops to the depressant but not to the excitant effects (Babbini & Davis, 1972). This excitatory effect of morphine intake is then inhibited by AMPT at a dosage which inhibited brain eatecholamine content by 50%. This suggests that the excitant effects of morphine are dependent upon normal availability of brain catecholamines (Davis, Babbini, & Khalsa, 1972). AMPT also has been shown to block the development of self-administration of both morphine and amphetamine in the rat (Davis & Smith, 1972). These authors suggested that AMPT acted to block the reinforcing aspects of morphine administration. Could the reinforcing and activating aspects of morphine be mediated by a different mechanism than the analgesic effects? If so, perhaps morphine, in conjunction with AMPT, can produce analgesia without addiction. This hypothesis remains to be tested in the human.

The serotonergic system: The neuroanatomic system of serotonin-containing neurons has been linked to the ability of morphine to produce physical dependence, as well as analgesia. Brain serotonin levels can be lowered by the administration of parachlorophenylalanine (PCPA) or reserpine. PCPA is a competitive inhibitor of tryptophan hydroxylase, the enzyme which controls the rate-limiting step in the production of serotonin (see Chapter 2). As was previously mentioned, reserpine causes the release and eventual depletion of several amines, including serotonin. The development of tolerance to morphine can be blocked by maintaining an animal on either PCPA or reserpine, while giving daily injections of morphine in quantities large enough that tolerance would normally develop. The effect of reserpine or PCPA on morphine tolerance can be reversed by injecting serotonin into the ventricular system to restore the normal level of brain serotonin. Systemic injections of serotonin have no effect because serotonin does not cross the blood-brain barrier. Five-hydroxy-tryptophan, which is the immediate precursor of serotonin, does cross the blood-brain barrier and once inside the brain is converted into serotonin. Systemic injections of 5-hydroxytryptophan also reverse this effect of reserpine or PCPA on morphine tolerance. This indicates that it is the influence of PCPA or reserpine on the function of serotonergic neurons that is important in the inhibition of the development of tolerance to morphine (Contreras & Tamayo, 1967; Ho, Loh, & Way, 1973; Ho, Lu, Stolman, Loh, & Way, 1972).

Further evidence for the involvement of serotonergic neurons in the development of tolerance to morphine stems from studies showing that when rats are made tolerant to morphine by chronic morphine injections, their rate of serotonin synthesis doubles when compared to control animals who are not morphine dependent. Simultaneous injection of morphine and naloxone, a morphine antagonist, does not lead to the development of morphine tolerance and no change in the rate of serotonin production results from this procedure. This suggests that there is a relationship between serotonin production and the development of tolerance to morphine such that an increase in serotonin production is necessary for the development of morphine tolerance (Shen, Low, & Way, 1969).

It is possible to reduce the serotonin levels in the brain by lesioning the raphe nucleus of the brainstem (as well as by administering reserpine or PCPA). This nucleus contains the cell bodies for most of the serotonin-containing neurons in the brain. Raphe lesions have been found to reduce the analgesic effect of morphine (Samanin & Bernasconi, 1972) and the effects of morphine on body temperature (Samanin et al., 1971). While lesions of the raphe nucleus reduce the total brain concentration of serotonin, stimulation of this nucleus increases the level of serotonin in the brain. If decreased serotonin content in the brain decreases the analgesic action of morphine, then an increase in serotonin due to raphe nucleus stimulation would be expected to potentiate morphine-induced analgesia; and this has been found (Samanin et al., 1971).

Summary: There appear to be certain preliminary conclusions that can be reached based on these data. First, it appears likely that receptors critically involved in the analgesic action of morphine are located in the midbrain. It is also likely that receptors involved in the analgesic and other aspects of morphine's effects are also located elsewhere in the brain. These effects include the sedation, excitation, euphoria, physical dependence, and tolerance that one sees with the narcotic drugs. The extent to which all or several of these actions are different aspects of a unitary action or process remains unclear. With respect to biochemical processes, cholinergic drugs share to some extent the analgesic properties of the narcotics, while noradrenergic and serotonergic systems both seem also involved in analgesia. It would appear that drug-induced analgesia is a complex process involving, to some extent, all three of the predominant brain biochemical systems. There may be a variety of subsystems involved in analgesia (as well as euphoria, sedation, excitation, tolerance and dependence), and these subsystems may involve all three primary biochemical transmitter systems.

Clinical uses of morphine (analgesia). Morphine is a very effective analgesic, with a 10-mg dose (by injection) bringing relief from pain in most clinical situations. The relief from pain and suffering brought about by morphine, in combination with its sleep-inducing and euphoric properties, make it an almost ideal preparation for postoperative pain. Morphine relieves not only the pain, but also the dread and anxiety often accompanying surgical procedures. This relief from dread and anxiety also makes morphine popular as a preanesthetic medication to help relieve the worry a patient often feels before major surgery. Only its side effects prevent morphine from realizing its full potential as a panacea in situations involving aversive stimulation or the threat of aversive stimulation. Many of the nonanalgesic effects of morphine also find usefulness in the clinical situation although an effect useful in one situation may be harmful in another.

Although morphine is a powerful analgesic, it has equally powerful side effects. It is, therefore, used primarily in situations where the less potent analgesics, with correspondingly less dangerous side effects, are not effective. The most common clinical use of morphine is for the relief of postoperative pain. Morphine is a nearly ideal drug for this type of pain which contains a large affective component. The sleep-inducing and euphoric effects of morphine bring relief not only from the pain which often follows surgical procedures, but also from the many unpleasant emotional responses associated with convalescence.

Morphine has always been a vital element in the military doctor's kit. The suffering due to wounds inflicted in battle is quite effectively relieved by morphine. Morphine has often been abused in this situation and after the American Civil War, morphine addiction was called the "soldier's disease" because it was so commonly seen in returning soldiers. Under most circumstances, an analgesic is needed only for a short period of time and the risk of addiction is, therefore, quite low.

Morphine is the most effective agent known for the relief of pain and suffering due to terminal cancer. Here, relief from dread is as important as the relief of pain. Addiction is considered a minor side effect in cases of terminal illness, but the dosage is held as low as is consistent with relief from pain in order to retard the development of tolerance. Even when the use of morphine is held to a minimum, severe tolerance will develop over a period of months and care must be exercised to insure that as the symptoms worsen, effective analgesia will still be obtainable. Occasionally, toward the end of a terminal illness when tolerance has developed to morphine, psychosurgery is the only remaining method which will produce effective analgesia.

Morphine is sometimes used in the clinic to reduce the pain of childbirth. However, morphine administered to the mother crosses the placental barrier and produces effects in the newborn. Among the effects of morphine on the newborn is a depression of respiration, which can cause serious complications. For this reason, morphine is not now commonly used during childbirth.

Other effects of morphine. As can be seen, morphine has many side effects which must be carefully considered before morphine is prescribed in any given situation. In the following section, the side effects of morphine will be examined in greater detail.

Euphoria: This is probably one of the most discussed effects of the narcotic drugs. Opium smoking for the purpose of producing euphoria has had a long history and the morphine content of opium is the responsible agent in the production of euphoria. It is probably for its euphoric effect that opium was first used. The sleepy (Morpheus is the Greek God of dreams), relaxed, "high" feeling often attributed to the intake of narcotics is not, however, a universal phenomenon. Most people who are not in pain find the effects of morphine either neutral or dysphoric (unpleasant). Only about 10% of the normal population who take morphine find it euphoric (Beecher, 1966). As many as 40% of the population find it to be dysphoric, with the remainder (50%) reporting a neutral experience. Many narcotic addicts report that their first experiences with narcotics were unpleasant and that they had to learn to appreciate the euphoria (Ray, 1972).

In considering the analgesic and euphoric effects of morphine and the other narcotics, one is led to wonder whether these two effects have a common mechanism. Euphoria is found primarily in those who are in pain, and thus benefiting from the analgesic activity of the narcotics. Euphoria is said to be produced by narcotics in only about 10% of the normal population (those not in pain). Perhaps a psychological pain is relieved in this group. Pain is certainly the supreme aversive stimulus and we have some knowledge of the aversion system of the brain. The periventricular system (PVS) traveling from the medial-dorsal midbrain to the thalamus has been implicated as a potent aversion system. It could be that the narcotics depress the aversion systems of the brain (such as the PVS) and that this selective depression of neural firing is responsible for both the analgesia and the euphoria found in humans who are suffering, whether due to illness or difficulties with life in general. Major advantages of this hypothesis are its parsimony and the unitary conceptualization of centrally mediated analgesia and euphoria. Such an inhibition of the aversive PVS system would enable an unopposed MFB reward system to become more active than normal. Such reciprocal relations between the MFB and PVS have been demonstrated (Olds & Olds, 1964).

Nausea: The primary cause of a dysphoric response to morphine is nausea. Nausea occurs as a result of morphine injection in about 40% of the normal population. In immobilized, bedridden patients, the incidence of nausea is much lower. It has been suggested that there is a strong vestibular effect on morphine-induced nausea and that the bedridden patient avoids nausea by virtue of the decrease in vestibular input resulting from his decreased motility (Jaffe,

1970b). The nausea and emesis produced by the narcotics seem to result from an action on certain structures in the medulla of the brainstem. Most morphine derivatives produce a degree of nausea equal to that produced by morphine in an equal analgesic dose (Jaffe, 1970b).

Respiratory depression: Death from an overdose of morphine, heroin, or any narcotic is almost invariably a result of the respiratory depression produced by these drugs. This respiratory depressant effect is mediated by a direct action on the brainstem respiratory centers. This depression of respiration typically begins within minutes of an intravenous dose of morphine and lasts from 2 to 5 hours. Narcotic analgesics do not depress the voluntary control of breathing and if the patient remains conscious, breathing may be maintained by simply periodically asking him to breathe. In severe poisoning, where consciousness is lost or severely impaired, artificial respiration is necessary to prevent death from hypoxia.

The respiratory depression produced by morphine is primarily a result of a decrease in the sensitivity of medullary centers which are sensitive to elevated carbon dioxide levels in the blood. Therefore, administration of pure oxygen may deplete the carbon dioxide level of the blood to the point where these centers are no longer stimulated and the patient stops breathing. Pure oxygen is, thus, not recommended for narcotic poisoning (Jaffe, 1970b). Caffeine is effective in reducing respiratory depression caused by morphine (Murphree, 1971). The cup of coffee invariably offered to the victim of a narcotic overdose in the movies is, therefore, a somewhat effective antidote for morphine poisoning. The best physiological antidote for morphine poisoning is pain (Jaffe, 1970b). Painful stimulation, by arousing the patient, will cause some return of consciousness, allowing voluntary breathing to be resumed (Jameson & Hasbrouck, 1971).

Although most of the morphine derivatives possess respiratory depressive activity in direct relation to their analgesic potency, the morphine antagonists (cyclazocine and levallorphan) have been found to produce analgesia without the severe respiratory depression found with the other morphine derivatives. These drugs will be discussed separately as they have many properties which distinguish them from the narcotic analgesics.

Antitussive action: Morphine inhibits the cough reflex and has been used as an antitussive in the relief of pathological cough. This antitussive action can be dissociated from the analgesic and respiratory effects of morphine; morphine derivatives, such as dextromethorphan, which are nonnarcotic and have no respiratory effects, are available as cough suppressants.

Pupil response: Morphine has a miotic (constricting) effect on the pupil. Pinpoint pupil is one obvious sign of morphine poisoning and, unfortunately, masks other pupillary signs which might be due to neurological disturbance. For this reason, morphine is often not used when head injury is present or when damage to the central nervous system is suspected. The use of morphine in these situations would invalidate one of the neurologist's most useful indices of nervous system function. Tolerance does not develop to the miotic effects of morphine and constricted pupils result from doses of narcotics too small to have a noticeable behavioral effect in the tolerant person.

Gut action: Morphine has a strong effect on the digestive system. Doses smaller than those necessary to produce analgesia, will produce constipation. This results from a decrease in the parastaltic motion of the stomach and intestines together with constriction of the pyloric and anal sphincters. The result is a delay in the passage of food through the system. This will cause constipation as a side effect in the normal person or will correct diarrhea in a person suffering from this disorder. In the past, relief of diarrhea has been one of the main uses of opium alkaloids. Tolerance to the constipating effect of morphine is slow to develop, leading to constipation as a chronic complaint of the narcotic addict (Jaffe, 1970b).

Other side effects: Two extremely important side effects of morphine are tolerance and addiction. These will be treated separately, later in this chapter, as they relate to all of the narcotic analgesics. The various effects of morphine on the body are summarized in Table 7.2. It should not be surprising that the mechanism of action of morphine on the body is not well understood, if for no reason other than the sheer number of morphine effects.

Contraindications: Due to its depressive effect on respiration, morphine is contraindicated in conditions where respiration is compromized. Morphine interacts with drugs affecting catecholamine and indolamine metabolism. These include MAO inhibitors, phenothiazines, tricyclic antidepressants and amphetamines. Caution is, therefore, required when treating patients who have been pretreated with these rather commonly used drugs. Many deaths, which have been classified as having been due to heroin overdose, have in fact been due to the interaction of heroin with other drugs. One of the greatest dangers of the so-called street drugs stems from the common practice of multiple drug usage. A notable example is the common use of methamphetamine by heroin addicts. Methamphetamine has been shown to significantly reduce the lethal dose of heroin in animals. The additive effects of morphine and alcohol in producing severe respiratory depression are well known; yet, death from this drug combination is quite common (Dubas, Lundy, Calhoun, & Parker, 1972; Jaffe, 1970a).

The Other Narcotic Drugs

Morphine is only one of the narcotic analgesics. A description of the behavioral and pharmacological effects of morphine has been presented in detail because it is representative of the entire class. We will now briefly examine a few of the other more common narcotic analgesics. These will include another opium alkaloid (codeine), a semisynthetic narcotic (heroin), and two synthetic narcotic analgesics (meperidine and methadone).

TABLE 7.2

Effects of Morphine

On	Effect
Higher CNS structures	Analgesia a. elevation of the pain threshold b. dissociation of pain perception from reaction to pain
Other areas of the CNS	Nausea and vomiting (medulla) Suppression of coughing Miosis (oculomotor nucleus) Respiratory depression (medulla)
Behavior	Euphoria/dysphoria Excitation/depression
Cardiovascular system	Depression of heart rate Postural hypotension Flushing of skin
Smooth muscles	Contraction of sphincters a. constipation b. urinary retention
Metabolism	Hyperglycemia
The skin	Triple response (intradermal injections only) Itching and sweating

Codeine

Raw opium is composed of about 0.5% codeine. The pharmacology of codeine is similar to that of morphine with two notable exceptions: (1) Codeine is much less powerful than morphine on a dose for dose basis (Table 7.3). (2) The ratio of oral to parenteral effectiveness for codeine is higher than that for morphine. Codeine retains about two-thirds of its effectiveness when taken orally as compared to parenterally. Morphine, on the other hand, retains only about one-thirtieth of its potency when taken orally.

It has often been stated that codeine is less addicting than morphine, but if equal analgesic doses are used, there is no difference in the addictive properties of the two drugs (Jaffe, 1970b). There is, therefore, no reason to use codeine over morphine if the route of administration is parenteral. The higher oral to

TABLE 7.3

Relative Analgesic Potency
of Some Morphine
Derivatives

Drug	Potency
Morphine	1
Methadone	1
Heroin	3
Phenazocine	3
Hydromorphine	3.5
Levorphenol	4
Desomorphine	10
Oxymorphine	10
M99	1,200
M183	1,500
Meperidine	1/10
Codeine	1/12

parenteral efficiency ratio of codeine has led to its use in orally administered analgesics and antitussives. For the relief of minor pain and coughing, relatively small amounts of codeine are effective and present little addictive liability. For this purpose, codeine is often compounded with other non-narcotic analgesics such as aspirin. The combination of these two drugs (codeine and aspirin) gives greater analgesia than that produced by either drug alone.

Heroin: A Semisynthetic Narcotic

Heroin is a semisynthetic narcotic which is formed from morphine by the addition of two acetyl groups to the morphine molecule. Chemically, it is diacetyl morphine. Heroin itself has little pharmacological activity but is converted in the brain first to monoacetyl morphine and then to morphine. It is these two metabolic products rather than the heroin which are responsible for the analgesic and other narcotic properties for which heroin is known (Way, 1968).

If the primary active product of heroin is morphine, one might ask how there could be any differences in action between the two drugs. In particular, why is heroin known to be more powerful than morphine on a dose for dose basis? Earlier, it was mentioned that there is a barrier between the blood and brain such that morphine does not easily enter the brain. This barrier is much less effective against heroin, allowing it to enter the brain much more rapidly and possibly in greater concentration than morphine. For this reason, heroin is a more potent drug than morphine and its faster onset of action results in a "rush" which is valued by the narcotic addict. Since there is no difference between the action of morphine and heroin on pain perception, but there is an increased addiction risk for heroin, heroin is not used for medical purposes (at least in the United States). In Great Britain heroin is used in clinical medicine and there are reports that it is more effective than morphine for certain uses (for example, to achieve postoperative analgesia in children). The potency and rapid onset of action with heroin, however, make it the choice for illicit use in both the United States and Great Britain (Jaffe, 1970a, 1970b).

The history of heroin use begins in 1874 when it was first synthesized from morphine. In 1898, it was placed on the market by the Bayer Company of Germany as a nonaddicting substitute for morphine. Early studies published in the New York Medical Journal in 1900 indicated that it was a relatively safe drug with only minor addicting properites. Within a few years, however, the true addicting properties of heroin became known (it is, if anything, more addicting than morphine). This information together with the Harrison Act of 1914, which made the unauthorized possession and sale of narcotics a criminal offense, removed heroin use from the medical sphere to the underworld (Ray, 1972).

Presently, except for research purposes, heroin is available in the United States only through illegal channels. The pusher prefers heroin to morphine because it is approximately three times as potent on a gram-for-gram basis (since more of it penetrates the blood-brain barrier in comparison to morphine); for that reason, smaller amounts need to be smuggled into the country. The user prefers heroin to other narcotics because of its more rapid onset of action (because of more rapid blood-brain barrier penetration).

Pharmacology. As morphine is the primary active metabolite of heroin, the pharmacology of heroin is essentially that of morphine with three primary differences, all of which can be traced to the differences in blood-brain barrier effects of the two drugs. These differences are: (1) a more rapid onset of action for heroin, (2) a higher peak analgesic action for heroin, and (3) slightly more rapid elimination of heroin from the body with withdrawal symptoms appearing approximately 4 hours after a heroin injection as opposed to 5 hours after a morphine injection (Jaffe, 1970b).

Meperidine

Meperidine (Demerol or Pethadine) is a synthetic analgesic with little chemical resemblance to morphine. It has the structure pictured in Figure 7.4. Meperidine was originally prepared as a result of attempts to create an atropinelike drug. During testing, one of the synthetic drugs was found to have analgesic properties similar to morphine. Due to meperidine's chemical dissimilarity to morphine, it was hoped that it might not possess some of the undesirable side effects of the morphinelike drugs. Subsequent experimentation revealed that despite the chemical differences between morphine and meperidine, the physiological effects of the two drugs were almost identical. It is now clear that the same receptor mechanism is acted upon by morphine and meperidine.

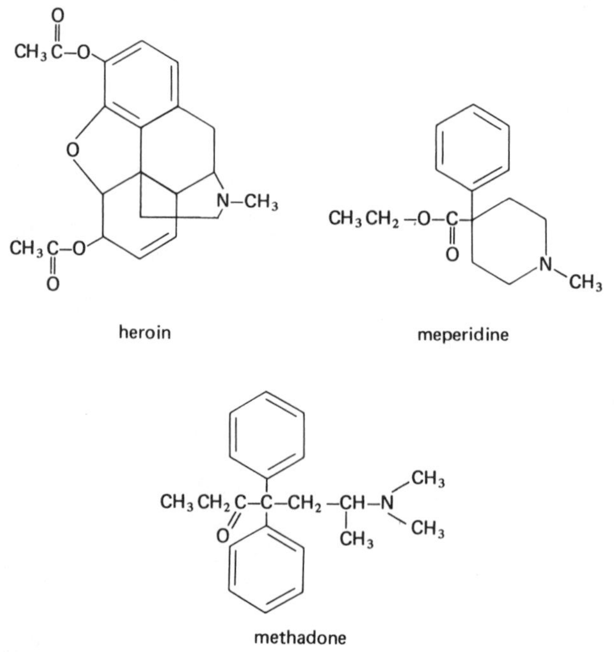

FIGURE 7.4.   Some semisynthetic and synthetic narcotic analgesics.

Meperidine may be taken orally or parenterally with parenteral administration being approximately twice as effective as oral administration. One-hundred milligrams of meperidine taken parenterally is equal analgesic to ten mg of morphine. Meperidine is faster acting than morphine and peak analgesia is reached in about 15 minutes following intravenous administration. The analgesic activity declines rapidly over the next 2 hours, giving meperidine a short period of action. Most of the meperidine is hydrolized by the liver but about one-third is N-demethylated to produce normeperidine. This metabolic product is a mild convulsant and when tolerance develops to meperidine's analgesic effect, an increase in the dose which would then be required to produce effective analgesia could result in tremor and convulsions. Apparently, tolerance does not develop to the convulsive effects of normeperidine. This problem is aggravated when an MAO inhibitor is used in conjunction with the narcotic (normeperidine is a monoamine and is detoxified by monoamine oxidase).

The hydrolized end products of meperidine and normeperidine are finally secreted into the urine and eliminated. The physiological effects of meperidine are similar to those of morphine with the exceptions of a shorter period of action and a lesser constipating effect from meperidine (it is ineffective in the treatment of diarrhea).

Although tolerance and physical dependence are slower to develop with meperidine than with morphine, they do occur. The timing of withdrawal symptoms is different than that found with morphine withdrawal, with the syndrome developing more rapidly and lasting for a shorter period of time.

Meperidine is used as an analgesic in place of morphine when a shorter duration of action is needed. It has also been found to produce less depression of respiration in the newborn when used to reduce the pain of labor and is often used in place of morphine for childbirth (Jaffe, 1970b; Murphree, 1971).

Methadone

Methadone is a synthetic narcotic analgesic developed by the Germans near the end of the Second World War. Methadone bears little chemical resemblance to morphine as can be seen in Figure 7.4. Although it is somewhat similar to morphine in action, methadone has some very important differences.

Methadone can be administered orally or parenterally and is only about twice as potent parenterally as orally. The onset of action is slow with peak analgesia occurring after one or two hours. Methadone is detoxified in the liver primarily by N-demethylation. A considerable amount of its metabolites can be found in the feces, which is the primary route of excretion for methadone. The metabolism of methadone is slower than that of morphine and a gradual buildup of methadone occurs with repeated dosages. Under some conditions, significant amounts of the active drug are still present in the body 72 hours after the last injection.

The clinical use of methadone includes its use as an analgesic which, due to its high oral to parenteral ratio, can be given orally for the control of moderate to severe pain. It is also used in the treatment of heroin addiction where either of two different procedures may be employed. The first procedure involves transferring dependence from heroin to methadone, which produces milder withdrawal symptoms and then withdrawing the person from methadone. The second involves transfer of the dependence from heroin to methadone and then maintaining the addict on oral methadone rather than parenteral heroin.

Other Synthetic Agents

The previously mentioned narcotic analgesics are the most important ones in terms of their clinical application. They are not, however, the only strong narcotic analgesics available. Some of the other synthetic analgesics are several times as powerful as morphine, while others are relatively weak. Unfortunately, all of these drugs have side effects similar to those of morphine, with the less potent analgesics (ethoheptazine and propoxyphene) demonstrating rather mild side effects and the powerful analgesics producing equally powerful side effects. It appears that the analgesic, euphoric, and addicting properties of the centrally acting analgesics cannot be separated, suggesting a unitary basis for these three actions. The only analgesics not subject to this problem are the peripherally acting ones, such as aspirin.

THE SEARCH FOR A POTENT NONADDICTING ANALGESIC: THE NARCOTIC ANTAGONISTS

Following the isolation of morphine and the determination of its chemical structure in 1925, many morphinelike compounds have been synthesized. By altering various parts of the morphine molecule, pharmacologists hoped to produce a synthetic compound which would retain the analgesic potency of morphine, but lack the serious side effects which accompanied the narcotic analgesics then available. The results of this effort to improve upon morphine were hydromorphine, metopon, oxymorphine and many other compounds, several of which were more powerful on a dose-for-dose basis than morphine. Unfortunately, the increased analgesic potency of these drugs was paralleled by increases in the severity of their side effects, including their addiction liability (Eddy, 1967).

At the present, the most promising area of research involving the separation of addiction and analgesia is in the development of a group of drugs called the *narcotic antagonists*. The narcotic antagonists are so named because they are effective in counteracting many of the effects of the narcotic drugs. They are thought to act as competitive inhibitors for the narcotic receptor area of the neuron. This means that they become attached to the same area of a neuron where narcotic drugs such as morphine would normally attach themselves. By occupying this site, the narcotic antagonist prevents the active part of the morphine molecule from making contact with the neuron and thereby prevents the narcotic from affecting that neuron. The narcotic antagonists are actually attracted to the morphine receptor site more strongly than is morphine itself. Thus, they will displace morphine molecules already bound to the receptor site and, thereby, render them ineffective. In order to be attracted to the morphine receptor site on the neuron, the narcotic antagonist must be similar in structure to the active part of the morphine molecule. Most of the narcotic antagonists are, therefore, similar enough in form to the narcotic drugs that they possess some morphinelike activity. These drugs are sometimes called agonist-antagonists.

Some narcotic antagonists, such as nalorphine, have very little morphinelike activity while others, such as pentazocine, have strong morphinelike effects. One compound, naloxone, appears to be without any morphinelike effects and may be a pure narcotic antagonist. The chemical structures of the five best known narcotic antagonists are shown in Figure 7.5. The physiological and psychological effects of the narcotic antagonists vary with the amount of morphinelike activity of the drug. Naloxone, which has essentially no morphinelike effects, does not produce any obvious physiological or psychological effects other than in its role as a morphine antagonist. It will, however, reduce

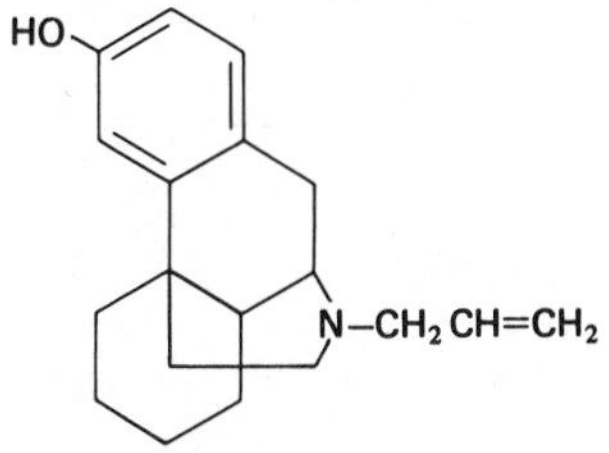

levallorphan
(nalorphine analog)

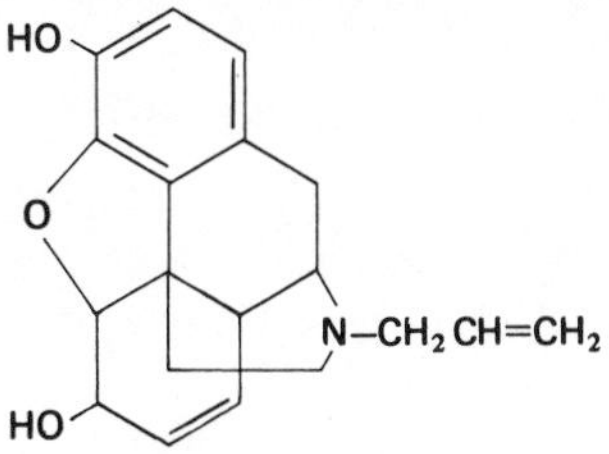

nalorphine

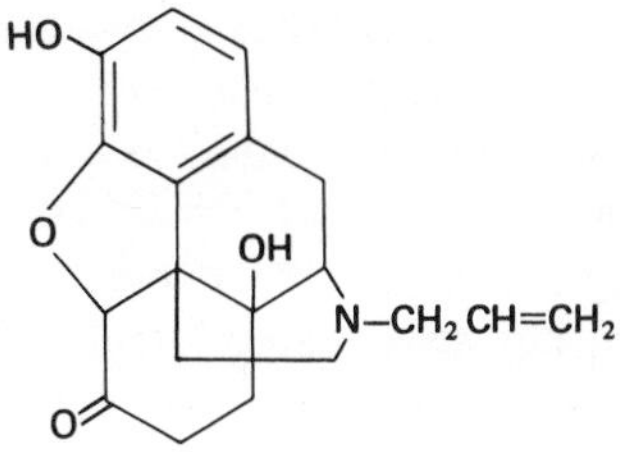

naloxone

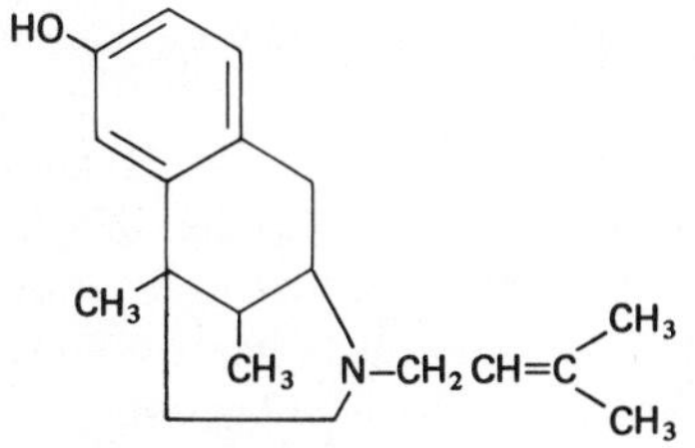

pentazocine

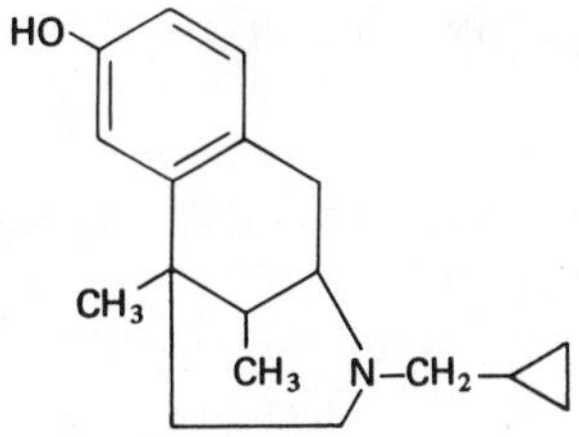

cyclazocine

FIGURE 7.5.   Structures of some narcotic antagonists.

the physiological and psychological effects of morphine if given before the morphine, and will precipitate a withdrawal syndrome if given to a person who is dependent upon a narcotic analgesic. Pentazocine, on the other hand, has strong morphinelike effects and produces physiological and psychological effects (in nondependent individuals) similar to those of the narcotics. The physiological and psychological effects of nalorphine, levallorphan, and cyclazocine are similar. Levallorphan is the most powerful of the three when given by injection. It is approximately ten times as effective as a narcotic antagonist on a dose-for-dose basis as is nalorphine or cyclazocine. Both nalorphine and levallorphan lose much of their strength when administered orally. Cyclazocine is the strongest of the three drugs when administered orally and is almost as effective by this route as by injection (Jaffe, 1970b).

Uses of the Narcotic Antagonists

The primary use of the narcotic antagonists is in the treatment of acute narcotic intoxication. The respiratory depression produced by the narcotic analgesics is rapidly reversed by the narcotic antagonists. For example, the respiratory depression in the newborn, which is sometimes caused by morphine administration to the mother during labor, can be reversed by the administration of a narcotic antagonist to the mother immediately prior to delivery, or to the newborn immediately after delivery. The narcotic antagonists may also be used for the reversal of clinical narcosis by morphine. Major surgery has been performed using morphine as the primary anesthetic agent. By the administration of a morphine antagonist following the surgery, recovery from the anesthetic depression is quite rapid. Morphine has been used as an anesthetic where a general anesthetic is contraindicated due to the poor physical condition of the patient (Jameson & Hasbrouck, 1971).

Although the narcotic antagonists do reduce the respiratory depression produced by the narcotic drugs, they are not respiratory stimulants and do not increase respiration that has been depressed by agents other than narcotics. In fact, the morphinelike activity of many of the narcotic antagonists will cause further depression of respiration just as would a small dose of morphine. The respiratory depression is related to the narcoticlike action of these drugs and naloxone, which has no narcotic action, does not produce respiratory depression. For this reason, naloxone is the drug of choice when there is some question whether the respiratory depression has been produced by a narcotic drug. If the respiratory depression is not due to a narcotic drug, the other narcotic antagonists might actually cause further depression through their morphinelike activity. Naloxone, in this situation, would have no effect (Jaffe, 1970b).

Narcotic antagonists have also been used in the diagnosis of narcotic dependence. When a narcotic antagonist is administered to a person who is physically dependent upon narcotic drugs, an abstinence syndrome will be precipitated. This procedure for the diagnosis of narcotic dependence by the precipitation of a withdrawal syndrome may be dangerous in persons with a high degree of dependence. A severe withdrawal syndrome may develop that cannot be alleviated even by high doses of morphine and death may result. Due to the severity of the withdrawal response that results from the administration of a narcotic antagonist to a dependent person, this procedure is seldom used. It should be noted at this point that the withdrawal syndrome produced by the administration of a narcotic antagonist to a person dependent upon narcotic drugs is more severe than that produced by simply withdrawing the person from the narcotic drug. This is probably due to the rapidity with which the antagonist reduces the effective concentration of the narcotic drug at the receptor site. When drugs are withheld, the concentration in the body gradually decreases, allowing some time for adjustment. When an antagonist is administered, its effect is almost immediate (Foldes, 1964; Jaffe, 1970b).

Another related use of the narcotic antagonists is in the control of narcotic addiction. Long lasting, orally administered antagonists, such as cyclazocine, can be given daily and will block the euphoria and other effects of subsequent narcotic intake. This technique is possible due to the development of tolerance to the narcoticlike action of cyclazocine, but not to the narcotic antagonist effects. Thus, the mild analgesic, respiratory depressant, and euphoric consequences of cyclazocine disappear entirely once the dose has been stabilized, but the narcotic antagonizing effect remains (Jaffe, 1970b). This effect will be discussed further in the section on rehabilitation of the narcotic addict.

A clever use of the narcotic antagonist, nalorphine, involves including it in narcotic preparations intended to be taken orally. A chronic problem with the medical use of narcotic analgesics is the difference between their oral and parenteral effectiveness. An oral dose of morphine capable of reducing pain can be converted into 30 parenteral doses capable of producing euphoria. This is clearly a profitable enterprise for the illicit dealer. Nalorphine has a much more potent action when taken parenterally than orally. Thus, the addition of a small amount of nalorphine to the morphine will have essentially no effect if the compound is taken orally (as intended by the prescribing physician), but the compound will be completely ineffective when taken by injection. In fact, it will produce an abstinence syndrome in a dependent person who injects it! This makes the narcotic compound useless to the illicit dealer and could considerably reduce the temptation to steal oral narcotic drugs if they were protected by the addiction of a small amount of nalorphine (Maugh, 1972). Narcotic antagonists have been investigated as possible analgesics but, with the possible exception of pentazocine, which is a weak antagonist with strong morphinelike effects, the range between the effective analgesic dose and the dose causing unpleasant psychotomimetic effects (see section entitled "Psychotomimetic effects") is too small for clinical usefulness (Jaffe, 1970b).

Side Effects of the Narcotic Antagonists

There are three primary side effects of the narcotic antagonists. The mild depressive effects upon respiration have been previously discussed. The other two are the development of a physical dependence, which differs from that produced by the narcotic drugs and a psychotomimetic effect.

Physical dependence.   Tolerance to the morphinelike effects of the narcotic antagonists develops rapidly and a withdrawal syndrome appears when the drug is discontinued. The withdrawal is much less severe than that from the narcotic drugs but includes some reactions not commonly found with narcotic withdrawal. Itching and brief periods of lightheadedness, described as *electric shocks* occur during withdrawal from narcotic antagonists, but not during withdrawal from narcotic drugs themselves. During the withdrawal of a narcotic antagonist, the drug craving commonly found during and after withdrawal from the narcotic drugs does not occur. This may be due, in part, to the frequently unpleasant psychotomimetic effects of the narcotic antagonists.

Pscyhotomimetic effects.   Most of the narcotic antagonists produce a dysphoric psychotomimetic effect in direct proportion to the strength of their morphinelike effects. The effect involves unpleasant and fearful hallucinations. Nightmares often occur, accompanied by parasympathetic side effects, such as sweating. Most persons find the experience quite unpleasant and, for this reason, there appears to be little danger of widespread abuse of the narcotic antagonists. This quality also limits their use as analgesics and none of the narcotic antagonists have been found suitable for analgesic use.

Contraindications

With the exception of naloxone, all of the narcotic antagonists possess some morphinelike action. This "agonistic" action, when an antagonist is given alone, results in a slight respiratory depression similar to that caused by a small dose of morphine. Although they do counteract the severe respiratory depression caused by an overdose of morphine, they do not reduce the respiratory depression caused by other drugs such as the barbiturates. In fact, the slight depression cuased by the morphinelike effects of the narcotic antagonists will increase the degression of respiration cuased by nonnarcotic drugs. Only naloxone, which is a pure narcotic antagonist devoid of narcotic effects, avoids this danger.

All of the narcotic antagonists are capable of precipitating a strong withdrawal syndrome when administered to persons dependent upon narcotic drugs, and care should be exercised in administering narcotic antagonists to persons suspected of being dependent upon narcotic drugs. For this reason, it is advisable to give only small quantities in order to improve respiration without the danger of causing an abstinence syndrome (Jaffe, 1970a; 1970b).

Summary

The narcotic antagonists are a group of drugs which are produced by altering the physical-chemical structure of a narcotic drug in such a way that it will bind to the narcotic receptor site but will not be active at that site. By occupying the narcotic receptor site on a neuron, the narcotic antagonist prevents the active part of a narcotic drug molecule from making contact with the receptor site and thereby prevents the narcotic from having an effect on the occupied site. Most of the narcotic antagonists are not completely inactive and the the narcotic activity of these compounds results in a slight morphinelike effect. The narcotic antagonist naloxone appears to be free of morphinelike activity and does not appear to be active at the narcotic receptor site.

The side effects of the narcotic antagonists are a result of the small morphinelike effect of these compounds and include a slight depression of respiration, unpleasant psychotomimetic effects, and a withdrawal syndrome which appears upon discontinuance of the narcotic antagonists. Their primary use is in the treatment of acute narcotic intoxication and some experimental investigations are pursuing the question of their use in the treatment of narcotic addicts.

PROBLEMS OF THE USE AND ABUSE OF NARCOTIC DRUGS

Three of the most serious complications resulting from the chronic intake of narcotic drugs are: the development of tolerance to these drugs, necessitating an ever increasing dosage in order to create the same effect; the production of physical dependence upon narcotic drugs, with the resultant withdrawal syndrome upon discontinuance of the drugs; and the creation of a strong craving for the continued use of narcotic drugs, following the development of tolerance and physical dependence. These three side effects of the narcotic analgesics are related and comprise the syndrome often described as *narcotic addiction*. Some authors include the strong desire for continued intake of narcotic drugs as a symptom of physical dependence and use the term physical dependence in place of addiction (Clouet, 1971; Jaffe, 1970a).

Tolerance and Physical Dependence

Tolerance to a drug may be defined as the decreased responsiveness to the pharmacological effects of that drug which follows previous experience with that drug or a related one. The degree of tolerance may vary from partial tolerance, involving a slight decrease in the drug's effectiveness, to complete tolerance, where the drug no longer elicits a measurable effect. The development of tolerance to some drugs can occur within a few minutes of the first administration of the drug. This rapidly acquired tolerance is called *acute tolerance* or *tachyphylaxis*. Tachyphylaxis probably occurs to a certain extent with the narcotic analgesics (Clouet, 1971), but is of little importance when compared to the effects of long term narcotic tolerance. Figure 7.6 shows the course of tolerance to morphine and heroin in former addicts. Note that over a 19-day period, the effective dose of morphine increased from 18 to 180 mg. One experimental addiction study produced a patient with an intake of 1,380 mg of morphine over a 24-hour period. This is well above the lethal dose in a nontolerant person. A 3-month period was required to produce this high degree of tolerance (Murphree, 1971). Tolerance develops much more rapidly and lasts longer than was once thought and has been demonstrated as much as 15 months after a single large injection of morphine (Murphree, 1971). Tolerance presents a special problem to the illicit user of narcotic drugs who, as tolerance develops, must increase his intake in order to ward off the withdrawal syndrome. If he then abstains from narcotic intake for a period of time sufficient to decrease his tolerance, he can then be killed by the same dose of narcotic that previously was only effective in warding off the withdrawal syndrome for a few hours in his tolerant state. Addicts have been known to enter treatment centers and go through withdrawal, simply to reduce their tolerance and, therefore, the expense of their habit. These persons often return to their drug-taking behavior only to reenter the treatment center again when, due to their increased tolerance, they

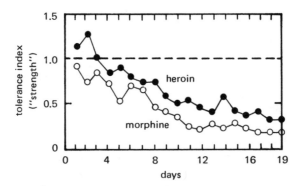

FIGURE 7.6. Course of development of tolerance to heroin and morphine. Eight addicts were studied. Heroin or morphine was administered intravenously four times daily. Morphine dose was increased gradually from 18 mg on the first day to 180 mg on the 19th day. Heroin dose was increased from 7.2 mg to 76 mg. Subjects were asked to estimate the "strength" of the drug, and these estimates were converted to a "tolerance index."

The tolerance index is the ratio of dose that would be required in a nontolerant subject to dose actually administered to achieve the same estimated effect in the tolerant subject. An index of zero would represent complete tolerance. (Reprinted by permission from W. R. Martin and H. F. Fraser, A comparative study of physiological and subjective effects of heroin and morphine administered intravenously in postaddicts. *Journal of Pharmacology and Experimental Therapeutics*, 1961, **133**, 388–399. © 1961 The Williams & Wilkins Co., Baltimore.)

can no longer afford the large quantities of narcotic drugs needed to sustain them.

As tolerance to the effects of the narcotic analgesics develops, the dose required to produce a noticeable effect increases and the body gradually develops a physical dependence upon narcotic drugs. This physical dependence is manifested by the appearance of a set of symptoms called the *withdrawal* or *abstinence syndrome* upon sudden discontinuance of the narcotic drugs. Several of the symptoms which comprise the withdrawal syndrome are listed in Table 7.4. It can be seen that many of the symptoms of withdrawal from the narcotic drugs represent a reversal of the drug's original effect. Thus, the analgesia produced by morphine is replaced during withdrawal by aches and pains and the somnolence by hyperactivity and arousal.

The development of physical dependence is a poorly understood phenomenon, which appears to be related to the development of tolerance. Physical dependence upon a given drug does not develop in the absence of tolerance to that drug, but tolerance may develop in the absence of physical dependence. The anticholinergic drugs, atropine and scopolamine, are examples of drugs to which tolerance develops without the appearance of a withdrawal syndrome when these drugs are discontinued.

The mechanism for the development of tolerance and physical dependence upon narcotic drugs is not presently known. Currently, several theories are under

TABLE 7.4

Sequence of Appearance of Some of the Abstinence
Syndrome Symptoms

Signs	Approximate hours after last dose		
	Heroin	Morphine	Methadone
Craving for drugs, anxiety	4	6	12
Yawning, perspiration, running nose, tearing eyes	8	14	34–48
Increase in above signs plus pupil dilation, goose bumps (pilo-erection), tremors (muscle twitches), hot and cold flashes, aching bones and muscles, loss of appetite	12	16	48–72
Increased intensity of above, plus insomnia; raised blood pressure; increased temperature, pulse rate, respiratory rate and depth; restlessness; nausea	18–24	24–36	
Increased intensity of above, plus curled-up position, vomiting, diarrhea, weight loss, spontaneous ejaculation or orgasm, hemoconcentration, increased blood sugar	26–36	36–48	

Note. Reprinted by permission from O. S. Ray, *Drugs, Society, and Human Behavior.* Rev. ed. Copyright 1974 by C. V. Mosby.

investigation. These include the inhibition of certain enzyme systems, an increased rate of synthesis of catecholamines, an immune reaction to morphine, increased serotonin synthesis, an increase in the number of narcotic receptor sites, and an increased neuronal sensitivity due to a process similar to denervation supersensitivity (Jaffe, 1970b). Of the above theories, the enzymatic change and immune reaction have received some support. Studies have shown that, in the blood, morphine combines with protein to form a morphine-protein conjugate. Antibodies are then formed in the body against this foreign substance (the combination of a normal body protein and a morphine molecule is recognized by the immune system as a foreign protein). This antibody might inactivate the morphine-protein complex resulting in tolerance to morphine (Cochin, 1971). Morphine becomes bound to protein in the brain and remains for an extended period of time after the morphine has disappeared from the blood. This suggests that tolerance and physical dependence may develop as a result of biochemical changes occurring due to the presence of the morphine-protein complex in the brain (Misra, Mitchell & Woods, 1971). The involvement of a morphine-protein interaction is further strengthened by studies showing that inhibition of protein synthesis slows the development of tolerance and that extracts of a small protein from the brains of morphine—tolerant rats imparts tolerance to mice when injected systemically (Misra et al., 1971).

Tolerance may not occur equally to all aspects of a drug's action on the body. While tolerance to the analgesic, euphoric and respiratory effects of the narcotic analgesics develops rapidly, no tolerance develops to their miotic (pupil-constricting) or convulsive effects, and only little to their constipating effects (Murphree, 1971).

The development of tolerance and physical dependence are both centrally mediated. They both can be produced by intraventricular injections of morphine, which are much smaller than the systemic injections required to produce dependence. Typical doses range from less than 1 mg at the beginning of the dependence-producing procedure to perhaps 10 mg at the end of the procedure. These are much smaller than the doses needed to produce the same degree of tolerance and physical dependence following systemic administration (Eidleberg & Barstow, 1971). Further evidence for the central nature of tolerance and physical dependence is available from studies demonstrating that rats made dependent upon morphine by systemic injection will show an abstinence syndrome when a narcotic antagonist is microinjected into the medial thalamus and other selected brain areas (Wei et al., 1972).

In summary, the available evidence suggests that the development of tolerance and physical dependence occurs as a result of the presence of a narcotic drug in the brain. The area surrounding the ventricles (medial thalamus) may be of special importance. The presence of protein bound morphine in the brain for an extended time following a morphine injection and the inhibitory effect of protein synthesis inhibitors upon the development of tolerance and physical dependence suggest that a biochemical change involving protein takes place in the brain as a result of chronic intake of narcotic drugs, and that this biochemical change may be responsible for the production of tolerance and physical dependence. The mechanism of this effect remains unknown.

Addiction to Narcotic Drugs

Probably the most serious consequence of the chronic intake of narcotic drugs is the development of a strong desire to continue taking these drugs, even in the face of severe hardship resulting from the drug intake. This exceedingly strong drive for the continued intake of a drug is often termed *addiction* or *physical dependence*. The physical dependence or addiction resulting from the chronic intake of narcotic drugs should be differentiated from the psychological dependence resulting from the intake of some drugs, such as the distorting drugs (LSD, etc.), where a withdrawal syndrome does not appear on discontinuance of the drug. The drug-taking behavior in the psychologically dependent person may be supported by the positive reinforcing effects of the drug, while the drug-taking behavior of the physically dependent person may also be supported by the removal of an aversive stimulus (the abstinence syndrome), as a result of drug intake. It is quite probable that both psychological and physical dependence result from the continued use of narcotic drugs and it is, thus, not too surprising that discontinuing the use of these drugs is extremely difficult.

Many of the psychological effects of the narcotic drugs suggest that they may act directly on the periventricular gray area of the brain which has been described by L. Stein (1964) as a punishment area. The narcotic drugs may act by inhibiting neural activity in this area and by thereby reducing the punishing effect of pain or other psychologically noxious stimulation. The withdrawal symptoms might be partially explained under this theory as a rebound effect (when the punishment area of the brain recovers its functions it may overreact). Clearly, the removal or amelioration of the unpleasantness of all noxious stimuli would be a strongly reinforcing event in the life of a troubled person. The reduction in the motivating strength of noxious stimulation (from such diverse sources as fear, hunger, and lack of sexual satisfaction) in addicts has led some investigators to suggest that the stimuli associated with the intake of a narcotic drug may become powerful secondary reinforcers, and that the desire for narcotic intake can then be triggered by any increase in the aversiveness of the environment. Under this model, a desire for narcotic drugs would be elicited by hunger, thirst, or any other unpleasant event. This conditioned drive for the intake of narcotic drugs could then be lessened by presenting the narcotic drug without allowing it to have its drive-reducing effect (extinction). This method is currently being investigated (Davis & Smith, 1972; Jaffe, 1970a).

After a review of the symptoms shown by detoxified narcotic addicts, Dole (1972) suggested that a permanent metabolic change takes place during the addiction process, resulting in a continued need or drive for the intake of narcotic drugs. Consistent with this proposal is the discovery of persisting signs of the abstinence syndrome many months after detoxification of narcotic addicts (Martin & Jasinski, 1969).

A ray of hope exists in the otherwise gloomy prognosis for detoxified addicts. There is some evidence that as middle age is reached, a significant number of narcotic addicts gradually reduce their intake of narcotic drugs and eventually cease narcotic intake altogether, without going through the withdrawal syndrome and without maintaining a high drive to resume drug intake. This process of maturing out (Ray, 1972), is dependent upon the addict reaching middle age, which is a difficult task for the chronic heroin user, who must contend with impure drugs, unsterile needles, and the need for a high monetary outlay in order to maintain relief from the monkey on his back.

Studies of narcotic addiction in animals. Attempts to determine the conditions necessary for the production of compulsive drug intake in lower animals have been centered on the conditions under which the intake of narcotic drugs acts as a reinforcer. In particular, scientists are interested in the effect of previous experience with narcotic drugs on their efficiency as reinforcers. The three primary questions are: Will drug naive animals begin the spontaneous intake of narcotic drugs? Are narcotic drugs effective reinforcers for animals who have been made physically dependent upon them? Will animals who have been previously dependent upon narcotic drugs show drug-seeking behavior following detoxification? These three conditions could be likened to the drug naive person, the addict, and the exaddict.

Drug naive animals: Early studies on drug naive animals showed that species other than man simply do not spontaneously take narcotic drugs (Cohen, 1970). Some of these early studies involved oral administration of the drug (morphine was made available in water). However, considering the bitter taste of the narcotic drugs, this result is not too surprising. More recent studies, in which the drug was administered intravenously following an operant response by the animal have offered partial support of the earlier studies. Dogs will not perform an operant response to obtain intravenous morphine and under most circumstances, neither will rats. Monkeys, however, will press a lever in order to obtain morphine injections (Jones & Prada, 1973). Even monkeys, who respond more strongly than other species to morphine, do not show strong evidence that morphine intake is reinforcing. Perhaps these results are not so surprising when one considers that most humans find their original experiences with narcotic drugs to be unpleasant (only about 10% report euphoria). As with the human, the situation changes drastically when animals are made physically dependent upon morphine by chronic administration.

Drug dependent animals: In a classic study by Spragg (1938) chimpanzees were trained with fruit reinforcement to assume a position in which they could easily be injected. Following this training, morphine injections were given daily for 13 months. This resulted in the development of physical dependence. As dependence developed, the animals began engaging in drug-soliciting behavior. They would lead the experimenter to the morphine and hand him the injection syringe. Even when they were food deprived, the chimps consistently chose a morphine injection in preference to a food reward. These results have been repeated for many different species and morphine is generally regarded as a potent reinforcer for the physically dependent animal (Jaffe, 1970a; Jones & Prada, 1973; Seevers, 1967). So far, the results of animal studies have closely paralleled those from studies on the human. The remaining question concerns the responses of previously dependent animals who have been detoxified. Will they, like the human, tend to revert to their drug-taking behavior?

Previously dependent animals: A serious consequence of narcotic dependence in the human is the strong tendency to return to drug-taking behavior following detoxification. Attempts to duplicate this effect in lower animals have met with mixed results. Spragg (1938) found that once his chimpanzees were detoxified, they no longer displayed drug-soliciting behavior. These early results promoted speculation that the human might be the only species to exhibit relapse to drug solicitation following detoxification and that this relapse must, therefore, be due to a "mental weakness" on the part of the addict. More recent studies have shown that most animals will return to drug-soliciting behavior following detoxification, and that this, therefore, is not a purely human trait (Cohen, J., 1970; Jones & Prada, 1973).

The results of both human and animal experiments indicate that the desire expressed by many former addicts to return to the use of narcotic drugs may be a result of either learning or a direct physiological effect of the narcotic drugs upon the brain. The exact nature of this effect is unknown. The suggestion that self-administration of the narcotic drug is an important aspect in the subsequent development of addiction and the finding that persons given morphine for the relief of pain seldom become addicted even though large doses are required, suggests that an element of learning is certainly involved (Jaffe, 1970a; Jones & Prada, 1973). We will now examine some of the techniques which have been used in attempts to treat the person abusing narcotic drugs.

Rehabilitation of the Narcotic Addict

Addiction to the narcotic analgesics has been a major social problem for centuries. Much of the research into the mechanism of action of these drugs has been prompted by a desire to find a "cure" for narcotic addiction. It was once hoped that simple withdrawal of the person from narcotic drugs, by eliminating the threat of withdrawal symptoms, might be enough to halt drug-taking behavior. This has turned out to be a false hope; estimates of the relapse rate following withdrawal approximate 90% (Kurland, 1969; Regush, 1971). The addict continues to feel a strong desire for narcotic drugs long after he has been detoxified and is no longer physically dependent upon them. The mechanism of this continued "craving" for narcotic drugs is not presently understood, but recent work (Dubas et al., 1972) suggests that it may involve persistent biochemical changes resulting from the presence of narcotic drugs in the brain, as well as learning that narcotic drugs make you feel better. A successful rehabilitation program must, therefore, either prevent the drug craving by physiological methods or involve powerful reinforcers for drug abstinence. These two approaches may be classified as physiological and psychological.

Physiological methods. One method of reducing the craving for narcotic drugs in persons who have become physically dependent on them is to satisfy that craving. This can be accomplished by maintaining the person on a controlled intake of a narcotic drug. This method has been used for several years in Great Britain, where heroin maintenance is a common form of treatment for narcotics addiction. In this system, the addict is not required to abstain from all intake of narcotic drugs, but is, instead, allowed a controlled dose of heroin. This is sufficient to prevent the onset of the withdrawal syndrome and blocks the strong desire for narcotic drugs. This program has been notably effective and British narcotic addicts number in the hundreds rather than in the hundreds of thousands. Brecher (1972) has suggested that the effectiveness of the British system has stemmed from the lack of publicity surrounding heroin use. Furthermore, the ability of the addict to buy inexpensive heroin eliminates the need for the acquisition of large sums of money which can lead to criminal activity by the addict and, at the same time, removes the profit from the black market sale of heroin. Why pay several dollars on the black market for a drug which you can buy for a few cents at the local drugstore?

A similar method is used in the United States, where methadone is substituted for the heroin. A great advantage of the methadone maintenance plan is that methadone can be taken orally rather than by injection; it is also a longer-lasting narcotic than is heroin, eliminating the need for several doses per day. The desired result of the maintenance programs is the stabilization of narcotic drug use by the addict at a low level, which will allow a relatively normal life. There appear to be relatively few serious complications to the chronic intake of a stabilized dose of the narcotic drugs, and once a stable rate of drug intake is reached, tolerance to the effects of the narcotic drugs occurs, and they have little noticeable effect upon the addict.

The primary objection to this type of therapy is that the underlying fault (addiction) is not being treated and that the person on a maintenance program is still an addict. The findings that persons on heroin or methadone maintenance can lead normal, productive lives are, however, points in favor of this approach. It has been pointed out that the diabetic is just as much dependent upon insulin as the addict is upon heroin or methadone. For a critique of the methadone program, see Lennard, Epstein, & Rosenthal (1972).

Psychological methods. The psychological approach to drug abstinence can take several different forms. Some suspected underlying cause of the addiction may be sought and removed; strong reinforcement can be offered for drug abstinence, or a process of extinction can be used in which the person is allowed to engage in drug-taking behavior while the effects of the drug are blocked physiologically. The last two methods will be discussed briefly.

Synanon: A program which focuses upon reinforcement of drug abstinence is Synanon. The Synanon program takes the approach of restructuring the addict's social situation so that it incorporates strong rewards for the abstinence and strong social disapproval for drug-taking behavior. In this program, the old behavior patterns are no longer socially accepted and behavior gradually changes to meet the new social demands. During his stay at the Synanon Center, the addict is brought into a program where attempts are made to change his self-perception and increase his emotional maturity to the point where he can control his desire to take narcotic drugs. He is asked to always remain in contact with the therapeutic Synanon community and preferably remain in the community. The primary drawback to this program is that if the addict (they say once an addict, always an addict) returns to his old enivronment, the old reward contingencies are again in effect and he may suffer a relapse. Some question the morality of a program which moves a person out of his normal environment and makes him dependent upon an artificial social system. However, the low relapse rate found in Synanon patients suggests that the program is effective (Jaffe, 1970a).

The relatively high success rates (60%-90%) which are often reported by the therapeutic communities may present a distorted picture of their success. These figures do not usually include those who were not qualified for the program or those who dropped out of the program. These two groups may account for a vast majority of the drug users. Furthermore, little followup information is available for those persons who do leave the therapeutic community and what information is available suggests that there is an extremely high relapse rate once the person leaves the protective environment of a community such as Synanon (Brecher, 1972).

Extinction: A technique which is in the experimental stage at the present time involves extinction of the drug-taking behavior. It has been argued that the continued desire for narcotic drugs in a previously dependent person stems from the fact that he has not unlearned his previous mode of responding. This unlearning (extinction of the responses involved in drug-taking behavior) can be brought about by having the person engage in the drug-taking behavior without this behavior being followed by a reinforcer. This can be accomplished by blocking the effect of narcotic drugs by a narcotic antagonist (Jaffe, 1970a) or possibly by AMPT (Davis & Smith, 1972). It was originally hoped that by administering a long-lasting narcotic antagonist such as cyclazocine the addict could be returned to his normal environment where if he engaged in drug-taking behavior, the usual reward (euphoria) would not occur and the behavor would extinguish. As this program is still in the experimental stage, the results are not known but preliminary studies have shown that few persons remain in this program for an extended period of time. Apparently, the desire for the effects of narcotic drug intake are too high and the patients discontinue the narcotic antagonist and return to heroin (Dole, 1972).

Syndrome X

Recently, detailed studies of deaths that were reported to have resulted from heroin overdose have failed to find evidence of elevated levels of heroin or morphine (the active metabolic product of heroin) in the blood of many of the "overdose" victims. The commonly observed syndrome of cardiovascular collapse and pulmonary edema, resulting in death, can occur apparently as a result of the injection of relatively small doses of heroin. Syndrome X, as it has been called, may account for a high percentage of the deaths which have been labeled "heroin overdose." The mechanism behind Syndrome X is not known, but it has been suggested that an allergic response to the heroin or to the adulterants commonly mixed with the heroin found on the street may be responsible. Whatever the causative agent, the response is extremely rapid and victims are often found with the needle still in their arm. The rapidity of the response, its unknown etiology and apparent occurrence following small doses of narcotic drugs is quite unexpected; the possible causes of this phenomena are now under study. There is also growing evidence that many apparent heroin suicides may have been the unexpected consequence of a normal dose of heroin (Brecher, 1972).

Summary

The outlook for the narcotic addict, while improved from a few years ago, remains serious. The mechanism behind the continued craving for narcotic drugs is not well understood but appears to involve a long-lasting metabolic change. Simply removing the threat of the withdrawal syndrome is not enough, as the desire for drug intake remains. The accepted methods of the learning theorist including extinction and counterconditioning do not appear to be effective and at present, the most successful program seems to involve maintaining the addict on a controlled dose of narcotic drug which enables him to function relatively normally in society. Even this method is far from completely successful. Work is progressing to further our understanding of the principles behind addiction to the narcotic drugs and this understanding will hopefully lead to its prevention or cure.

8
STIMULANT AND
ANTIDEPRESSANT DRUGS

Barry J. Krikstone and Robert A. Levitt

The drugs to be discussed in this chapter are the "uppers," the stimulants and the antidepressants. The stimulants typically enhance the excitation of the nervous system. Many of them show some selectivity, primarily stimulating cerebral, brainstem, or spinal functions. Stimulants have a long and interesting history. Yet, for many of their previous uses they have been replaced by newer and safer drugs. The major drugs to be discussed are: the cerebral stimulants—cocaine, caffeine, and methylphenidate; the brainstem stimulants—picrotoxin, pentylenetetrazol, and nikethamide; and the spinal stimulant—strychnine. Several important stimulants have been treated in previous chapters. These are the adrenergic stimulants (amphetamines, Chapter 3) and the cholinergic (nicotine) and anticholinergic (atropine) stimulants (Chapter 4).

The antidepressants primarily excite the nervous system and behavior of sedated or depressed humans or animals. There are two types of antidepressants: the MAO inhibitors and the inhibitors of presynaptic reuptake. The presumed biochemical bases for the therapeutic effectiveness of these agents have previously been discussed (Chapter 2).

CNS STIMULANTS

Many drugs of psychopharmacological interest have a stimulating effect on the CNS. These drugs are relatively nonspecific in their sites of action; although a major effect may be seen in the cerebral cortex, brainstem, or spinal cord, stimulant and excitatory effects are also seen at other neural levels. This lack of neural specificity often precludes therapeutic use, except in cases where other

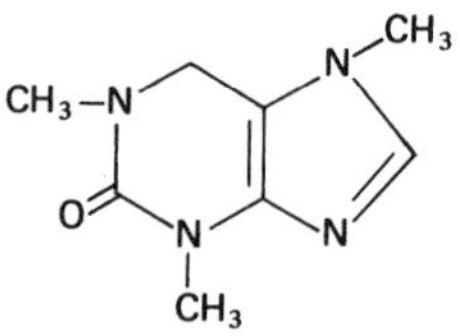

caffeine

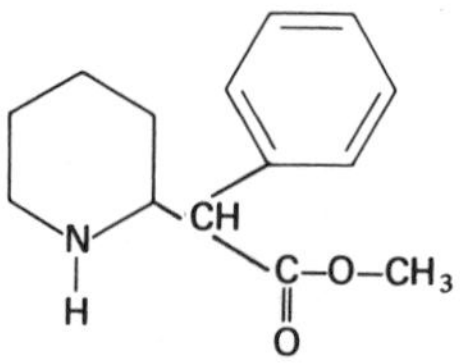

methylphenidate

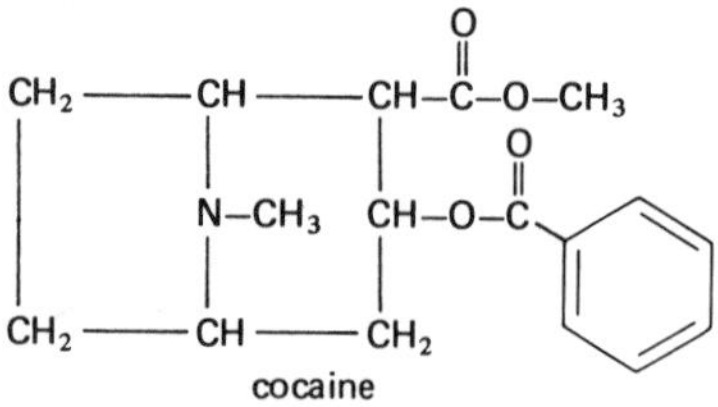

cocaine

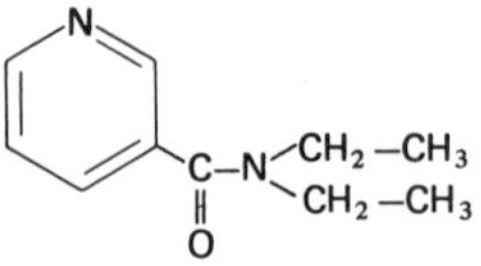

nikethamide

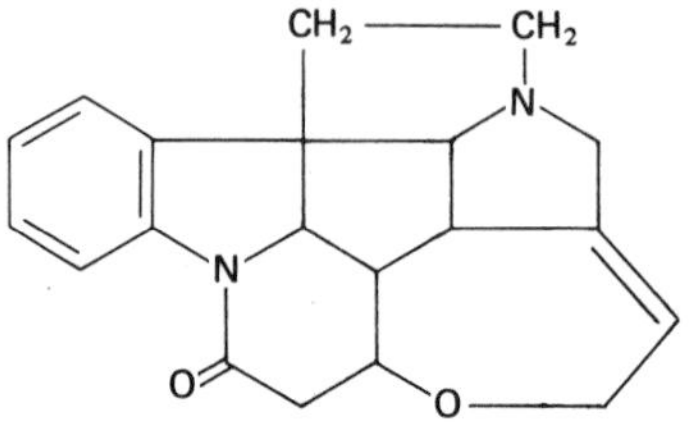

strychnine

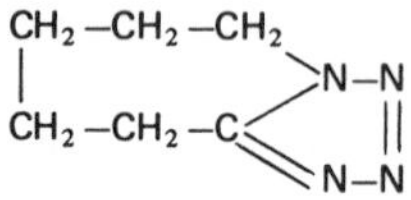

pentylenetetrazol

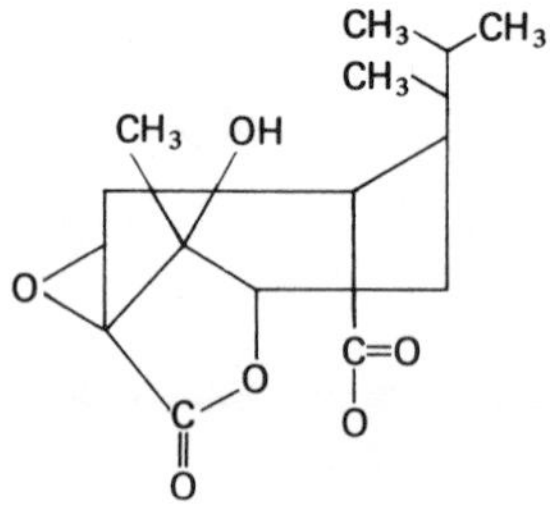

picrotoxin

FIGURE 8.1. Structural formulas of some CNS stimulants.

medical and pharmacological techniques have failed. Even though the CNS stimulants usually have a generally diffuse, excitatory, and stimulant effect, they have tended to be classified by their dominant site of action. This classification is used for convenience in discussing and cataloging these drugs, but should not be viewed as an attempt to rigidly classify the drugs according to neuroanatomical site of action. (Figure 8.1 shows the structural formulas for representative stimulants.)

CEREBRAL STIMULANTS

This group of drugs includes the amphetamines (Chapter 3), the xanthine derivatives (caffeine, theophylline, theobromine), methylphenidate, and cocaine. These drugs, as a class, usually cause wakefulness, talkativeness, and increased random motor behavior. The drugs included in this group have diverse effects and probably act via diencephalic nuclei and the ascending reticular activating system (ARAS). For instance, electrical stimulation of the ARAS and amphetamine ingestion produce similar arousal effects on the EEG. Drugs in this class given in toxic doses produce hallucinations, manic excitement (mania), and uncoordinated, uncontrolled movements, which may end in convulsions and death. The potential for abuse is high and this subject will be discussed for each drug.

The Xanthine Derivatives

The xanthines are three of the oldest stimulants known to humanity. *Xanthine* itself is a Greek word meaning yellow; this is the color of the residue left by the xanthines if heated with acid. The three xanthine drugs, caffeine, theophylline, and theobromine, are closely related chemicals that occur in plants found throughout the world. From earliest times, people have made beverages from extracts of these plants. Theophylline, meaning "divine leaf," is found in the leaves of *Thea chinensis,* which is used for brewing tea. Theobromine, meaning "divine food," is the primary active ingredient in cocoa, which is obtained from the seeds of the chocolate tree, *Theobroma cacao,* and is found in cocoa drinks and chocolate bars. Caffeine is the xanthine stimulant that has been most carefully studied and is obtained from the seeds of *Coffea arabica,* cola (*Cola acuminata*), and tea. Maté, the national drink of many South American countries, contains caffeine, and many of the soft drinks so popular in the United States contain caffeine because they are made from extracts of cola nuts (the nuts contain about 2% caffeine).

Mythology.   The earliest history of the xanthine-related beverages is lost, but a considerable mythology has grown around their initial uses and the discoveries of their stimulant properties. The best-known legend about the beginning of coffee is the tale about the Arabian shepherd, Kaldi, who found his goats jumping and hopping around the hillside. He followed them up the mountain one day and ate some of the red berries they were munching. Soon Kaldi began jumping and hopping around the hillside with the goats. Kaldi reported the event to a local holy man, who joined him and his goats on the hillside; soon the holy man and Kaldi and the goats were jumping and hopping around the hillside. Legend then has it that Mohammed told the holy man to boil the berries in water and have the brothers in the monastery drink it so they might remain awake for their prayers.

The legend surrounding tea is neither as boisterous nor as exuberant as that of Kaldi and the goats. One tale tells us of Daruma, the founder of Zen Buddhism. He fell asleep one day while meditating, and to prevent this from ever happening again, he cut off both eyelids. From the spot where his eyelids touched the ground, a new plant grew whose leaves, when brewed with water, would prevent one from falling asleep.

The chocolate tree, according to Aztec legend, was given to humanity as a gift from paradise by Quetzalcoatl, the Aztec god of the air. Linnaeus remembered this legend when he named the cocoa tree, *Theobroma,* food of the gods. (For a more complete history of the xanthine drugs, see Ray, 1972.)

Absorption and metabolism. The xanthines are readily absorbed after oral, rectal, or parenteral administration: the specific effect depends on the specific drug chosen and the route of administration. The oral route is most convenient and peak blood levels are reached after 30 to 60 minutes. Maximal CNS effects are usually seen within 2 hours, but the onset of effects may be noticed as soon as 30 minutes after ingestion. Oral ingestion of the xanthines often produces variable results because absorption may be erratic. This may be due to the poor solubility of the xanthines in water. The side effects of the xanthines include gastric irritation, nausea, and vomiting. Because of this, the xanthines are sometimes administered via rectal suppository or enema, or orally, by using a xanthine salt, which is absorbed more readily and has less irritating side effects. Although the specific enzymes responsible for the biodegradation of the xanthines are not known, in the body the xanthines are partially demethylated and oxidized and are excreted as methyluric acids or methylxanthines.

CNS effects. The central nervous system stimulatory effects of the xanthines form the basis of much of their use. Caffeine is a powerful CNS stimulant; theophylline is less of a stimulant, and theobromine has relatively little CNS excitant properties. Since caffeine is the most powerful as a CNS stimulant, the majority of xanthine research has used this drug; hence the discussion which follows refers to caffeine, unless the other xanthines are specifically mentioned.

All levels of the central nervous system are affected, with the cortex being the first, then the medulla, and finally, after very large doses, the spinal cord. At a dose of 150 to 250 mg (about 2 cups of brewed coffee or 3 cups of instant coffee) the cortex shows an EEG of arousal, i.e., low voltage, rapid waves, and a person reports mood elevation and difficulty in going to sleep. There is a strong relationship between the extent to which the caffeine produces an elevation of mood and its capability to prevent and disturb normal sleep patterns. Ritchie (1970b) states that the action of caffeine is to

> produce a more rapid and clearer flow of thought, and to allay drowsiness and fatigue. After taking caffeine one is capable of a greater sustained intellectual effort and a more perfect association of ideas. There is also a keener appreciation of sensory stimuli, and reaction time to them is appreciably diminished. . . . In addition, motor activity is increased; typists, for example, work faster and with fewer errors. (p. 359)

In addition to cortical stimulation, caffeine also stimulates the medullary, respiratory, vasomotor, and vagal (cranial nerve X) areas. This stimulatory action is therapeutically useful when the medullary centers are depressed (as they are by morphine or many other drugs). However, the dose of 150 to 250 mg caffeine taken orally produces little or no respiratory stimulation. If oral doses are to be used, then about twice this dosage (or about 500 mg) must be ingested to obtain the respiratory stimulation. Parenteral administration of 150 to 250 mg of caffeine, however, will stimulate the respiratory areas of the medulla. Large doses of caffeine and theophylline produce an excitation not only at the cortical and medullary levels, but virtually throughout the CNS, including the spinal cord. Reflex excitability is increased, and in animals this has led to convulsions and death. The cellular mechanism of action for the xanthines is unclear. However, the most plausible proposals include a facilitation of cyclic AMP and the release of calcium from binding sites (Ritchie, 1970b).

Tolerance and dependence. A large degree of tolerance and cross-tolerance may develop to the xanthines. This is seen with respect to their diuretic (increased urine flow) and vasodilator actions, but little or no tolerance develops to the CNS stimulation effects. There is no doubt that a certain degree of dependence may develop to caffeine. This is true in both the habitual user and in the person who just takes a cup or two of coffee in the morning to wake up. The feeling of well-being and alertness and the increased "energy" seem to produce no harm, and anyway, the morning cup of coffee seems to have become so ingrained into American life that few would look upon it as a drug habit. Dependence on caffeine, however, is real.

A pathological dependence on caffeine is called *caffeinism* and a typical case history of a patient addicted to caffeine is described by Dr. Hobart A. Reimann of the Hahnemann Medical College. The patient was a 39-year-old housewife and waitress who had been running a slight fever for 6 months, lost 20 lb so that she now weighed 107 lb, and complained of occasional flushing, and chilliness, insomnia, irritability, and lack of appetite. She was placed in the hospital when antibiotics failed to bring down her temperature, and during her 5-day stay in the hospital, her temperature went down to normal and remained there. The case history of the patient reports that she smoked a pack or more of cigarettes a day and drank between 15 and 18 cups of brewed coffee between 8 a.m. and 4 p.m. When she left the hospital and again resumed her coffee drinking habit, her temperature began to rise again. Warned that coffee might be producing the symptoms, she stopped drinking the coffee. From then on her sleep improved, her appetite improved, her temperature went back to normal, and she began gaining weight. Caffeinism, Dr. Reimann notes in his conclusion, "is said to be current among intellectual workers, actresses, waitresses, nocturnal employees, and long distance automobile drivers. Illness otherwise unexplained may be caused by excessive ingestion of the xanthine alkaloids, including those in coffee, tea, cocoa, and those in some popular (cola) beverages" (Reimann, 1967).

Is caffeine addicting? Ask 20 experts that question and you will probably get 20 different replies. First, one feature of an addiction is the tolerance which builds up to the drug. Tolerance builds to heroin, barbiturates, and ethanol. A tolerance (and cross-tolerance) also develops to the xanthines and this is seen most with respect to both the vasodilator and the diuretic properties of the drugs. Secondly, a withdrawal syndrome and physical dependence are symptoms of an addiction. The withdrawal syndromes from heroin, barbiturates, and ethanol are well known, but those produced by caffeine are not clear. There are some symptoms produced by caffeine withdrawal, i.e., a CNS depression that follows the caffeine-produced excitation. However, the addiction liability of the xanthines is clearly much lower, and the withdrawal syndrome much milder than for the depressants and narcotics. The difference is so great, that we consider it grossly misleading to use the same term, *addiction,* to describe the dependence problem with these various drug classes.

Toxicity. When taken in large doses, caffeine may be a potent poison. Fatal doses given to animals produce convulsions that resemble strychnine-produced convulsions, and death from respiratory failure. A fatal dose in humans is presumed to be about 10 g or about 100 cups of brewed coffee. However, no human fatalities have been reported from an oral overdose of caffeine. The central stimulant and toxic effects can be counteracted by the CNS depressants (Chapter 6; and Peters, 1967a). Large doses of caffeine given to animals produce often bizarre and shocking results, as evidenced by the fact that rats fed massive doses of caffeine (Peters, 1967b) became aggressive and in many instances launched physical attacks against other animals. In some cases, the caffeine-crazed rat may bite and mutilate itself until it dies from hemorrhagic shock.

Methylphenidate

Methylphenidate (Ritalin) is a mild CNS stimulant that counteracts physical and mental fatigue, while having only a slight effect on blood pressure and respiration. In potency, the drug is more effective than caffeine, but less effective than the amphetamines. The mechanism for the stimulant action of methylphenidate is unknown. There has been little research on the subject. However, the similarity between its actions and those of the amphetamines leads one to suspect an interaction with brain bioamine transmitters.

Therapeutically, the drug has received extensive testing for the relief of depression, in the treatment of barbiturate overdose and for the relief of slowness and fatigue from numerous causes. However, the most important current use of the drug is in the management of hyperkinetic children. Methylphenidate is the drug of choice in such cases. Well-controlled studies (Knights & Hinton, 1969) have clearly demonstrated that the drug can improve both behavior and learning ability in children with poor attention spans. Millinchap and Fowler (1967) note that in a comparison of methylphenidate and amphetamine, 84% of the patients showed a reduction of hyperactive behavior when methylphenidate was used and 69% showed improvement when amphetamines were used. They also report annoying side effects in 15% of the patients regardless of which drug was used. Neither the physiological basis for the hyperkinetic behavior nor the physiological mechanism of action of methylphenidate is known, but empirically it has been shown that methylphenidate (or amphetamine) treatment is the best available psychopharmacologic tool in controlling this very difficult syndrome. (See Wender [1971] for a discussion of this syndrome, which Wender calls *minimal brain dysfunction*, and of its pharmacological management.)

Cocaine

Cocaine is a chemical obtained by extraction from the coca plant native to Peru (*Erythroxylon coca*). It has a long history of use in South American countries as a CNS stimulant, and today it is estimated that 2 million Peruvians living in the Andean Mountains consume approximately 90,000 kg of cocaine annually (Jaffe, 1970a). These people have a long history, going back for centuries, of chewing coca leaves for recreation. It is noteworthy that these highlanders characteristically abandon the use of cocaine when they come down from the mountains. After years of continuous use, they do not become addicted to the drug.

Absorption and metabolism.   Metabolism of cocaine is very rapid, and the duration of its effects may be for no more than minutes after intravenous injection. The drug is absorbed from all sites of application, including mucous membranes. In fact, cocaine reduces mucous membrane swelling. This action no doubt stimulated the idea of sniffing the drug—a not uncommon method of use today. Most of the ingested cocaine is destroyed by the liver but some may be excreted unchanged in the urine.

CNS effects.   The most important chemical action of cocaine is to block nerve conduction upon local application—hence its use as a local anesthetic. However, the most striking systemic effect is that of a general CNS stimulant. Small doses of cocaine have a major cortical effect. The first symptoms seen in humans include talkativeness, restlessness, and excitement. Cognitive abilities do not seem to be debilitated; in fact, they may be heightened. Motor activity is usually well coordinated, and an inhibition in this sphere is usually not seen until higher doses are reached. There are effects at lower levels of the nervous system and these get progressively more serious as the dose of the drug is increased. Medullary actions seen include an increase in respiration and also increased activity of the medullary control areas for vomiting and vasomotor activity. Vomiting is not uncommon after cocaine ingestion (Ritchie, Cohen, & Dripps, 1970). The cellular mechanism for the stimulant action of cocaine, discussed in Chapter 2, appears to involve inhibition of the presynaptic reuptake of bioamine transmitters.

Behavioral effects.   The subjective effects of cocaine include a mood elevation that is even greater than that seen after the amphetamines. Jaffe (1965) has stated:

> It produces a marked decrease in hunger, an indifference to pain, and is reputed to be the most potent antifatigue agent known. The user enjoys a feeling of great muscular strength and increased mental capacity and greatly overestimates his capabilities. (p. 298)

After the stimulating effect, however, cocaine produces a pronounced depresssion. In many cases the depression then leads the user to another cocaine injection and hence, another stimulation effect, and then another depression, etc.

The contrast between the euphoria produced by the cocaine and the depression following use often leads users to increase the dosage to toxic levels. If toxic dose levels are reached, a syndrome resembling schizophrenia is often seen, characterized by paranoid ideation, persecutory delusions, and visual, auditory, and tactile hallucinations.

The psychoanalyst.   Freud, who was himself a user of cocaine for over 3 years, and described it as "a magical drug" in a letter to his fiancee, Martha, wrote once that "a small dose lifted me to the heights in a wonderful fashion. I am just now busy collecting the literature for a song of praise to this magical substance" (Jones, 1953, p. 84).

Freud later described a psychosis in his friend (Dr. von Fleischl-Martow) who had been taking 1 g of cocaine per day—a major symptom was the hallucination of "white snakes" creeping over his skin. A peculiar characteristic of the hallucinations seen in cocaine toxicity include "formication"—the hallucination that ants, or insects, or snakes are crawling along the skin or under it. After this frightening experience with Fleischl, Freud no longer glorified cocaine and became intensely against it (see also Brecher, 1972, pp. 272–277).

Who done it?   Another early user of cocaine is described in the following passage:

> [He] took his bottle from the corner of the mantlepiece, and his hypodermic syringe from its neat morocco case. With his long, white nervous fingers he adjusted the delicate needle and rolled back his left shirtcuff. For some little time his eyes rested thoughtfully upon the sinewy forearm and wrist, all dotted and scarred with innumerable puncture-marks. Finally, he thrust the sharp point home, pressed down the tiny piston, and sank back into the velvet-lined armchair with a long sigh of satisfaction.
> "Which is it today," I asked, "Morphine or Cocaine?"

The user in this tale is none other than Sherlock Holmes and the questioner is the faithful Dr. Watson (Doyle, 1938, pp. 91–92).

Tolerance and dependence.   Cocaine dependence differs from ethanol, opiate, or barbiturate addiction in two major areas. First, the physical effects of cocaine withdrawal are mild. The major symptoms are depression, fatigue, and weariness, which develop almost immediately after the drug is removed. This leads to the second major difference—the speed with which the depression develops after the cocaine has been removed. The delirium tremors of ethanol and barbiturate addiction and the bizarre behavior following opiate withdrawal take hours and, in some cases, days to appear.

There is no sure way to understand why some users develop an intense craving for cocaine and a need to continually escalate the dose. There are currently three views available. One view insists that there is an "addictive personality," i.e., the user must possess specific personality characteristics (dependence, insecurity, etc.) which lead to the need for a drug crutch. The other two explanations are more psychopharmacologically oriented. First, there is the view that a genetically determined biochemical difference, perhaps enzymatic, predisposes some to revert to drug use. The final explanation relates to the dosage and the frequency of use. In those who are heavy users, and who continually increase the dose to maintain a constant euphoric state, dependence may result. In those users, like Freud, who are occasional low-dose users and find no need to increase the dosage to maintain the "high," excited state, dependence does not result and there is little danger of reaching the toxic dose range. Probably, the abuse potential for an individual is based on some combination of these (personality, biochemistry, frequency, and size of dose) and other factors.

The effects of cocaine were known in medical circles by 1890. Subsequently, in 1914 federal laws classifying cocaine as a narcotic were passed regulating the possession, sale and use of the drug. This is clearly a misclassification, since cocaine is not at all like the addicting narcotic analgesics (see Chapter 7). Use of cocaine had continually decreased until in the 1960s its black market sale was relatively small. However, law enforcement cannot be credited for the decrease in cocaine use—instead the cocaine user found a new drug which would produce similar effects, was cheaper and was available—the amphetamines. Late in the 1960s when law enforcement officials cracked down on amphetamine sales, the smuggling and black market sale of cocaine increased.

BRAINSTEM STIMULANTS

This group of drugs includes picrotoxin, pentylenetetrazol, and nikethamide. Each acts throughout the cerebrospinal axis and large doses produce convulsions and death. All are drugs that have been used in research. Rarely have they been subject to abuse.

Picrotoxin

Picrotoxin comes from the *Anamirta coculus,* a climbing shrub native to the East Indies. The drug is contained in the fruit of the vine, called *fishberries*—so called because if the bruised fruit is thrown into the water, fish consume it, become immobilized, die, and float to the surface. Picrotoxin itself is inactive, but it can be broken down into two derivatives, picrotoxinin and picrotin. Picrotin is also inactive but picrotoxinin possesses powerful CNS stimulant capability. Mild doses given to humans produce little effect but larger doses (20 mg) produce convulsions. The convulsions seen in response to picrotoxin are repetitive and uncoordinated. Tactile or auditory stimulation may trigger the convulsion as with strychnine (discussed in the section entitled "A Spinal Cord Stimulant: Strychnine"). Accompanying the convulsion are salivation, a rise in blood pressure, and frequent vomiting (Esplin & Zablocka-Esplin, 1970).

The major clinical use of picrotoxin is as an antidote to barbiturate poisoning or as an aide in increasing respiration which has been depressed by any number of drug agents.

The neurophysiological action of picrotoxin has been extensively investigated, and research has shown the drug to block several different inhibitory synapses. Picrotoxin has been shown in mammals to selectively block a type of inhibition called presynaptic inhibition. However, the role of presynaptic inhibition in motor excitability remains unclear. Thus we see a stimulant-convulsant action because the nervous system has lost its capability to inhibit neuronal discharge. The blocking action of picrotoxin is inhibited by GABA (gamma-aminobutyric acid) and research indicates that GABA is a neurotransmitter at inhibitory synapses in the central nervous system (Elliot & Florey, 1956; Robbins & Van der Kloot, 1958).

Pentylenetetrazol

Pentylenetetrazol (Metrazol, Cardiazol) is a synthetic CNS stimulant which has potent convulsive properties and is primarily used in research, although it has previously had clinical trials for various uses. The convulsions produced by small doses of pentylenetetrazol are different from those produced by strychnine or picrotoxin. Where the latter two drugs mainly produce convulsions characterized by limb and body extension, small doses of pentylenetetrazol produce convulsions reminiscent of petit mal epileptic seizures—the righting reflex is not lost and the animal maintains a sitting posture with forelimb and jaw extension. With larger doses, asynchronous repetitive seizures are seen.

The mechanism of action of pentylenetetrazol is unclear. The drug does not block either presynaptic or postsynaptic inhibition. It does not appear that the stimulant action is due to direct neuronal depolarization, but there is evidence that it may work through a decrease in neuronal recovery time. Scientists have observed a decrease in the relative refractory period of nerve tissue tested in vivo (Eyzaguirre & Lilienthal, 1949), and also a decreased recovery time for monosynaptic pathways in the spinal cord (Lewin & Esplin, 1961) after treatment with pentylenetetrazol. There is little evidence on the interaction of this drug with any of the putative neurotransmitter systems.

Pentylenetetrazol has been used briefly for many different clinical conditions. Originally, the drug was used as a cardiovascular stimulant, but it proved of little value for this specific purpose. At one time it was used as an agent in shock treatment for depressed patients. Due to inferior results and a high incidence of fractures and other side effects, insulin and electric shock are preferred for this purpose. With the new antidepressant drugs available, the use of shock treatment is also gradually declining (although with patients depressed to the point of being suicidal, electric shock is still the treatment of choice).

Nikethamide

Nikethamide (Coramine) is primarily used as a respiratory and cardiac stimulant. Generally, the drug produces an excitation over all of the cerebrospinal axis. The mechanism of action of the drug is unknown. However, it produces respiratory stimulation at doses that do not produce general CNS excitement, and this may be via direct stimulation of brainstem respiratory areas. The major use of the drug is in cases of respiratory failure or depression usually due to excessive use of central depressants.

A SPINAL CORD STIMULANT: STRYCHNINE

The only spinal stimulant we will discuss is strychnine, a drug that has no demonstrated therapeutic value, but a drug which has greatly advanced the knowledge of neurophysiology. Strychnine acts at the level of the spinal cord in the gray matter, which makes up the core surrounding the central canal. Of all the central nervous system stimulants, strychnine is probably the drug that is best understood. Chemically, it is an alkaloid found in nux vomica, the seeds of a tree native to India, *Strychnos nuxvomica.* The seeds of the tree were introduced into Germany in the 16th century as a rat poison and its use as a poison continues to this day in many parts of the world.

CNS Effects

Strychnine is a powerful central nervous system stimulant that acts by selectively blocking neuronal inhibition. It enhances and exaggerates incoming sensory information by removing inhibitory influences from the information processing pathways. Sensory input, then, is shunted throughout the central nervous system in cycles, increasing and decreasing, not according to the sensory input, but rather, relative to the increases and decreases of the neuronal refractory periods.

The strychnine convulsion is powerful and has a characteristic motor pattern. Because the drug is a disinhibitor, that is, it inhibits inhibition, the form of the convulsion will follow the relative strength of antagonistic muscles at the joints. Only the most powerful muscle at each joint will take part in the convulsion. Typical strychnine convulsions occur in spinal animals, and strychnine exerts a marked stimulant effect when applied directly to the spinal cord. For this reason, the convulsions are often termed *spinal convulsions.* Strychnine only affects those areas of the CNS that possess inhibitory nervous connections. Certain areas of the cerebellum and the autonomic ganglia are not stimulated by the drug because they lack the concentration of inhibitory connections.

The characteristic effects of strychnine to enhance ongoing neural activity and to exaggerate the effects of evoked activity are manifest on many portions of the CNS, not just the spinal cord. Therefore, use of the term *spinal stimulant* is a misnomer. It is only that the spinal actions are the most striking and easiest to observe.

The blockade of spinal inhibition was first demonstrated by Bradley, Easton, and Eccles in 1953. Strychnine specifically blocks postsynaptic inhibition—a type of inhibition presumed to be due to a specific chemical transmitter (GABA). This inhibitory transmitter produces inhibition through binding with the postsynaptic membrane. Presynaptic inhibition is not inhibited by strychnine, but there is growing evidence that picrotoxin may act via a disinhibition of presynaptic inhibitory influences. An example of postsynaptic inhibition is found in the functioning of the Renshaw cells of the spinal cord. These interneuronal connections are excited by collaterals of the motor neuron axons of the ventral horn cells. The excitatory transmitter to the Renshaw cell is known to be acetylcholine. Strychnine blocks the inhibitory impulses from the Renshaw cell (via GABA), which would feed back and inhibit the ventral horn motor activity, but it does not inhibit the cholinergic collateral-Renshaw synapse. The synaptic site of action of strychnine has not been determined. It may act postsynaptically to alter the membrane or compete with the transmitter, or it may block the presynaptic release of the transmitter.

Strychnine Poisoning

Despite the fact that chemical preparations with strychnine are not generally available, there are still several cases of strychnine poisoning each year. Suicides by means of strychnine have declined as the barbiturates have grown in popularity. Symptoms of strychnine poisoning in humans resemble those behaviors seen in animals. First, there is a stiffening of the neck and facial muscles, and soon there is a heightened reflex excitability. Any stimulus may provoke a violent motor response, which at first may be a coordinated extensor thrust, but then develops into a full repetitive convulsion. The body is arched in a hyperextension so that only the heels and top of the head may be touching the ground. All voluntary muscles are in full contraction and respiration may cease.

Treatment of the poisoning is based on preventing the convulsions and aiding respiration. CNS depressants (usually the short-acting barbiturates) will inhibit the tetanic spasms and only the extensor thrusts will continue (which are not fatal). Effective respiration will now be possible. It is important throughout the treatment to minimize tactile and auditory stimulation to the patient. The increased reflex excitability may last for as long as 24 hours after strychnine ingestion.

ANTIDEPRESSANTS

Depression, as is the case with most of the behavioral disorders, is a complex and confusing condition. Depression is a mood that most everyone experiences at one time or another. No "normal" individual lives in a state of perpetual euphoria, and minor variations in mood are seen as healthy signs. Normal individuals will become depressed, for example, at the death of a loved one, a failure at school or business, or a grave illness. Typically, these depressions pass, and soon the individual regains a productive role in society. However, when the depression does not pass, it is advisable to consult professional help.

Types of Depression

Depression cannot be precisely defined; to some it represents a symptom of a more general disease, and to others it is a disease in itself. This confusion about the very nature of the disorder has hindered its treatment. The symptoms are probably most clearly described as an unjustified and profound sadness and diminished emotional participation in interpersonal situations. Jarvik (1970) has provided a concise account of the various classes of depression, and the following is a brief summary of that classification.

When a neurotic disorder is present, the depression may be long lived and exaggerated, and it may be incapacitating. When this occurs, and the precipitating event can be identified, it has been called a *reactive* or *neurotic depresssion*. These depressions may be quite severe and may last for a long time.

There is a second group of persons who seem to be constantly in a state of depression; they are unable to experience happiness in their daily living (*constant depression*). Social interaction and interpersonal relationships are deficient: their self-esteem is chronically low. This is commonly seen in the alcoholic, the narcotic addict, and the sociopath.

A third major group of persons are those who exhibit depressed behavior patterns, but these depressions do not seem to be attached to any significant external event. Such people are usually older and the depressions are said to be *endogenous* (of unknown cause, and not related to any particular precipitating events). Often these depressions occur cyclically and may be characterized by quiet feelings, marked retardation, and autonomic signs such as decreased appetite, constipation, and weight loss. Some experts use the term *endogenous depression* to label this group of persons, while others use the terms *psychotic depression* or *involutional depression*.

Treatment of Depression

This diverse group of depressed behaviors may represent a single neurophysiological malfunction or they may represent separate neurophysiological or biochemical alterations. The etiology of the disorder is open to question at this time. Due to the uncertain nature of the disorder, a variety of psychotherapeutic techniques have been employed to deal with the depressed patient. Individual and group psychotherapy, family counseling, hospitalization, electroconvulsive shock treatment (ECT), and antidepressant drug therapy are today the most widely used treatment procedures. Many times the treatments are used singly, but more often the treatments are combined.

Until the middle of the 1950s the major treatment for severe depression was ECT. In cases where there is high suicidal risk, when a quick reversal of the depression is imperative, ECT is usually still employed. Also in cases where prior treatment with antidepressants has proven ineffective, or when the patient refuses to take medication, ECT is still recommended. However, when ECT is not indicated, drug treatment with the antidepressants may be employed.

Depressive illnesses are associated with the highest rate of suicide (attempted or completed) of all the behavioral disorders. In addition, a depressed person may be dangerous to others and capable of homicide. Since suicide or homicide is a possibility, it is important to bring the depression rapidly under control. The rapid onset of antidepressant action for ECT, and the fact that some antidepressant drugs take a week or two to become effective, leads to a preference in severe and potentially dangerous cases for immediate initial use of ECT, followed by attempted drug maintenance.

There are two major classes of drugs that we shall examine: the monoamine oxidase (MAO) inhibiting chemicals and the agents that are tricyclic in chemical structure (see Figure 8.2 for representative formulas). As we shall see in our investigation of these two classes of antidepressants, there is definite evidence to show the efficacy of drug treatment in the depressions; but as Ray (1972) notes,

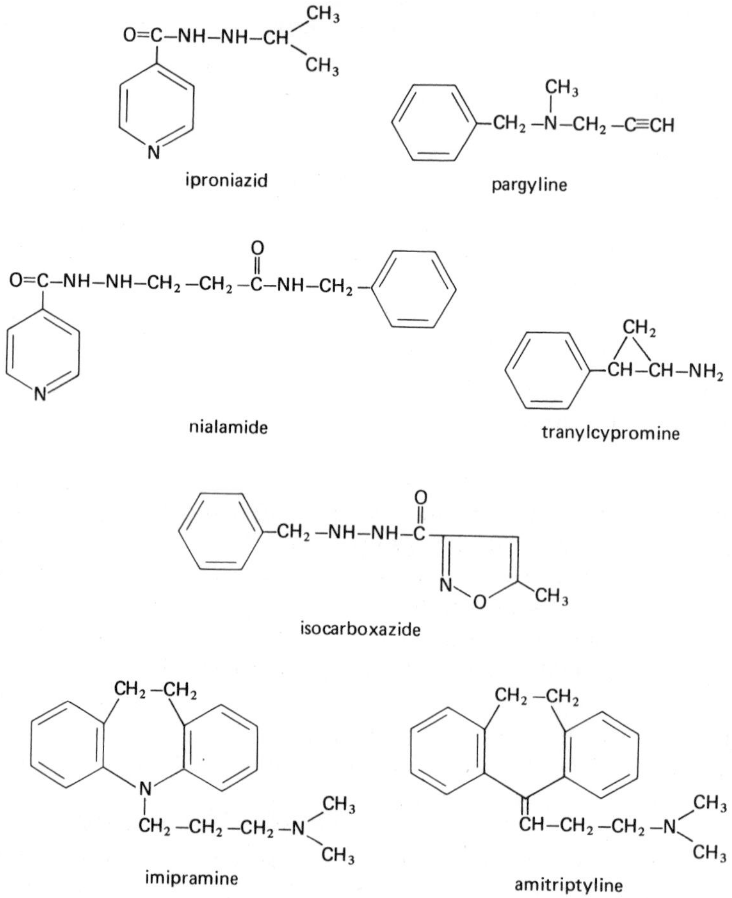

FIGURE 8.2. Structural formulas of some antidepressants.

ECT is probably still the most effective treatment for the depressed patient. Klein and Davis (1969) reviewed several studies comparing the effects of ECT and antidepressant drugs to a placebo treatment. They found that in seven of eight studies, ECT was the most effective treatment for depression. They also point out that, in four studies, ECT was more effective than the antidepressants and in three other studies, the two treatments were of equal effectiveness. One factor which makes ECT the more effective treatment is the amount of time before the depression is reversed. With the antidepressant drugs, long latencies (often 3-4 weeks) are common, whereas for ECT, the effects may be seen immediately. Spontaneous recovery from depression usually occurs in 20% to 25% of depressed patients. Placebo treatment may increase the recovery rate to between 25% and 60% and an effective antidepressant drug may increase the recovery rate to 50 to 75% (Lehmann, 1966).

MAO Inhibitors

The MAO inhibitors are a group of drugs that have in common the ability to block the action of the enzyme, monoamine oxidase, which deaminates the endogenous amines. This has the indirect effect of increasing the concentration of adrenergic transmitter substances. However, it must be pointed out that the relationship between this neurobiochemical effect of the MAO inhibitors and the mood-elevating properties of the drugs is not firmly established in the scientific literature.

History.   Like so many drugs used in the treatment of behavioral disorders, the MAO inhibitors were initially tested and used in the treatment of an unrelated condition. The mood-elevating properties of isoniazid, a drug used in the treatment of tuberculosis, were noticed in 1951; and in 1952; Delay, Laine and Buisson (1952) reported on the antidepressant properties of the substance.

The story of isoniazid in the treatment of tuberculosis, however, goes back to 1945 when Chorine reported the "tuberculostatic" actions of nicotinamide; it was later found that pyridine derivatives related to nicotinamide also possessed the tuberculostatic effects (isonicotinic acid and the thiosemicarbazones, for example). Isoniazid and its isopropyl derivative, iproniazid, were soon synthesized and found to be potent antituberculosis agents as well as mood-elevating agents. There was a question, however, as to the genesis of the elevated mood—was it from direct CNS effects or from a reversal of a bacterial infection? Early research by Zeller (1952) indicated the strong MAO-inhibiting action of iproniazid and called attention to the profound changes in catecholamine metabolism that this drug caused. In 1956, Brodie, Pletscher, and Shore confirmed this fact by showing increased levels of serotonin and norepinephrine after iproniazid administration. Due to its marked stimulant and euphoric effects, the drug was discontinued as an antitubercular treatment. Three independent teams of psychiatrists, Klein and his colleagues at Rockland State Hospital, Crane at Montefiore Hospital, and Scherbel and his collegaues at the Cleveland Clinic, simultaneously investigated the antidepressant effects of the drug and in 1957 it was introduced into psychiatry as an aid in the management of depressed patients (see Remmien, 1962). It was Kline (1959) who first attributed the euphoric drug effects to the inhibition of MAO and the subsequent increase in cerebral serotonin and norepinephrine. He further contrasted the mood-elevating effects of iproniazid and the increased concentrations of the monoamines to the quieting or sedating effects of reserpine and the correlated decrease in cerebral serotonin and norepinephrine concentrations. Kline referred to iproniazid as a *psychic energizer* and soon it was used in psychiatric hospitals for the treatment of psychotic depression, and also in nonhospitalized outpatients suffering from neurotic depression. The glowing reports of iproniazid-induced mood elevation prompted biological and pharmaceutical chemists to develop many new related compounds that also possessed the MAO-inhibiting properties.

Because of a high tendency toward toxicity, many of the MAO inhibitors are no longer available for clinical use. Iproniazid, although the initial MAO inhibitor used in psychiatric patients, proved to be very toxic and was soon replaced with other, less toxic derivatives. Drugs that have been introduced but are no longer available include iproniazid (Marsilid), pheniprazine (Catron), and etryptamine (Monase). At present, the drugs marketed for use in the treatment of depression include isocarboxazid (Marplan), nialamide (Niamid), phenelzine (Nardil), and tranylcypromine (Parnate). Tranylcypromine was withdrawn from general use for several months in 1964 but was later reintroduced.

Chemistry. The first MAO inhibitors used in the treatment of depression were derivatives of hydrazine, a substance highly toxic to the liver. Chemical alterations, however, have produced many useful compounds, which are not so toxic; the MAO inhibitor antidepressant drugs being one such drug group.

Two compounds which were synthesized in an attempt to reduce the toxicity of iproniazid were isocarboxazide and nialamide. Isocarboxazide was synthesized in an attempt to increase the MAO-inhibiting and antidepressant properties of iproniazid and to reduce the liver toxicity. While the new substance has been shown to possess increased MAO-inhibiting power and less toxicity than the parent compound, iproniazid, increased antidepressant properties have not been definitively demonstrated. The aim of the synthesis of nialamide was similar. The isopropyl substituent of iproniazid was replaced with a complex chemical substitution that reduced toxicity and increased MAO-inhibiting capacity. However, this chemical substitution also reduced the antidepressant properties of the drug.

The second major group of MAO-inhibiting antidepressant drugs are derivatives of amphetamine. Structural changes in the original phenylethylamine skeleton of amphetamine resulted in tranylcypromine, the prototype antidepressant drug. Tranylcypromine has amphetamine like CNS stimulant properties, in addition to a potent ability to inhibit MAO. Pargyline is another nonhydrazine MAO inhibitor. It is commonly used as an antihypertensive drug, but also has marked MAO-inhibiting properties and practically no liver toxicity; some clinical findings suggest that it may have antidepressant properties.

Metabolism. Although these drugs are typically prescribed orally, the presently available MAO inhibitors are readily absorbed regardless of the route of administration. The absorbed MAO inhibitor is taken up by sites where MAO is found (liver, heart, brain). The ability of these compounds to penetrate the brain is directly related to their lipid solubility. Due to the long latency until a behavioral effect is seen, the drugs are not administered parenterally.

Biochemical and neurophysiological effects. The role of the MAO enzyme is to catalyze the oxidative deamination of endogenous and exogenous monoamines (see Chapter 2). The primary activity of the MAO inhibitors is to block this catabolic pathway of the monoamines. Not only do the MAO-inhibiting drugs produce an increase in the endogenous monoamines, they also cause precursors of these chemicals to have marked stimulant effects. In addition, the MAO inhibitors potentiate the action of the indirect sympathomimetic stimulant drugs like amphetamine or tyramine.

Early studies by Schallek and Kuehn (1960) failed to show any changes in the EEG after iproniazid treatment, but more recent data have shown electrophysiological changes at several levels of the CNS (Himwich, 1965; Schallek and Kuehn, 1965).

Behavioral effects. The behavioral effects of the MAO-inhibiting drugs may best be viewed in a two-stage sequence. The first stage is that produced by the direct action of the MAO-inhibiting drug on the CNS. The second stage is correlated with the subsequent buildup of endogenous adrenergic chemicals. Administration of the MAO-inhibiting drugs alone produces either minor changes in the behavior of animals or no change at all. Physiologically, we may see alterations in endogenous monoamine concentrations, but behaviorally there may be little or no change from predrug baseline levels. However, when the MAO inhibitors are given in combination with other drugs, there are often marked behavioral changes. Typically, precursors of the monoamines are administered with the MAO inhibitor. After administration of an MAO inhibitor together with 5-hydroxytryptophan, the precursor of serotonin, there is a marked potentiation of the tremor produced by the drug, and after combination treatment with dihydroxyphenylalanine (DOPA), the precursor of norepinephrine, there is a potentiation of central excitement. These studies (see Ban, 1969) have shown that all three of the hydrazine derivatives, isocarboxazide, nialamide, and phenelzine, were from 15 to 20 times more potent behaviorally, than iproniazid, and it has been suggested that the increased potency of these drugs is a direct result of the degree of inhibition of the MAO enzyme.

The combined administration of an MAO inhibitor with tetrabenazine or reserpine (these drugs free the bound vesicular forms of the monoamines and thus make them available for synaptic transmission and for oxidative deamination by the MAO enzyme) has been extensively investigated. Tetrabenazine typically produces a depression and a blockade of conditioned avoidance responding. Pretreatment with any of the MAO inhibitors will reverse this effect. Among the many reserpine effects that are counteracted or reversed by the MAO inhibitors are depression, sedation, decrease in motor activity, catalepsy, hypotension, and the prolongation of ethanol sleeping time.

Clinical use. The MAO inhibitors have two major effects for which they are used in clinical medicine, an antianginal effect, which is considered to be a function of coronary artery dilation. Second is their antidepressant action which is useful in the treatment of behavioral depression and phobic anxiety states (and which has been the major use of these drugs). With those antidepressants which have been synthesized from phenylethylamine, the mood elevation is preceded by an amphetaminelike behavioral stimulant action. Continuous administration of the MAO inhibitors may lead to agitation, talkativeness, hypomania, or even manic reactions.

The most frequently used clinical procedure in the administraion of the MAO inhibitors is continuous therapy. Usually there is a 2-to-3-week latent period before the antidepressant effects are seen, but after this period the dosage of the drug may be reduced. The usual beginning dose of isocarboxazide is 20 to 30 mg a day, with the first therapeutic response seen in 2 to 3 weeks. Tranylcypromine is usually given in the same dose, but has the advantage that antidepressant effects may be seen in 2 to 4 days. The usual starting dose for nialamide is 75 to 100 mg per day, and phenelzine is usually started between 40 and 60 mg per day. The duration of the treatment is dependent upon the condition. For slight transient depression, the duration may be a month or 6 weeks; but for recurrent depression, drug treatment may go on for several years. Because of the marked cardiac effects of the drugs, termination is usually a slow tapering off process rather than an abrupt discontinuation.

Contraindications and side effects. The MAO inhibitors depress the ability of the body to metabolize both endogenous and exogenous monoamines. A particularly serious problem concerns tyramine, an indirect-acting adrenergic stimulant similar to amphetamine. Tyramine is naturally found in fermented foods such as cheese, beer, and wine. If a patient taking an MAO inhibitor ingests these foods, the liver may not be able to properly oxidize the tyramine, leading to a dangerous level of adrenergic stimulation. There are several reported cases of death due to a stroke from just this combination of MAO inhibition and adrenergic stimulation. Obviously, a patient taking an MAO inhibitor must be very carefully and strongly cautioned about these dietary restrictions.

The MAO inhibitors not only inhibit the enzyme, monoamine oxidase, but also inhibit other oxidative enzyme systems of the liver microsomes. For this reason, not only are the effects of the adrenergic and serotonergic drugs facilitated; but the actions of the tricyclic antidepressants, the narcotic analgesics, and barbiturates and other sedatives are also potentiated. In general, no other drug should be administered to a patient being treated with one of the MAO inhibitors; this restriction further limits their usefulness.

The MAO inhibitors produce a number of other potentially dangerous side effects. These include a manic reaction, suicide attempts, and exteriorization of delusional processes. The increased probability of suicide during the first days of treatment (also found with the tricyclics) is attributed to an amelioration of the psychomotor inhibition before the mood is elevated. Other serious side effects include damage to the blood-forming organs and liver damage. Since the MAO inhibitors are so toxic and also generally considered less effective than ECT or the tricyclics, they are usually not used until these other treatments have failed. Although some tolerance may develop, these drugs are not addicting; neither physical dependence nor a withdrawal syndrome has been demonstrated.

The Tricyclic Antidepressants

In addition to the MAO inhibitors, a second class of drugs, those that are tricyclic in chemical structure, has been shown to be effective in relieving depression. These are now the most widely used of the antidepressant drugs.

History. In 1889, Thiele and Holzinger synthesized iminodibenzyl and described its chemical properties. However, it was not until more than half a century later, in 1951, that its pharmacological properties were investigated and catalogued. Haefliger (1959) synthesized more than 40 derivatives of iminodibenzyl and tested them for their possible use as antihistamines, sedatives, analgesics, and antiParkinsonian drugs. Following careful screening experiments in animals, several drugs, including imipramine (Tofranil) were selected for therapeutic trials.

Imipramine is closely related chemically to the phenothiazine tranquilizers. However, Kuhn (1958) reported that unlike the phenothiazines, imipramine was relatively useless for calming the agitated psychotic patient, but instead was beneficial in depressed patients who were withdrawn and inactive. Since then, further evidence has accumulated and imipramine and its chemically related compounds—amitriptyline (Elavil), desmethylimipramine (Norpramin), and desmethyl amitriptyline (Aventyl)—have been the drugs of choice for depression, because they have been shown to be safer than the MAO-inhibiting agents and easier to apply than ECT.

Chemistry. The close structural relationship between the tricyclic antidepressants and the phenothiazines (see Chapter 5) is easily seen. Structurally, in the phenothiazine ring, a sulfur atom connects the two benzene rings; whereas in the tricyclic antidepressants, an ethylene linkage (CH_2-CH_2) provides this connection. Amitriptyline is similar to imipramine but a carbon atom replaces the nitrogen in the center ring and the chain is attached to the ring by a double bond.

Biochemical effects. The basic pharmacology of imipramine and amitriptyline is quite complex. This class of drugs does not inhibit the MAO-enzyme system, but instead has anticholinergic, antiserotonergic, and antihistaminic actions. It has been shown that an adequate catecholamine store in the CNS is a prerequisite for tricyclic antidepressant activity. If brain catecholamines have been depleted, imipramine does not antagonize the sedation produced by other drugs. When the catecholamine levels are restored to normal physiological levels, imipramine counteracts the sedation.

At an NIMH pharmacology workshop in 1966, the blockade of the reuptake of norepinephrine was suggested as the mechanism of action for the tricyclic antidepressants. In addition to increasing brain norepinephrine potency, the tricyclic antidepressants also enhance the action of injected norepinephrine or epinephrine at peripheral sympathetic receptor sites. It is tempting to speculate that the commonality which underlies the functioning of both the MAO-inhibiting drugs and the tricyclic antidepressants is the high levels of norepinephrine in the brain.

Some investigators (Cairncross, Gershon, & Gust, 1963; Mandell, A. J., Markham, Tallman, & Mandell, M., 1962) have preferred to view the anticholinergic properties of imipramine as the salient feature in the treatment of depression. Mandell, for instance, draws a close comparison between Parkinsonism, cholinergic activity, and the imipramine effects. These scientists found that Parkinsonian patients were significantly more depressed than normals, and it is not uncommon to find suicidal tendencies also present in these patients. Although a brain deficit in dopamine has been demonstrated, it is possible that an adrenergic-cholinergic imbalance exists. It has been suggested that an increase in cholinergic levels is present in this condition, since cholinomimetic drugs aggravate the patient's behavior and anticholinergics are often quite helpful in treating the condition. Imipramine administration to these patients improved the rigidity and alleviated the depression, although the tremor became more serious. The most convincing evidence, however, for an anticholinergic mechanism of action for these drugs is the numerous atropinelike side effects which often accompany their use.

Neurophysiological effects. Just as the biochemical correlates of these drugs are complex and many-sided, so are the neurophysiological effects that may be seen. There is no single neural site of action, but many researchers believe that the drugs affect several subcortical structures with little or no cortical effects.

The autonomic nervous system effects seen after tricyclic antidepressant administration are related to the previously discussed anticholinergic action of the drug. Some effects that may be seen include blurred vision, dryness of the mouth, constipation, and urinary retention. Sigg (1959) has demonstrated that imipramine produces such atropinelike effects as interference with pilocarpine-induced salivation, interference with bradycardia following vagus nerve stimulation, and a decrease in the acetylcholine-induced activity of isolated intestine.

It has been found that the tricyclic antidepressants have neurophysiological effects on the reticular-activating system, the hypothalamus, and several limbic-diencephalic structures. The tricyclic antidepressants depress the electrical activity of the ascending reticular-activating system; however, this must be viewed carefully, for the other group of antidepressants (MAO inhibitors) actually increases the electrical activity of the ARAS. This implies that the mode of action of the drugs is not the exclusive result of ARAS effects.

EEG studies (Fink, 1959) have shown that imipramine not only decreases total electrical activity, but decreases the percentage time of alpha waves and increases both theta and beta (fast) waves. Other neurological effects seen after imipramine administration include an increased rate of self-stimulation with electrodes in the lateral area of the hypothalamus (Olds, 1956), inhibition of the septal area as seen by decreased duration of afterdischarges, a slight increase in the excitability of the amygdala, and convulsant brain wave patterns in the hippocampus.

Behavioral effects. Despite its clinical utility as an antidepressant drug, imipramine produces a depression in spontaneous motor activity in laboratory animals, a prolongation of barbiturate sleeping time, and of ethanol-induced sedation. It also decreases body temperature and causes motor incoordination (ataxia). The depressant action of the tricyclic antidepressants is also seen in a decrease in conditioned avoidance responding. Imipramine is also capable of stimulating several behaviors in animals. Dews (1962) has shown that the speed with which a pigeon pecks for a grain reward increases after imipramine or desmethylimipramine administration, but is slowed by chlorpromazine injection.

The ability of imipramine to act synergistically with other chemicals has been suggested as a possible mechanism of action. It has been found that imipramine increases the amphetamine effects of increased operant responding (Carlton, 1961b) and also increases hypothalamic self-stimulation (Stein & Seifter, 1961). The facilitation of operant behavior by methylphenidate (a CNS stimulant) is also potentiated by imipramine, amitriptyline, and their desmethyl analogues.

Even though the tricyclic antidepressants are helpful in depressed patients, they do not appear to stimulate normal adult volunteer subjects. Rather, they tend to produce fatigue and side effects which very much resemble the effects of atropine. Ban (1969) states:

> A self experimenter has described that, after a latent period of about 30 minutes, 50 or 100 mg. of imipramine caused a sense of tiredness along with the feeling of growing distance between himself and his surroundings. This was followed by an inner restlessness, which he described as "inner-quivering." The overall effect was characterized as a feeling which one experiences when tired and unable to get to sleep. Another introspectionist reported that after a short phase of pleasant relaxation he felt an inner-harmony and increased vitality, but without an urge for action "similar to that which one experiences under the influence of amphetamines." (p. 277)

Clinical use. Since the introduction of the tricyclic antidepressants, they have been used widely and with much success in the treatment of depressions, and for several other psychological disturbances ranging from enuresis (bed wetting), to alcoholism, to neurotic disturbances.

The manner in which the drugs produce their effects on the patient is not clear. Cole (1964) has described the effect as a dulling of the ideation of the depressive, rather than the euphoriant response produced by the MAO inhibitors. However, there are some reports of a manic excitement and euphoria following imipramine administration. The definitive experiment to isolate the major behavioral mechanisms is yet to be done.

Since the nature and etiology of depression is still an open question, there is much semantic bickering over which and what kind of depression seems to respond best to which drug. It appears that many clinicians believe that a depression where the symptoms are experienced as physical ailments responds best to the tricyclic antidepressants. These are patients whose behavior is characterized by sleeplessness, headache, pressure on the chest, and loss of appetite. In the endogenous depressions, including the manic-depressive type, the tricyclic antidepressants have been shown to be superior to a placebo or to no drug treatment. Lehmann (1966) reviewed the data from over 130 studies involving about 10,000 depressed patients and found that imipramine and amitriptyline produced improvements of between 15% and 100%.

The question of when to use the psychopharmacological agents or to use other means of treatment must be taken into consideration. The most important variable is the potential for suicide on the part of the depressed patient. If the patient is suicidal, the fastest-acting treatment should be employed and this is still considered to be electroconvulsive shock treatment (ECT). If the patient is not suicidal, a less severe treatment regime would be recommended. Since the average latency for the tricyclic antidepressants to take effect is anywhere from 3 days to 6 weeks, the patient must be monitored and doses varied according to the response. Usually a patient's treatment is begun with one-third the average optimal daily dosage and this is increased until a behavioral effect is seen, and the optimal dose is reached. The patient must continue taking the medication for continued effects since the effect of the drug wears off rapidly. Because of this consideration, discontinuation of treatment is usually done slowly, permitting monitoring of the behavior brought about by decreasing the drug treatment.

The antidepressants are also used in cases of schizophrenia where there are affective problems and in the depressive hypochondriacal states of some chronic paranoid schizophrenics. In some cases these drugs have proven useful in treating childhood syndromes like nail biting, hair pulling, tantrums, school phobias, and enuresis.

These drugs are not appreciably toxic and are relatively safe for chronic use. Furthermore, little tolerance develops and they are not addicting (there is no craving or withdrawal syndrome). Although different investigators favor different members of the group, research does not permit a choice between them.

The introduction of the antidepressants has been an important impetus to psychiatric medicine, for now drugs are available that, when prescribed in adequate dosage, will decrease the length of depression in a high percentage of cases. The availability of this group of drugs permits many people to remain in society during depressive stages and prevents them from being admitted to a mental hospital where the care may be more custodial than therapeutic. The drugs also protect from relapse a large number of people who have suffered a depressive stage.

SUMMARY AND CONCLUSIONS

Some of the stimulants are primarily of toxicological and experimental interest. These drugs include picrotoxin and strychnine. Pentylenetetrazol and nikethamide have had some use in the treatment of respiratory depression, especially that resulting from poisoning with the depressant drugs. Cocaine has previously been used as a local anesthetic, but is now of interest because of its recreational use. The amphetamines (Chapter 3) are similar in action to cocaine and are of importance for several reasons: therapeutic usefulness, recreational use, and use in experimental research. Caffeine and nicotine are primarily of importance because of the prevalence of their use in the form of beverages and tobacco, respectively. Methylphenidate is now the drug of choice for certain of the behavioral problems of children (the so-called hyperkinetic syndrome), although the amphetamines have also enjoyed some success in the treatment of this condition.

The tricyclic antidepressants are the drugs of choice in the treatment of depression, although ECT is still favored by many. Most observers consider the inhibition of adrenergic presynaptic reuptake to be responsible for the antidepressant properties of these drugs. The MAO inhibitors would appear to be a last resort treatment for depression because of problems of toxicity, contraindications, and side effects. However, the phenylethylamine MAO inhibitors, which also have an immediate amphetaminelike stimulant action, are being increasingly used for short-term treatment because of their immediate amphetaminelike onset of action, accompanied by the delayed onset MAO inhibition.

Some of these drugs can be dangerous and are quite toxic: the brainstem stimulants—picrotoxin, pentylenetetrazol, and nikethamide; the spinal stimulant—strychnine; and the MAO inhibitors. However, these drugs are not generally used in suicide attempts. They are also not addictive, although in many cases tolerance does develop; physical craving and a withdrawal syndrome are not seen. However, there is usually a short-lived depression following rapid withdrawal of stimulants or antidepressants. It seems improper to describe these effects with the same term, *addiction,* which is applied to the depressants (including the minor tranquilizers) and the narcotic analgesics.

9

DISTORTING DRUGS

Barry J. Krikstone and Robert A. Levitt

INTRODUCTION

In this chapter we will discuss a group of drugs used to achieve effects that are considerably different from those of most of the drugs previously discussed in this book. These are the "distorting drugs," which have been used for centuries as means of attaining a religious or mystical experience and which presently are used to escape the world in either a religious or a recreational setting. These uses differ from those of most drugs discussed up to this point, which have been used in either a research or a therapeutic setting. Rarely have the distorting drugs been used in either a research or a therapeutic setting (the one major exception is LSD, which has been used in the United States and in Europe as an adjunct to psychotherapy).

The content of this chapter will not be limited to a purely psychopharmacological analysis of these drugs. Instead, to give a full appreciation of this class of drugs, we must include some additional material. We will look at the historical uses of the drugs in order to better appreciate their current status. In addition, we must, of necessity, use much introspective, subjective accounting of the specific drug effects. Finally, we will discuss the moral and ethical issues that surround the use of these drugs. We hope to provide knowledge of the specific psychological and biological facts, and also an appreciation of the critical social issues, so that the reader will be able to make informed decisions relating to the use of these drugs.

Terminology

We have chosen the term *distorting drugs* to describe the chemical agents discussed in this chapter. Traditionally, numerous semantic labels have been attached. Humphrey Osmond (1957) has used *psychedelic* to describe this class of drugs because he wished to emphasize the "mind-manifesting" or "mind-expanding" properties of the drugs. Others have used the term *psychotomimetic* (Efron, 1970). Since this term implies that the drugs are mimicking a psychotic state and since evidence indicates gross differences between a psychotic break and a drug "high," we do not feel this is an accurately descriptive term. Yet, the phenothiazines and butyrophenones are very effective specific antidotes for the "states" induced by most of the distorting drugs (including LSD, psilocybin, mescaline, and related chemicals); chlorpromazine is generally the drug of choice in such emergencies. Thus, there must be some basic underlying biological commonality between schizophrenia and the states induced by these drugs. The similarity between the effects of these distorting drugs is also pointed to by the large amount of cross-tolerance that one of them produces for the effects of the others.

A third term that has been popular is *hallucinogen*; however, the basis for this term must also be questioned. In a true hallucination, the sensory experience does not exist outside the "mind" or brain. Psychotic patients may genuinely experience hallucinations. The psychotic may see God talking to him or have the feeling of snakes or ants crawling over his body. In contrast, the drug user may see distortions, but generally he perceives what is there. He may modify the external sensory world so as to perceive it kaleidoscopically or as a wavering, distorted form, but he rarely hallucinates (imagines or manufactures perceptions). Instead, the drug user perceives a distorted version of what is in the environment. Dr. Jerome Levine (1966; cited by Brecher, 1972, p. 348) has recommended that we call the drug-induced perceptions *pseudo-hallucinations* to distinguish them from the psychotic state, but we feel a more operational term is needed. We have therefore chosen the term *distorting drugs* to describe more accurately the effects of these agents. We do not believe that this term will solve all the different problems of nomenclature and ideological views, but we do believe that it allows a fresh start into a very complicated (and often emotionally charged) subject area.

Classification

There are a large number of chemical agents which may act as distorting drugs. These agents have been classified in a number of ways. One is into groupings of major and minor drugs. According to Tart (1969) the major and minor drugs can be distinguished according to the following four criteria: the amount of volitional control maintained while experiencing the drug actions; the duration of the distorting effect; the amount of aftereffects resulting from the drug experience; and the degree to which users are likely to become proselytizers of drug-induced euphoric states. Frankly, we do not favor this admittedly appealing division into major and minor drugs because we believe it to be both simplistic and inaccurate. For example, while marijuana is seen by some as a minor drug, its active ingredient (THC) could qualify as a major drug. Thus, dose, form, and route of administration may influence the characterization of a drug as possessing major or minor actions.

We favor, at least for the present, a biochemical classification of the distorting drugs. According to current knowledge these agents seem to alter the biochemical balance of brain functions that exists between adrenergic, serotonergic, and cholinergic activity. It may not be simply a matter of some pattern of facilitation or inhibition of synaptic transmission. Instead, the distorting drugs seem to alter or "distort" transmitter systems in some aberrant manner. The chemical structures of most of these distorting drugs also are similar to those of the major putative neurotransmitters (D, NE, 5HT, ACh), or to the other drugs which influence these neurotransmitter systems.

Some of the distorting drugs may seem mild because one has to ingest or smoke a large amount of a particular mushroom, leaf, or seed, to achieve the drug effect; yet, this is a misleading situation. In their most concentrated forms, and by their most effective routes of administration, these agents all are active at quite low doses and produce major effects.

The Basis for Recreational Drug Use

It is not only important to realize that these drugs are toxic; it is the toxicity itself that is responsible for their use. These agents do not simply favor adrenergic functionings biochemically. Their biochemical consequences seem to be abnormal, toxic, and distorting to brain biochemical transmitter processes. The cognitive (introspective) consequences of these distortions of normal brain functioning happen to be ones that are perceived by human beings as pleasurable or rewarding. These rewarding perceptions seem to primarily involve a distortion of sensory awareness and of emotional or motivational feelings (such as changes in arousal, "happiness," hunger, or sexual feelings). These biological, cognitive, and introspective alterations also have important behavioral manifestations that may be studied.

As we have said earlier in this book, we do not consider the physiological, or the cognitive, or the behavioral to be primary, or of primary importance. They are equally important, but each allows the investigation of the underlying biological events at a different analytical level.

Euphoria vs dysphoria. An important point here, which may stand reemphasis, is that the particular drugs that humans choose to take recreationally are those whose actions are perceived as pleasant. Many drugs have both pleasant (euphoric) and dysphoric, or aversive, actions. Sometimes, these coexist, with one or the other being predominant. With other drugs, predominant stages with euphoric and dysphoric consequences may occur sequentially. The particular balance between euphoria and dysphoria may be a result of dose, route of administration, set, individual differences among takers, or a host of other factors. This balance achieved by the drug taker will, of course, be a major determining factor in whether or not he or she will choose to continue the recreational use of a distorting drug or of other such drugs.

The moral issue. At this time, the dangers of this type of drug use, for the individual user, and to the society, are much debated, but are still quite unclear. The biological dangers themselves are unclear, and only now are attempts being made to establish them. The religious, moral, and cultural implications of such recreational drug use are also now being debated (aside from the biological consequences) and are subject to much controversy and disagreement. We believe this is a subjective topic involving the ethical code and value system of the individual and the society. Therefore, although we can present some biological and psychological information that would influence your judgment and can make up our own minds on this subject, we will not attempt to make up your mind for you. We will, therefore, keep our personal moral or ethical opinions to ourselves.

Outline of the Chapter

We will begin this review of the distorting drugs with LSD, perhaps the most discussed and certainly the most studied of these agents. We will then discuss a number of other distorting substances which are chemical relatives of LSD. These include psilocybin (from the mushroom called teonanacatl by the Mexican Indians), ololiuqui (the seeds of certain plants that can be classified as morning glories and contain chemicals that are derivatives of LSD), and dimethyl-tryptamine (DMT, a short-acting tryptaminic distorting drug). We will conclude this section with *Amanita muscaria* (fly agaric), which may also depend on an alteration in serotonergic activity for its recreational use.

We will then discuss the distorting drugs that possess some similarity in chemical structure to the catecholamines. These include mescaline (from the cactus called peyote), DOM (also called STP), and myristicin (from nutmeg). We will conclude with a discussion, first, of marijuana and then, of the banana skin hoax.

Although we will separately discuss these drugs in detail and give many different examples of their individual effects, they do seem to have much in common. The sensory distortions, alterations in arousal, and motivational or affective changes produced by these agents are quite similar. They do differ, however, in the patterning of these actions and in the balance that is achieved of euphoric to dysphoric effects. These differences may be based not only on generic differences between the drugs, but also on such factors as dose, set, and route of administration.

It is important to realize that although tolerance (and cross-tolerance) develops to these drugs, they are clearly not addicting. There is no physical dependence or craving, and a withdrawal syndrome does not result from their discontinuance. Moreover, deaths directly attributable to their use in the human are rare. As a matter of fact, it is not clear that any cases have been reported in the modern literature of death resulting directly from the toxic effects of a lethal dose. However, accidental or "suicidal" deaths have been reported that may be considered as indirectly caused by actions of these agents.

LSD

LSD (lysergic acid diethylamide) is probably the best known and most researched of the distorting drugs. LSD is a synthetic chemical that is not found endogenously in plants or animals, even though it is chemically related to the ergot alkaloids (from the fungus, *Claviceps purpurea*) which produce the disease ergotism (see section on St. Anthony's Fire that follows). LSD is also the most pharmacologically potent of all of the distorting drugs, with effective doses being calculated in millionths of a gram (micrograms), rather than the more traditional milligram dosage.

Saint Anthony's Fire

The earliest history of LSD must begin with the disease technically known as *ergotism* but through legend known as St. Anthony's Fire. Ergotism is caused by eating an infectious mold which grows on grain, especially rye. Grain that is infected by the fungus is easily identifiable and is normally destroyed immediately. However, during times of great famine, often the grains are not destroyed, but instead are used to feed the hungry. Between 945 and 1600 A.D. there were at least twenty outbreaks of ergotism.

The disease usually takes one of two forms. The first is a syndrome of tingling sensations in the skin, accompanied by muscle spasms that may develop into convulsions; the victim also experiences insomnia and disturbances in thinking and consciousness. The second form of the affliction is gangrenous ergotism, in which the limbs suddenly swell up and become inflamed; the individual usually experiences a burning pain before the area becomes numb. Often a limb will fall off at a joint (knee or elbow). The following account describes such a case:

> The separation of the gangrenous part often took place spontaneously at a joint without pain or loss of blood. It is related that a woman was riding to the hospital on an ass, and was pushed against a shrub; her leg became detached at the knee, without any bleeding, and she carried it to the hospital in her arms. (Barger, 1931, p. 30)

The disease may move very rapidly. Sometimes only 24 hours will pass between the first signs of pain and the onset of gangrene. The gangrene is caused by contraction of the blood vessels to the extremities, which limits the blood supply to them.

During the 12th century, ergotism became associated with St. Anthony, although the reasons for this are unclear. Some suggest that the hospital for treating ergotism was built near the shrine of St. Anthony because he was afflicted with a mild case of the disease and some believe that the demons he reported battling were a result of the disease (Hordern, 1968). Others believe that the name came from the fact that those who journeyed to Egypt, where St. Anthony had lived, were cured of the disease. No matter which legend is true, it is a fact that those entering the hospital and those making the pilgrimage to Egypt were cured of the disease. This is probably due, however, to a change to a diet that did not include the ergot-infected grains. Although the cause of the illness was established before 1700, only symptomatic treatment exists. There have been no recent reports of ergotism infection.

The Discovery of LSD

On April 16, 1943, Dr. Albert Hofmann, a chemist at the Sandoz Pharmaceutical Laboratories in Basel, Switzerland, became ill and later recorded the following account of his symptoms:

> Last Friday . . . I had to interrupt my laboratory work in the middle of the afternoon and go home, because I was seized with a feeling of great restlessness and mild dizziness. At home, I lay down and sank into a not unpleasant delirium, which was characterized by extremely excited fantasies. In a semiconscious state, with my eyes closed (I felt the daylight to be unpleasantly dazzling), fantastic visions of extraordinary realness and with an intense kaleidoscopic play of colors assaulted me. After about two hours this condition disappeared. (Reprinted from Hofmann, 1968, pp. 184–185, by courtesy of Marcel Dekker, Inc.)

At the time of this experience Dr. Hofmann and his colleague, Dr. W. A. Stoll, had been working on derivatives of ergot (which could not itself have produced these bizarre symptoms). A derivative nicknamed LSD-25 had earlier been synthesized and given this name because it was the 25th compound to be synthesized in the series. Initial animal testing revealed that it was not of interest. It was put on the shelf without human testing, to remain there for 5 years. Three days after he wrote the first account in 1943, to find out if this drug could have produced the bizarre effects, Dr. Hofmann ingested what he thought was a small amount (about 0.25 mg) and made the following record in his notebook:

> *April 19, 1943*: Preparation of an 0.5% aqueous solution of d-lysergic acid diethylamide tartrate.
> *4:20 P.M.*: 0.5 cc. (0.25 mg. LSD) ingested orally. The solution is tasteless.
> *4:50 P.M.*: No trace of any effect.
> *5:00 P.M.*: slight dizziness, unrest, difficulty in concentration, visual disturbances, marked desire to laugh . . . (Hofmann, 1968, p. 185)

Dr. Hofmann had begun what now is called an *LSD trip* and he was in for a disturbing, exhausting 6-hour period. After his recovery he noted:

> The last words could only be written with great difficulty. I asked my laboratory assistant to accompany me home as I believed that my condition would be a repetition of the disturbance of the previous Friday. While we were still cycling home, however, it became clear that the symptoms were much stronger than the first time. I had great difficulty in speaking coherently, my field of vision swayed before me, and objects appeared distorted, like images in curved mirrors. I had the impression of being unable to move from the spot, although my assistant told me afterwards that we had cycled at a good pace. . . .
> By the time the doctor arrived, the peak of the crisis had already passed. As far as I remember the following were the most outstanding symptoms: vertigo, visual disturbances; the faces of those around me appeared as grotesque, colored masks; marked motor unrest, alternating with paresis; an intermittent heavy feeling in the

head, limbs, and the entire body as if they were filled with metal; cramps in the legs, coldness and loss of feeling in the hands; a metallic taste on the tongue; dry, constricted sensation in the throat; feeling of choking; confusion alternating between clear recognition of my condition in which state I sometimes observed, in the manner of an independent, neutral observer, that I shouted half insanely or babbled incoherent words. Occasionally I felt as if I were out of my body.

The doctor found a rather weak pulse but an otherwise normal circulation.

... Six hours after ingestion of the LSD-25 my condition had already improved considerably. Only the visual disturbances were still pronounced. Everything seemed to sway and the proportions were distorted like the reflections in the surface of moving water. Moreover, all objects appeared in unpleasant constantly changing colors, the predominant shades being sickly green and blue. When I closed my eyes, an unending series of colorful, very realistic and fantastic images surged in upon me. A remarkable feature was the manner in which all acoustic perceptions (e.g., the noise of a passing car) were transformed into optical effects, every sound causing a corresponding colored hallucination constantly changing in shape and color like pictures in a kaleidoscope. At about 1:00 o'clock, I fell asleep and awakened next morning somewhat tired but otherwise feeling perfectly well. (Hofmann, 1968, pp. 185–186)

The amount of LSD that Hofmann ingested is about five to eight times the normal effective dose for producing the distorting state. This account of Hofmann's experience is most valuable because his experience was uncontaminated with preconceived notions about the drug experience or with specially stimulating environments (like piercing music, bright posters, and flashing strobe lights). Subsequent to these initial experiments with LSD, scientists in Europe and the United States explored the possibility that LSD was somehow related to the neurophysiological substrates underlying the "mental disturbances" like the schizophrenic disorders. Since such a small quantity of LSD (0.03 to 0.05 mg) is effective in producing bizarre behavior reminiscent of psychotic behavior patterns, it was only reasonable to consider the possible link between the two. The search began and to this very day the search continues for the neurophysiological link between LSD and the schizophrenic disorders.

Current Legal Status

The history of the experimental and recreational use of LSD began only two decades ago (for an excellent review of the history of LSD, we suggest *Licit and Illicit Drugs* by Edward Brecher, 1972). The first experimental study of the drug occurred in Zurich, Switzerland in 1947; in North America, the first report of the use of the drug in humans was in 1949. Sandoz Laboratories applied to the Food and Drug Administration to study the effects of the new drug and in the early 1960s they distributed large quantities to qualified scientists who performed biochemical and animal behavior research with the drug. In 1966, for a variety of reasons, Sandoz recalled the LSD it had distributed and withdrew its support from LSD research. The company continues to manufacture the drug, but the federal government, through the National Institute of Alcohol, Drug Abuse and Mental Health, and the Food and Drug Administration is now the distributing agent. It should be emphasized at this point that the scientific data collected and published are based on pure LSD. The effects detailed in the scientific literature may be slightly different from rumors about "street drug" effects because in many instances LSD purchased on the street is not pure. Some of it even contains no LSD at all, but an amphetamine (or even strychnine) substitute.

Pharmacology

LSD is an extremely potent crystalline chemical which is tasteless, odorless, and colorless. It has been estimated that one ounce of the compound is sufficient to produce 300,000 human adult doses. The typical method of ingestion is orally (usually the drug is dropped onto a sugar cube), although some feel it is necessary to administer the drug intravenously. In any case, the drug is rapidly absorbed and is widely distributed throughout the body. Half of the blood-LSD is metabolized every 3 hours and seems to be broken down in the liver and excreted as 2-oxy-LSD (Axelrod, Brady, Witkop, & Evarts, 1957).

Neurology. Studies utilizing radioactively tagged LSD have indicated that the drug is concentrated in the liver with relatively little in the brain. However, that portion of the drug that does enter the brain is highest in the visual areas, parts of the limbic system, and reticular formation. Many attempts have been made by using the EEG to localize a specific neural site of action for LSD. The drug has been reported to increase the low voltage, fast activity of the rabbit EEG, and this also has been reported in the human. Purpura (1956) has demonstrated a blockade of the cortical response to repetitive thalamic stimulation, a "recruitment block." Brücke (cited in Longo, 1972) has demonstrated that the firing of neurons in the hippocampus is almost completely inhibited after intravenous administration of LSD. The relationships between these neurophysiological findings and the distorting effects of the drug, however, are still a mystery and must await further research for clarification.

One of the major neurological effects of LSD is to increase the sensitivity of the sensory collaterals that feed into and activate the reticular formation. This is not a similar effect to that of amphetamine, however. LSD lowers the threshold for sensory input into the reticular formation but does not directly increase the sensitivity of the reticular formation itself. Due to the increased sensitivity of the collaterals, stimulation that normally would not get into this information processing system now is processed and directed to the cortex. Although LSD does not activate the sensory centers themselves, it probably functions to increase the sensory input by increasing the size of the sensory signal reaching cortical areas. This may offer a tentative explanation of the vivid sensory displays and distortions experienced after LSD ingestion.

Biochemistry. There have been two major theoretical notions as to the mechanism of action behind the LSD effect. The first of these stresses the sympathomimetic nature of many of the responses and the second has attempted to relate the LSD behavioral effects to the antiserotonergic biochemical effects of the drug.

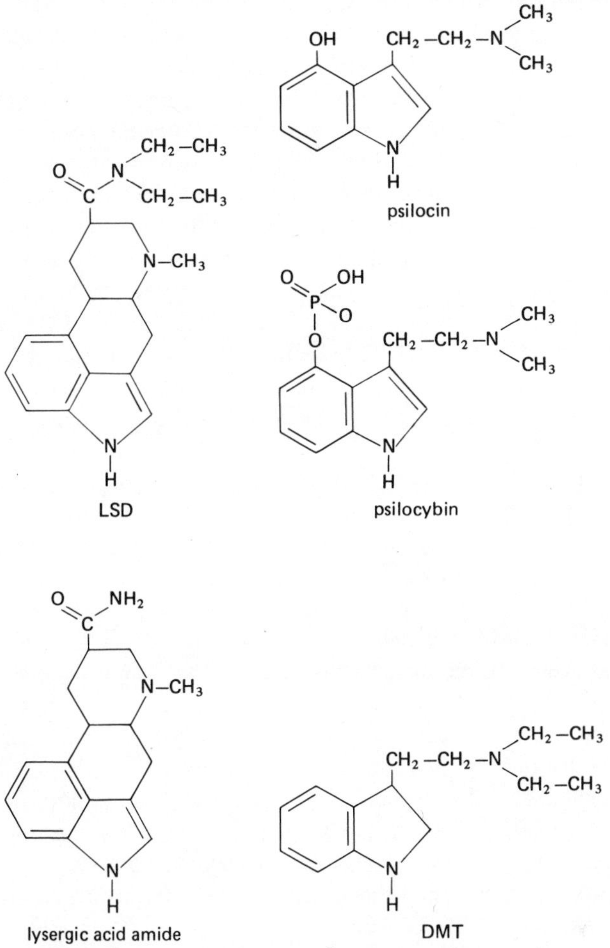

FIGURE 9.1. Chemical structures of some of the distorting drugs that possess an indole nucleus.

The sympathomimetic nature of this drug is evident not only from its behavioral effects but also from its chemical structure (see Figure 9.1). Chemically, it is a sympathomimetic compound because of the presence of the phenylethylamine within its structure. The signs of acute intoxication, such as motor excitation and increased body temperature, are very similar to some of the signs of sympathetic nervous system arousal. These comparisons have led some to postulate a sympathetic mechanism of action.

The second theory postulates an antiserotonin action to account for the LSD effects. In 1954 Gaddum and Hameed demonstrated that LSD was a powerful antagonist of serotonin in vitro and suggested that this blocking property may be responsible for the effects on the brain. Many studies have tried to correlate antiserotonin effects with the distortion properties of various drugs, but the results have not been conclusive. Brom-lysergic acid diethylamide and l-methyl-lysergic acid butanolamide, two drugs closely related chemically to LSD, both have strong antiserotonin activity, but possess relatively little and inconsistent hallucinogenic action (Isbell, 1959). The exact nature of the serotonin effect is unknown, but there is evidence that suggests LSD occupies the receptor site for serotonin since it acts as a potent inhibitor of serotonin uptake by cells, and inhibits the central nervous system actions of serotonin. Ray (1972) has suggested that LSD probably competes with serotonin at the receptor site since lowered levels of serotonin usually lead to an increase in LSD effectiveness, and increased serotonin levels (following MAO inhibitors) usually lead to decreases in LSD effects.

Tolerance and addiction. Both human beings and monkeys develop a tolerance to the behavioral effects of LSD, and this usually occurs within a few days. Cross tolerance has been noted between LSD, mescaline, and psilocybin, as well as with other lysergic acid derivatives. The development of physical dependence or addiction has not been shown for any of the distorting drugs.

Toxicity. LSD has proven to be one of the most toxic of all the synthetic derivatives of lysergic acid. The toxic dose varies from species to species with mice tolerating the highest dose and rabbits being the most sensitive (lethal dose 0.3 mg/kg i.v.) of all laboratory animals. The most sensitive species to date has been the elephant. At the Oklahoma City zoo 0.1 mg/kg was enough to kill this huge animal (West, Pierce, & Thomas, 1962). The drug is also active in lower vertebrates not commonly studied in the laboratory. It causes deviant behavior in insects, mollusks, and fish. Siamese fighting fish (*Betta splendens*) placed in water containing 0.2 mg/liter lose their aggressiveness; spiders spin disorganized and very unsymmetrical webs; and the mystery snail shows motoric disruption.

An antidote. Many of the actions of LSD (as well as mescaline and psilocybin) can be effectively counteracted in both humans and other species with chlorpromazine and the other phenothiazine derivatives. Reserpine, on the other hand, exacerbates the LSD effects.

The Distorting Effects of LSD in Humans

Dr. Timothy Leary (1968), the former Harvard psychologist, probably started the "psychedelic era." It was Dr. Leary and his colleague, Dr. Richard Alpert, who, while at Harvard from 1960 to 1963, conducted experiments on the effects of LSD. Leary became interested in distorting drugs when he ate mushrooms containing psilocybin during a trip to Mexico in 1960. He later said it was then he realized the old Timothy Leary was dead and the "Timothy Leary game" was over. Leary and Alpert discussed the drug effects with Aldous Huxley (who had written in *The Doors of Perception* [1954] of his own experiences with mescaline in the early 1950s) and soon began their scientific studies.

The early investigations at Harvard were well-controlled experimental studies done in the laboratory under the guidance of a physician, in case any drug side effects should occur. Soon, however, the physician was eliminated and many of the scientific, experimental controls were dropped. Leary began taking the drugs with his subjects, for he thought this would permit him to communicate with them better. Later the experiments were moved outside the laboratory to various off-campus dwellings. As early as late 1961, there were official complaints about Dr. Leary and the conduct of his experiments, but no action was taken. Finally, in 1963, both Leary and Alpert were dismissed from the University and Leary quickly became the guru of the 1960s. He retired to an estate in Millbrook, New York, owned by a wealthy follower of his, and was subsequently arrested there for illegal possession of marijuana. He has repeatedly stated since 1963 that drugs are not necessary to open up the mind or have a full religious experience; they only help. They act as a key to help in opening up one's inner self.

Stages of the LSD experience. The effects of LSD may be divided into an autonomic stage and a central stage. Houston (1969) has analyzed the distorting effects (the central stage) of the LSD drug experience and has broken them down into four categories; the sensory level, the recollective-analytic level, the symbolic level, and the integral level. Figure 9.2 is a hypothetical curve showing how increased doses of LSD lead to increased effects. The first stage of autonomic effects is experienced with the minimum dosage. These symptoms include chills, sweating, dilation of the pupils, nausea, headache, and a dry mouth. The following four stages are primarily central in nature and range from the kaleidoscopic visual displays of the sensory level to a feeling of oneness and unity with God in the final stages.

In the sensory stage, which is reached by almost all users, there are distortions in the perception of almost everything. Colors, sounds, tastes, and tactile experiences all take on a different perspective. There is also the phenomenon of synesthesias in which sense modalities seem to be crossed. Colors evoke musical

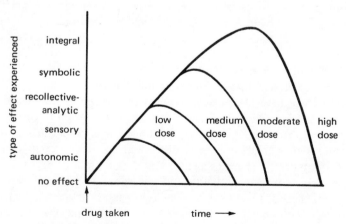

FIGURE 9.2. Hypothetical dose- and time-response curve for LSD. (Reprinted by permission from O. S. Ray, *Drugs, Society, and Human Behavior.* Rev. ed. Copyright 1974 by C. V. Mosby.)

melodies and rhythms, and a Beethoven symphony or Rolling Stones album elicits a free form of colors and textures, constantly changing and entertaining the subject. If the subject stares at his own hand, it changes before his eyes. It is a slow, continuous change in which the outline of the hand gradually becomes distorted and wavy (Longo, 1972).

The third stage in the LSD syndrome is the recollective-analytical level of consciousness. This is the first stage in which thought disorders are seen, and the hallmark of this stage is that the subject begins to look at himself in an evaluative context. One sees himself in his own history and personality. When one is forced to confront himself, many times this is met with panic and fright. One also during this stage often better appreciates his hopes and aspirations.

The final stages of the LSD effect have been labeled the symbolic and integral levels. These have been described as explorations of our true selves. At the symbolic level there is an appreciation of our oneness with the universal concepts expressed in myths. To experience the integral level has been likened to a religious conversion, that is, the sudden awareness that we have been accepted by God and are saved. At this level the individual feels a unity with God and/or with the essence of the universe.

Situational factors. There are three factors that interact to produce any given LSD effect: the environmental setting, the use of the guide, and the dose of the drug taken. It is well known that the more stimulating and exciting the environment, the greater will be the effect of the drug. It is probably because of this that laboratory studies into the LSD effect produce different results from rumored street use. Another important variable is the presence or absence of a guide to aid in monitoring and leading a new drug user through his initial experiences. How should one react to the new experiences? the distorted perceptions? and the synesthesias? It is the function of the guide to help the novice through these initial stages of drug experience. It is a common practice to have one person in the group stay "straight" and refrain from any drug use in order to monitor and guide the other participants. The length and extent of the drug experience is directly related to the dose of the drug. As the dose increases, the depth of the experience also increases, but the autonomic and sensory effects seem to be present at even the most minimal doses.

LSD art. There have been many attempts to analyze art drawn under the influence of LSD. Figure 9.3 is a picture of a man drawn under the influence of LSD. Notice the distorted perceptions of the fingers, eyes, nose, and mouth. The entire picture is an example of sensory distortion. The series of self-portraits in Figure 9.4 illustrate the changing perceptions during the LSD experience. The first picture depicts the subject before LSD ingestion. As the pictures progress, and the LSD begins to distort the perceptions to a greater degree, the completeness and the detail of the portraits begin to wane. The eyes become unfinished and in the third picture even begin to look wild. The final picture was drawn 9 hours after LSD ingestion, and the subject was less pleased with this portrait than with the initial picture.

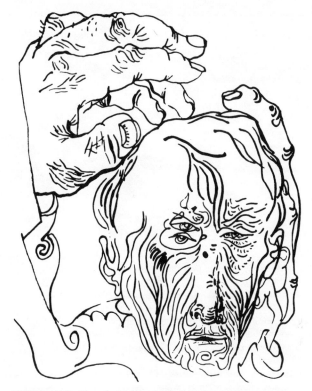

FIGURE 9.3. The phenomenon of alteration in the appreciation of the body extremities is illustrated in a sophisticated
way by a professional painter. This drawing was executed by
a well-known Czech artist after recovery from LSD intoxication. (Courtesy of Panorama Sandoz.)

Adverse Effects and Hazards of LSD

As LSD became more and more popular in the 1960s, the adverse effects and
hazards of the drug also began to increase (or at least seemed to increase). In a
study surveying most of the legal investigations in the United States, Cohen
(1960) reported relatively few side effects and complications from LSD. Data
were reported from over 25,000 doses in 5,000 patients. In experimental
subjects receiving LSD or mescaline 0 out of 1,000 attempted suicide, 0 out of
1,000 completed suicide, and 0.8 out of 1,000 reported a "psychotic reaction"
lasting over 48 hours. In patients undergoing psychotherapy 1.2 out of 1,000
attempted suicide, 0.4 out of 1,000 completed suicide, and 1.8 out of 1,000
reported a "psychotic reaction" lasting over 48 hours. In 1963 Cohen and
Ditman reflected on these data:

> The actual incidence of serious complications following LSD administration is not
> known. We believe, however, that they are infrequent. It is surprising that such a
> profound psychological experience leaves adverse residuals so rarely. (p. 479)

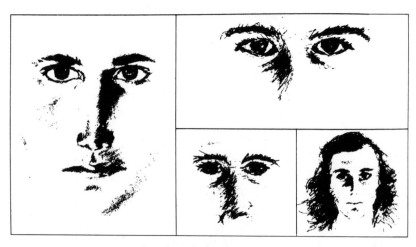

FIGURE 9.4. This series of self-portraits was drawn by an artist at several points during the course of an LSD experience. (*Left*) the first self-portrait was completed just prior to taking the drug; he said that this picture reflects his soul as he saw it. (*Top right*) the next self-portrait was executed three hours after he had ingested LSD. His desire and ability to concentrate had decreased, and he had begun to "feel paranoid" about his artistic ability. As a result, he frantically sketched this picture "to recapture the person I knew I was." (*Bottom left*) three hours later the next portrait was attempted. At this point he was almost totally distracted by hallucinations; he could not concentrate, and had no desire to draw. He described this portrait as a "futile attempt." (*Bottom right*) his final picture of the series was done nine hours after taking the LSD; at this point its effects were wearing off. He diligently attempted a self-portrait, but was less satisfied with this picture than with his initial effort above. He explained that the sketchiness of the drawing "was directly attributable to the paranoia generated by my artistic insecurity." (Reprinted by permission from *Psychology Today: An Introduction* [2nd ed.]. Del Mar, Calif.: CRM Books. Copyright 1972 by Communications Research Machines, Inc.)

The study of the adverse reactions to LSD is an emotional area and is one of complexity due to individual differences and also to variations in the drug. Brecher (1972) lists twelve reasons for the adverse effects that may be seen:

1. Increased expectation of adverse effects. When an individual attempts to take an LSD trip and has anxiety or apprehension over the experience, trouble may result. The nationwide warnings about LSD in 1962 and 1967 may have contributed to the increase in side effects by suggesting some to naive users.

2. Unknown dosages. Patients and those receiving the drug from a legally registered researcher usually received properly and accurately measured doses; however, when the drug is bought on the street in a sugar cube or a capsule there is no guarantee as to the precise dose of the drug contained. Related to this also are

3. Contamination of the drug and

4. Adulteration of the drug. Early drug doses were chemically pure and were known to be high-grade LSD. In some street sales, the LSD is prepared in

impure containers and various side effects may be the result of these impurities. Also, many times the drugs purchased as LSD really are adulterated with other drugs (STP, DMT, mescaline, amphetamine); it is impossible to state if adverse effects are the result of the LSD, the adulterating chemical, or some interaction of the two.

5. Mistaken attribution. A substantial number of LSD users experiencing adverse reactions have used other drugs, either at the same time or at other times. Again, it is impossible to attribute the side effects to any specific drug in these cases.

6. Side effects of law enforcement. In some cases an individual having a bad trip is imprisoned instead of having a guide help him through the ordeal. In one example, several people in the San Francisco Haight-Ashbury area had bad trips on LSD distributed at a celebration in a park. Thirty-two users were treated at a local clinic and were returned home or to the care of a friend. Seven others were detained by the police and imprisoned, and later taken to San Francisco General Hospital. A physician commented that the adverse reactions were due not to the "intensity of the reaction but to its management." The person under the influence of LSD should never be left alone. There is need for supervision, and a guide should always be present. As LSD became more available on the black market, this safeguard was often ignored and people were unable to cope with the drug experience.

7. Lack of supervision.

8. Mishandling a panic reaction and

9. Misinterpretation of reaction. In many cases, early tales of side effects came from hospital emergency rooms. Subjects brought in often had their stomachs pumped in order to remove the drug from the system. This is a noxious experience in any case, but probably that much worse under the influence of LSD. In other cases, the patients were labeled as *psychotic* and were taken to the psychiatric wards with other psychotic patients.

10. Flashbacks. One of the early publicized adverse effects was the phenomenon of flashbacks, that is, the sudden recurrence of the LSD experience days, weeks, or months after the drug had been ingested. This led some to immediately claim permanent brain damage. Dr. Cohen, in the study quoted earlier, did not report any incidence of flashbacks, and as late as 1967 only 11 cases of flashbacks were reported in the medical literature. An explanation has been offered that suggests that all intense emotional experiences produce flashbacks. Whether these are LSD-induced or not, people who have intense emotional experiences (the death of a loved one, the moment of falling in love, the moment of an automobile crash) have flashback experiences that may last a week, a day, months, or years depending on the intensity of the emotional experience.

11. Preexisting pathology: a major cause of the adverse effect is the widespread availability of the drug to everyone, to adjusted as well as maladjusted persons, to normals, as well as undiagnosed psychotics. It would

appear that the LSD experience may be too strong for those personalities bordering on the edge of collapse.

12. A final reason for adverse reactions is that some people take the drug unknowingly. It is given as a prank or a practical joke. The unwitting receiver may not be ready for the sudden experience and may panic and suddenly not know what is happening around him. This most definitely would be a traumatic experience.

PSILOCYBIN

The history of the Mexican mushrooms is very interesting and closely intertwined with the early Aztec and Mexican cultures. The mushrooms had been used by these early cultures for religious ceremonial purposes; large stone mushrooms with god figures carved on the stems, dating back to before 9000 B.C., seem to signify the importance of the mushroom to these societies. In the 16th century, the use of these drug-containing plants was banned. The mushrooms had been named *teonanacatl*, which can be translated as *god's flesh* or *sacred mushroom*. In the late 1930s it was clearly shown that these mushrooms were still being used by natives in Mexico. For more detailed accounts of the historical aspects of psilocybin and the other distorting drugs treated in this chapter, we suggest that the reader consult Brecher (1972) or Ray (1972).

One of these Mexican mushrooms is *Psilocybe mexicana* (Figure 9.5), and the active distorting drug that has been isolated from it is psilocybin. The drug was isolated in 1958 by Albert Hofmann and was later synthesized. Early use of the drug was by ingesting the natural mushrooms, but now modern experimental usage and "tripping" are both almost entirely with the synthetic chemical. Before Hofmann synthesized the chemical, he ate 32 of the mushrooms (which is an average dose) and reported the following effects:

> Thirty minutes after taking the mushrooms the exterior world began to undergo a strange transformation. Everything assumed a Mexican character. As I was perfectly well aware that my knowledge of the Mexican origin of the mushroom would lead me to imagine only Mexican scenery, I tried deliberately to look on my environment as I knew it normally. But all voluntary efforts to look at things in their customary forms and colors proved ineffective. Whether my eyes were closed or open I saw only Mexican motifs and colors. When the doctor supervising the experiment bent over me to check my blood pressure, he was transformed into an Aztec priest and I would not have been astonished if he had drawn an obsidian knife. In spite of the seriousness of the situation it amused me to see how the Germanic face of my colleague had acquired a purely Indian expression. At the peak of the intoxication, about 1½ hours after ingestion of the mushrooms, the rush of interior pictures, mostly abstract motifs rapidly changing in shape and color reached such an alarming degree that I feared that I would be torn into this whirlpool of form and color and would dissolve. After about six hours the dream came to an end. Subjectively, I had no idea how long this condition had lasted. I felt my return to everyday reality to be a happy return from a strange, fantastic but quite really experienced world into an old and familiar home. (Hofmann, 1968, p. 176)

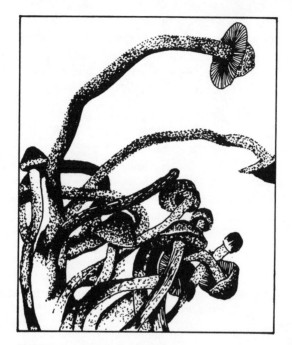

FIGURE 9.5. *Psilocybe mexicana*, grown in the laboratory. A handful of these mushrooms, ingested raw,
induces the hallucinogenic experience.

Pharmacology

The dried mushrooms contain from 0.2% to 0.5% of psilocybin, and the distorting effect experienced is dose dependent. Hofmann's laboratory established the effective dose for an adult at between 6 and 12 mg. Doses at this level (and sometimes even less) produce a pleasant experience and relaxation. Higher doses of about 25 mg or more produce the perceptual distorting effects, which in some individuals include hallucinations. Along with the psychological distortions there are sympathetic nervous system effects seen with psilocybin.

Isbell (1959) has investigated the psychological effects of both psilocybin and LSD, and under experimental conditions, the distorting effects are similar. The first period is rather unpleasant, characterized by dizziness, nausea, and general sympathetic disturbances, and lasts about 1/2 hour. Following this is a second 1/2 hour, usually characterized by further sympathetic complaints, coupled with some impairment in cognitive control and attention. The following 4 to 12 hours is characterized by the typical euphoric and distorting effects. The larger doses will produce the longer periods of hallucinogenic or distorting actions. Following this period is a stage of quietness, lassitude, and headache. This later stage is not typical of the LSD effect. In addition to the similar effects of the psilocybin and LSD, there is a cross-tolerance which develops between

LSD, psilocybin, and mescaline. This cross-tolerance suggests that these three drugs share common properties (Isbell, Wolbach, Wilker, & Miner, 1961).

It has been suggested that the effects of psilocybin are due to a biochemical breakdown to psilocin. This chemical is present in the mushroom, but only in trace amounts. The greater effects from psilocin may be due to its increased lipid solubility and, hence, the relative ease with which it may cross the blood-brain barrier and affect the central nervous system. The chemical formulas for both psilocybin and psilocin are shown in Figure 9.1. Both are indole chemicals closely related to LSD.

Research with psilocybin on animals has indicated that it does not produce the excitatory actions seen with LSD nor the convulsive actions seen after large doses of mescaline. In some animals (cats) hypertension is seen, whereas in others (dogs) hypotension is noted. The neurological effects of psilocybin are similar to that of mescaline, but differ from those of LSD. Low doses of psilocybin activate the EEG tracings, while higher doses usually induce the appearance of slow waves. Psilocybin, like many of the distorting drugs, markedly decreases hippocampal electrical activity (Longo, 1972). The drug interferes with the performance of learned tasks, particularly complex activities where discriminations are required (Adey, Bell, & Dennis, 1962; Baran & Longo, cited by Longo, 1972).

OLOLIUQUI

Ololiuqui is another substance used by the South American Indians as an intoxicating and distorting drug. The pharmacological agents come from the seeds of the morning glory plant, *Rivea corymbosa*. The identification of the active ingredients in the seeds was made by Hofmann and Tscherter in 1960 and they reported finding several chemically similar alkaloids, including lysergic acid amide (Figure 9.1), a chemical about one-tenth as potent as LSD (the presence of the amide in the seeds was quite surprising to botanists because the drug had previously been isolated only from much more primitive plants like the ergot fungus).

In 1955, Humphrey Osmond reported "a strange mental state" after ingesting 100 seeds that had been ground to a powder and swallowed with water. Apathy, withdrawal, and sedation were reported with few, if any, visual or sensory distortions. A similar response was reported by Hofmann and Cerletti (cited by Longo, 1972, p. 141), who self-experimented with an extract of the seeds. At a drug workshop held in 1969, Osmond reported during one of the discussions:

> I had a curious experience while taking *ololiuqui* when it was supposed to be an inactive substance and I was still not sure about it. I was listening to the music of Gesualdo, a nobleman of the Italian Renaissance whose works I usually find somewhat repugnant. This time, however, I really listened to the music and enjoyed it greatly. I have no doubt about that. And after listening to it since without *ololiuqui* it has continued to be of interest to me. I am not musical and normally this

very complicated music is beyond me, but it was as if my perception of the music had in some way been altered or possibly reorganized, and this persisted afterwards. (Osmond, 1970, p. 319)

It is difficult to compare and analyze the psychotropic effects of the different distorting drugs. Longo (1972) has postulated that perhaps in early times when these chemicals were used in combination, the psychic experience may have been a distinct result of the mixture of the various components. Using this concept, Isbell and Gorodetsky (1966) compared the effects of morning glory seed extract, a synthetic mixture of the alkaloids, and LSD. The drugs were given to six healthy male, ex-opiate addicts. The effects of the crude extract and the synthetic mixture were similar, but both were different from LSD. Symptoms seen included nausea, headache, increased blood pressure, apathy, and sleepiness. There were no reports of hallucinations or sensory distortions. Thus it does not seem that these drugs induce the "trip" syndrome, but act more like sedatives or tranquilizers.

Fink, Goldman, and Lyons (1966), on the other hand, have reported hallucinations and sensory distortions after ingestion of morning glory seeds in hospitalized, maladjusted patients. We must be careful in analyzing these results, however, because the subjects in both the Isbell and the Fink studies had been taking a variety of other drugs. In the Isbell study, the men had been opiate addicts, and this may have unknown biochemical effects that could influence their reaction to the ingestion of other drugs. In the Fink study, the patients were hospitalized and could have a long history of previous drug use.

Most of the morning glory seeds available in the United States are believed to lack the alkaloid drug concentration that these South American plants are known to possess. A word of caution is also in order because other substances besides the lysergic acid-like alkaloids are found in morning glory seeds. The isolation and testing of such a compound is described by Cook and Keeland (1962), and administration to rabbits at a dose of 30 mg/kg proved fatal.

DMT

DMT (dimethyltryptamine), an effective psychoactive compound, is probably one of the most popular worldwide, if not in the United States. The drug naturally occurs in many plants and is relatively easy to synthesize. It is an important ingredient in cohoba snuff, which is used by some South American and Caribbean Indians. Usually the drug is inhaled via snuff or smoking, or it may be injected; it is ineffective when taken orally. In some instances the chemical is prepared in a liquid form, then parsley, tobacco, or marijuana is dipped into it, and then smoked in a pipe or a cigarette.

Lingeman (1970) has labeled the drug "the businessman's lunchtime high" because the euphoric, distorting state lasts for only about 30 minutes. DMT administered in moderate doses (50-100 mg) induces a number of disturbances which have been described by Szara (see Garattini & Ghetti, 1957) who self-experimented with the drug. These effects included hallucinatory components, distorted perceptions, euphoria, autonomic responses, and motor disturbances in the form of choreiform compulsive movements.

The effects are not as severe or complete as the effects of LSD are. With LSD they last several hours; with DMT, they are seen for only 30 minutes to an hour. The delusions and sensory distortions caused by LSD include the entire sensory range—visual, auditory, olfactory, tactile and taste; with DMT the sensory disturbances are confined mainly to the visual system. The chemical structure of the drug is shown in Figure 9.1. Notice the structural similarity between DMT, psilocin, and psilocybin.

AMANITA MUSCARIA

As the Mexicans had their mushrooms containing psilocybin, so too the Siberians had a mushroom with perceptual distorting properties. *Amanita muscaria* has been used for centuries in Russia and Scandinavia as a hallucinogen, and some (Wasson, 1967) have suggested that it will take its place next to alcohol and tobacco as "outstanding inebriants used by *Homo sapiens*." The mushroom is also called *fly agaric*, partly because it has been used as an insecticide. It doesn't kill the flies outright but rather, after the flies suck the mushroom, they go into a stupor for two or three hours, then die. Other authorities have suggested that the name *fly agaric* came from a medieval legend in which madness was associated with being possessed and infested by flies. The fly was a sign of insanity. When successfully treated, a fly was supposed to emerge from the patient's nostril, and when this happened, a cure was proclaimed.

Wasson (1967) has outlined the characteristics of *Amanita muscaria* intoxication, which are based on his own use and on that of his friends. He found a few mushrooms sufficient to produce the psychic effects. The plants can be eaten raw, their pressed juice can be drunk, or they can be eaten toasted or in soups or other foods. The effect may be broken down into two phases. In the first phase the subject reports a depression and a sleeplike or trancelike state. This stage usually begins 15–20 minutes after drug ingestion. The second phase is one of elation and excitement, and it is during this phase that the subject may experience perceptual distortions and imagery. A recent article by the famous ethnobotanist R. E. Schultes (1969) summarizes many of the effects of the drug:

Effects of *Amanita muscaria* vary appreciably with individuals and at different times. An hour after the ingestion of the mushrooms, twitching and trembling of the limbs is noticeable with the onset of a period of good humor and light euphoria, characterized by macroscopia, visions of the supernatural and illusions of grandeur. Religious overtones—such as an urge to confess sins—frequently occur. Occasionally, the partaker becomes violent, dashing madly about until, exhausted, he drops into a deep sleep. (p. 246)

The Siberians discovered that the drug was not only potent but also reusable. It seems that the active drug substances are not destroyed during metabolism, but are excreted unchanged in the urine. Hence, ingestion of the urine of someone who consumed the mushroom would lead to another drug-induced trip.

An interesting legend concerning the drug has to do with the Norse warriors of old, whose ferocious rage and unbridled violence were said to be due to their consumption of some of the mushrooms before battle. There is considerable doubt over the validity of this legend, however.

Pharmacology

The pharmacology of *Amanita muscaria* is not known for certain, although its study goes back more than a century. Many chemical substances have been identified as present in the mushroom. Among these are muscarine, choline, acetylcholine, atropine, hyoscyamine, and bufotenine (N,-N-dimethyl serotonin). Bufotenine has an indole chemical structure, but the evidence that this substance is responsible for the psychoactive properties is far from clear. Since bufotenine (as well as atropine and hyoscyamine) are present in the mushroom in very small quantities, it is difficult to see how they could be the dominant psychoactive agents. It is interesting to note that if bufotenine should prove to be the active chemical, it could have been the important ingredient in the witches' brew in the opening scene of Shakespeare's *Macbeth*, since the toad skin, a part of the cauldron's brew, has a fair amount of bufotenine. In 1964, three other substances were isolated from the mushroom: ibotenic acid, muscimol, and muscazone (see Eugster, 1967). The chemical structures of these substances are shown in Figure 9.6.

Muscimol and ibotenic acid have been studied pharmacologically and found to have central neural effects. Actions included arousal, dilated pupils, and

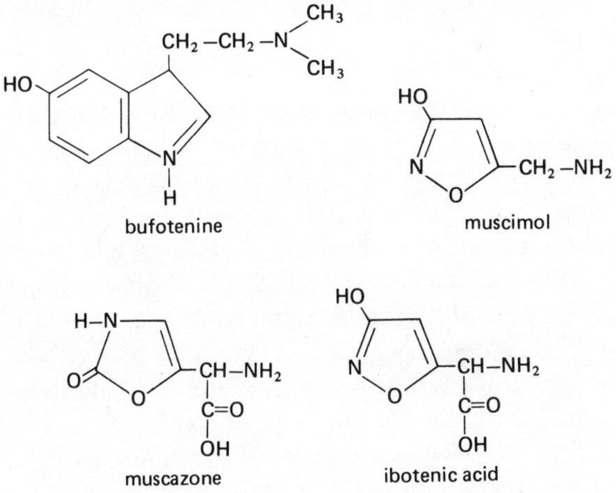

FIGURE 9.6. Some substances found in *Amanita muscaria*.

cramps, followed by sedation. Other effects were antiemetic and antitussive properties, as well as dose-related EEG changes. Theobald (1968) has demonstrated a synchronizing effect at low doses of muscimol (0.5 mg/kg), and a spiking effect at higher doses (2–5 mg/kg). Waser and Bersin (1970) reviewed the effects of ibotenic acid and muscimol on endogenous levels of monoamines in the brain. They state that these two substances have effects similar to LSD in relation to norepinephrine, dopamine, and serotonin concentrations in the brains of mice and rats. All three drugs produce an increased serotonin concentration in the hypothalamus and midbrain. This biochemical change may or may not be the neurophysiological substrate for the behavioral psychoactive properties.

MESCALINE

Mescaline is one of the alkaloids that may be extracted from the peyote cactus. This cactus was previously botanically labeled as *Anhalonium williamsi* or *A. lewini* (after Lewin, the German pharmacologist who performed the initial pharmacological studies of the chemical). Its botanical designation, however, has been changed to the current *Lophophora williamsi* or *L. lewini*. The drug has a long history of religious ceremonial use by the early Mexican Indian cultures (the Mescaleros, hence the derivation of its name) and is used even now by the Native American Church during rituals and ceremonies of prayer.

The peyote cactus is a small plant that grows in the desert regions. Much of the plant is underground, and only the part that is above ground is easily edible. Figure 9.7 shows the cactus plant. The entire plant contains the psychoactive compounds, but the top part of the plant is typically sliced into small discs and dried. These dried slices remain psychoactive indefinitely, and are known as *mescal buttons*. When the buttons are ingested, they are first put into the mouth and soaked until soft. They then are taken into the hand and formed into a small ball and swallowed. This method of ingestion has been followed for centuries.

Early Use

The European community was made aware of the use of peyote at the time of the Spanish conquest in the early 1500s. When Cortez came into Mexico, the Christian missionaries with him had the job of bringing God and religion to the heathen cultures. Many of the ancient religious ceremonies (including those using the peyote cactus) were then forced underground, but Dr. Francisco Hernandez, the court physician to King Philip II of Spain, was able to compile much of the lore about the early Mexican drugs and herbs. He described the peyote cactus in the following manner: "the root is of nearly medium size, sending forth no branches or leaves above the ground. . . . Both men and women are said to be harmed by it . . . it causes those devouring it to be able to foresee and predict things . . ." Other reports from this period indicate that ". . . those who eat or chew it see visions either frightful or laughable . . ." and ". . . see

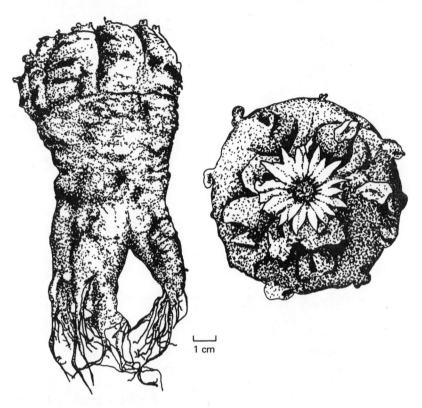

FIGURE 9.7 The cactus peyote. (*Left*) the shape of this small plant resembles that of a molar tooth, since it exhibits a crown and a forked root. The light green crown is hemispherical, with several grooves. (*Right*) the cactus in bloom. Note the patches of whitish hairs; these hairs, particularly evident in the dry plant, suggested the name of the drug; in the local dialect, *peyote* means "white fuzz"

visions of terrifying sights like the devil . . ." (see Ray, 1972, p. 215). Early reports state that in the pre-Columbian Mexican culture, the Aztec, Huichol, and other Mexican Indians ate the plant and experienced profound sensory and psychic distortions which led these early cultures to use it religiously (LaBarre, 1964).

Pharmacology

The initial research on the psychoactive agents in the peyote cactus was carried out in Germany at the end of the 19th century. These investigations (Heffter, 1897, cited by Longo, 1972; Lewin, 1888) confirmed the excitatory nature of the chemical extract and subsequently identified many of the alkaloid substances present in the cactus plant. Heffter also came to the conclusion that mescaline (Figure 9.8) was the single alkaloid responsible for the hallucinatory

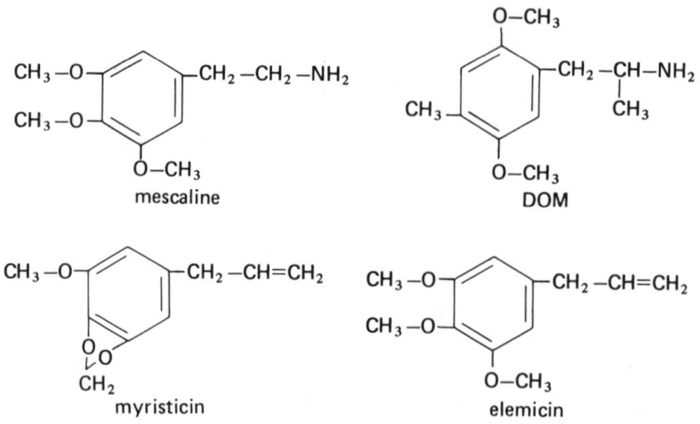

FIGURE 9.8. The catecholaminic type distorting drugs.

effects. In subsequent studies, no less than 30 alkaloids have been isolated, and again mescaline has been found to be the only alkaloid having psychoactive properties.

Metabolism and excretion. The drug is readily absorbed when taken orally, and maximum brain concentrations of mescaline are reached after 30 to 120 minutes. Low doses of the drug, about 3 mg/kg (200 mg in a 150-lb human), are effective in producing the full hallucinatory effect. About half of the drug is excreted in 6 hours, but there is evidence that some of the drug remains in the brain for up to 9 to 10 hours after ingestion. The drug is mostly excreted in the urine unchanged; however, the metabolites thus far identified have proven to be inactive.

Neurology. Neurophysiological data on mescaline are not complete. According to Speck (1958), low doses of mescaline (50 mg/kg) increase the low-voltage, fast-wave activity of the rat EEG, and high doses (200–400 mg/kg) induce a spiking EEG pattern. Monnier and Krupp (1960) and Baran and Longo (1965; cited by Longo, 1972) described EEG activation after 25 mg/kg doses of mescaline in the rat.

Affective responding. The performance of a learned response also seems to be disrupted by mescaline. In an early study (Sivadjian, 1934; cited by Longo, 1972), rats trained in an avoidance learning paradigm showed a disruption in their responding after 100 mg/kg of mescaline. They responded to the sound signal as if it were the noxious shock stimulus to be avoided. This hyperemotional responsiveness has been replicated for rats and extended to dogs (Bridger & Gantt, 1956). Chorover (1961) found that mescaline (25 mg/kg) produced an immediate suppression in the extinction of a conditioned-avoidance behavior.

Toxicity. Mescaline is relatively nontoxic, i.e., large doses will be tolerated in animals. Given intraperitoneally to rats, the median lethal dose is 370 mg/kg, far above the minimum dose necessary for psychoactive effects. The intoxication seen after this huge dosage may be conveniently divided into two phases, the first characterized by mild autonomic disturbances and the second by generally depressive CNS effects. Experimental research has indicated that during this second phase, dogs and cats become docile and tame (Sturtevant & Drill, 1956), rats become inactive, stare into space, and become hyperexcitable to sudden noises (Speck, 1957), and mice indulge in compulsive scratching (Garattini & Ghetti, 1957). Like many of the other distorting drugs (LSD, for example), the effects may be countered by chlorpromazine.

Tolerance and addiction. Tolerance does develop, but no addiction has been reported with mescaline, and there appears to be no abstinence or withdrawal syndrome when the drug is discontinued.

Religious Use

Peyote began as a ceremonial, religious drug in the pre-Columbian Mexican Indian cultures. It is currently used in the United States in the rites and ceremonies of the Native American Church, a congregation of various Indian tribes estimated to number about a quarter of a million people. For an analysis of the early and modern religious uses of peyote see Ray (1972).

The Native American Church originated in 1918, when the Indian tribes of Oklahoma organized and chartered the Peyote Church, a composite of old Mexican rituals, Christian ceremonies, and local customs. Changing its name to the Native American Church, it stated its basic beliefs and dedication to the use of peyote in its articles of incorporation, as quoted by LaBarre, McAllester, Slotkin, Stewart, and Tax (1951):

> The purpose for which this corporation is formed is to foster and promote religious beliefs in Almighty God and the customs of the several Tribes of Indians throughout the United States in the worship of a Heavenly Father and to promote morality, sobriety, industry, charity, and right living and cultivate a spirit of self-respect and brotherly love and union among the members of the several Tribes of Indians throughout the United States ... with and through the sacramental use of peyote. (p. 582)

Since 1918, there has been much confusion, argument, and discussion over the use of peyote by the Native American Church. Those involved include the Indians, the United States Congress, a Secretary of the Interior (Harold Ockes), and numerous scientists. In 1951, LaBarre and four other anthropoligists issued a statement on peyote which concluded:

> ... the Native American Church of the United States is a legitimate religious organization deserving of the same right to religious freedom as other churches; also, that peyote is used sacramentally in a manner corresponding to the bread and wine of white Christians. (p. 582)

The Distorting Effects of Mescaline in Humans

The major effects of peyote are to induce visual sensory distortions and to diminish one's sense of hunger and thirst. Usually, unpleasant autonomic side effects accompany the psychic effects. These typically include nausea, vomiting, goose flesh, and dilation of the pupils. Longo (1972) has described the visual distortions as color hallucinations, generally agreeable in nature. Sensory illusions and transposition of sensorial excitation are also present: ordinary objects appear marvelous and strange, in beautiful and brilliant colors; sounds or noises are "seen" in color. In comparison, the impressions of everyday life seem pale and static. (p. 103)

One of the early investigators into the effects of the peyote cactus, Dr. Weir Mitchell, described his psychic experience:

The display which for an enchanted two hours followed was such that I find it hopeless to describe in language which shall convey to others the beauty and splendor of what I saw. Stars, delicate floating films of color, then an abrupt rush of countless points of white light swept across the field of view, as if the unseen millions of the Milky Way were to flow in a sparkling river before my eyes . . . zigzag lines of very bright colors . . . the wonderful loveliness of swelling clouds of more vivid colors gone before I could name them. (From DeRopp, 1957, p. 34)

Another early experimenter in the area, Havelock Ellis (1902), described his experience in these words:

On the whole, if I had to describe the visions in one word, I should say that they were living arabesques. There was generally a certain incomplete tendency to symmetry, the effect being somewhat as if the underlying mechanism consisted of a large number of polished facets acting as mirrors. It constantly happened that the same image was repeated over a large part of the field, though this holds good mainly of the forms, for in the colors, there would still remain all sorts of delicious varieties. Thus at a moment when uniformly jewelled flowers seemed to be springing up and extending all over the field of vision, the flowers still showed every variety of delicate tone and tint. (p. 59)

In addition to the written accounts of the visual displays, there has been much research on the effect of the various distorting drugs on artistic expression. Marinesco (1933) published a drawing of a hand (Figure 9.9) done under mescaline intoxication. It is interesting to note the distortions in body image under the influence of the drug. Some mention should be made about the validity of these artistic expressions while under the influence of a distorting drug. Artists generally have been dissatisfied with the paintings and drawings done in this manner. They typically report that the representations are not accurate accounts of the distorted visual activity. It appears as if the subject cannot carry on a hallucination and make an artistic representation simultaneously. When the subject begins a period of visual disturbance, he typically stops the artistic expression and continues only when the hallucination period is over (Longo, 1972).

We believe that these introspectionistic, subjective data must be evaluated very carefully and very selectively. The essence of any scientific understanding is the replicability and public nature of the phenomenon. With personal, introspective, and subjective accounts of drug experiences, we necessarily lose some measure of objectivity and replicability, and hence must proceed with caution.

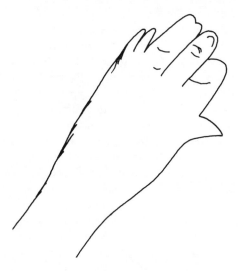

FIGURE 9.9. Drawing of a hand like one made under the influence of mescaline, illustrating the phenomenon of megalo- and macropsia. (After Marinesco, 1933.)

DOM

DOM, or STP, is most certainly a very powerful psychoactive distorting drug; it has even been labeled a *megahallucinogen* (by Wells, 1973). This label does not deter many; rather, in some cases, it probably attracts the young drug user in search of a new experience. DOM is an abbreviation of the formal chemical name, 2-5-methoxy-4-methyl-amphetamine. The psychic distorting properties of the drug were probably discovered by some San Francisco–based hippie in the early 1960s. Some believe that because of the elation, excitement, and powerful distorting qualities of the drug-induced experience, the drug became known on the street as STP (the name of a popular fuel additive—Scientifically Treated Petroleum). Others believe that STP stands for "Serenity, Tranquillity, and Peace," the teaching of Timothy Leary, a leader of the 1960s drug cult. Whichever derivation is correct, the experience of this drug is probably closer to a fuel injection than to the serenity and tranquillity of a peaceful summer day. The drug was very popular on the street, although very little was known scientifically about its effects. In the late 1960s government officials purchased some of the street substance, and it was then chemically identified and used in experimentation (Snyder, Faillace, & Hollister, 1967).

Pharmacology

It was found that moderate doses of the drug (10-15 mg) produced an elation and excitement similar to the effects of mescaline, but with more marked euphoria and excitement. Lower doses (2 mg) produced an amphetaminelike arousal and hyperactive state, but not the euphoria and excitement associated with larger doses. This makes DOM about 100 times as potent as mescaline, but only about one-thirteenth as strong as LSD. The chemical structures of both DOM and mescaline have a catechol nucleus (Figure 9.8). The similarity of the effects of DOM and mescaline, and of the sympathomimetic compounds, is no doubt due to this close biochemical structural similarity. Ray (1972) points out that in one study, out of 23 mescaline purchases on the street, none was mescaline, but several were DOM. It appears that pushers are able to substitute DOM for mescaline because of the similar behavioral effects.

It was once thought that chlorpromazine, the phenothiazine tranquilizer that successfully halts or diminishes the psychoactive, distorting effects of many of the distorting agents, was not effective in countering the euphoric state induced by DOM. However, scientific studies have failed to prove this point. It appears that there are two distinct stages of the DOM trip; the first stage, seen with low doses, includes a sympathetic arousal, and the second, seen with high doses, includes motor dysfunctions and convulsions (Florio, Lipparini, Scotti-Decarolis, & Longo, 1969). Small doses of DOM (0.5 mg/kg) in rabbits produced pupillary dilation, startle reactions to external stimuli, and lacrimal, salivary, and bronchial hypersecretion. Searching and exploratory periods in the cage alternated with stuporous, catatonic behavior. This behavior was accompanied by cortical and subcortical EEG activation with pronounced hippocampal involvement.

With higher doses (2-3 mg/kg) motor dysfunctions and convulsions appeared, first localized in the limbs and accompanied by a grinding of the teeth, and later progressing to a general convulsion involving the entire body. These convulsions usually continued for a long time, leading to a state of exhaustion and eventually death. The EEG during this stage resembled that of the grand mal epileptic attack. Chlorpromazine administered during this second stage was not effective in halting or reducing the convulsive state. However, chlorpromazine administered after the low dosage of DOM was effective in controlling the sympathomimetic responses; the EEG showed slow waves, the animal calmed down, the pupils constricted, and only the hypersecretions remained. The earlier notion of chlorpromazine failure to counteract the DOM state may have been due to the large doses of DOM traditionally sold on the street (about 10 mg in each pill).

In a study showing the stuporous effect of the drug and the disruptive effect it has on learned behavior, Florio et al. (1969) taught cats to press a bar for food reward on the discriminative cue of a buzzer sound. After administration of DOM (0.25 mg/kg) the cat maintained a catatonic posture with panting and pupillary dilation. These researchers also report evidence of hallucinatory behavior (with animals given 0.5 mg/kg), as the animals showed a fixed stare and would suddenly leap from one place to another as if to catch imaginary objects. The research story is still very incomplete on this potent distorting drug, and until we can be sure exactly why and where the chemical is acting, we should proceed with great caution, for we really do not know the full power of this substance that has the same name as a fuel additive.

NUTMEG

Who would have thought that the ground nutmeg on the Christmas eggnog, the spice in the applesauce-spice cake, or the taste in the rice pudding would turn out to be a mind-distorting, hallucinogenic substance? Well, it may be true. That can of nutmeg on mother's shelf could be a can of mind-distorting chemical.

Nutmeg is actually the dried seed kernel of an East Indian evergreen tree, *Myristica fragrans*. There are other plant members of this group that contain various distorting drugs (Schultes, 1969), and the alkaloid common to all and believed to be the active ingredient is myristicin, or perhaps a very similar chemical called elemicin (Longo, 1972; see Figure 9.8). Nutmeg is probably one of the weakest distorting drugs of the group and certainly is much less potent than any of the drugs discussed in the previous sections.

The amounts needed to feel the effects of nutmeg are huge by any pharmacologic standard; generally 10 g, or about 1/3 oz, is needed to achieve relatively mild effects. Increasing the dosage will increase the effects, but will also increase the probability of poisoning. Hoffer and Osmond (1967) have summarized some data concerning nutmeg trips; they found generally that the drug typically produces an unpredictable and, in many ways, unpleasant experience.

The problem appears to be in the ingestion of the drug. The sheer quantity of drug necessary to experience a pleasant effect makes ingestion a noxious experience. Usually the drug is mixed with juice or hot water and drunk; once this is done, the subject must struggle to keep the concoction down and fight off the first autonomic effects of continuing waves of nausea and weakness. These unpleasant autonomic effects continue until the euphoria and feeling of well-being take over. Finally, one loses the ability to concentrate and think in coherent patterns. In many instances, individuals never experience the euphoric and perceptual distortions because of the very strong, unpleasant autonomic feelings immediately following the drug's ingestion.

The use of the drug has usually been restricted to young people looking for "kicks" from new experiences. Nutmeg has rarely, if ever, been used for religious or ceremonial purposes, and legends and tales of use and abuse are rare. Apparently the experience of waves of nausea and vomiting from a single dose of the chemical is enough to vastly decrease the subject's use of nutmeg as a distorting drug.

MARIJUANA

Marijuana, more than any other psychoactive agent, has typified the drug culture of the 1960s and 1970s. Not only do teenagers, college students, and so-called dropouts use marijuana, but many "straight" adults in business and the professions commonly use the drug in a recreational sense. What follows is a summary of the marijuana story. For a detailed discussion of the history, sociology, and cultural implications of marijuana use, see Brecher (1972), which recommends the legalization, or at least the decriminalization, of marijuana. A slightly different point of view is found in Ray (1972). Nahas (1973) is a quite detailed analysis of the history, botany, chemistry, pharmacology, toxicology, and social aspects of marijuana. Nahas also provides quite a different point of view regarding the legalization of marijuana; read his book for the negative position with respect to legalization. Then you hopefully will be able to knowledgeably arrive at your own position on this issue. It is our opinion that the position of these people, and of many others, (both those in favor of and those opposed to legalization), is founded more on philosophy and ideas about social systems and human rights and privileges than on pharmacology. Thus, this matter seems more a philosophical/political than a psychological or pharmacological issue, and we will therefore not try to convince you one way or the other.

Historical Considerations

The first recorded use of *Cannabis* as a remedy was in China nearly 4,000 years ago by Shen Nung, a mythical Chinese emperor and pharmacist, who advocated its use as a sedative and an all-purpose medication. The plant was not used as a hallucinogen in China; however, its medical use spread throughout India and Asia several centuries before Christ.

On the Indian subcontinent the plant came to be regarded as holy and played an important role in early ceremonial rituals. It is referred to in the Sanskrit literature as *food of the gods*, *glory*, and *victory*. While the priestly class knew of the intoxicating qualities of the plant, it is difficult to pinpoint the precise time that the common class found out about its inebriant qualities.

After the plant spread to India, the next region to discover the psychological effects of this drug was the Middle East. Legends abound but one of the most popular concerns Haider, a seclusive monk. Robinson (1925) states:

> One burning summer's day when the fiery sun glared angrily upon Mother Earth as if he wished to wither up her breasts, Haider stepped out from his cloister and walked alone to the fields. All around him lay the vegetation weary and without life, but one plant danced in the heat with joy. Haider plucked it, partook of it, and returned to the convent a happier man. The monks who saw him immediately noticed the change in their chief. He encouraged conversation, and acted boisterously. He then led his companions to the fields, and the holy men partook of the hasheesh, and were transformed from austere ascetics into jolly good fellows. (pp. 29–30)

The Arab invasions of the 9th through the 12th centuries introduced *Cannabis* into North Africa, from Egypt to Tunisia, Algeria, and Morocco. The tales of the *Arabian Nights*, written between 1000 and 1500 A.D., refer often to the marvelous properties of hashish (a concentrated form of marijuana). Perhaps the authors were flying on their magic carpets when they were composing the stories!

Hashish and marijuana didn't find their way into Europe until the middle of the 19th century, and the first report of their use was in 1845 by Moreau, who has been called the father of psychopharmacology. After ingesting *Cannabis*, he described the effects of the intoxication. Moreau experimented with the drug and encouraged many of his friends to also experiment with it. It was during the middle of the 19th century that a group of French artists gathered monthly to use drugs. The club known as *Le Club des Hachischins* ("The Club of the Hashish Eaters") included such notable people as Theophile Gautier, Charles Baudelaire, and Alexander Dumas. Gautier (1846; cited by Nahas, 1973) described his experiences in a magazine article:

> Hallucination, that strange guest, had set up its dwelling place in me. It seemed that my body had dissolved and become transparent. I saw inside me the hashish I had eaten in the form of an emerald which radiated millions of tiny sparks. All around me I heard the shattering and crumbling of multicolored jewels. I still saw my comrades at times but as disfigured half plants half men. I writhed in my corner with laughter. One of the guests addressed me in Italian which hashish in its omnipotence made me hear in Spanish. (p. 5)

These recollections are obviously tinted with a little poetic license taken by a talented writer enthusiastic about this new drug experience. Charles Baudelaire (1858), another member of the club, but one not as enthralled with the drug as Gautier, also wrote of his drug experiences in the book, *The Artificial Paradises* (reprinted in Baudelaire, 1971):

> the uninitiated . . . imagine hashish intoxication as a wondrous land, a vast theatre of magic and juggling where everything is miraculous and unexpected. That is a preconceived notion, a total misconception . . . the intoxication will be nothing but one immense dream, thanks to intensity of color and the rapidity of conceptions; but it will always preserve the particular tonality of the individual . . . the dream will certainly reflect its dreamer . . . he is only the same man grown larger . . . sophisticate and ingénu . . . will find nothing miraculous, absolutely nothing but the natural to an extreme. The mind and body upon which hashish operates will yield only their ordinary, personal phenomena increased, it is true, in amount and vitality, but still faithful to the original. Man will not escape the fate of his physical and mental nature: to his impressions and intimate thoughts, hashish will be a magnifying mirror, but a true mirror, nonetheless. (pp. 41–43)

Cannabis came to the United States as a fiber crop of the early American settlers. George Washington grew the plant on his farm, not to smoke, but to use in making ropes. Marijuana and hashish were unknown to the early settlers for their inebriant qualities. They were used in the 19th century by physicians as all-purpose medications but did not become "distorting drugs" until the early part of the 20th century. Marijuana, as a pleasure-inducing drug, began coming into the United States around 1910 from Mexico, when Mexican farmers started to smuggle it into Texas. After World War I, marijuana smoking began to spread among the poor black and Mexican farm workers in Texas and Louisiana. New

Orleans became the major port of entry for illegal marijuana; in 1926 the *New Orleans Morning Tribune* published a series of articles denouncing the "marijuana menace" and linking use of the drug with crime. In 1936, *Scientific American* (Marihuana menaces youth, 1936) stated that marijuana "produces a wide variety of symptoms in the user, including hilarity, swooning and sexual excitement. Combined with intoxicants, it often makes the smoker vicious, with a desire to fight and kill" (p. 151). Even with this publicity the majority of United States citizens were unconcerned about marijuana. The Federal Bureau of Narcotics, led by Harry Anslinger, was concerned about the harmful effects that *Cannabis* might have on the individual and on society. In 1937 the Marijuana Tax Act was passed, which banned cultivation, possession, and distribution of the plants. Only the birdseed industry, which used 2,000,000 tons of *Cannabis* seed every year, escaped the ban; they were permitted to use sterilized seed incapable of germination.

After the tax act was passed, there were reports of an almost immediate decline in violent crimes committed under the influence of marijuana, and the price of the drug increased rapidly. In 1938, the mayor of New York, Fiorello LaGuardia, questioned the effects of marijuana and wondered about their seriousness. He recalled two army studies on the use of marijuana by soldiers in the Panama Canal Zone, both of which found the drug to be an innocuous agent; the association with increased crime seemed due to the effect of mixing marijuana and alcohol. The report of the LaGuardia Commission, issued in 1944, concluded:

> It was found that marijuana in an effective dose impairs intellectual functioning in general . . . Marijuana does not change the basic personality structure of the individual. It lessens inhibition and this brings out what is latent in his thoughts and emotions but it does not evoke responses which would otherwise be totally alien to him. It induces a feeling of self-confidence, but this expressed in thought rather than in performance. There is, in fact, evidence of a diminution in physical activity . . . those who have been smoking marijuana for a period of years showed no mental or physical deterioration which may be attributed to the drug. (Solomon, 1966, p. 408)

The report was met with challenges left and right. The federal government disapproved, and the American Medical Association labeled it as "unscientific" and "uncritical." The challenges to the LaGuardia report were based more on emotional grounds than on intellectual foundations, and to date no evidence has proven the report wrong.

The 1950s, 1960s, and 1970s have marked a turning point in the history of marijuana. The amount of research has been continually increasing as has the amount of everyday, or "street," usage. The use of other distorting drugs has declined, and today marijuana is probably the major distorting drug used throughout the world. Table 9.1 lists the names and composition of the *Cannabis* preparations used in various countries.

TABLE 9.1

Names and Compositions of *Cannabis* Preparations in
Various Countries

Country	Name	Composition
Indian subcontinent	Bhang	Dried mature leaves
Indian subcontinent	Sawi (green-leaved)	Dried mature leaves
Indian subcontinent	Ganja	Flowering tops
Indian subcontinent	Charas	Resinous material
Arabia, Iran, Middle East	Kannabis and cannabis	Entire plant
Arabia, Iran, Middle East	Banji	Entire plant, mostly leaves
Arabia, Iran, Middle East	Hashish	Resinous material and flowering tops
Israel	Shesha	Entire plant
Turkey and Iran	Esrar	Resinous material with flowering tops
U.S.S.R. (southern)	Anascha	Resinous material and flowering tops mixed with leaves
Egypt	Hashish	Resinous material and flowering tops
Morocco and North African coast	Kif	Resinous material mixed with leaves and flowers
West coast of Africa	Dimba	Entire plant
Congo, Central Africa	Suma, dacha	Entire plant
South and Southwest Africa	Dagga	Entire plant, mostly leaves and flowering tops
Zulu, Swazi	Lebake	Entire plant
East Africa	Njemu	Entire plant
Madagascar	Vongony	Entire plant
United States, Canada, Mexico	Marihuana	Leaves and flowering tops
Brazil	Machona	Entire plant with leaves

Note. Reprinted by permission from *Marihuana—Deceptive Weed* by G. G. Nahas.
© 1973 by Raven Press, New York.

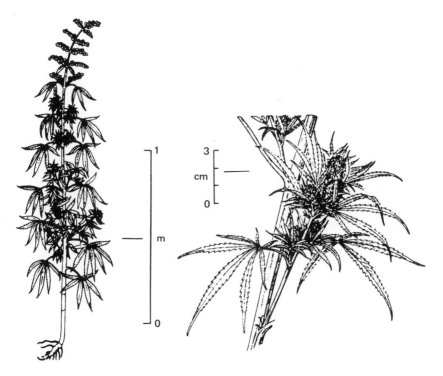

FIGURE 9.10. *Cannabis sativa.* (*Left*) male plant, (*right*) female plant. (Reprinted by permission from *Marihuana–Deceptive Weed,* by G. G. Nahas. © 1973 by Raven Press, New York.)

Botany

Cannabis sativa is a plant that is widely distributed throughout the temperate and tropical zones of the world. It is not a single plant but one with as many as 100 known varieties. In Latin, the word *Cannabis* means hemp and denotes the genus of the plant group. *Sativa,* the species name, means planted or sown. The adjectives *indica* or *americanes* indicate the geographical location where the plant is grown, *indica* meaning India and *americanes* meaning America. Since the plant has spread to so many different geographical locations, these two adjectives no longer have much meaning. The plant has been cultivated for centuries for the hemp in its stem, the oil in its seeds, and the psychoactive substance in its flowering tops.

The *Cannabis sativa* plant has a separate male and female plant; both manufacture the psychoactive chemical in usable amounts. The female plants have a heavy foliage up to the top, while the male plant is characterized by sparse leaves (Figure 9.10). The male plant is not as hearty as the female, and withers sooner. In some cases the males are weeded out to harvest a better crop of female plants. The female flower clusters are larger and more densely packed than the male's, and they do not project beyond the leaves. The male plant is taller than the female but dies after its pollen is shed. The female plant survives until killed by frost or until the seeds have matured. The female plants also have a strong, pungent odor and secrete a resin that may be so thick as to appear like dew in the middle of the day. It has been suggested that this resin acts to protect the maturing seeds from the hot sun and any lack of moisture.

There appear to be two different types of the plant. One is the fiber type, which has been cultivated as a fiber source; this plant contains little of the psychoactive substance. The psychoactive type has been cultivated for the resin and contains from 1% to 5% of the psychoactive chemical. Most of the *Cannabis* grown in the United States is of the fiber variety and contains little, if any, active drug. The word *marijuana* (also spelled marihuana) comes from a Spanish word meaning intoxicant and refers to the smoking preparation of leaves, flowers, and stems of either male or female plants. Table 9.2 shows the amounts of active chemical found in nine marijuana samples from the United States. It should be noted that the only sample containing enough drug to produce behavioral effects by smoking was the Illinois 1968 sample, which contained approximately 11 mg of active substance in a 1,000 mg cigarette. Nahas (1973) has stated:

> The recent North American experience of *Cannabis* intoxication appears to be to a great extent limited to the casual use of the home-grown fiber-type marijuana with little psychoactive material, or to mixtures of imported weeds in which cannabinoid content varies widely. In fiscal year 1970, analysis of all the marijuana seized in the

TABLE 9.2

Concentration of Active Chemical (Delta-9-THC) in Native
United States Marijuana

Origin	Type of plant	Delta-9-THC in a 1000-mg cigarette	
		Percent	Milligrams
Minnesota, 1968	Fiber	.07	.7
Minnesota, 1968	Fiber	.07	.7
Minnesota, 1969	Fiber	.05	.5
Minnesota, female seed (Bract)	Fiber	.05	.5
Minnesota, female leaves	Fiber	.04	.4
Iowa, 1968	Fiber	.06	.6
Iowa, 1968	Fiber	.07	.7
Illinois, male, 1968	Psychoactive	1.10	11.0
Laboratory grown	Fiber	.19	1.9

Note. Reprinted by permission from *Marihuana–Deceptive Weed*, by G. G. Nahas. © 1973 by Raven Press, New York.

United States by the Federal Bureau of Narcotics and Dangerous Drugs indicates that 12.2% of the samples did not contain any intoxicating material. In addition, there were seasonal variations; 14% of the specimens analyzed in the first quarter were negative for cannabinoid content, 16% in the second quarter, 77% in the third and 12% in the fourth. In Ontario, Canada, similar observations were made: 33% of the samples of "marijuana" collected from smokers did not contain any cannabinoid. "Some of it appeared literally to be grass lawn clippings; some of it looked like hay and smelled like hay." (p. 76)

It is clear that a substantial amount of the marijuana that is purchased on the street is liberally stretched with many additives—grass, oregano, or inactive pieces of stem—thus making the sale of the drug a very lucrative (although illegal) enterprise.

Chemistry

The chemistry of *Cannabis* is very complex, and even today isolation and extraction techniques are difficult and require a trained technician. Before 1964 the active ingredients were unknown, but in that year Gaoni and Mechoulam first isolated the major biologically active substance in *Cannabis sativa*, delta-9-THC (delta-9-tetrahydrocannabinol). In 1966 Hively and his colleagues isolated the second naturally occurring psychoactive substance in the plant, delta-8-THC (delta-8-tetrahydrocannabinol). The total amount of delta-8-THC and delta-9-THC varies widely from one sample of *Cannabis* to another. Growth, harvesting, curing, and, of course, the plant type determine the amount of active ingredient found in the plant. Two other cannabinoids have been isolated from the plant, cannabidol (CBD) and cannabinol (CBN). Loewe (1950) reported that cannabidol potentiated the sedative-hypnotic effects of barbiturates. The chemical structures of these substances are shown in Figure 9.11.

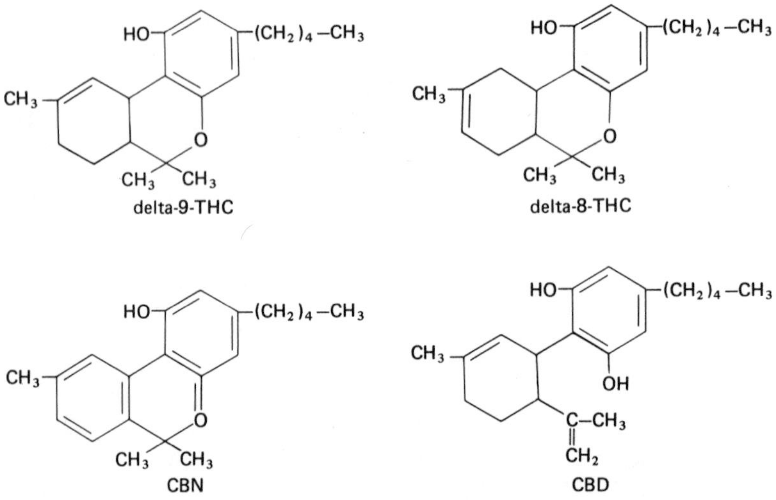

FIGURE 9.11. Chemical structures of some of the constituents of marijuana.

In addition to the four chemicals already described, there are other cannabinoids present in *Cannabis*. These include cannabigerol, cannabicyclol, cannabichromeme, and cannabidivarin. None of these alone appears to be psychoactive, but it is not known to what extent, if any, each interacts with delta-8-THC or delta-9-THC to produce psychoactive effects.

In summary, we should make several points: (1) *Cannabis* is one of the oldest plants known to humanity. From its early beginnings in China and India, it has spread to virtually every temperate and tropical region of the world. (2) *Cannabis* is a single species with many variants. Two major types have been most frequently used, the fiber variety and the psychoactive variety. (3) Concentration of psychoactive drug in a marijuana cigarette is a function of several factors including growth, harvest, curing, and type. (4) The majority of the *Cannabis* grown in the United States is of the fiber type, which has minimal THC content. Drug-type marijuana, however, is increasing in successful cultivation. (5) The major active substance in *Cannabis* is delta-9-THC, a unique chemical not found anywhere else in nature. (6) The molecular structure of the chemical is related to the other distorting drugs—LSD and psilocybin. (7) The biological activity (or inactivity) of the other cannabinoids isolated from the *Cannabis* plant has not been fully explored.

Pharmacology

Early studies of the pharmacology and toxicology of marijuana must be viewed with skepticism. Before 1968 it was most difficult, if not impossible, to accurately quantify and measure the amount of the psychoactive agent that had been administered, since the major route of administration had usually been by inhalation. However, the recent availability of synthetic delta-9-THC and delta-8-THC has given the psychopharmacologists new precision in their studies of the effects of marijuana. We must, however, add a note of caution at this point. Experimental studies employing chemically pure delta-9-THC on animals cannot be generalized to human use, which has primarily been by smoking impure marijuana preparations. Surely, marijuana when smoked is a mixture of the cannabinoids mentioned in the previous section, as well as the tar, carbon monoxide, acids, aldehydes, and other impurities of the cigarette wrapping. We must be cautious in generalizing from the studies employing pure delta-9-THC until we know more fully how this specific agent interacts with the other cannabinoids in the normally used marijuana smoking mixture.

Metabolism. The recent availability of radioactively tagged THC has permitted studies of its metabolism and distribution (Agurell, Nilsson, Ohlsson, & Sandberg, 1970; Dingell, Wilcox, & Klausner, 1971; Klausner & Dingell, 1971). Generally, after ingestion the drug shows no preferential accumulation in the brain, but rather is concentrated in organs of metabolism and absorption (liver, lung, spleen) and of excretion (liver and kidney).

The biotransformation of delta-9-THC is quite complex and many different metabolites are formed. While many of the metabolites are inactive and are eventually excreted in the urine or feces, there is evidence to indicate that some of the metabolites may be psychoactive (Agurell et al., 1970; Truitt, 1970; Truitt & Anderson, 1971). These investigators have suggested that 11-hydroxy-delta-8- or delta-9-tetrahydrocannabinol may be active metabolites.

Very little delta-9-THC is left unchanged in the body. Much of the drug is excreted as metabolites in the urine and feces. In the rat, 80% of the excretion is in the feces (Agurell, Nilsson, Ohlsson, & Sandberg, 1969), whereas in the rabbit most of the metabolites are excreted in the urine (Agurell et al., 1970).

Neurology. The distribution of delta-9-THC and its metabolites was studied in the brain of squirrel monkeys by McIsaac and his colleagues in 1971. The animals were given between 2 and 30 mg/kg of labeled THC, and general behavior was measured in addition to specific neural loci that showed drug accumulation. The dose-response relationship was similar to that seen in humans. Low doses had a euphoric, quieting effect with little perceptual disruption; moderate doses produced excitement, stimulation, lack of coordination, and some evidence of hallucinations. High doses were accompanied by severe psychomotor incapacitation. A correlation was made between the different structures showing labeled THC and the behaviors. High concentrations were noted at various times in limbic system structures and also in various neural structures related to visual information processing. Neurological and neurobiochemical studies of the actions of marijuana are just getting under way, however. We currently have very little knowledge of these actions, but can expect an avalanche of data to appear in the next few years.

General physiological actions. In a report on the effects of marijuana, the U.S. Department of Health, Education, and Welfare (1971) stated:

> Physiological changes accompanying marijuana use at typical levels of American social usage are relatively few. One of the most consistent is an increase in pulse rate. Another is reddening of the eyes at the time of use. Dryness of the mouth and throat are uniformly reported. Although enlargement of the pupils was an earlier impression, more careful study has indicated that this does not occur. Blood pressure effects have been inconsistent. Some have reported slightly lowered blood pressure, while others have reported small increases. Basal metabolic rate, temperature, respiration rate, lung vital capacity and a wide range of other physiological measures are generally unchanged over a relatively wide dosage range of both marijuana and the synthetic form of the principal psychoactive agent delta-9-THC. . . .
>
> There is evidence that the drug in large amounts can slow gastrointestinal passage of an experimental meal and relax an isolated intestine although it is not constipating. The sometimes reported enormous increase in appetite following marijuana smoking may also be related to effects in the gastrointestinal tract. . . .
>
> Because smoking is the typical mode of use of marijuana in America, studies of its effects on lung function are of considerable potential importance . . . even though preliminary experiments have not shown this form of smoking to be as damaging as tobacco smoking. . . . (pp. 9–10, 94, 173–174)

Toxicity, tolerance, and addiction. The lethal dose of *Cannabis* has not been determined for humans, and there have been no reports of death due to an overdose of marijuana. However, experts (as noted in Ray, 1972) have estimated the lethal dose to be about 40,000 times the effective dose of THC. *Cannabis* is not addicting and there do not appear to be any adverse symptoms when the individual stops using the drug. Tolerance, however, is still an issue subject to debate. It has been shown in animal studies and in some human reports. Yet, the question of whether the tolerance is psychological or physical has not been resolved. Wilson and Linken (1968) reported from England that a few users tend to increase the dosage with continued use. Miras (1969) reports that hashish smokers he has known in Greece for 20 years are able to smoke at least 10 times as much as other people. If a beginner smoked the same quantity he would collapse.

A candid report from Israel (Freedman & Peer, 1968), studying the *Cannabis* habits of pimps and prostitutes ranging in age from 18 to 42 (median=28), reported the development of tolerance. Seven of the 21 subjects reported a need to increase the dose. "When your body gets used to it you want it stronger, the body needs more and more. . . . You start off with a small cigarette, then a big one, then a water pipe." These comments are typical of the report. It should be pointed out that many of the 21 subjects also had a history of an opium habit, and that the interactions of these two drugs are far from clear.

The data from animal studies also indicates the development of tolerance (Black, Woods, & Domino, 1970; Harris, 1971; McMillan, Harris, Frankenheim, & Kennedy, 1970), and the concept of "reversed tolerance," as suggested by Weil and his colleagues (1968), is probably incorrect. The concept of a reversed tolerance comes from the reports by many users that after the initial few trials of marijuana smoking they require less of the drug to reach the same heights. As a result, they do not feel that it is necessary to increase the dosage in order to obtain greater experiences. Nahas (1973) has suggested that this reversed tolerance may be due to a combination of enzymatic induction necessary for the production of "active metabolites," and also to a conditioned reinforcement from the smoking process. In any case, the phenomenon is short-lived. As the drug intake increases, the half-life of the metabolites decreases and the amount excreted by the kidney increases, a "metabolic tolerance." Also as the dose increases there is probably some "tissue tolerance" (also called "functional tolerance") that develops at receptor sites. As Nahas (1973) concludes, "The combined development of metabolic and functional tolerance in chronic users of *Cannabis* will eventually predominate over psychological conditioning and increments in drug intake will be required to obtain the desired effects."

Behavioral and Clinical Effects of *Cannabis*

As we have reviewed earlier, the symptoms of *Cannabis* intoxication have been known for centuries. The recent discovery of delta-9-THC as the active substance, and the development of techniques of synthesis and extraction, now permit the psychopharmacologist to begin dose-response studies to attempt to more objectively quantify the euphoric and distorting effects. Most contemporary writers delineate three stages in the process of learning to smoke marijuana

(Becker, 1963). It is important that these writers believe that an individual must *learn* to experience the effects of the THC, that the response patterns are not innate, genetically precoded, and released by the chemical agent.

The first stage in the process of learning to smoke marijuana is learning to deeply inhale the smoke and hold it in the lungs for 20 to 40 seconds. The second stage is learning to identify and control the effects, and the final stage is learning to label these effects as pleasant. Because of this process the new user of the drug rarely feels "high" or "stoned," as he or she may have expected. The great effect of learning on the marijuana experience only serves to underline the fact that setting and environmental stimuli to a large degree determine the extent of the drug experience.

The first clinical study of the psychological effects of *Cannabis* using synthetic chemical was performed by Isbell and his colleagues in 1967. They confirmed the older observations of Moreau (1845) about the hallucinogenic properties of the plant. Isbell included *Cannabis* among the hallucinogens and concluded his report: "The data in our experiments definitely indicate that the psychotomimetic effects of delta-9-THC are dependent on dosage and that sufficiently high dosage (15-20 mg. smoked, 20-60 mg. ingested) can cause psychotic reactions in any individuals." Two subsequent studies (Crancer, Dille, Delay, Wallace, & Haykin, 1969; Weil, Zinberg, & Nelson, 1968) did not take such a hard line; in fact, they labeled the drug a "mild intoxicant" whose effects were not dose related, and which did not impair performance of chronic users. They also suggested the concept of reverse tolerance.

From then until the present day, people have debated whether *Cannabis* is or is not a hallucinogen. Should it be classed with LSD, mescaline, and psilocybin or should it be classed separately?

The effects experienced by the marijuana smoker have been described in detail by Moreau (1845). These experiences have generally been confirmed by more recent introspectionist reports. Tart (1970) has summarized the effects of marijuana, based on subjects' reports:

> Sense perception is often improved, both in intensity and in scope. Imagery is usually stronger but well controlled, although people often care less about controlling their actions. Great changes in perception of space and time are common, as are changes in psychological processes such as understanding, memory, emotion, and sense of identity . . . to the extent that the described effects are delusory or inaccurate, the delusions and inaccuracy are widely shared. It is interesting, too, that nearly all the common effects seem either emotionally pleasing or cognitively interesting, and it is easy to see why marijuana users find the effects desirable regardless of what happens to their external behavior. (p. 704)

At the level of social intoxication, various responses are seen. One of the most pronounced is a tachycardia (increased heart rate), which appears to be dose related and to last throughout the period of intoxication. There is also impairment in cognitive and psychomotor tests. In the Weil (1968) study, naive users reported fewer subjective effects but showed greater decrements in test performance than did experienced users. One effect consistently seen is alteration in short-term memory. The user who is intoxicated many times cannot recall information he was told just minutes or seconds earlier: this perhaps could be a reason for the broken, fragmented discussion seen during drug intoxication. This short-term memory disruption also produces changes in the individual's time sense; she or he markedly overestimates the time that has passed. This, probably more than any other effect, has been the most consistently reported. Melges and his coworkers (1970) have postulated that distorted time sense is the basic effect of THC and that the other effects seen are results of it.

Many users report increased sensitivity to sensory events, but these effects have not been replicated in the laboratory. This may again be due to setting and the response to specific sensory input, and not to a change in the perceptual characteristics of the individual. Generally a state of euphoria and carefreeness predominates but, in some individuals, fear, anxiety, and trepidation persist. These may be due to the individual's inability to cope with the time distortions, short-term memory disruption, stimulus sensitivity, and tachycardia, and are probably not the result solely of the drug.

Summarizing the effects of *Cannabis* on human behavior is a difficult task, because most of the points are still debatable. (1) The early studies of Moreau (1845) and the effects he reported have generally been replicated and confirmed in the 20th century. (2) Marijuana seems to be viewed as a mild intoxicant by some researchers and as a potent hallucinatory substance by others. The true place of the drug is not known as yet, and when emotional argument gives way to rational discourse, we will properly be able to classify the active substances. (3) It appears that a marijuana "high" has to be learned; thus it is questionable whether the entire experience is an effect of the drug. Some actions may be the result of psychological tuning or manipulations within the environmental setting. (4) The drug does impair short-term memory, which is demonstrated in conversations and by the general time distortion reported after use. An overestimation of time is common.

Some Additional Considerations

Not all the effects experienced after marijuana smoking are pleasant. The adverse effects are complex and vary from acute toxic psychosis (Kaplan, 1971) to impotence in the male (Kolodny, Masters, Kolodner, & Toro, 1974). Many factors influence these reactions including dose, prevailing mood of the subject, environmental setting, and the length of time the subject has been using the drug.

Panic reactions. The panic reaction is probably one of the most common side effects seen on the initial trial of marijuana use. The subject is overcome with fear and anxiety and is confused and disoriented. However, he or she will respond to a guide, and realizes that the effects are due to the drug and not some mental breakdown. The following case, reported by Weil (1970), is an example of the panic reaction:

A 37-year old housewife was persuaded by her 15 year-old daughter to "turn on" by eating candy made with hashish. She had never tried *Cannabis* before and agreed to do so out of curiosity although she was very apprehensive. The daughter ate three times as much candy as the patient and became "pleasantly high" for about 6 hours. The patient, 1 hour after ingesting the candy, felt her heart racing and thought she was going to have a heart attack. She became panicky and lay down without telling her daughter what was wrong. Shortly afterward she felt "flushed and dizzy" and became convinced that she was poisoned. Finally, she got the daughter to call a family physician, who persuaded the patient to take a taxicab to a nearby emergency ward. When the physician arrived at the hospital, he found her in a state of nervous collapse with a regular heart rate of 140. He ordered an intramuscular injection of chlorpromazine and had her admitted to a psychiatric bed. She remained agitated and depressed for 4 days and was discharged on the fifth with no aftereffects. The daughter, who had taken three times the dose of hashish, had a "good time" that lasted about 6 hours. (pp. 998–999)

Toxic psychosis. Administration of *Cannabis* preparations may cause a toxic psychosis, which is a "temporary malfunction of the brain" (Nahas, 1973). The clinical symptoms seen in such a case include confusion, prostration, disorientation, derealization, and periodic visual and auditory hallucinations. In the LaGuardia report, 6 subjects were reported to have had "toxic episodes." Talbott and Teague (1969) reported cases of toxic psychosis in 12 soldiers in Vietnam. One of them shot his comrade and boasted afterward that he had killed Ho Chi Minh.

Many do not believe that the degree of disorientation should be labeled as psychotic. Grinspoon (1971) takes a more permissive view of the subject. He believes that certain "susceptible" subjects may experience the adverse effects described, but that they should not be considered in the same class as the psychotic reactions of the schizophrenic. Whatever the outcome of this debate, it is clear that certain individuals will experience very severe reactions to marijuana. Most of the patients recover from this syndrome in a few days; however, in rare cases phobias and inhibitions may develop during these episodes that may last for extended periods.

Male impotence. Recent (Kolodny et al., 1974) data indicate that plasma testosterone levels are depressed by chronic marijuana use. Twenty men (ages 18–28 years) who had smoked marijuana a minimum of 4 days a week during the preceding 6 month period were subjects in this study. They were individually matched with control subjects who were like them in all respects except that the controls did not smoke marijuana. The plasma testosterone levels of the experimental subjects were lower than they were in the controls (see Figure 9.12). The effect seemed to be dose related, and abstention from marijuana or stimulation with human chorionic gonadotropin during continued marijuana use produced marked increases in testosterone levels. There appears to be a contradiction between the subjective reports by males of increased sexual excitement following the use of marijuana and these data, which show decreased testosterone levels in the blood. Further research is needed.

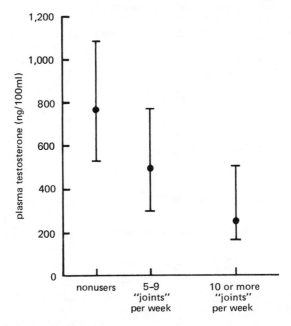

FIGURE 9.12. Relationship of plasma testosterone levels to marijuana use by men, means and ranges.

The amotivational syndrome. The prolonged use of marijuana may lead to a syndrome characterized by a lack of motivation, an "I don't care" attitude, and an inability to make decisions. The individual may become depressed, lazy, lax, and may go about her or his daily routine in a starry-eyed, expressionless manner; this has been described by Moreau earlier, but West (1970) gave it the current name *amotivational syndrome.* Scientists in India and Egypt have described similar states in chronic users: lethargy, social deterioration, and drug preoccupation (Chopra & Chopra, 1967; Souief, 1967). Smith and Mehl (1970) have described the syndrome as a loss of desire to work, to compete, to face challenges. Interests and major concerns of the individual become centered around marijuana, they said, and drug use becomes compulsive. The individual may drop out of school, leave work, ignore personal hygiene, experience loss of sex drive and avoid social interaction.

The case of a college freshman (reported by Kolansky & Moore, 1971) will serve as an example:

A 19 year-old college freshman arrived on time for psychiatric consultation dressed in old, torn, dirty clothes. He was unkempt, with long hair that was uncombed, and disheveled. He talked in a slow, hesitant manner, frequently losing his train of thought, and he could not pay attention or concentrate. He tried hard to both talk and listen, but had difficulty with both. He had been an excellent high school athlete and the highest student in his class in a large city. He was described as neat, orderly, and taking pride in his appearance, intellect and physical fitness. During the last half of his senior year, he began casual (one or two marijuana cigarettes each weekend) smoking. By the time of the evaluation in the middle of his first college year, he was smoking several marijuana cigarettes daily. While in college, he stopped attending classes, didn't know what his goals were, and was flunking all subjects. He partook in no athletic or social events, and was planning to drop out of college to live in a young, drug-oriented group. (p. 490)

This syndrome of dropping out is very often reported and may be the result of an interaction of drug effects with the individual's personality.

Conclusion

Marijuana is a drug. It is a drug that has been used for religious means and recreation for centuries, but we must always remember that drugs have both beneficial and adverse effects, and, even if the pharmacologist cannot explain the neurophysiological actions of the drug, each individual must be responsible for his or her own use of these substances. There is no cop-out or walking away from the drug's effects. If one wants the euphoria, excitement, and relaxation produced by marijuana use, then one must also be ready for the possibility of the adverse effects discussed in the last section.

BANANA SKINS

Another recent, rather faddish excerpt in the story of distorting drugs is the use of banana skins as hallucinatory agents. However, it is not sufficient to ingest a large quantity of bananas; a specific preparation is needed. The inner layers of banana skins are scraped and then slowly dried in a warm oven. The dried remains are then rolled into a cigarette or put into a pipe and smoked.

The exact effect of the mixture is open to debate. Lingeman (1970) claims that when the skin burns, it produces a distorting chemical, which may produce effects reported as a mild high. However, other investigators have labeled the phenomenon *the great banana hoax* (Borrzetti, Goldsmith, & Ungerleider, 1967), and agencies having control over drugs and drug abuse have said that the banana does not contain hallucinogenic chemicals. (However, we do know that bananas are very rich in serotonin.) Whatever the true nature of the chemical content of banana skins, their use is not a subject of major concern and seems to have been a tangential effect of the drug scares and drug cultures of the 1960s.

CONCLUSION

Rather than providing a summary here, we refer you back to the introduction to this chapter. You will find there our analysis and discussion of the central issues regarding these distorting drugs.

10
LEARNING AND MEMORY

Robert A. Levitt and George D. Goedel

Much of the behavior of humans and other species is altered as a result of earlier experiences. Therefore, the information or knowledge resulting from these previous experiences must be acquired (learned), retained, and utilized during an organism's lifetime. Because of the importance of these experiences in determining an organism's actions, the processes of learning and memory have come to occupy a central position in the study of behavior. Although we still remain a long way from understanding the essential nature of these processes, great strides have been made in recent years. Many of these advances have resulted from psychopharmacological investigations. These studies have directed our attention toward (a) the biochemical events in the brain, which may be the substrates of learning and memory, and (b) the manner by which various drugs affect these biochemical reactions (and thus affect learning and memory).

In this chapter we will first review the processes of registration, retention, and retrieval—the three separate abilities necessary for learning and memory to occur. We will point out that there appear to be two stages of retention, short-term and long-term. Short-term retention appears to be based upon the patterned firing of specific groups of neurons. The patterned neural firing, if sufficiently organized and widespread, will result in some permanent biochemical change in the involved neurons. This biochemical change will remain, long after neural firing has returned to "normal." The biochemical changes now mediate retention, and this is called the long-term stage of retention or memory. The development of long-term memory from short-term memory is called consolidation.

Numerous investigators have studied the biochemical basis of long-term retention. This biochemical basis appears to involve brain macromolecules;

however, theories attributing a long-term memory function to proteins, RNA, or DNA alone have not received support. A reasonable alternative theory now appears to be one which attributes long-term retention to (a) the derepression of previously repressed gene function (DNA) by patterned neural firing, (b) the manufacture of RNA from this newly functioning DNA, and (c) the manufacture from this new RNA, of proteins that change cell functioning.

THE STATES OF MEMORY:
THREE SEPARATE ABILITIES

Registration, retention, and retrieval are three abilities that may logically be veiwed or studied as separate states in the memory process. *Registration* refers to the input or encoding of experience by the organism. If one were to learn the names of the first 32 presidents of the United States, the registration of this information would be considered the first "state" in the learning and memory process. The second state is *retention*. If the names of the presidents are to be remembered, they must be retained, i.e., there must be some permanent neurological record of this experience. For retention (memory) to be possible, some permanent change in the chemistry or physiology of the organism must take place in order to preserve the experience. Research efforts to determine the chemical basis of the permanence of memory have generally been focused upon this state of the process.

Retention has frequently been separated into two stages, *short-term* and *long-term*. An example of short-term retention is when one goes to the telephone book, finds a specific number, memorizes it, and then makes a phone call. One usually finds that there is no long-term retention ("memory") of the phone number at some later time. Long-term retention, however, if formed, may remain with the organism for decades. One usually remembers well his name, address, phone number, and even social security number. Behavioral, physiological, and pharmacological evidence has generally tended to support this distinction between short- and long-term retention processes.

The third state of memory, *retrieval*, is the process whereby information or experience, previously registered and retained, can be made accessible to the organism, enabling it to successfully interact with the environment. To continue with the example of the memorization of the list of the presidents, we may view the testing of this information and its successful retrieval as a third and separate state within the processes of learning and memory. All three states are, of course, essential for the neural processing of information and the performance of behavior based on previous experience.

In this regard, two additional important points should now be mentioned. First, we cannot view the states of learning and memory as a single process that is going on only once. Several experiences may contribute to an individual memory. The processes resulting from these various experiences may simultaneously be in the states of registration, retention (short-term and long-term storage), and retrieval. For example, we may administer a number of trials in a learning paradigm (say 10 trials a day for 5 days). On Trial 6 of Day 2, the information from the Day-1 trials may be in long-term retention, Trials 1 through 5 of Day 2 may be in short-term retention, while Trial 6 of Day 2 is in the state of registration. Therefore, it is wise to view memory as a set of parallel processes, each happening at many different times and each overlapping with the others.

A second very important question remains as to whether these states are merely temporal distinctions of the same ongoing process, or whether each state may involve different chemical or physical changes that overlap to form the basis of memory. If different changes occur within each of these states, and if these changes are chemical in nature, then scientists should be able to selectively alter one state in the memory process without affecting the others. For instance, it may be possible to accelerate registration without affecting retrieval or to facilitate retrieval without affecting the permanence of the experience being retrieved. In fact, these things are possible, and it appears that registration, retention, and retrieval are dependent on separable neural processes.

THE NATURE OF MEMORY

Early theories of memory were generally based upon the assumption of an electrical process occurring during learning and remaining active in widespread neural circuits for some time (*reverberatory circuits*) (Gerard, 1955; Hebb, 1949). A reverberatory circuit is presumed to be a pathway of neurons which eventually feeds back on itself. Neural firing in such a recurrent or self-exciting pathway would tend to reverberate through the neural chain. Hebb (1949) referred to this type of reverberatory circuit as a cell assembly.

Consolidation Theory

A related popular notion was the consolidation theory first proposed at the turn of the century (Müller & Pilzecker, 1900). This theory separated the basis of memory into the two previously discussed stages, short-term and long-term. The first stage was proposed to consist of electrical activity occurring in reverberatorylike circuits, while long-term retention, the second stage, was proposed to include some sort of permanent physical change occurring as a result of the preceding memory stage. Consolidation was conceived as the development of long-term retention (a biochemical change) from the short-term retention (reverberatory circuits). Retrieval was thought to occur from either the short- or long-term process (Grossman, 1967, Ch. 14).

Post-traumatic amnesia. Evidence supporting such a theory has come from clinical observations of amnesia resulting from concussive head injuries. Accompanying cerebral trauma, there is usually a period of unconsciousness followed by a state of confusion. This phenomenon, which has been called *post-traumatic amnesia*, may last from a few minutes to weeks. Drug treatment (usually a barbiturate) may reduce the effect of the post-traumatic amnesia.

The following hypothetical case (a fictionalized account based on cases discussed by Russell & Nathan, 1946) illustrates post-traumatic amnesia. A student motorcyclist on his way to class was involved in a severe accident. When questioned by police officials several hours later concerning the incident, his earliest recollection was that of being carried on a stretcher into an ambulance. The actual time of this experience was about a half hour after the accident occurred, which was when the ambulance finally arrived. The second thing he could recall was someone mentioning that he would need stitches. This comment had been made by a doctor when he arrived at the hospital nearly a half hour after he was first placed in the ambulance (this retrieval was occurring according to our model, out of short-term retention).

He was questioned again by his insurance investigator about one week after the accident. At this time he could no longer remember being placed in the ambulance and his earliest memory was the comment made by the doctor about stitches. In fact, he reported that his memory of the entire day of the accident was quite vague, but the police reports of the first examination revealed his memory for the events of the day to have been rather good.

Some improvement in memory was noted, however, upon administration of the drug thiopental (a barbiturate). Under the influence of the drug he could once again recall being lifted on the stretcher into the ambulance, as well as part of the ride to the hospital. He could also remember the doctor remarking that he would need stitches although his memory of the medical examination, given when he was admitted to the hospital, continued to remain quite vague. One explanation for this efficacy of the barbiturate as an aid to retrieval involves state-dependent learning (to be discussed). The concussion and the barbiturate may depress or alter neural firing in somewhat similar manners, so that there is greater retrieval transfer between these two states than between either one and a normally functional state. We now see that part of the failure of memory was not due to a loss of retention but to a disturbance in retrieval out of long-term retention stores. This case nicely points out the difficulty in determining the basis of a performance decrement.

Retrograde amnesia. A loss of memory (or, more accurately, retrieval capacity) for events preceding the trauma (*retrograde amnesia*) is also almost always found to occur. These effects are most severe on recent memory with recall of the oldest memory recovering first and most recent events last. Memory for events a few moments prior to the trauma may never return. Retrograde amnesia may occur as a result of physical trauma, mental trauma, anesthesia, and in some cases, as an accompanying symptom of chronic alcoholism (Korsakoff's Syndrome; see Chapter 6) (Talland, 1965). Since much or all of the memory may recover, the difficulty seems to be with access to the memory (retrieval). However, since older memories are retained, there appears to be an interaction with consolidation processes. It may be that memories continue to become more resistant to disruption for weeks, months, or years after the original experience.

ECS. The consolidation theory has been supported by studies of the effects of electroconvulsive shock (ECS) (Glickman, 1961; McGaugh & Herz, 1972). It appears that the major effect of ECS is to prevent the formation (consolidation) from short-term retention of the storage system responsible for long-term retention. Following administration of electroconvulsive shock in humans, memory for events immediately preceding the shock is permanently lost (an effect on retention). Experimentally, electroconvulsive shock has been employed with animals to produce similar effects. If a strong convulsant electric current is administered to a subject shortly after it has learned a habit, it performs poorly on retention tests. Most of the experimental data are on animals, but in the few studies using humans as subjects, the effects have been similar. In one such study the subjects were trained on a paired-associate list of words (seeing one word as the stimulus should produce the response of the word that had been paired with it) and were given the electroconvulsive shock treatment immediately following training or some hours later. The ECS immediately following registration impeded retention, but later ECS had no effect (Williams, 1950; Zubin & Barrera, 1941). However, at the same time that the subjects do not remember the recently presented information, they are capable of learning another task, and are also able to demonstrate the retention of older habits. Therefore, the ECS selectively destroys retention, leaving registration and retrieval processes unaffected. Studies have generally shown that the severity of the impairment in retention varies inversely with the time between learning and shock administration.

Other factors have also been shown to be important in determining the amount of retention disruption. Among these are the difficulty of the task to be learned, the strength and mode of delivery of the ECS, and the strength of the reinforcer, such as foot shock (Ray & Barrett, 1969; Ray & Bivens, 1968). For example, the more difficult the task, the longer the habit takes to consolidate; the stronger the ECS, the more likely memory will be disrupted; and the stronger the foot shock, the faster the habit will consolidate.

REM sleep. One recent experiment has led to the suggestion that memory may be transferred from short-term to long-term stores during the rapid eye movement (REM), dreaming, phase of sleep. Mice were deprived of this phase of sleep (called *paradoxical sleep* in animals) for 48 hours following a learning session. At the conclusion of this deprivation period, the mice were subjected to ECS. The ECS eliminated the memory, although ECS did not have this effect 48 hours after learning in nondeprived mice. These data suggest that the memory was kept in a short-term store and prevented from consolidation into long-term retention during the deprivation of paradoxical sleep (Fishbein, McGaugh, & Swarz, 1971). Could it be that consolidation occurs normally during REM, or paradoxical, sleep?

Temperature. Other experimental techniques have also been used to disrupt electrical brain activity. Several investigators have reported memory deficits from anoxia (lack of oxygen) similar to those produced by electroconvulsive shock treatment (Hays, 1953; Meier, 1971; Thompson & Pryer, 1956). Altering the temperature of the organism is another means of changing electrical activity in the brain (Pepler, 1971). In work with goldfish, heat narcosis (anesthesia) has been produced by raising the temperature at varying intervals following learning. These treatments, in turn, resulted in retention deficits (Cerf & Otis, 1957). The effects of cooling on retention are unclear, depending to some extent on the species employed. Some investigators (using rats) have reported retention deficits and others (using hamsters) have found no effect (Mrosovsky, 1963; Ransmeier & Gerard, 1954). One effect of lowering body temperature which has been consistently reported, however, is a prolongation of the time following learning during which electroconvulsive shock is an effective disruptor of memory (Agranoff, Davis, & Brink, 1965; Gerard, 1955). Cooling may act to slow down consolidation by slowing down the chemical processes that are required for registration or by slowing down the consolidation of long-term retention from short-term retention.

Drugs. Administration of a number of chemical agents, including both stimulants (see Chapter 8) and depressants (see Chapter 6), has been found to produce amnesia (Grossman, 1967, Ch. 14; Pearlman, Sharpless, & Jarvik, 1961). It appears that after training, any major change in the pattern of neural firing (either an increase or a decrease) that disrupts the organized activity produced by a learning experience, disrupts the consolidation of that experience into memory storage. However, although consolidation is prevented, it has recently been shown that short-term memory itself is not destroyed. Although animals receiving ECS immediately after acquisition do not remember 24 hours later, they remember quite as well as control animals a few minutes or hours later. This continuing short-term retention is supposedly based on the persistence of short-term memory (McGaugh, 1970). Therefore, ECS may disrupt the consolidation of long-term retention from short-term retention without destroying the short-term retention; the reverberatory circuits may continue, but be prevented from inducing the biochemical changes (according to our model of memory).

A Biochemical Basis for Long-Term Memory

It appears certain that there is, following learning, a period of variable length during which the consolidation of experience is susceptible to disruption by altering the electrical activity of the brain. However, attempts to disrupt electrical brain activity after this period has passed have no observable effects upon retention. Thus, while a theory encompassing ongoing neural activity as the basis of memory may plausibly account for short-term storage (retention), it cannot account for long-term storage (retention). The consolidation of long-term retention from short-term retention is disrupted by electroconvulsive shock treatments, cooling, heating, and certain drugs (stimulants or depressants), but long-term retention (once formed) seems immune to these drastic changes in neural firing. Long-term retention must involve some ECS-resistant permanent physical or chemical change, and this change must occur somewhere in the nervous system. Recent efforts to establish the locus of memory have tended to direct our attention toward the chemical aspects of the nervous system.

The Search for the Location of Memory

Now that we have decided that long-term retention is based on some permanent biochemical change in the nervous system, let us discuss the question of where these changes are taking place. What is the locus of memory? This question of where our experiences are stored is an intriguing one, which has stimulated research in many directions and on many different levels. One method of study is to examine different brain structures for their role in the memory process. Two major techniques employed in this area include (1) clinical observation of patients with brain damage and (2) surgical lesioning (removing tissue or cutting pathways) in animals. A pioneer in the use of lesioning techniques was Karl Lashley, who accumulated a considerable amount of data to suggest that the memory trace, or *engram* as it has been called, is usually widely spread throughout the brain. Although certain areas of the cortex, such as the temporal lobe, and certain limbic system structures, such as the hippocampus and amygdala, have been implicated as being directly involved in the memory process (Milner, 1970), no one area or structure has been consistently found to be indispensable. In fact, Lashley commented from his extensive study, *In Search of the Engram* (1950), that "in reviewing the evidence on the localization of the memory trace, the necessary conclusion is that learning just is not possible." However, in a more serious mood he declared that "it is not possible to demonstrate the isolated localization of a memory trace anywhere in the nervous system. Limited regions may be essential for learning or retention of a particular activity, but . . . the engram is represented throughout the region." The phenomenon of state-dependent learning, discussed next, also points out the general diffuseness of the memory trace.

State-dependent Learning

When an animal or human learns to perform a particular behavioral sequence in the presence of a particular stimulus situation, a great deal is learned in addition to the behavioral response. The subject learns about the environment or stimulus situation that triggers the behavior, which may include such things as many different types of external sensory inputs (visual, auditory, tactile, etc.) as well as many different types of internal stimuli representing the animal's motivational state (blood glucose, tissue osmolarity, hormone levels, temperature, etc.). The various patterns of neural firing reflecting external and internal stimulus conditions become a part of the memory trace so that any change in an external or internal stimulus will lead to a pattern of neural firing differing to some degree from that present during the initial sequence of experiences. Therefore, learning (and memory of what is learned) may be state dependent. This means that a particular behavioral response learned in the context of specific external and internal environmental cues may not be recalled if the stimulus complex is varied.

The phenomenon of state-dependent learning has been demonstrated with several drugs (Overton, 1971). Drugs such as curare, the depressants (ethanol, the barbiturates, and anesthetics), or the antischizophrenic tranquilizers (for example, the phenothiazines), when given to an animal or human, have a profound effect on the pattern of neural firing. It has been found that if an organism is taught a particular behavioral sequence under the influence of one of these drugs and then tested without the drug, the retention of the behavior is seriously retarded. However, if the drug is once again administered and the organism is tested under its influence, retention is high (Girden & Culler, 1937). Likewise, if an organism is trained under a no-drug condition, retention is low if tested with a drug, but high when tested with the original environmental cues (i.e., no drug).

There also appears to be good transfer between drugs possessing similar pharmacologic properties. An animal may be trained under one phenothiazine tranquilizer and show high retention when tested under another phenothiazine, but may show low retention when tested after administration of a barbiturate or another kind of drug. Thus, retrieval of information that was stored while the organism was in one state may be difficult or even impossible if the organism is in another state. Information stored while the CNS is in a specified state is most easily retrieved when the same state is again imposed. State dependency, however, is not found for all drug classes. For example, this phenomenon has not been demonstrated with the adrenergic stimulants or the CNS stimulants, which may even facilitate retrieval when the drug has worn off.

One explanation for the phenomenon of state-dependent learning is that the alteration in neural firing patterns produced by a drug is a part of the total environmental stimulus complex and consequently becomes incorporated into the engram, or memory trace. Do not forget that neural firing patterns and changed neural firing patterns result from the activity of large numbers of particular neurons. Therefore, the memory, or an organism's performance of a learned task, is a reflection of the totality of events going on in the central nervous system at the time of learning and of retrieval. These neural firing patterns that form the basis for an engram must be widespread and diffuse. However, regardless of the diffuseness of memory, the next section shows that changes in synaptic function would seem to be indispensable.

The Synapse

If memory is diffusely represented in the nervous system and if the state of the organism must be controlled in order to investigate memory, one might wonder where a search for memory could be undertaken and, perhaps more importantly, what the nature of the substrate providing the basis for memory might be. Investigation of the memory process at the molecular level may provide the answer. If it can be agreed that behavior is ultimately the result of nervous system activity and that synaptic transmission is an important aspect of this activity, then it would be reasonable to choose the synapse as a likely interface between memory and performance and a logical place to pursue the memory process. Furthermore, since transmission at the snyapse is known to be chemical, it follows that memory may be chemical in nature. If this is true, the use of chemical agents should be able to provide some insight into the mechanisms of memory.

The cholinergic system.   During the last decade, there have been a number of studies suggesting that neural transmitter substances may be involved with the memory trace (Koelle, 1971). The majority of these studies have employed indirect approaches in attempting to assess the role of the chemical transmitters in memory. A variety of experiments, which we shall now briefly review, allow us to conclude that brain acetylcholine has an important role in determining the efficiency of learning and memory processes. Perhaps the most promising and elaborate set of studies along this line have been those conducted by several investigators at the University of California, Berkeley (Bennett, Diamond, Krech, & Rosenzweig, 1964; Rosenzweig, 1970; Rosenzweig, Krech, & Bennett, 1960). Their initial work in this area was an attempt to correlate measures of acetylcholine (ACh) in the brain with measures of behavior. Some studies have measured levels in homogenized whole brain, while others have used only certain brain regions for biochemical analysis. However, even in these last studies subtle synaptic biochemical changes would be masked by homogenization of brain fragments. The genetic background of the organism was found to produce correlated differences in maze learning and in ACh and acetylcholinesterase (AChE). In many studies AChE has been measured, since it is more easily studied than is ACh. The AChE concentrations of rats which had been bred for several generations according to their maze-learning ability (the Tryon maze-bright and maze-dull strains) were found to differ, with the maze-bright rats having higher levels than the maze-dull. This evidence led these investigators to suspect a relationship between learning capacity and the neurotransmitter.

Another important observation to come out of these studies was the marked influence early environmental experience had upon cortical growth as well as on ACh and AChE levels. It was discovered that rats raised in a complex, "rich," environment had thicker and heavier cerebral cortices along with greater cortical ACh and AChE as adults than did their litter mates (used as controls) raised in an "impoverished," or intermediate, laboratory environment. These studies have provided evidence that the neurotransmitters may possibly be part of the neurological substrate for learning and memory. It appears that different brain levels and distributions of ACh as well as the other neurotransmitters and enzymes may result from both genetic and experiential influences. These biochemical differences may then account, to some degree, for differences in problem-solving ability and "intelligence," even in humans.

Anticholinergics: Other evidence has accumulated to suggest that the cholinergic transmitter does indeed play a role in the memory process. Several reports have indicated that anticholinergic drugs (which diminish the effectiveness of acetylcholine), when administered to humans in low dosage, tend to produce sedating and amnesia effects (Longo, 1966). Scopolamine, for instance, is used to produce "twilight sleep" during birth and tends to produce an amnesia for the delivery. Scopolamine and atropine, when given in high doses, however, have been reported to produce restlessness, excitement, and confusion. The effects of these drugs on learning are rather complex and depend to a large extent upon such factors as the level of training, type of procedure used, species, dose, and route of administration. For instance, it has been reported that application of atropine to the reticular nuclei of the thalamus of rats impairs the acquisition of discrimination or avoidance tasks. Application of the drug to the midline nuclei of the thalamus, however, facilitates acquisition of both tasks (Grossman, S. P., & Grossman, L., 1966; Grossman & Peters, 1966; Grossman, Peters, Freedman, & Willer, 1965). Thus, while scopolamine and atropine have generally been found to retard acquisition in a variety of tasks and procedures, some reports of enhanced responding and increases in performance can be found with the use of these agents. When administered following training, however, the most consistent results reported are transient impairment or disruption of responding (Carlton, 1963, 1969; Carlton & Markiewicz, 1971).

Anticholinesterases: Somewhat complementary results have been reported with anticholinesterase agents (Deutsch, 1971). These drugs slow down the destruction of ACh by combining with cholinesterase, the enzyme that inactivates ACh, and thus produce an increased availability of the endogenous cholinergic transmitter. When conduction across a synapse is at a low level, such a drug would be expected to facilitate transmission, since the destruction of ACh would be slowed. However, when conduction is at a high level, transmission may be hindered by such a drug, since it would allow ACh to accumulate to an excessive amount and would overload the synapse. According to this model, therefore, there is an optimal level of ACh for normal functioning. Too little ACh fails to fire the postsynaptic neuron, while too much ACh overloads the enzymatic capacity of AChE (producing a depolarizing blockade; see Chapter 4). The postsynaptic neuron is then maintained in a depolarized (nonfunctional) state because there is insufficient AChE to remove the ACh from the receptors on the postsynaptic membrane. Behavioral data consistent with this model have been gathered. Injections of the anticholinesterase drug diisopropyl fluorophosphate (DFP) intracerebrally into rats have been found to block the recall of a well-learned task shortly after training (high level of ACh and transmission) but facilitate recall of the task when the response had been nearly forgotten (low level of ACh and transmission). Similar time-dependent effects have also been obtained with intraperitoneal injections of the anticholinesterase physostigmine.

These amnesic effects produced by anticholinesterase agents have been found to be only temporary, however; this fact contributes to the idea that the amnesia is produced by a synaptic block (there is an inhibition of retrieval, but no effect on retention). If, during testing, trials are spaced, allowing time for the excess ACh that is producing a transmission block to be cleared away, amnesia is minimal, while amnesia is most severe when a massed practice procedure is employed.

Nicotine: Finally, the effects of nicotine and other cholinomimetic drugs on learning have provided some additional evidence to support the likelihood of the involvement of cholinergic mechanisms in learning and memory processes (McGaugh & Petrinovich, 1965). Nicotine has been found to produce a facilitating effect on acquisition of an avoidance task with rats. The influence of genetic variables is important here, since this facilitation has been found to be greater for rats bred for low avoidance-learning ability as compared to those bred for high ability. Although initial results indicating facilitation were thought to be due to the state-dependent learning phenomenon discussed earlier, later results have tended to show that learning and retention are enhanced by nicotine and that the drug has its effects by acting directly upon the central memory process.

Stimulant drugs. A popular approach in assessing the chemical nature of the memory process has been that of administering a drug and observing its effects upon learning and memory (McGaugh & Petrinovich, 1965). Early studies along these lines employed substances such as thiamine, glutamic acid, barbiturates, and amphetamine. Today a large number of compounds are being screened for possible memory effects. One of the major problems encountered by such an approach is to distinguish the effects these drugs have on learning and memory from those on other processes such as motivation, attention, sensation, perception, etc. Thus, much of the effort in this direction has been an attempt to refine experimental procedures and look for consistent effects of drugs over a variety of learning tasks such as maze learning, discrimination learning, avoidance conditioning, and classical conditioning. In general (with some exceptions) it has been reported that anticholinergic agents, barbiturates, and other compounds with depressant actions tend to impair learning or retention, while anticholinesterase agents, stimulants, and convulsant drugs, *given in subconvulsive doses*, tend to facilitate learning or storage of the memory trace. A common feature among many of the substances that have been found to have a facilitative effect on learning and memory is that they tend to increase the excitatory action of the central nervous system, although their mechanisms of action may be quite different. When given at convulsive doses, however, drugs such as pentylenetetrazol or strychnine are as effective as ECS in disrupting consolidation (Bohdanecky, Kopp, & Jarvik, 1968; Jarvik & Kopp, 1967).

Administration prior to training: The typical procedure employed to test the effects of a chemical agent on learning or registration is to administer a subconvulsive dose of the agent to the organism some 10 to 20 minutes prior to training on a learning task. In some studies, training may be continued for several days using this procedure, while in others, all of the training may take place during one session. The chemical agent strychnine has been found to facilitate acquistion under this procedure for a number of species (cats, monkeys, rats) and a variety of tasks (discrimination learning, escape and avoidance learning, classical conditioning, maze learning, and delayed-response tasks). Similar effects have also been obtained with pentylenetetrazol. Some have interpreted such results as indicating an enhancement of learning due to the action of these substances on the neural processes involved in memory. However, such an interpretation is suspect, due to the possibility that the enhancement may be due to sensitization (Cholewiak, Hammond, Seigler, & Papsdorf, 1968) or altered attention during learning (McGaugh, 1966, 1969, 1970; McGaugh & Petrinovich, 1965).

Administration following training: An alternative procedure that has been employed in the attempt to divorce the effects these substances have on memory storage from those on other processes has been to administer these agents at various intervals following training on some task. With this procedure, any effect of the drug would appear to be on consolidation processes occurring subsequent to the learning trial. Using this post-training procedure, several stimulants such as strychnine, picrotoxin, and pentylenetetrazol have been found to facilitate the learning of a number of tasks by several species (Breen & McGaugh, 1961; Hudspeth, 1964; Krivanek & McGaugh, 1968; McGaugh, 1961; Zerbolio, 1967).

Maze-bright and maze-dull rats: The enhancement in learning appears to be due to an increase in consolidation and has been demonstrated very nicely in experiments employing maze-bright and maze-dull rats. It has been noted in experiments with these two strains of rats that differences in their performance can be eliminated by training the animals over an extended period of time (spaced training) as opposed to a concentrated training session (massed training). This suggested that the differences in their maze-learning ability might be due to differences in the amount of time needed for consolidation. It was found that if substances such as strychnine or picrotoxin were administered to both maze-bright and maze-dull animals, the group differences in trials to criteria with massed trials disappeared and both strains learned in about the same number of trials. There was a negligible effect seen in the maze-bright rats; however, there was a marked improvement in the maze-dull rats, such that the genetic differences between the two strains became of little consequence (McGaugh & Petrinovich, 1965; McGaugh, Thompson, Westbrook, & Hudspeth, 1962). Could rapidity of consolidation account to some extent for differences in learning, problem-solving ability, and "intelligence" in other species, including humans?

A BIOCHEMICAL BASIS FOR MEMORY

Each of the approaches to the study of memory thus far discussed has contributed much to our understanding of this most complex process. Registration, short-term retention, and consolidation, especially, are now better understood. Nevertheless, the approaches detailed up to now have yielded little in helping to explain the permanence of memory (long-term retention). It is in the final approach to be discussed here, the one most molecular in nature, that information pertinent to this goal of understanding long-term retention may be realized. This approach has focused its attention upon the macromolecules of the cell, proteins and nucleic acids (DNA and RNA), as possible candidates for the substrate of learning and memory. Beginning in the 1950s with some investigators speculating as to the possible role these molecules might play in the memory process (Katz & Halstead, 1950), this approach has since attracted widespread interest (Bogoch, 1968; Gaito, 1963; Gaito & Zavala, 1964; Grossman, 1967, Ch. 16). Perhaps the most important factors responsible for this surge of interest are the recent discoveries made in the field of molecular biology concerning the genetic code and the fundamental role played by the nucleic acid, deoxyribonucleic acid (DNA). Since DNA contained the genetic material or the genetic memory of an organism and directed the biochemical reactions of the cell, it seemed reasonable to postulate that a similar mechanism might account for individual (or experiential) memory.

Before a molecule can be given serious consideration as the substrate of memory, there are several criteria that it would have to meet besides the obvious ones of being present in the nervous system and having a role in neural metabolism. First, it would have to be *labile*, which means that extraorganismic agents must be able to affect the molecule such that information in the form of input to the central nervous system could be processed and stored. Second, the molecule must be either stable or replicable. Thus, information, once stored by a change in the molecule, would remain permanent due to its stability or due to the molecule's ability to replicate itself. Last, the molecule must be capable of encoding complicated information within itself; therefore, it should be of some size and complexity. DNA, ribonucleic acid (RNA), and protein molecules seem to fulfill these criteria. They are sufficiently complex to adequately store the most complicated information, are highly replicable to insure permanence, and, with the possible exception of DNA, are labile to change resulting from environmental influences (Gurowitz, 1969).

Prior to discussing the evidence which suggests these substances as potential memory molecules and the relative importance each has been given in the memory process, we would like to present a model of the biochemistry of learning and memory, which we believe best encompasses the data. This model, called the derepression hypothesis, is based on current knowledge of the genetic control of cellular processes. For a review of these processes, see one of the following references: Grossman (1967); Gurowitz (1969); John (1967); Watson (1970).

The Derepression Hypothesis

Basic to the understanding of this hypothesis is knowledge of the manner in which RNA is synthesized from a DNA template in the nucleus and the manner in which cell protein manufacture is controlled by RNA. A type of RNA (called messenger RNA) is formed from DNA segments in the nucleus of a cell and travels out of the nucleus into the cytoplasm until it contacts a structure called a *ribosome*. The messenger RNA–ribosome complex then manufactures a protein by assembling amino acids from the cytoplasm according to a coded message specified by the messenger RNA. *Operator* is the term applied to a segment of DNA located on adjacent regions of the chromosome. The operator (a gene) functions as a unit to manufacture an RNA molecule that controls some cellular function. An operator is capable of only two states, either open or closed. When the operator is in the open state, it synthesizes messenger RNA, which then is responsible for the formation of some cellular protein. When the operator is in the closed state, the synthesis of messenger RNA by this DNA segment is prevented. The operator is placed in the closed state by a cytoplasmic substance (the product of a regulator gene) called a *repressor*. Repressors are most likely to be the enzymatic proteins that regulate various metabolic processes in the neuron.

The regulator genes, in turn, are controlled by the concentration of other specific ions or metabolites, called *effectors*, which are related to cellular firing and may be found in the cytoplasm of the cell. Therefore, it has been proposed that effectors can ultimately control the synthesis of particular proteins by either activating or inactivating repressors. In this way, changes in the concentration of certain substances in the cytoplasm of a cell can either initiate or terminate protein synthesis through effects on nuclear DNA (see Figure 10.1). This sort of scheme would provide a homeostatic type of feedback system, from the cytoplasm to the nucleus and back again to the cytoplasm, for the regulation of protein synthesis. Protein synthesis would then be effectively controlled by either increasing or decreasing the concentration of effectors that activate repressors or those that inactivate repressors.

Effectors. It has been proposed that the state of regulator genes and the manufacture of repressor substances may be influenced by two different types of substances that act as effectors: (1) metabolites of low molecular weight, such as ions (sodium, potassium, chloride, and calcium are possibilities), and (2) high-molecular-weight proteins (such as the enzymes involved in the metabolism of the neurotransmitters). However the possibilities are not limited to transmitters. Proteins or lipids that form part of the cell wall, especially in presynaptic and postsynaptic regions, might also be manufactured in increased amounts. This might increase the sensitivity of this neuron to selected input (presynaptic cell wall buildup) or the ease with which this neuron fires certain other neurons (postsynaptic cell wall buildup), especially if the cell wall buildup is selective, as it certainly might be. Such a system would allow ionic changes as a result of neural activity to produce long-lasting and stable changes in the concentration of particular proteins which then change the functioning of the cell, and also maintain this new changed condition by inhibiting a regulator gene. The key to this idea is that the proteins (enzymes) produced at the ribosomes both change cellular functioning and act as effectors.

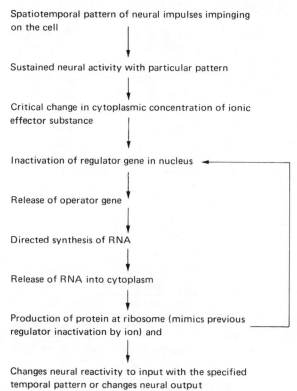

Spatiotemporal pattern of neural impulses impinging
on the cell

Sustained neural activity with particular pattern

Critical change in cytoplasmic concentration of ionic
effector substance

Inactivation of regulator gene in nucleus

Release of operator gene

Directed synthesis of RNA

Release of RNA into cytoplasm

Production of protein at ribosome (mimics previous
regulator inactivation by ion) and

Changes neural reactivity to input with the specified
temporal pattern or changes neural output

FIGURE 10.1. The derepression hypothesis. (Reprinted by permission from E. R. John, *Mechanisms of Memory*. Copyright 1967 by Academic Press.)

In proposing the derepression hypothesis to account for the neural basis of memory formation, we must assert that the storage of information cannot be accounted for by changes in the structure of DNA or RNA or by changes in the synthesis of protein. We argue that changes in the structure of DNA are virtually impossible, since DNA synthesis is completely determined by the structure of the DNA molecule from which it is formed. With the possible exception of mutagenic influences, the DNA molecule is extremely stable and resistant to changes. Furthermore, since RNA is synthesized from a DNA template, fairly rigid restraints are placed on the structure of this substance. Finally, proteins are built up from amino acids whose structure is determined by instructions from messenger RNA.

Therefore, it has been reasoned that some other mechanism must mediate information storage and that such a mechanism may be found in the rate of protein synthesis and in the concentration of proteins in the cytoplasm of the cell. Specifically, the derepression hypothesis contains three major tenets. First, it assumes that the potential for the synthesis of many substances by way of DNA is, for the most part, repressed and that derepression must occur for this potential to be realized. Second, it assumes that derepression, resulting in the subsequent synthesis of substances in the cytoplasm, can be brought about by a shift (*critical shift*) in the concentration of existing cytoplasmic materials as a result of sustained neural activity. This period, during which there is a critical shift in the intracellular concentration of some ion, would seem to correlate with the period of sustained electrical firing of the neurons (the firing of a reverberatory circuit) and with short-term retention. Third, the derepression hypothesis assumes that the substrates (proteins, probably enzymes) synthesized as a result of this derepression are responsible for long-term retention and have two features: (1) the ability to mimic the derepression action the of initial ionic effectors, thus continuing synthesis independently of the metabolic state originating derepression and (2) the ability to alter the reactivity of the neurons to input or to alter the output of the neuron.

Motivation and reinforcement. We would now like to make two additional important points. First, motivation and reinforcement appear to have a special role in learning and memory. In the section on state-dependent memory (really, state-dependent retrieval) we pointed out that the motivational state at the time of registration becomes a part of the engram and that retrieval would be maximized by reestablishing that motivational state. It may be that registration processes, retention processes, and/or retrieval processes are also specially dependent upon a reinforcer for their activation.

Comparator. The second important point concerns the comparator mechanism, which is responsible for the retrieval of memory. How is a particular memory retrieved and what is the cause of this particular memory being activated? Probably the most reasonable, yet simplistic model of this function is that a memory is retrieved when it has a large degree of overlap with the spatiotemporal pattern of cell firings produced by the present total sensory situation (internal and external environment). This sensory situation could certainly include internally generated "thought processes." This "stream of consciousness" appears normally to follow patterns of relatedness or relevance.

Such a model as this can incorporate much of the data on memory, both electrophysiological and biochemical. It not only helps to integrate much of what is already known about the memory process into a more organized system but also should stimulate new research by providing a different framework within which memory may be investigated.

EVIDENCE FOR A MEMORY MOLECULE

By far, the majority of research in this area has tended to focus upon one or another of the major nitrogen-containing molecules (DNA, RNA, proteins) as forming the basic substrate for the long-term retention of memory. This does not preclude, however, the possibility that the memory substrate may be somewhat more complex, involving DNA, RNA, and the proteins interacting together.

We shall now review the theories suggesting a role for DNA, RNA, and proteins in long-term retention. The first three sections will review the evidence pertaining to theories proposing that DNA, RNA, or proteins are the substrate of long-term retention. With respect to DNA, we will see that experience has little effect on the amount of this material or the structure of the DNA molecules.

The data pertaining to RNA and proteins, each under consideration as a long-term retention molecule, are quite complex. In general, these molecules seem to have some role in long-term retention, but the flaw in the early theories is that RNA or proteins do not seem to work alone. The fourth section reviews the data on the interanimal transfer of memory by injecting material from the brains of trained "donor" animals into untrained "recipient" animals.

You should keep the derepression hypothesis in mind during the reading of this material. In this theory, no new DNA is produced. Instead, DNA that was already present, but whose functioning was previously repressed, becomes active as a function of experience. The newly functioning DNA causes the manufacture of RNA, which causes the manufacture of a protein, which alters the function of the cell (and thus mediates long-term retention). We believe that this theory comes the closest to properly incorporating the data on long-term retention.

DNA

Initially, the molecule receiving the most attention was DNA. This molecule, due to its role in the encoding and transmission of genetic information, appeared to be a likely candidate for the encoding of experiential information. It fulfilled the requirements of being highly stable and of sufficient size to encode information. However, a variety of experimental manipulations have failed to produce a change in the quantity or activity of DNA. Such a change would seem to be necessary for the molecule to encode experiential information. The use of mechanical stimulation of neurons, electroconvulsive shock, or the administration of narcotics have all failed to produce changes in DNA metabolism. Furthermore, the amount of DNA also appears to be invariant across species and resistant to change by any normal means. Only through the use of a *mutagenic agent* (radiation or irritative chemicals that physically alter the structure of the gene) can DNA be changed by chemically altering its component parts, thereby replacing one or more of its normal components by one not normally occurring in DNA. Such a process would appear an unlikely basis for memory, since brain DNA molecules possessing an abnormal structure have not been found to date. Therefore, by itself, DNA does not seem to hold much promise as the biochemical substrate of memory. This does not, however, rule out the possibility that some modification of DNA's action may play a role (Gurowitz, 1969, Ch. 4). The derepression hypothesis, for example, requires no change in the amount or structure of DNA, only the start of active functioning by previously nonfunctional DNA molecules.

RNA

RNA, on the other hand, has been supported by many as a molecule responsible for experiential memory (Booth, 1967b). Logically, it can be argued that stimuli which act upon a cell do so at its outer surface and, if the stimuli alter the chemical constituents of a cell, they probably alter those substances in close proximity to the surface. The presence of RNA in the cytoplasm of cells readily suggests this as the substance that is modified. Neural excitation due to natural or artificial (mechanical, electrical, etc.) stimulation has generally resulted in an increase in the level of RNA in the neurons affected. Similarly, decreases in the levels of RNA have generally been found following neuronal inhibition, produced by either exhaustion or drug-induced narcosis, by amobarbital, sodium, or ethanol (Gurowitz, 1969, Ch. 5; Pevzner, 1966; Talwar, Goel, Chopra, & D'Monte, 1966).

Effects of learning on RNA. In addition to demonstrations of altered RNA synthesis as a result of neural stimulation and inhibition, a number of studies have shown increases in RNA synthesis as a function of learning. Typically, this approach involves the establishment of a new behavior in an organism and subsequent analysis of molecules in the brain to determine whether or not the synthesis of specific types of molecules can be correlated with the learning process. Such an approach has been undertaken by Hydén and others in an effort to provide evidence linking RNA with learning and memory (Hydén, 1970). Their experiments have included training rats on various tasks, such as walking up a tightwire or learning to use a nondominant paw to obtain food. Changes in the structure of RNA as well as increases in the absolute amount of RNA have been reported. These structural changes were found to be localized to the vestibular nuclei in the first experiment and the contralateral paw area of the cerebral motor cortex in the second. Data such as these have often led to the assumption that changes in the structure of RNA may be the key to how memory is encoded. This assumption must be made with extreme care, however, since oftentimes adequate controls are lacking in these experiments. In fact, some evidence indicates that structural changes may not be specific to learning but rather, a result of stimulation or activation in general. According to the derepression hypothesis the changes in the amount and structure of RNA that can be measured are not the result of direct actions on RNA. Instead, newly functioning DNA by manufacturing RNA is altering the amount and type of RNA measurable because it is newly producing a particular RNA molecule.

Effects of drugs on RNA and learning. Another avenue of approach in the study of RNA and its role in learning and memory has been the administration of various drugs in an effort to either facilitate or inhibit RNA synthesis and thereby possibly enhance or interfere with memory. The drugs that have been used as inhibitors are essentially antibiotics. Antibiotics are generally employed to combat invading bacteria at a dose that leaves the host cells relatively healthy while inhibiting the cell metabolism of the bacteria. Used at higher doses, these agents can be administered either systemically or intracerebrally to inhibit cell protein or RNA metabolism during learning.

8-Azaguanine: The drug 8-azaguanine has often been used to inhibit RNA synthesis. This drug is a derivative of one of the normal constituents of DNA and RNA, called guanine, and as such is incorporated into the RNA molecule, rendering the molecule metabolically inert (Creaser, 1956). Injections of this drug into rats have been reported to interfere with the learning of a water maze without affecting motor performance or the retention of previously learned mazes (Dingman & Sporn, 1961). Although this evidence has fostered the conclusion that RNA is involved in the encoding or registration process and not the retention process, the fact that this drug also affects biochemical processes not related to RNA synthesis must not be overlooked. Such a conclusion may also appear to be premature in the face of conflicting experiments, which have found no effect of this agent on learning or retention (Chamberlain, Rothchild, & Gerard, 1963). This contradictory evidence may be due to a number of factors, perhaps the most important being the route of administration of the drug. Since intraperitoneal injections have been used by those reporting no effects of this drug on learning, there is some question as to how much of this substance, if any, crosses the blood-brain barrier into the brain. It appears that registration is retarded when 8-azaguanine is administered directly to the CNS.

Actinomycin-D: The antibiotic actinomycin-D has also been used as an inhibitor of RNA synthesis. This substance has been found to bind with the guanine constituents of DNA, thereby blocking RNA synthesis (Reich, 1963). In this respect the actions are quite specific, blocking the formation of new RNA, while having no direct effect on existing RNA or protein synthesis. Research with this drug has been somewhat limited by its toxic effects. When injected into mice systemically at a dose inhibiting approximately 95% of cerebral RNA synthesis, the animals develop irreversible illness within a few hours after injection. In general, this drug has been reported to have no detrimental effect on learning or retention with rats or mice under a variety of doses (75-95% cerebral RNA synthesis inhibition) using both active and passive avoidance tasks (Barondes & Jarvik, 1964; Cohen & Barondes, 1966). While such evidence suggests that the manufacture or synthesis of RNA during learning is not essential to the registration or retention of a task, other evidence suggests the contrary. Actinomycin-D has been shown to be quite effective in permanently disrupting memory in goldfish when injected intracranially immediately after training on a discrimination avoidance task (Agranoff, 1965, 1967). The basis of this conflict between the effect of actinomycin-D in mice and rats vs goldfish is unclear.

Magnesium pemoline: A drug that has commonly been used to facilitate RNA synthesis is magnesium pemoline (Cylert) (Glasky & Simon, 1966). Pemoline alone is a central nervous system stimulant that has been used clinically as an antifatigue agent. Magnesium pemoline, the mixture of pemoline and magnesium hydroxide, has been used experimentally in attempts to improve learning and memory, since it has been shown to stimulate RNA metabolism in vitro. Although initial studies showed better learning and retention by rats on active avoidance tasks following various oral doses of this drug (Plotnikoff, 1966, 1969), later studies have shown that such results may be due to the drug's general alerting and stimulating effects rather than to an effect on learning and memory (Beach & Kimble, 1967; Talland, 1966). Performance on a passive avoidance task, for instance, has been shown to be worse following the administration of this drug, which would be expected if the drug has stimulating effects. Research with humans using a variety of tasks, such as verbal or motor learning, visual reaction time, auditory and visual short-term memory, classical conditioning, arm-hand steadiness, and tasks requiring continuous attention, have shown this drug to have no effect on learning or retention except for those tasks involving sustained attention, thus demonstrating its general alerting effects (Smith, 1967). Furthermore, tests of this drug on patients with Korsakoff's Syndrome (memory impairment as a result of alcoholism) have yielded no evidence of memory improvement (Talland, Hagen, & James, 1967). Recent reports that magnesium pemoline has no effect on RNA metabolism in vivo following intraperitoneal injections (Morris, Aghajanian, & Bloom, 1967) would seemingly rule out the systemic use of this drug as a means of investigating the role of RNA in the learning process (Smith & Baker, 1969; Talland, 1969). It appears likely that the positive reports of memory enhancement were due to the drug's CNS stimulant properties.

Planaria transection and ribonuclease: Several other approaches have been employed in the investigation of learning and memory and the possible role RNA may play in these processes. One such approach has included the use of naturally occurring enzymes, such as ribonuclease, to interfere with RNA synthesis. Small intraventricular injections of ribonuclease into cats have been reported to temporarily disrupt performance on pattern discrimination tasks. It has been difficult to determine whether or not such effects are due solely to the destruction of brain RNA since intraventricular injections of calcium salts have been found to be equally disruptive (Cameron, Kral, Solyom, Sved, Wainrib, Beaulieu, & Enesco, 1966).

Another set of studies along these lines has involved the training, transection, and regeneration of planaria. Planaria are flatworms that have been found to be capable of learning a conditioned response to light. Following training, these animals can be transected and will regenerate new heads and tails with both halves retaining the conditioned response (McConnell, Jacobson, & Kimble, 1959). The effects of ribonuclease have been tested by allowing the transected halves of these animals to regenerate in ribonuclease solutions and by comparing their retention of the response with halves allowed to regenerate in natural pond water. The results have been that both halves (heads and tails) regenerated in pond water have retained the response, but in the ribonuclease solution only the head halves growing new tails retained the response (Corning & John, 1961). These results have been interpreted to suggest that ribonuclease does not enter into existing RNA molecules but destroys the manufacture of RNA during regeneration. Since the major portion of the nervous system of this animal is in the head section, destruction of RNA during regeneration of a new tail would not interfere with retention, while destruction of RNA during the regeneration of a new head would. In extending these results to a hypothesis implicating RNA in the memory process, a number of factors would suggest some caution. These factors include the nature of the supposed conditioned response to light in planaria, which may be the result of sensitization rather than conditioning, as well as the possibility that the observed effects may be due to factors other than RNA destruction, such as abnormalities in regeneration or altered receptor sensitivity (Halas, James, & Knutson, 1962).

Yeast RNA: On the assumption that an increase in available RNA may facilitate learning and retention, an RNA extract from high-RNA-yielding substances such as yeast has been administered to subjects and the effect of the RNA on behavior has been observed. There are several clinical reports of improvements in memory in aged human patients given either oral or intravenous doses of yeast RNA. The discontinuance of such treatment has usually resulted in a recurrence of memory deficits (Cameron et al., 1966).

Often, however, such reports are difficult to interpret, since necessary controls may be difficult if not impossible to obtain in research with human patients. Thus, much of the evidence pertinent to this approach has been obtained from experimental work with animals. These studies have generally found that improvements in learning and retention are limited to certain treatment conditions and dose levels. Although improvements have been noted in tasks such as active avoidance pole-climbing with rats, little or no effects have been reported with other tasks using different response modalities or reinforcement procedures. Several factors have combined to make it difficult to draw any conclusions concerning this approach and the possible role of RNA in memory. Any attempt to attribute memory improvement to increases in RNA availability via this technique may be faulty, since the components of the RNA molecule, rather than the RNA molecule itself, may be responsible for some of the effects obtained (Gurowitz, 1969, Ch. 5). Also, the possibility that yeast may be of some nutritive value cannot be overlooked, as well as the fact that certain impurities often in yeast RNA may contribute to its effects. Finally, as with 8-azaguanine, there is some question as to whether or not this compound can cross the blood-brain barrier. Recent evidence has suggested that it does not cross the barrier into the brain and thus may not be capable of having any direct effect on learning (Eist & Seal, 1965).

Summary. To summarize these data on the possible role of RNA in the retention of memory is a difficult task. The amount and structure of RNA molecules are clearly influenced by stimulating or depressing the subject. Changes in the amount and structure of neural RNA have even been found to follow the learning of particular tasks; and these changes appear to be localized in parts of the CNS which seem to be important for the task. However, the specific dependence of the changes on the fact that the task involved learning and memory is unproven. The effects of drugs that may interfere with RNA (such as 8-azaguanine or actinomycin-D) or facilitate RNA (magnesium pemoline) on the registration, retention, and recall of memory are also unclear. It may be that ribonuclease interferes with the transfer of memory in planaria from a transected tail to a regenerating head, but this is also unclear, as is the effect of yeast RNA on humans and animals. All the data taken together suggest that RNA has some role in learning and memory functions; however, the nature of the role and its mechanism is unclear. The data are consistent with the depression hypothesis, which would require either the appearance of a new species of RNA or an increased amount of an RNA already present to occur, following learning, in the neurons responsible for long-term retention.

Protein

Two lines of evidence suggest that proteins may play a central role in long-term information storage basic to the memory process (Barondes, 1965). Research pointing to protein as the memory molecule responsible for long-term retention comes primarily from studies using drugs and those showing transfer of behavior between animals via brain extract. There have been few studies of the effects of learning on proteins. There are so many proteins found in the brain that one does not know which to investigate. However, you may reread the previous section on brain acetylcholine and behavior to see the current situation with respect to the most thoroughly investigated brain amine.

Three drugs that have effects on proteins and learning will be discussed: puromycin, AXM, and TCAP.

Puromycin. Perhaps the drug that has been most widely used to disrupt protein synthesis and evaluate subsequent effects on memory is the antibiotic, puromycin. This agent has been found to disrupt protein synthesis by essentially blocking the incorporation of the amino acids carried by transfer RNA in the formation of proteins (Yarmolinski & de la Haba, 1959). The growth of the protein is interrupted or "cut short" by incorporating this molecule instead of the appropriate amino acid (Dackin, 1964; Nathans, 1964). This action by puromycin apparently does not affect the synthesis of RNA and its effects are therefore independent of RNA synthesis mechanisms. Although initial studies reported no effect of this agent on memory when injected subcutaneously in mice, more recently memory deficits have been reported with intracranial injections.

Memory deficits in mice trained to criterion on a shock-avoidance Y-maze task have been observed with bilateral temporal lobe injections of puromycin 24 hours after training. Intracranial injections have been found effective in eliminating memory 11 to 43 days following training, only if given in the frontal and ventricular regions of the brain as well as in the temporal lobe. Such results have suggested the possibility that different anatomical regions of the brain are differentially important in the consolidation and storage phases of memory. Further studies of the effects of puromycin on mice have revealed that the memory deficit obtained appears to be specific to the training received and not a general impairment of the memory process. Animals trained to criterion still show retention from 10 to 20 hours after injection, after which time memory appears to be permanently lost. This suggests that short-term retention is not affected, but that consolidation into long-term retention is prevented, an effect that may be similar to that of ECS. In addition, injections given prior to training have no observable effect upon registration as compared to saline-injected controls (puromycin must be active during the consolidation phase that follows training, not during registration) (Barondes & Cohen, 1966; Flexner, L. B., Flexner, J. B., & Roberts, 1967).

Injections of puromycin in yet another species, the goldfish, have also been reported to produce memory deficits. Goldfish trained to swim to either the light or dark end of a tank to avoid shock showed retention deficits following intracranial injections (over the brain, but not into it) of puromycin shortly before training. An important difference that has been noted between the effects of puromycin in these two species is that no deficit in memory can be obtained in goldfish if the drug is administered an hour or more following training. It is interesting to note, however, that the period following training, during which memory is susceptible to puromycin disruption in the goldfish (less than an hour), can be lengthened somewhat by retaining the animal in the training situation. This would suggest that the consolidation process may not commence until experience in the training situation has ended (Agranoff, 1965, 1967).

This evidence on the effects of puromycin has generally been taken to indicate that *while registration and short-term retention may not require protein synthesis, the long-term retention of information does*. The fact that puromycin disrupts protein synthesis, however, may not be enough to support such an assumption. Studies in mice have shown that bilateral temporal lobe saline injections have restored memory previously lost following puromycin injections (Flexner, L. B., & Flexner, J. B., 1968). These results leave open the possibility that interference with protein synthesis may not affect the retention of memory but rather may disrupt retrieval processes (if any treatment, such as these saline injections, can restore memory, then retention could not have been prevented). Furthermore, puromycin has been found to also alter the activity of cholinesterase by depressing its synthesis. Reports of a similarity in the time course of the amnesic effects produced by anticholinesterases and puromycin suggest that puromycin's effects on memory may be related to effects on a particular protein, cholinesterase (Deutsch, 1971).

AXM. Another antibiotic drug that has been found to inhibit protein synthesis in a somewhat different manner from that of puromycin, is acetoxycyclohexamide (AXM). Whereas puromycin has its effect by substituting for an amino acid in the formation of a protein, AXM slows down the rate at which the amino acids are joined together. The effects of this drug on memory are somewhat unclear. Several experiments with mice have shown that while this drug is a powerful inhibitor of protein synthesis, its effects on memory, unlike those of puromycin, are either temporary impairment or none at all. The effect of joint puromycin and AXM injections has been a reduction in the amnesia effects of puromycin alone (Barondes & Cohen, 1967; Flexner, L. B., et al., 1967). By slowing down polypeptide formation, AXM may reduce the amount of substrate available for puromycin to act upon.

However, other investigators have demonstrated memory deficits as a result of AXM injections. When given to goldfish, the effects on memory are similar to those reported with puromycin (Agranoff, 1967). In addition, AXM injections given to mice prior to training, both intracerebrally and subcutaneously, have been found to produce memory deficits similar to those observed with puromycin, if training is limited (not carried to criterion) (Flexner, L. B., et al., 1967). It has been proposed that a high level of training may permit memory formation by the small amount of protein synthesis not disrupted, since AXM does not inhibit protein synthesis completely.

Different mechanisms of action on memory have been proposed for puromycin and AXM. It has been found that puromycin produces changes in the electrophysiological activity of the hippocampus, while AXM does not (Cohen & Barondes, 1967; Cohen, Ervin, & Barondes, 1966). Thus, some investigators have suggested that puromycin may produce seizure activity sufficient to impair memory formation, without affecting registration (Bohdanecka, Bohdanecky, & Jarvik, 1967). Although puromycin has been found to potentiate pen-tylenetetrazol-induced convulsions in both mice and goldfish, providing some support for a seizure hypothesis of puromycin action, other data have been inconsistent with such a proposal. A more toxic derivative of puromycin, PAN (puromycin aminonucleoside), which doesn't appear to inhibit either RNA or protein synthesis, has also been found to potentiate pentylenetetrazol con-vuslions, but has no effects on memory in either mice or goldfish (Farnham & Dubin, 1967).

TCAP. Some agents have been used in attempts to enhance protein synthesis. One drug that has been used for this purpose is tricyanoaminopropene (TCAP). Since TCAP has been found to facilitate RNA synthesis as well as protein synthesis, having a somewhat stronger effect on the latter, it is difficult to interpret any behavioral result as supporting one or the other of these molecules as responsible. Rather, the effects of this agent are generally related to the joint facilitation of both. Although the effects of this drug have been somewhat less than consistent, it does appear to have some facilitative effect on learning ability. In general, facilitation of avoidance learning in rats has been reported, while no effects have been noticed for some maze learning tasks (Chamberlain et al., 1963). It has been suggested that the duration of drug administration may be a factor, since chronic administration of the drug has generally resulted in facilitation, while acute administration has not. TCAP has also been found to somewhat counter the disruptive effects of electroconvulsive shock (Essman, 1966), thus indicating that its effects may primarily be on the speed of consolidation. It is interesting to note that the effect of this drug in possibly speeding up consolidation is analogous to that observed with strychnine, a convulsive agent discussed earlier. A parallel increase in RNA synthesis has often been noted to accompany the increased neural activity brought about by strychnine injections. Thus, it has been implied that the effects of strychnine, and possibly other agents similarly affecting consolidation, are mediated by RNA synthesis. Although further work along these lines would be necessary before any conclusions could be drawn, this possibility would not seem unreasonable.

Interanimal Memory Transfer

Three types of studies have dealt with this question. The planaria cannibalism studies were the first in the area. Then came studies in rats, in which brain extracts from trained animals were administered to naive animals. Last, we will discuss studies in which drug tolerance or habituation was transferred between animals.

Cannibalism. A group of experiments commonly referred to as the *cannibalism studies* have involved the use of planaria that have been conditioned to respond to light, are cut up, and then fed to naive planaria (McConnell, 1962). These naive planaria, after ingesting their comrades, have been reported to show the conditioned response when compared to other planaria that were fed nonconditioned worms. It has been assumed that, since the digestive system of planaria is quite rudimentary, it is possible that cannibal worms are capable of ingesting the tissue of donor worms without altering the molecular structure very greatly, thus being able to, in a sense, swallow memory. Such a contention appears quite farfetched and these studies have been subjected to severe scrutiny and criticism. Not only has the capability of this organism to learn a conditioned response been questioned, but many other aspects of the experimental procedure, such as the handling and maintenance procedures, as well as the lack of appropriate controls have been criticized (Hartry, Keith-Lee, & Morton, 1964). Evidence has been reported to show that the mere ingestion of other planaria, whether they be subjected to light alone, shock alone, unpaired light and shock (pseudoconditioning), both light and shock in a conditioning procedure, or only handling results in some observable response transfer (Hartry et al., 1964). Such evidence emphasizes the possible nutritional factors and changes in sensitization, not related to memory transfer, which may account for some of the findings.

Brain extracts. Another approach that has been employed is to attempt to transfer learned behavior from one animal to another by extracting RNA and/or brain proteins from the brains of trained animals and then injecting these substances into untrained animals. Some success has been reported in transferring complex responses, such as approaching a food cup, lever-pressing, and maze-learning, all in rats (Jacobson & Schlecter, 1970; Rosenblatt, Farrow, & Rhine, 1966). McConnell, Shigehisa, & Salive (1970) have found that brain RNA extracts from partially trained rats facilitate instrumental bar-press learning by recipient rats. However, failures to obtain such results using this technique have been far more frequent (Hartry et al., 1964; Byrne et al., 1966).

Since the extract used in these studies often contains a variety of substances, it is difficult to evaluate those instances where transfer has been obtained, in terms of RNA's role in such transfer (Frank, Stein, & Rosen, 1970). In fact, several findings suggest that the role played by RNA may be minimal (Frank et al., 1970). In cases where transfer has been obtained, subjection of the extract to the enzyme ribonuclease prior to injection has had no effect (Rosenblatt, Farrow, & Herblin, 1966). Furthermore, in experiments where radioactive RNA extract has been injected intraperitoneally, little evidence of this extract in the brain or bloodstream has been found (Enesco, 1966; Luttges, Johnson, Buck, Holland, & McGaugh, 1966; Sved, 1965). In addition, several studies have found no transfer effects with direct injection of RNA extract into the brain (Luttges et al., 1966). Generally, in those studies where transfer has occurred, a better case has been made for protein as the responsible agent, rather than for RNA (Rosenblatt, Farrow, & Herblin, 1966).

Drug tolerance and habituation. Nevertheless, the possibility that learned material may be contained in some chemical brain substance transferable between animals, thereby transferring experience, is an intriguing one and continues to receive much attention. Although the data on the transfer of specific instrumental responses is considered suspect by many, recently other alterations in behavior have been successfully transferred between animals. For instance, it has been demonstrated that tolerance to drugs such as morphine and response habituation to stimuli such as a tone or an airblast can be transferred by means of intraperitoneal injections of brain homogenates from trained animals to naive animals both within species (mice) and between species (dogs and rats to mice) (Ungar & Cohen, 1965; Ungar & Irwin, 1967; Ungar & Oceguera-Navarro, 1965). Increases in the amount of substance injected have been found to result in increases in transfer.

In one related study, brain substance from fish embryos was injected into the brain region of other embryos. When mature, those subjects with the augmented brains that survived the procedure showed some improvement in learning when compared to untreated fish (Bresler & Bitterman, 1969). Here, a transfer of specific material is not involved, but this study perhaps suggests the ability to improve behavior by simply increasing the amount of brain substance.

Summary. As striking as the results may seem, it would be well to remember that replication is often difficult and many times impossible. Many reported attempts to transfer experience between animals, by means of extracting and injecting brain substances, have not been successful (Byrne et al., 1966). Such reports have only added to the present skepticism of many regarding the transfer of behavior by such methods. In addition, in order for such reported transfer phenomena to attain a degree of plausibility, it would have to be demonstrated that injected substances do indeed enter the brain of recipient animals and are incorporated into the cells of brain tissue. Studies that have radioactively tagged such substances have, for the most part, failed to substantiate such a requirement (Luttges et al., 1966). Thus, the evidence currently available in this area is difficult to evaluate. The chemical and behavioral procedures used by different investigators are grossly variable. This lack of standardization has surely contributed to the abundance of disparate findings. Although the number of positive transfer reports appears to be growing, thus suggesting that memory may be chemical in nature and that protein substances may be involved, a great deal of research remains to be done.

CONCLUSIONS

At this point we might well reflect upon the evidence and try to determine whether or not a molecule for memory exists. Perhaps the safest conclusion we can make is that the evidence to date neither confirms nor denies the existence of such a molecule. From the vast amount of research that has been done it would seem reasonable to believe that memory, or at least long-term retention, is chemical in nature and that one or more of the molecules considered may be involved. Although the evidence would seem to favor some role for protein or RNA over that of DNA, none of these molecules can be reasonably denied some potential role in the memory process.

Current notions concerning the molecular basis of memory are far removed from the idea of a single memory molecule. Instead, models are being constructed that include complex interactions between various molecules. A representative model of this sort, the DNA derepression hypothesis (John, 1967), was presented earlier. This model draws upon the work of Lashley and Hebb, and is favored by the present authors.

The belief that a biochemical approach may provide insight into the mechanisms of information storage seems more dominant today than at any time in the past, despite the numerous technical and procedural problems that have been encountered. Such a belief has been greatly encouraged by the tremendous strides made in molecular biology and genetics, providing the brick and mortar from which biochemical theories on memory may be built. Nevertheless, the extent of our knowledge still remains severely limited. The questions of the where, what, and how of memory that have persisted down through the ages are still with us today. We have by no means unraveled the mystery of memory. We can only hope that continued research in this most promising area will bring us closer to that goal.

As far as the future is concerned, one can only speculate. The implications of unlocking the secrets of information storage seem to be unlimited. On the basis of experimentation going on now, it would seem likely that the therapeutic treatment of learning and memory disorders through the use of chemical agents may be possible in the near future. If the transfer-of-behavior studies presently being undertaken in various laboratories prove more reliable than they have been in the past, one might envisage similar transfer in humans, or even the synthesis of knowledge in an encapsulated form that could be swallowed, thus reducing present forms of learning to things of the past. As fantastic as these things may sound, even more fantastic may be the possibility of imparting knowledge before birth by genetic manipulation. Whether all these things and more may be possible or just the stuff of science fiction, only time will tell.

11
BEHAVIORAL ENDOCRINOLOGY

Robert A. Levitt and James Y. O'Hearn

Up to this point in the book we have selected for study drugs whose principal sites of action are in the nervous system. The reason for this selection is that it is primarily these drugs that influence behavior and are, therefore, of most interest to the psychologist. This chapter and the next one will now concentrate on a second class of chemical agents that is of considerable interest to psychologists. These chemical agents are the hormones normally found in the body.

Hormones have critical roles in the maintenance of homeostasis. They also profoundly influence the psychological state and behavior of the individual. These behavioral influences (because of effects on neural processes) become especially obvious in cases of glandular disease when circulating levels of a particular hormone may become either deficient or excessive. Drugs may be used to replace the missing hormone in cases of hypofunction of a particular gland. These drugs may simply be the natural hormone, usually extracted from animals, or they may be a synthetic preparation of the hormone. For hyperfunction of a gland, in certain cases, there are drugs that block or depress hormone manufacture or activity, and these agents may be used to combat the symptoms of the disease. Examples of each of these types of drugs will be found in this and the next chapter.

This chapter will include a brief review of the structure, function, pathology, pharmacology, and behavioral actions of each of the endocrine glands, with the exception of the gonads. Gonadal (sexual) functions have been particularly well studied and are thus treated separately and in more detail in the next chapter.

INTRODUCTION: CLASSIFICATION
OF CHEMICAL AGENTS

Hormones

Hormones are chemicals synthesized by specialized ductless glands (endocrine glands) and carried by the circulating blood throughout the body. The hormones then facilitate particular physiological actions by acting on a variety of target tissues. Endocrine glands can be distinguished from the exocrine (or ducted) glands, such as the salivary and lacrimal glands, which secrete chemicals into particular localities via specialized ducts. Ducted glands are located close to their targets and their secretions have very localized and specialized actions. In contrast, endocrine glands may be located at great distances from their targets, their secretions are carried from the gland to the target tissue via the circulatory system, and the hormones evoke widespread physiological adjustments.

Neurohumors

The hormones should also be distinguished from two other classes of chemical agents that share some of their properties. These chemicals are the neurohumors and the neurohormones. The *neurohumors* are the synaptic transmitters that are synthesized and secreted by nerve cells and then travel very short distances over the synaptic gap to affect the firing of other, adjacent, nerve cells.

Neurohormones

The neurohormones share some of the properties of neurohumors and also some of the properties of hormones. Neurohormones, like the neurohumors, are manufactured and released by nerve cells. However, unlike neurohumors, neurohormones do not act via the synapse on adjacent neurons, but instead are released into the circulatory system, as are hormones. Therefore, *neurohormones* can best be considered as a subclass of hormones; they are hormones manufactured by neurons.

Some neurohormones are first held in storage sites and then released into the bloodstream. Examples of this type of neurohormone are ADH and oxytocin, which are manufactured in the supraoptic and paraventricular nuclei of the hypothalamus and then carried within the axons of the neurons that produced them to the posterior lobe of the pituitary gland (for storage). These two neurohormones are then separately and individually released from the posterior lobe into the circulatory system when they are needed to produce particular physiological and behavioral adjustments.

Other neurohormones, also manufactured by hypothalamic neurons, are called *releasing factors*. These releasing factors are secreted into a part of the circulatory system called the *hypothalamic-pituitary portal system*. The releasing factors are then carried in the bloodstream (via the portal system) to the anterior lobe of the pituitary gland where they regulate the secretion of anterior lobe hormones.

NEUROENDOCRINE RELATIONSHIPS

The nervous and endocrine systems do not act independently. Instead, there are feedback loops between these two systems. For instance, sympathetic preganglionic neurons stimulate the release of hormones from the adrenal medulla. Releasing factors produced in hypothalamic neurons stimulate the release of hormones from the anterior lobe of the pituitary gland, while other hypothalamic releasing factors inhibit anterior pituitary hormone release. We, therefore, see that the nervous system can influence the endocrine system in two ways: by neural firing (neurohumors) and by neurohormonal release.

In the opposite direction, many hormones influence nervous system functioning. Hormones produced by the thyroid, adrenal cortex, and sex glands increase or decrease the firing of neurons in certain brain areas, and the release of neurohormones by the brain. These interactions between the nervous and endocrine systems have led to the conceptualization of a unitary neuroendocrine system functioning to maintain biological homeostasis by producing physiological and behavioral adjustments.

Hypothalamic Releasing Factors

A clearer understanding of neuroendocrine relationships has been reached due to the discovery of a group of chemical messengers known as the *hypothalamic releasing factors* (Schally, Arimura, & Kastin, 1973). It has long been known that destruction of parts of the hypothalamus leads to significant abnormalities of endocrine function; however, only recently, has evidence developed showing that the hypothalamus exerts direct control over the release of hormones from the pituitary gland. Because the pituitary gland secretes hormones that stimulate many of the other endocrine glands, we can see that this hypothalamic-pituitary interaction can serve as a principal link between the nervous and endocrine systems for the integration of complex patterns of behavior.

The hypothalamic releasing factors themselves are neurohormones produced by neurosecretory cells originating in the hypothalamus (Figure 11.1). These neurohormones are deposited near capillaries in a region of the hypothalamus called the *median eminence*. The releasing factors are then carried to the anterior lobe by a system of blood vessels called the *pituitary portal system*. In this manner, the hypothalamic releasing factors are able to influence the secretions of the anterior pituitary.

For at least three pituitary hormones there is a dual system of hypothalamic control, one system being inhibitory and one being stimulatory. The need for hypothalamic inhibitors, as well as stimulators of growth hormone, prolactin, and melanocyte-stimulating hormone can be explained by the absence of negative feedback products from their target tissues. In the case of corticotropin, thyrotropin, luteinizing

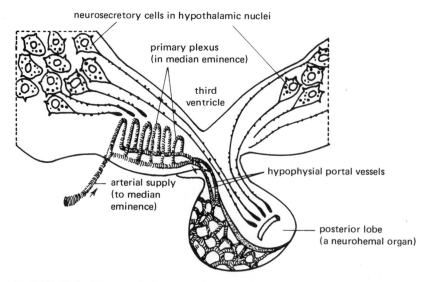

neurosecretory cells in hypothalamic nuclei

primary plexus
(in median eminence)

third
ventricle

hypophysial portal vessels

arterial supply
(to median
eminence)

posterior lobe
(a neurohemal organ)

FIGURE 11.1. Diagram of the anatomic connections between the hypothalamus and the pituitary gland. Neurosecretory cells are present in certain hypothalamic nuclei: some of the secretory axons pass down the infundibular stalk and terminate near blood vessels in the posterior lobe, others terminate in close proximity to the capillary loops of the median eminence. The hormones of the posterior lobe (vasopressin and oxytocin) are the products of hypothalamic neurosecretory cells and are stored and released from the posterior lobe (a neurohemal organ). The pituitary portal venules convey blood downward to the anterior lobe. There are strong indications that the hypothalamic axons of the median eminence liberate multiple releasing factors (probably peptide in nature) into the portal vessels and that these neural factors are concerned with the regulation of anterior pituitary functions. It is apparent that the whole pituitary gland is predominantly subservient to and partly evolved from the hypothalamic portion of the brain. (Reprinted by permission from C. D. Turner and J. T. Bagnara, *General Endocrinology* [5th ed]. Copyright 1971 by W. B. Saunders Company.)

> hormone, and follicle-stimulating hormone, hormones (corticosteroids, thyroxine, and sex steroids) from the target glands inhibit secretion of these anterior pituitary hormones by negative feedback action exerted on the pituitary, hypothalamus, or both. (Schally, Arimura, & Kastin, 1973, p. 341)

Thus, only stimulatory hypothalamic releasing factors appear to operate with respect to these last four hormones, while separate stimulatory and inhibitory releasing factors are thought to exist for each of the first three hormones listed.

Feedback Mechanisms

The neuroendocrine system can be viewed as a unit that functions to continually maintain a homeostatic balance within the organism, despite constant stresses from the environment. This maintenance of a constant optimal level of body function is accomplished by means of feedback loops in the face of a constantly and sometimes abruptly changing external environment.

In a simple negative feedback loop a hormone not only affects its target tissue, but also feeds back to inhibit its own secretion. If blood hormone levels are low, the negative feedback effect is also low, allowing for more hormone secretion. If blood hormone levels are high, the negative feedback effect is enhanced, and this causes an inhibition of hormonal secretion. The negative feedback mechanism is a highly efficient means of maintaining physiological homeostasis. Most hormonal feedback loops are actually more complex than this and include various intermediate steps. For example, the hormone of the thyroid gland, thyroxine, inhibits the release of the hypothalamic releasing factor for the anterior pituitary thyroid-stimulating hormone, thyrotropin. Thus, higher levels of circulating thyroxine lead to a reduction in the manufacture and release of thyroxine.

Positive feedback loops are not encountered as often as negative loops because stimulation would cause excessive amounts of hormone to be secreted. However, positive loops are found in certain situations in which another factor can override the positive loop. For instance, estrogen increases the release of LH from the anterior pituitary. High LH levels then lead to the secretion of even more estrogen and also of another hormone, progesterone, which has an inhibitory effect on LH production.

THE PITUITARY GLAND

The adult human pituitary (often called the *hypophysis*) weighs about 600 mg in the male and slightly more in the female. It is lodged in an impression in one of the bones of the skull and attaches to the base of the hypothalamus by a stalk called the *infundibulum.* The pituitary gland, its location, and its connections with the hypothalamus can be seen in Figure 11.1. We may speak of three divisions (lobes) of the pituitary gland, which are responsible for releasing a total of nine hormones (Table 11.1). The anterior lobe (adenohypophysis) manufactures and secretes six of these hormones, while the intermediate lobe manufactures and secretes one. The other two hormones are actually neuro-hormones that are manufactured by neurosecretory cells of the hypothalamus and are stored in, and later secreted from, the posterior lobe (neurohypophysis; Turner & Bagnara, 1971, Ch. 3).

The Anterior Lobe

The anterior lobe of the pituitary gland secretes six hormones. Five of these (thyrotropin, adrenocorticotropin, follicle-stimulating hormone, luteinizing hormone, and prolactin) are usually referred to as *trophic hormones,* as their primary actions involve influencing the secretion of specific hormones by certain other glands. The sixth is called *growth hormone* (or somatotropin). Growth hormone has a more general effect of facilitating protein synthesis and tissue buildup throughout the body, and so we may consider this agent as being trophic to organism growth and functioning in a general way.

TABLE 11.1
Hormones of the Pituitary Gland

Hormones	Principal actions
Anterior lobe	
Growth hormone (somatotropin, STH)	Growth of bone and muscle; promotes protein synthesis effects on lipid and carbohydrate metabolism
Adrenocorticotropin (ACTH)	Stimulates secretion of adrenal cortical steroids by the adrenal cortex; certain extraadrenal actions
Thyrotropin (TSH)	Stimulates the thyroid gland to form and release thyroid hormones
Luteinizing hormone (LH, ♀) or interstitial cell-stimulating hormone (ICSH, ♂)	Ovary: formation of corporalutea; secretion of progesterone; probably acts in conjunction with FSH Testis: stimulates the interstitial cells of Leydig, thus promoting the secretion of androgen
Follicle-stimulating hormone (FSH)	Ovary: growth of ovarian follicles; functions with LH to cause estrogen secretion and ovulation Testis: possible action on seminiferous tubules to promote spermatogenesis
Prolactin (lactogenic hormone, luteotropin, LTH)	Proliferation of mammary gland and initiation of milk secretion; may prolong the functional life of the corpus luteum—secretion of progesterone
Intermediate lobe	
Melanophore-stimulating hormone (intermedin, MSH)	Dispersion of pigment granules in the melanophores; darkening of the skin
Posterior lobe	
Antidiuretic hormone (ADH, Vasopressin)	Elevates blood pressure through action on arterioles; promotes reabsorption of water by kidney tubules
Oxytocin	Affects postpartum mammary gland, causing ejection of milk; promotes contraction of uterine muscle; possible action in parturition and in sperm transport in female tract.

Note. Reprinted by permission from C. D. Turner and J. T. Bagnara, *General Endocrinology,* (5th ed.). Copyright 1971 by W. B. Saunders.

Growth hormone. Growth hormone is also referred to as *somatotropin* or *STH*. It is a protein, but the particular amino acid sequence is slightly different in different species (Raben, 1962). For this reason, growth hormone from certain animals may be too different from human growth hormone to stimulate human growth processes. For example, growth hormone obtained from cattle or sheep is ineffective in humans, whereas that obtained from other primates will usually stimulate human growth processes.

An excess of growth hormone during development produces giantism in the human, characterized by excessive height and body size and by enlargement of most organs. Pituitary insufficiency in the young results in a failure to grow, but this is one of the rarer causes of dwarfism. Although growth hormone is essential for growth and development of most tissues of the body, it is not necessary for nervous system growth. Intelligence and personality do not seem to be greatly affected by growth hormone, since the development of the nervous system is not dependent upon it. Excess growth hormone, or an absence of the hormone, during animal development, has been shown not to influence the adult size of the brain or its rate of development. In one study of pituitary growth hormone, members of the African Pygmy tribe were found to secrete normal amounts of growth hormone (Greene, 1970, Ch. 20). This finding suggests that their small size is a result of a failure of the tissues to react normally to growth hormone. Although defects in growth hormone production produce striking effects on body size, growth hormone does not seem to be the factor controlling fetal growth and body size in normal individuals of varying size (instead, genetic influences seem to predominate).

Biologically, growth hormone has important influences on protein, fat, and carbohydrate metabolism. Its effect on growth processes results from facilitating the incorporation of amino acids into proteins. The specific mechanism of action of growth hormone is thought to be due to a promotion of amino acid transfer across cell membranes. Besides the effects already mentioned, growth hormone often operates in combination with other hormones. Certain of the effects of thyrotropin and the gonadotropins are enhanced when in combination with growth hormone. Growth hormone is used rarely in clinical medicine, but has found usefulness in the treatment of pituitary dwarfism in infancy and of pituitary insufficiency developing in adulthood.

Psychological considerations: Growth hormone has been shown to at least partially reverse the physiological and psychological effects of dietary restriction of isolation rearing in rats (Ray & Hochhauser, 1969; Zamenof, van Marthens, & Grauel, 1971). Data consistent with these animal studies have also been found in human infants suffering from "maternal deprivation". These children, usually from disturbed homes, although not food deprived, exhibit a "failure to thrive" and are dwarfed. Their growth hormone secretion is also found deficient. When removed to a hospital or foster home, they begin to grow and their growth hormone secretion returns to normal. We may speculate that in these cases of infants stress, growth hormone secretion is inhibited neurologically via the hypothalamic control of growth hormone releasing factors (Gardner, 1972; Patton & Gardner, 1963; Powell, Brasel, & Blizzard, 1967).

The trophic hormones. Adrenocorticotropic hormone (ACTH) and thyrotropic hormone (TSH) have their principal actions on the adrenal cortex and thyroid glands, respectively (see below, this chapter). Three of the trophic hormones of the anterior lobe of the pituitary gland primarily influence gonadal functions. These hormones are follicle-stimulating hormone (FSH), luteinizing hormone (LH), and prolactin. They have major roles in the reproductive and parental physiology and behavior of both sexes. For instance, FSH stimulates the development of an immature ova to maturity in the female and the manufacture of mature sperm cells in the male, whereas LH stimulates release of the mature ova (ovulation) in the female, and the production of male sex hormones (androgens) in the male. Prolactin stimulates the manufacture of milk in the breasts of the human female, but its normal role in human males is unknown (see the next chapter).

The Intermediate Lobe

The intermediate lobe of the pituitary gland produces melanophore stimulating hormone (MSH), which functions to stimulate skin pigment cells to produce a dark pigment called *melanin* (Novales, 1967). In cold blooded vertebrates, MSH is involved in rapid color changes, such as that occurring in chameleons. However, MSH does not play such an important role in the human, although there are situations in which color changes do take place. For instance, the skin darkening of the sunbather is due to the manufacture of additional melanin, partially due to the release of MSH from the intermediate lobe. Interestingly, it has been found that testosterone (male sex hormone) has influences on pigmentation. Castrated male humans do not tan well, and this abnormality has been shown to be due to the absence of testosterone. This suggests that the tanning produced by MSH also requires sex hormones (Greene, 1970, Ch. 18).

The Posterior Lobe

The posterior lobe of the pituitary gland is an extension of neurons originating in the central nervous system and this lobe functions as a neurohemal (hormone storage) organ. The hormones stored and released from the posterior lobe are actually produced in the supraoptic nucleus (SON) and the paraventricular nucleus (PVN) of the hypothalamus. These hormones reach the posterior lobe of the pituitary via axonal streaming and are then stored by and released from this organ. The two hormones of the posterior lobe, antidiuretic hormone (ADH; also called vasopressin) and oxytocin, are thought to be transported from the SON and PVN together in a protein complex called *neurophysis* (van Dyke, Adamsons, & Engel, 1957; van Dyke, Chow, Greep, & Rothen, 1942). Each of these hormones is an octapeptide, consisting of eight amino acids (Sawyer, 1963). ADH and oxytocin have overlapping effects, but their principal ones are different. Each of these hormones is selectively released from the posterior lobe, and it is thought that this selective function is either due to different types of excitatory neurons, or to the pituicites, a group of gliallike cells found in this region. Since pituitary gland removal causes only a minor depletion of posterior pituitary hormones, it is likely that the broken end of the pituitary stalk accumulates neurosecretory material and undergoes reorganization to form a miniature posterior lobe. Destruction of the SON and PVN, however, causes a nearly complete loss of these two hormones.

Antidiuretic hormone. This hormone has two general actions. The first type is to constrict the smooth muscle of blood vessels (hence the name vaso*pressin*). Blood vessel constriction, however, requires large amounts of vasopressin (ADH), and this function is normally controlled by other substances. The second and more important action of ADH is to increase the reabsorption of water by the kidneys. Destruction of the SON and PVN with a resultant loss of ADH causes *diabetes insipidus,* a disease characterized by the loss of large amounts of water through the urine (polyuria), and, consequently, the development of a profound water deficit, with the individual then drinking equally large amounts of water (polydipsia).

The SON and PVN appear to be sensitive to the osmotic pressure of the blood circulating in their regions (and thus, cells in these regions have been called *osmoreceptors*). Direct injection of hypertonic solutions into these hypothalamic nuclei has been shown to elicit the ingestion of water in several species of mammals (Andersson, 1952). An extract from the posterior lobe of the pituitary (containing ADH) may be used clinically as a replacement in cases of diabetes insipidus. The relief is only temporary, however, and lasts only so long as the extract is given.

Oxytocin. Oxytocin is present in both sexes, but its function in the male is unclear (it may have a role in the contractile spasms of the genital organs during orgasm in both sexes). In the female this posterior lobe hormone has been found to have several important functions. First, it acts to stimulate milk ejection from the mammary gland. This mechanism is called the milk-let-down reflex. Oxytocin does not actually increase the milk production by the mammary glands, but merely causes a rapid expulsion of milk by contracting the smooth muscle of the gland. Oxytocin also increases uterine contractions during parturition (birth) and thereby facilitates the expulsion of the fetus from the female tract. A possible third function of oxytocin is that of facilitating the ascent of spermatozoa in the female tract after intromission. A unitary mechanism of action can be seen for oxytocin in these three actions—that of stimulating the contraction of smooth muscles that are related to reproductive functioning. Oxytocin is used clinically to arouse or strengthen uterine contractions during parturition. A synthetic oxytocin called *syntocinon* has been used to induce milk ejection when this process is impaired (see the next chapter).

Summary

The pituitary gland sits at the base of the forebrain and attaches to the hypothalamus by means of the infundibulum. The gland can be divided into three lobes; the anterior lobe is controlled by hypothalamic releasing factors. The anterior lobe secretes six hormones; one, growth hormone has a general role in facilitating tissue growth. The other anterior lobe hormones function in neuroendocrine integration by communicating hypothalamic instructions to other endocrine glands (the thyroid, adrenal cortex and gonads). The intermediate lobe has a role in pigmentation. The posterior lobe hormones, ADH and oxytocin, have important roles in body fluid balance and blood pressure regulation (ADH), and in reproductive functions (oxytocin).

THE ADRENAL MEDULLA

The adrenal glands are located adjacent to and just above the kidneys. In mammals, they are composed of two functionally and morphologically distinct layers. There is an inner layer called the *adrenal medulla,* which develops embryologically in association with the nervous system and secretes cate-cholamines. The medulla is surrounded by an outer layer called the *adrenal cortex,* which develops in association with the genital system and secretes hormones that are chemically classified as steroids.

Biochemistry and Physiology

The cells of the adrenal medulla are modified postganglionic sympathetic nerve cells. They are of two types; one secretes norepinephrine, while the other secretes epinephrine. The difference between the two types of adrenal medullary cells is that in epinephrine-producing cells, the enzyme phenylethanolamine-*N*-methyl-transferase (PNMT) is present to convert norepinephrine into epinephrine. It is of interest that in animals whose adrenal cortex function has been impaired, a large reduction in the level of PNMT is found in the adrenal medulla (Axelrod, 1971). These data suggest that the presence of a functioning adrenal cortex is an important factor in the activity of the enzyme PNMT and, therefore, in the functioning of the adrenal medulla.

In the human fetus, the output of the adrenal medulla is almost entirely norepinephrine. As maturation takes place, an increasing percentage of epinephrine is produced until the adult human ratio of 20% norepinephrine and 80% epinephrine is reached (Coupland, 1965). This developmental trend, which may relate to the development of the adrenal cortex, implies that the PNMT enzyme system matures later than the other enzyme systems responsible for the production of catecholamines.

Like neural tissue, the adrenal medulla does not have the power of regeneration and, once destroyed, there is a permanent decrement in catecholamine secretion. This property is used to advantage in the preparation of demedullated animals. To create this preparation, the entire adrenal gland is removed except for a small remnant; the cells of the adrenal cortex then regenerate, while those of the medulla do not, resulting in an animal without an adrenal medulla (Pachkis, Rakoff, Cantarow, & Rupp, 1967). Demedullated animals can survive, but show a diminished ability to respond to stress (Danowski, 1962b). For example, demedullated animals cannot maintain their body temperature as well as normal animals and succumb sooner in a cold environment. They also exhaust sooner if made to walk on a treadmill or to exercise in other ways, since the normal cardiovascular changes that aid a human or animal in dealing with stress and emergencies do not occur as readily (see Chapter 3).

Neural Control of the Adrenal Medulla

The splanchnic nerve (the sympathetic nerve that innervates the adrenal medulla) seems to be the major controlling factor in the release of catecholamines from the adrenals (Guyton, 1971). Stimulation of the splanchnic nerve and the resulting discharge of epinephrine and norepinephrine from the adrenals may be triggered by stress, either physiological (such as immersion of the feet in ice water) or psychological (such as during a final exam). Mobilization of the body's energy stores results, producing an increase in the energy output of the body, which facilitates survival during brief stressful situations.

Pathology

Tumors of the adrenal medulla are called *pheochromocytomas* and cause an increase in the release of catecholamines. In the adrenal medulla an increase in epinphrine, norepinephrine, or both, may be found; while in extraadrenal neural tissue a pheochromocytoma usually causes an increase only in norepinephrine secretion (Danowski, 1962b). Unlike normal adrenal medullary cells, these tumorous cells may release catecholamines spontaneously, resulting in sudden increases in epinephrine and norepinephrine levels. These sudden increases in catecholamine levels may result in increased blood pressure, sweating, peripheral vasoconstriction and a feeling of anxiety. For this reason, persons with pheochromocytomas occasionally seek professional aid for an anxiety attack.

Psychological Considerations

The behavioral roles of the catecholamines, including epinephrine, were reviewed in detail in Chapter 3. Here we will concentrate on the role of adrenal medullary secretions in emotional behavior. The first question we might ask concerns the effect of stressful situations, which might be thought of as emotion-provoking, on adrenal medullary secretion. Levi (1968) has reported an important series of studies on the effects of a number of conditions on urinary excretion of epinephrine. A variety of psychic stressors was seen to increase urinary epinephrine excretion, sometimes to amounts seen in patients with adrenomedullary tumors (pheochromocytomas). Treatments have included simulated industrial work, public speaking by stutterers, films (such as *Paths of Glory* and *The Devil's Mask*) chosen to induce anxiety and aggressiveness, simulated aircraft flight, and simulated ground combat. Each of these conditions increased urinary epinephrine excretion. Interestingly, pleasant humorous stimuli are also capable of increasing epinephrine excretion. In addition, experimental stimuli evoking responses of calmness (such as bland nature scenery films) significantly lowered excretion rates below control levels. These data were taken as supporting the theory that adrenal medullary excretion is a response to level of psychic activation, irrespective of the type of stimulation; the secretions of the adrenal medulla may reflect the intensity, but not the type, of emotional arousal.

Consistent with this view have been the studies of Schacter (Schacter & Singer, 1962; Schacter & Wheeler, 1962). The basic question asked was the relative role of adrenal medullary epinephrine and of cognitive processes in the experience and expression of emotionality. Schacter concluded from these experiments that epinephrine was a major factor controlling the level of emotional arousal, but that cognitive situational factors regulated the type of emotion provoked. In one experiment, human subjects were injected with epinephrine or a control saline solution, and put into a situation where a "stooge" attempted to provoke anger or euphoria on the part of the subject. Schacter found that the epinephrine injection greatly facilitated the elicitation of an emotion, but that anger or euphoria could be equally elicited depending on the experimental situation. In another study, an epinephrine injection was also found to enhance the amount of amusement experienced by subjects in response to a humorous film. Thus, Schacter concluded that adrenomedullary excretion affected emotional intensity, but that cognitive factors controlled the type of emotion provoked.

Some investigators have suggested (in contrast to the views of Schacter) that the autonomic arousal pattern differs in different emotions, such as fear and anger. Wolf and Wolff (1947) studied the physiological reactions of the stomach wall in one human subject with a gastric fistula and reported two distinguishable patterns in fear and anger. Ax (1953) measured a number of autonomic indices in human subjects during the provocation of fear or anger. Both emotions were accompanied by heightened autonomic arousal, but there was a difference in the degree of activation on several indices. It should be pointed out, however, that it is not clear that the difference in pattern of autonomic arousal in the Ax study was due to the difference between the two emotions, fear vs anger, or to some other factors in the situations.

Most investigators consider the question of whether there are different peripheral nervous system concomitants of arousal in different emotional states as an open one. In any event, if there are differences they would seem to be rather subtle when compared to the large cognitive differences between the different emotions. Therefore, the level of adrenal medullary epinephrine secretion seems to be a reflection of arousal, whether emotional or not. Whether there are patterns of adrenal medullary function or autonomic arousal reflective of "the emotions" or differences between different emotions are open questions.

THE ADRENAL CORTEX

The adrenal cortex, which surrounds the medulla, secretes hormones that have two major types of influences. Certain hormones of the adrenal cortex primarily affect electrolyte balance and are called mineralocorticoids, while others primarily affect carbohydrate metabolism and are called glucocorticoids.

Steroid Chemistry

The hormones secreted by the adrenal cortex, testis, and ovary, and part of the hormonal production of the placenta have a similar chemical constitution. These steroid hormones have an extremely important position in endocrine biology. For this reason we will now briefly examine steroid biochemistry in preparation for discussions of these hormones in this and the next chapter. All steroids can be considered as derivatives of the parent basic steroid nucleus, called sterone, consisting of three 6-carbon rings, labeled A, B, and C, and one 5-carbon ring, labeled D (see Figure 11.2). Since sterone contains 17 carbon atoms it is referred to as a C-17 steroid.

The steroid hormones are commonly designated according to the number of carbon atoms present in the nucleus and side chains. Estrogenic hormones have an 18-carbon structure and are therefore, referred to as *C-18 steroids* (see estrone and estradiol in Figure 11.2). Similarly, androgens have a 19-carbon structure with methyl groups at the C-10 and C-13 positions, and are called C-19 steroids (for example, testosterone and androstenedione in Figure 11.2). Progestogens (progesterone) and the adrenocortical steroids (DOC, corticosterone, aldosterone, deoxycortisol, cortisol, cortisone) are all C-21 steroids. The probable pathways of steroid hormone biosynthesis in Figure 11.2 show that these hormones are synthesized from cholesterol (Dorfman, Forschielli, & Gut, 1963). The substrate for all hormonal steroids is thought to be pregnenolone (Kahnt, Neher, Schmid, & Wettstein, 1961). The chemical structures shown in Figure 11.2 are not presented for you to memorize, but rather, you should note the general structural configuration of steroid hormones and the *extremely close structural similarity of such physiologically diverse hormones as the corticosteroids, estrogens, progestogens and androgens.* The fact that progesterone is a structural intermediary in the manufacture of estrogens, androgens, and corticosteroids has important pathological implications (for example, the adrenogenital syndrome to be discussed later in this chapter).

Mineralocorticoids

Removal of the adrenal cortex results in death within a few days, due primarily to a depletion of sodium and chloride, which leads to a lowered cardiac output and eventually to shock. The administration of large amounts of sodium chloride solution will prolong life by correcting some of the symptoms, but the sodium chloride will not work indefinitely. Life can be prolonged

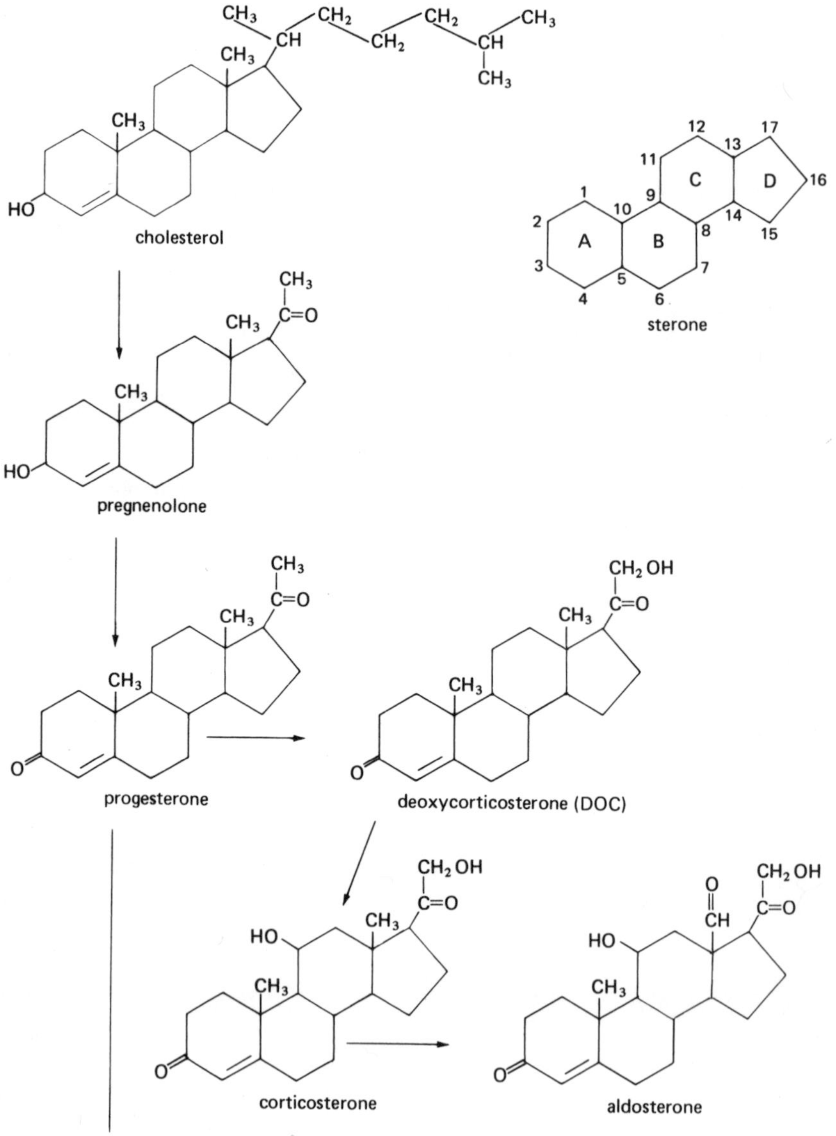

FIGURE 11.2. Some pathways of steroid biosynthesis.

indefinitely, however, by replacement therapy with mineralocorticoids. The most important of these mineralocorticoids is aldosterone. Others are corticosterone and deoxycorticosterone (DOC) (see Figure 11.2). The major influence of the mineralocorticoids is to decrease the excretion of sodium through the kidney tubules. An increased level of plasma sodium and a decreased level of plasma potassium result from increased mineralocorticoid activity. The retention

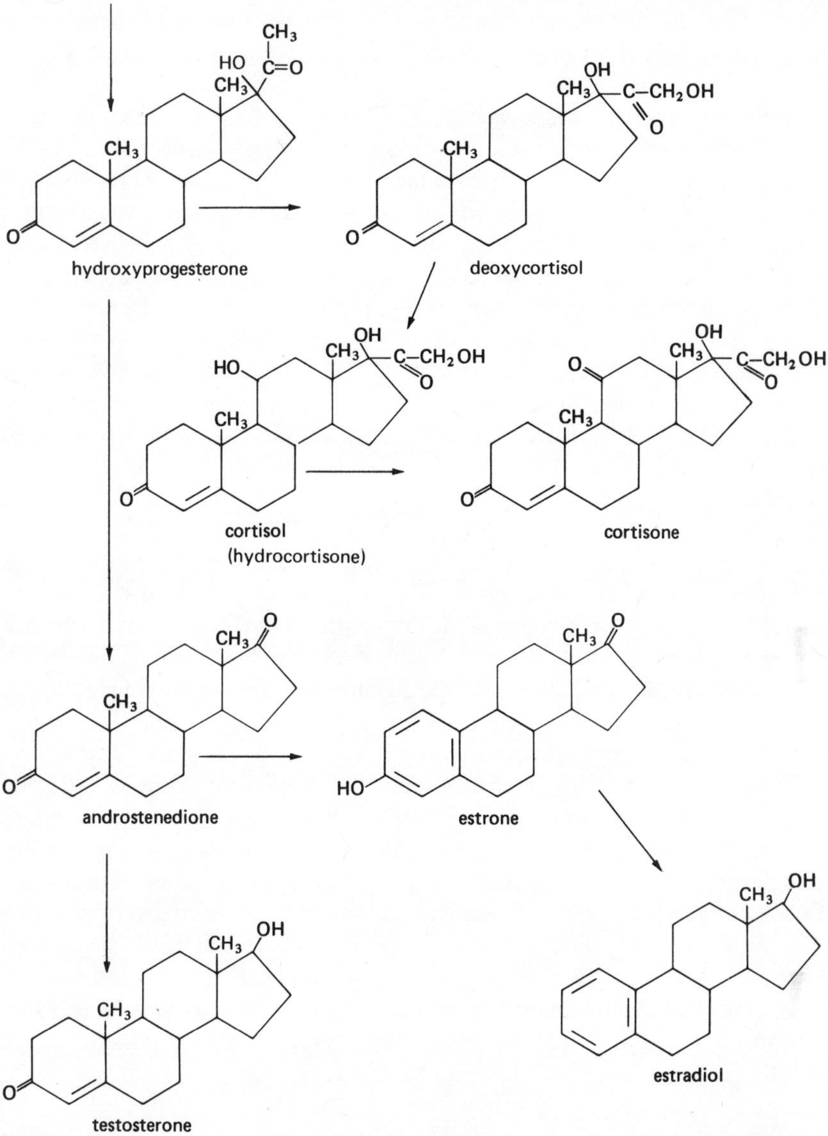

FIGURE 11.2. *(Continued)* Some pathways of steroid biosynthesis.

of sodium also causes a secondary retention of chloride and water (Guyton, 1971).

Drugs affecting mineralocorticoid function. Spironolactone is a synthetic steroid that antagonizes the effects of mineralocorticoid function by competing for the kidney tubular receptors involved in the sodium-potassium exchange. Triamterene is another drug that antagonizes aldosterone at the level of the renal tubules. However, it does not compete with aldosterone but has a direct effect on the renal tubules (not a competitive inhibitor), favoring sodium excretion and potassium retention (Hutcheon, 1971).

Factors controlling mineralocorticoid secretion. ACTH, which is the major factor controlling glucocorticoid release, seems to have little effect on the mineralocorticoids. Instead, three main factors have been postulated to stimulate mineralocorticoid release: (1) Solutions containing more than normal amounts of potassium or less than normal amounts of sodium when perfused directly into the adrenal artery cause an immediate release of mineralocorticoids, implying that these substances act directly on the adrenals. (2) Lowered extracellular sodium levels in the diencephalon may cause the release of a substance called *adrenoglomerulotropin* from an area near the pineal gland and this trophic releaser may act on the adrenal cortex to stimulate the release of mineralocorticoids. (3) The third mechanism involves the manufacture of a substance called *angiotensin-II.* When blood flow to the kidneys is reduced, renin is released by this structure. Renin is an enzyme which is then thought to act on a protein found in the bloodstream. This protein is called *renin-substrate* and is manufactured in the liver. This interaction between renin and renin-substrate produces angiotensin-I (a decapeptide), which is then converted to the physiologically active octapeptide, angiotensin-II, by another blood-born substance called *converting enzyme.* Angiotensin-II causes powerful arterial constriction, therefore elevating the blood pressure. Angiotensin-II also causes constriction of the uterine muscles, ADH release from the posterior pituitary, and aldosterone release from the adrenal cortex. This is often called the *renin-angiotensin-aldosterone* system, and seems of primary importance in hypovolemia, a condition characterized by a reduced volume of extracellular fluid and blood (Guyton, 1971). A major cause of hypovolemia is blood loss due to a traumatic accident or injury. This system ameliorates the low blood pressure by causing vasoconstriction. The system also helps to counteract the blood loss by reducing urine output of both fluid and sodium. In addition, injections of angiotensin have been shown to elicit water ingestion in experimental animals, including the cat and rat (Epstein, Fitzsimons, & Simons, 1969; Fitzsimons & Simons, 1969; Sturgeon, Brophy & Levitt, 1973). Systemic injection of renin or either systemic or CNS injection of angiotensin-II results in water ingestion.

Glucocorticoids

Following adrenalectomy, replacement therapy with a mineralocorticoid prolongs life, but does not bring the animal completely back to normal. This is because the adrenal cortex also regulates glucose metabolism via the glucocorticoids. The glucocorticoid steroids, as well as the mineralocorticoids, must be present for normal functioning of the body. The main glucocorticoids are *cortisol,* which comprises about 90% of the glucocorticoid output in the human, and *cortisone.* The pathway for glucocorticoid synthesis is shown in Figure 11.2 and it can be seen that the steps are similar to those for the mineralocorticoids.

Carbohydrate metabolism. Since the glucocorticoids, and also insulin, have their major effects on carbohydrate metabolism, a brief review should be helpful to an understanding of these hormones. In its most general sense, carbohydrate metabolism concerns the utilization of carbohydrate molecules by the body for a variety of purposes. A major portion of our diet consists of carbohydrates. Furthermore, about 80% of these carbohydrates are absorbed into the bloodstream as glucose (Guyton, 1971). After absorption, the glucose is carried through the bloodstream to all the cells of the body. The most notable tissues utilizing glucose are brain, fat and muscle. By following Figure 11.3 we can trace, in a simplified form, the pathways of glucose utilization. Aided by insulin, the glucose crosses the cell membrane and is immediately phosphorylated (a phosphate group is added) at position six (the carbon atoms of glucose are numbered 1 through 6). This reaction is aided by an enzyme called *hexokinase,* and the product is glucose-6-phosphate (G-6-P). From this point, the G-6-P has three possible fates. First, it may be temporarily stored as glycogen by the liver or the muscles. Second, it may be converted to fats, amino acids, or other types

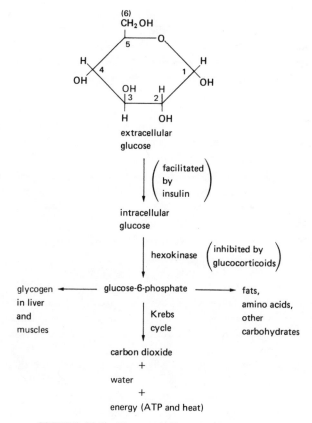

FIGURE 11.3. The metabolism of carbohydrates.

of carbohydrates (for storage or for use in tissue growth or rebuilding). Finally, it may be broken down to carbon dioxide and water with a resultant production of energy as both heat and ATP. Remember that when needed, the glycogen, fats, amino acids, and other carbohydrates can be converted back to G-6-P for energy utilization.

Mechanism of action. The major mechanism of action of the glucocorticoids is via an inhibition of the initial step in carbohydrate metabolism, the combination of glucose with phosphorus that is catalyzed by the enzyme hexokinase to form glucose-6-phosphate (Turner & Bagnara, 1971). This is the first step in the utilization of glucose and by slowing this step, less glucose is available for utilization. This inhibition of hexokinase produces three main secondary effects: (1) decreased carbohydrate utilization by the body tissues; (2) increased gluconeogenesis (the production of glucose from protein and fat) in the liver and muscles, and (3) increased deposition of glucose in the liver as glycogen (the storage form of glucose). The result of these three processes is to increase the levels of glucose in the blood and of stored glucose (glycogen), effects that function in opposition to those of the hormone, insulin, secreted by the pancreas. The high blood glucose level resulting from increased glucocorticoid secretion can result in "adrenal diabetes," which is unresponsive to insulin therapy (Turner & Bagnara, 1971).

The control of glucocorticoid secretion. Glucocorticoid release is primarily under the control of ACTH produced by the anterior pituitary. Homeostatic levels of glucocorticoids are maintained via a feedback loop in which increased output of ACTH results in an increase in the output of glucocorticoids. The glucocorticoids then act on the hypothalamus via the bloodstream to reduce the secretion of corticotropin releasing factor (CFR); this in turn results in a reduced output of ACTH by the pituitary (Turner & Bagnara, 1971).

Stress. This homeostatic system may be overridden in stressful situations when epinephrine released from the adrenal medulla acts to stimulate CRF release (at the median eminence, a site at which the blood-brain barrier is ineffective), and thus counteracts the effects on ACTH of a high glucocorticoid level (Turner & Bagnara, 1971). Therefore, ACTH release is maintained and the level of circulating glucocorticoids during stress is very high. The effect of the increased level of glucocorticoids is to increase resistance to stressors. When compared to laboratory animals, wild animals or animals kept in dense colonies show a large increase in the size of the adrenal cortex. These animals also show a greater resistance to stressors (Turner & Bagnara, 1971). Adrenalectomized animals, therefore, have a lowered resistance to most types of stress, which can be remedied by replacement therapy with the glucocorticoids.

Therapeutic use of glucocorticoids. The glucocorticoids and their synthetic derivatives are widely used in medicine because of their antiinflammatory and antiimmunological actions. The mechanism of action involves changes in cell membrane permeability and a decrease in lymphocyte and specific antibody formation by the organism. A part of the action involves a nonspecific stabilization of cellular and subcellular membranes. The dosage required to cause cellular stabilization, however, is 400 to 1,000 times the amount of glucocorticoids normally found in the organism, and it is, therefore, not clear whether this effect occurs as a result of normal increases in glucocorticoid levels due to stress. The benefits of glucocorticoid therapy are not without their price. The normal inflammatory reaction helps to prevent the spread of infection, and while glucocorticoids remove the symptoms of an infection, they actually speed its spread. This effect, plus the decrease in the immune response, create a situation where rapid spread of infection can go unnoticed. For a detailed discussion of the use of corticosteroids to treat allergic and inflammatory conditions and shock see Schumer and Nyhus (1970).

Pathology of the Adrenal Cortex

There are three general types of pathology of the adrenal cortex, involving reduced functioning, increased functioning, and altered functioning (adrenogenital syndrome and aldosteronism) of the gland.

Hypofunction of the adrenal cortex: Addison's disease. This disturbance may result from a lack of ACTH secretion due to anterior pituitary disorder or from a failure of the adrenals themselves. The symptoms include fatigue and loss of weight. There is a drop in blood pressure, and in severe cases circulatory collapse, shock, and death may ensue. Renal function is impaired and excess sodium and water are excreted. These symptoms result from an electrolyte imbalance caused by decreased mineralocorticoid function and also from defects in glucose metabolism caused by low levels of glucocorticoids. The CNS is partially protected against the effects of electrolyte imbalance by the blood-brain barrier. However, a general decrease in cortical excitability and a tendency toward depression has been found in Addisonian patients (Danowski, 1962b).

An interesting phenomenon present in almost all cases of adrenal hypofunction is an increase in the sensitivity of the sensory receptors. Thresholds for taste, smell, and hearing may be decreased a hundredfold or more during adrenal hypofunction. This seems to be due to the decreased glucocorticoid level, since replacement therapy with glucocorticoids, but not with mineralocorticoids, returns the sensory thresholds to normal. Glucocorticoid administration does not, however, alter sensory thresholds in normal persons. The increase in sensitivity is accompanied by a concomitant decrease in the information processing ability of the sensory systems in Addisonian patients (at least for hearing). Even though an Addisonian patient can report the presence or absence of a word presented tachistoscopically at a lower threshold level than a normal person, the ability to recognize the word is lowered so that the normal person will be able to name the word before the Addisonian patient (Henkin, 1970).

Hyperfunction of the adrenal cortex: Cushing's syndrome. Hyperfunctioning of the adrenal cortex usually results from the presence of increased levels of circulating ACTH, as a result of either pituitary dysfunction or ACTH therapy. Occasionally, hyperfunctioning results from a tumor of the adrenal cortex itself.

The symptoms constituting Cushing's syndrome are the result of increased mineralocorticoids, glucocorticoids, and adrenal sex hormones. Increased retention of sodium chloride (due to hypersecretion of mineralocorticoids) results in a puffiness of the lower face ("moon face") and in hypertension (high blood pressure). Decreased levels of potassium result in cramps and muscular weakness and in increased neural excitability. This is evidenced by an increase in the amplitude of shock-evoked potentials at the cerebral cortex (Danowski, 1962b). Behavioral symptoms—usually of an excitatory nature, including hallucinations, delusions, and mania—are common (Abrams, 1971; Danowski, 1962b).

The excess of glucocorticoids causes a redistribution of lipid tissue resulting in an enlargement of the trunk and thinning of the limbs. The excess glucocorticoids also increase the blood glucose level causing adrenal diabetes. Excess glucocorticoids also inhibit the inflammatory response, reduce the amount of lymphocytes, and inhibit blood antibody reactions, as well as increase stomach hydrochloric acid secretion. These actions serve to facilitate the spread of infection and the formation of ulcers.

Aldosteronism. Increased secretory activity may be restricted to the enzyme systems that produce aldosterone, resulting in aldosteronism. This condition may be due to a tumor or may be secondary to some other disease or condition. Secondary aldosteronism occurs naturally during pregnancy and in certain disease states such as congestive heart failure, liver disease, or kidney disease. The results of aldosteronism are due to high levels of circulating mineralocorticoids and include loss of potassium ion and excess retention of sodium and chloride ions. These electrolyte changes lead to weakness, periodic paralysis of the muscles, and hypertension. Often, adrenal diabetes occurs as a result of the glucocorticoid activity of aldosterone (which has up to 80% as much glucocorticoid activity as hydrocortisone) (Danowski, 1962b).

The adrenogenital syndrome. The adrenal cortex and gonads both develop from the same primitive embryological tissue and these structures contain similar enzyme systems. Figure 11.2 shows the pathway for the synthesis of gonadal hormones in the adrenal cortex (and in the gonads themselves). Note that the first steps are identical for all of the steroid hormones. The sex hormones of the adrenal cortex are manufactured under the control of ACTH and have effects identical to the hormones secreted by the gonads themselves. Under normal conditions the amounts of androgens and estrogens produced in the adrenal cortex are too small to produce noticeable physiological effects (although it has been suggested that in women adrenal androgens function as a libido hormone; see the next chapter).

In cases of metabolic disturbance due to a genetic defect or an adrenal tumor, large quantities of androgens, estrogens, or both may be produced. The chief metabolic disorder is a failure of the enzyme that converts hydroxyprogesterone to deoxycortisol (Figure 11.2). This results in above normal amounts of hydroxyprogesterone, and this excess is subsequently converted into adrenal androgens or estrogens (Turner & Bagnara, 1971). Decreased production of glucocorticoids also results, interrupting the ACTH feedback system and causing large amounts of ACTH to be released (in an attempt to bring the glucocorticoid level back to normal). Injections of a glucocorticoid may control the adrenogenital syndrome by lowering the ACTH level and slowing the synthesis of hydroxyprogesterone (Turner & Bagnara, 1971).

The adrenogenital syndrome may be congenital, that is, a pregnant female or the fetus itself may have a malfunctioning adrenal cortex, secreting high levels of androgen. This may result, with a female offspring, in the birth of a pseudohermaphrodite having masculinization of the genitals. In the case of a male offspring, there may be precocious development of the testes, penis, and secondary sexual characteristics (a so-called *Hercules infant*). When the adrenogenital syndrome develops in adulthood, there is a tendency to conversion to the secondary sexual characteristics of the opposite sex. Adult women with cortical hyperfunction develop male secondary sex characteristics, a condition called *adrenal virilism*. Adult males occasionally develop enlarged breasts and may begin milk production, a condition called *gynocomastia*.

Psychological Considerations

Development.   There is an inhibition by glucocorticoids of growth hormone secretion. It may be that the "maternal deprivation" syndrome, in which there is a reduction in growth hormone production (and growth) in infants, results from excessive glucocorticoid production due to stress. Neonatal administration of glucocorticoids to rats produces a retardation of development associated with an almost complete absence of growth hormone. This treatment also results in some improvement in performance on instrumental learning tasks (maze-learning or bar-pressing) later in life. It is worthwhile noting that human infants and children administered glucocorticoids for asthma or other allergic disorders also frequently exhibit retarded growth. Whether there are effects on adult learning, or other behavioral consequences in the human is unknown (Schapiro, 1971).

Euphoria.   One of the side effects of glucocorticoid treatment has been reported to be a mild euphoria. This euphoria may be related to the finding that glucocorticoids increase the rate of electrical self-stimulation in rats (Slusher, 1965; see also Chapter 3 in this book). The increased self-stimulation, and also the euphoria, indicate effects on brain biogenic amines. Glucocorticoids have been found to increase, and adrenalectomy to decrease, brain levels of tyrosine hydroxylase and of tryptophan hydroxylase, enzymes essential to the production of dopamine, norepinephrine and epinephrine, and of serotonin, respectively (McEwen, Zigmond, & Gerlach, 1972; also see Chapter 2 in this book).

Learning.   Removal of the adrenal cortex has been shown to inhibit the extinction of avoidance or appetitive learned responses (in rats), and to inhibit the habituation of electrocorticographic responses to novel stimuli (in humans; DeWied, Bohus, & Greven, 1968; DeWied, van Delft, Gispen, Weignen, & van Wimersma Greidanus, 1972; Endroczi, 1972; Levine, 1971). Glucocorticoid administration, furthermore, has been found to facilitate the extinction of avoidance responses (in the rat). These data have led to the hypothesis that the effects of these hormones on conditioning and extinction are due to direct actions of the glucocorticoids on some aspect of brain activity. DeWied's group has implicated the thalamic reticular area (1968, 1972). However, one recent study (Pfaff, Silva, & Weiss, 1971) has shown that the corticosteroids have effects on the firing of individual neurons in the rat dorsal hippocampus.

It should be emphasized that the effects of these hormones on conditioned behavior need not imply any specific role for the adrenocortical steroids in learning, habituation, or extinction. It may be that the effects on conditioning are secondary to carbohydrate mobilization factors and are related to the general role these hormones play in the response to stress. It has been found, for example, that a procedure which attenuates the performance of a conditioned emotional response in the rat (intracerebral injection of potassium chloride) also attenuates the corticoid mobilization in response to fear (Auerbach & Carlton, 1971).

Sensation. Many of the behavioral (conditioning) effects of the glucocorticoids may relate to an adrenocortical role in sensory processes. These data were discussed previously in relation to Addison's disease. Human patients with a surgical adrenalectomy or with hypoadrenalism (Addison's disease) show a marked increase in the ability to detect sensory signals over a variety of sense modalities, including taste, smell, hearing, and proprioception. In contrast, patients with hyperadrenalism (Cushing's disease) show a considerable impairment of sensory thresholds. It is possible that some of the conditioning changes discussed above are due to these altered sensory functions (Henkin, 1970).

THE PANCREAS

Were it not for the prevalence of diabetes mellitus, the pancreas might well be a relatively obscure gland. Because diabetes is so common, however, research concerning this gland has been greatly stimulated. Because of this research, diabetes, which only 100 years ago was incurable, is now fairly well controlled, and the diabetic can look forward to a relatively normal life.

Although Thomas Cawley thought as early as 1788 that the pancreas was related to diabetes mellitus (Grollman & Grollman, 1970), it was not until 1889 that removal of the pancreas was shown to produce the disease (Von Mering & Minkowski, 1889). Up to 1922, persons with diabetes mellitus were condemned to die of the disease. During that year, however, insulin was extracted from the pancreas and used therapeutically in humans (Banting, Best, Collip, Campbell, & Fletcher, 1922), dramatically revolutionizing the treatment of diabetes.

Structure

The pancreas is a long narrow gland which sits in the vicinity of the small intestine. It is actually both an endocrine and an exocrine gland. The exocrine portions secrete digestive enzymes through the pancreatic duct into the intestine. The endocrine aspects of the pancreas are termed the *islets of Langerhans*. There are about two million islets, but they only constitute about 1% or 2% of the weight of the pancreas. The islets become separated from the pancreatic duct during intrauterine life and contain two main types of cells called *alpha* and *beta*. The alpha cells produce glucagon and comprise about 10% to 40% of the islet cells. The more predominant beta cells produce insulin and, of course, constitute the remainder of the islet calls (Pachkis et al., 1967).

Physiology

Although the pancreas serves as both an exocrine and an endocrine gland, this discussion will only cover the endocrine aspects. It is interesting to note, however, that the exocrine functions, aiding in the digestion of foodstuffs, are related to the function of the endocrine portion of the gland. The two hormones of the pancreas, insulin and glucagon, have a variety of functions related to the metabolism of carbohydrates, principally glucose (carbohydrate metabolism was briefly reviewed earlier in this chapter).

Chemistry of insulin and glucagon. Insulin is a protein with a molecular weight of about 6,000. The amino acid sequence and structure of this molecule was the first protein to be so determined (Sanger, 1960). A few years later, insulin was synthesized in the laboratory and so also became the first naturally occurring hormone to be synthesized (Katsoyannis, 1967). Glucagon is a straight chain polypeptide. It has a molecular weight of 3,485 and is quite different from insulin (Bromer, Sinn, & Behrens, 1957). Like insulin, glucagon has also been synthesized in the laboratory (Wunsch, 1967).

Biosynthesis and control of insulin and glucagon. Insulin is formed in the beta cells as a single chain polypeptide called *proinsulin*. Proinsulin is biologically inactive (Levine, 1970, p. 295), but becomes active when split by intracellular proteolytic (protein destroying) enzymes, forming insulin (Antoniades, Bougas, Camerini-Davalos, & Pyle, 1964). The most important regulator of insulin secretion is the level of glucose in the bloodstream (Levine, 1970, p. 296). Various other carbohydrates, proteins, and amino acids may also cause insulin release (Floyd, Fajane, Knopf, Rull, & Conn, 1964; Rabinowitz, Merimec, Maffezzoli, & Purgess, 1966).

Insulin levels are elevated during pregnancy (Leake & Burt, 1962) and resistance to insulin develops during the last three months (Burt, 1956). It has been postulated that the increased insulin is due to this resistance and that increased amounts of the hormone are required to maintain a normal glucose level (Berson & Yalow, 1970). A placental hormone, human placental lactogen, has been implicated as a possible substance producing the insulin resistance (Kalkhoff, Schalch, Walker, Beck, Kipnis, & Daughaday, 1964).

The catecholamines, epinephrine and norepinephrine, have been shown to be capable of inhibiting insulin secretion. They are thought to act by increasing activity at the alpha adrenergic receptor sites (Porte & Williams, 1966). One of the more important classes of compounds that affect plasma insulin levels are the sulfonylureas, which are presently being used as oral antidiabetic drugs. These drugs, which have been found to increase plasma insulin levels in acute experiments (Williams, 1968b), are thought to act by directly stimulating the beta cells of the pancreas (Pfeiffer, Schoffling, Ditschuneit, Ziegler, & Gepts, 1969).

The production and control of glucagon, the hormone of the alpha cells, is still a relative mystery to researchers. Early studies with crude insulin preparations showed that a short hyperglycemia often preceded the hypoglycemic main effect of the insulin. Kimball and Murlin (1924) suspected that an impurity existed in the preparation and named it *glucagon.* Although this hormone was studied indirectly (as an insulin preparation impurity), it was not until the early 1950s that it was isolated in crystalline form (Staub, Sinn, & Behrens, 1953). Since that time, however, little has been learned about the biosynthesis or control of glucagon. The main reason for this failure of progress is lack of an adequate assay technique. This in turn is due to a variety of things including very small amounts present in the plasma, rapid degradation (especially in the liver), and the presence of glucagonlike substances in the intestinal mucosa (Turner & Bagnara, 1971). The evidence that does exist shows that glucagon secretion is increased during times of glucose need (Williams, 1968b) and is decreased after loading with glucose (Ohneda, Parada, Eisentraut, & Unger, 1968).

Effects of insulin. The most important effect of insulin is on the carbohydrates, especially glucose. Probably the most quoted statement about insulin is that it increases the body's utilization of glucose. Glucose can be used without insulin being present, but in the presence of insulin this process is much more efficient. The major manifestation of insulin is a decreased blood glucose level. This is accomplished not only by facilitating glucose utilization, but by simultaneously increasing the formation and storage of glycogen derived from glucose.

Insulin seems to have two main effects with respect to fat metabolism. First, it promotes the synthesis of fats, and second, it inhibits the breakdown of existing fat stores (Fain, Kovacev, & Scow, 1966). It is not known at present whether either of these effects are direct, or if they are due to insulin's actions on the carbohydrates. Since the presence of insulin leads to a greater energy yield from glucose, it is possible that the energy derived from fat metabolism is not needed, and thus fats are not metabolized. The effects of insulin on protein metabolism are similar to those on fats; increased insulin leads to increased protein synthesis and decreased protein degradation.

Insulin seems to exert most of its effects on skeletal muscle tissue and on adipose (fat) tissue, which together account for about 65% of the weight of the human body (Guyton, 1971). Its effects on glucose are also seen to a great extent in the heart and in some other types of smooth muscle organs. The places where insulin does not seem to be very effective include the intestinal mucosa, kidney tubules, brain cells, and the liver. It may seem strange that these tissues, which need efficient transport of glucose, are the very ones that cannot utilize insulin. However, research on the physiology of these tissues shows that there exist insulin-independent active transport mechanisms which greatly facilitate the passage of glucose into each of them.

Insulin: Mechanism of action. Insulin's specific mode of action has long been a puzzle to psychologists. Three general mechanisms have been postulated to explain the action of many of the hormones and include (1) direct action on particular genes, (2) an effect on intracellular enzyme systems, or (3) some type of cellular membrane regulation. The membrane hypothesis seems ideally suited for insulin (Park, 1956). Looking back to Figure 11.3 it is easily seen that if insulin just facilitates the entry of glucose into the cell (with subsequent change to G-6-P), then an entire series of reactions will be set into play. Not only will glucose metabolism be affected, but also fat and protein metabolism. However, there have been many studies in the last 10 to 15 years which show that many of insulin's effects can proceed in the absence of glucose (Mahler, Tarrant, Staffard, & Ashmore, 1963; Wool & Krahl, 1959; Zierler & Rabinowitz, 1964). Nevertheless, the membrane explanation is still the most probable one, and recent evidence shows that insulin may inhibit adenyl cyclase (Exton, Jefferson, & Park, 1966; Jungas, 1966; Sutherland, 1972), an enzyme implicated in the functioning of the membrane systems. Thus, what seems to be developing in this area is some combination of enzyme and membrane system regulation, probably at specific receptor sites.

Glucagon: Its functions and method of action. Recent evidence has shown that glucagon is an essential hormone (Sokal, 1966). Without glucagon, a fasting organism will often go into a hypoglycemic coma and die. Thus, the major effect of glucagon is to raise the plasma glucose level when it falls below the normal range. This hormone is thought to exert most of its effect by directly stimulating glucose formation in the liver (Sokal, 1970). Glucagon is thought to cause this glucose formation by way of cyclic AMP (Sutherland, 1972).

Pathology of Diabetes

The term *diabetes* may be used to refer to any of several abnormal conditions characterized by an excessive excretion of urine. The two most common types are *diabetes insipidus* and *diabetes mellitus*. Diabetes insipidus results from a loss of ADH and was discussed earlier. Diabetes mellitus is by far the most prominent of the diabetic pathologies. The word mellitus can be roughly translated from the Latin as *honeysweet* and refers to the *glycosuria* (sugar in the urine) characterizing this disease. Diabetes mellitus is a disorder of carbohydrate metabolism, resulting from inadequate secretion or utilization of insulin. Without insulin, glucose is not taken up by cells for use or for storage; thus, blood glucose levels are subject to great variability. This variability or lability is seen in the extremely high blood glucose level reached at a meal; then, because glucose is not stored, there follows a gradual reduction to very low glucose levels following an extended fast. The primary action of insulin is to enhance the ability of glucose (and other sugars) to enter the cell. When this action is suppressed (as in diabetes mellitus), the glucose does not enter the cell and is not phosphorylated to G-6-P. By following Figure 11.3 we can see clearly how this inhibition of G-6-P production manifests itself in the diabetic state.

First, the blood glucose level becomes elevated following a meal because the ingested glucose is not taken up by the cells. When this level goes from its normal concentration of about 90 mg/100 ml of blood to about 180 mg/100 ml of blood, the kidney tubules cannot reabsorb all the glucose and it begins to spill into the urine (glycosuria). The osmotic pressure of these glucose molecules pulls water along with it leading to an excess urine production (polyuria). The polyuria has two major effects. First, the fluid loss causes an intense thirst with a consequent large fluid intake (polydipsia). Second, the urine carries with it an excess of minerals and electrolytes causing an ionic imbalance.

The second major effect of G-6-P inhibition is an inability of the cell to utilize the glucose for the production of ATP. Not only does the organism lose this valuable energy source, but the various intermediates utilized in protein synthesis are no longer supplied. Thus any proteins broken down are not replaced efficiently. Finally, fatty acids are not synthesized. Since carbohydrates cannot be utilized by the cells, the existing fats become the sole energy source for the body. As these fats are broken down they begin to accumulate as free fatty acids (FFA), which are then broken down to acetyl coenzyme A (acetyl CoA). The most available metabolic pathway for the acetyl CoA is in the production by the liver of ketone bodies (such as acetone). These ketone bodies are then released and accumulate in the blood (ketonemia) and are seen in great quantity in the urine (ketonuria). Some of the excess acetone accumulates in the lungs and is secreted with the expired air, resulting in acetone breath, one of the most obvious signs of an untreated diabetic.

The diabetic symptoms include all of those previously mentioned, the most critical of which is the presence of the ketone bodies. The combination of the heightened levels of ketones (which are acidic) and the loss of sodium through the excessive urine causes an extreme metabolic acidosis. If corrective steps are still not taken, the acidosis will eventually depress the central nervous system. The person first becomes disoriented, followed by coma and eventually death. The treatment almost always includes immediate injection of insulin. Depending on what other symptoms are present, the patient may also be given sodium, potassium, or some circulatory agent such as whole blood or plasma.

Types of diabetes mellitus. Diabetes mellitus can best be broken down into two basic types. The first is juvenile-onset diabetes (*JOD*), while the other is mature-onset diabetes (*MOD*). Since both these conditions are termed *diabetes mellitus*, they share most of the characteristics that were described in the previous section. Nevertheless, there are various differences between JOD and MOD (Table 11.2).

JOD. The JOD patient develops diabetes early in life (usually before age 15) and is characterized by a lowered insulin level in both the pancreas and in the

TABLE 11.2

Juvenile-onset Diabetes vs Mature-onset Diabetes

	Juvenile-onset	Mature-onset
Percent of all diabetes	<5%	>75%
Family history of diabetes	Common	Less Common
Age at onset	<15	Adult (typically 40+)
Body size	Normal or thin	>50% obese
Rate of clinical onset	Rapid	Slow
Severity	Severe	Mild
Ketoacidosis	Common	Infrequent
Stability	Unstable	Stable
Insulin therapy required	Almost all	<25%
Insulin sensitivity	More sensitive	Less sensitive
Sulfonylurea response	Very few	>50%
Chronic manifestations (complications)	>90% in 20 years	Less common; slower developing

Note. Reprinted by permission from R. H. Williams (Ed.), *Textbook of Endocrinology* (4th ed.). Copyright 1968 by W. B. Saunders Company.

plasma. Although only about 5% to 15% (Forsham, 1970, p. 694) of diabetics have JOD, it is the more dramatic of the two forms. Its onset is usually fairly rapid, and it is much harder to control than MOD. The average life span of a JOD patient is about 10 to 20 years shorter than that of an average person (Forsham, 1970, p. 697). In most cases, the cause of death is some type of vascular complication. Almost all JOD patients require insulin after a while, although newly treated juvenile diabetics can often be stabilized for up to a year (after some initial treatment with insulin) by regulating their diet. Eventually, however, JOD diabetics require some form of continual insulin treatment which may be compounded with other medication, such as an oral antidiabetic drug. What seems to be manifested in the juvenile-onset diabetic is an inability of the pancreas to supply the body with insulin. This disease is genetically inherited and is due to a recessive gene. It has been estimated that this diabetic gene is present in 20% to 25% of the total population (Williams, 1968b). There are, however, other ways in which the beta cells of the pancreas can be destroyed, leading to a loss of insulin. Destruction of the pancreas by some type of accident, infection, or surgery will of course also lead to diabetes mellitus.

MOD. Although juvenile-onset diabetes clearly seems to result from a loss of insulin production, the mature-onset type just as clearly does not. The MOD patients, who comprise 80% to 90% of all diabetics, often have normal or even heightened insulin levels (Williams, 1968b). Since they require as much as 5 to 20 times as much insulin as a normal pancreatectomized human, even if their pancreas did function normally, they would need more insulin than it could produce. It is thought that MOD is due to a failure of the tissues to respond appropriately to insulin. One of the important characteristics of the MOD patient is the prevalence of obesity. There is also a positive correlation between the amount of obesity and the incidence of MOD (Williams, 1968b). It has not yet been shown, however, that obesity itself will cause diabetes, as it is possible that both conditions have a similar origin. It may be that some factor correlated with lifelong obesity leads to the production (or overproduction) of a substance that inhibits or antagonizes insulin or to an "exhaustion" of body cells and a subsequent deficiency in the ability of cells to utilize insulin. Fortunately, the oral antidiabetic drugs (which will be discussed later) have been found to be effective in the treatment of these patients. Also, both the acute and chronic manifestations of MOD are milder and slower to develop than in the juvenile type.

Other types of diabetes mellitus have also been described. Most of these can be classified with the juvenile-onset type since they are due to destruction of the pancreatic beta cells. Two of the most common ones are pituitary diabetes and adrenal diabetes. In each type, an overabundance of some hormone (possibly growth hormone or cortisol, respectively) causes an elevation of blood sugar levels. It is theorized that the increased sugar levels cause an increased insulin need, which may eventually overwork the beta cells and lead to their destruction.

Treatment of Diabetes

Diabetics generally take one of two types of medication—insulin or the oral hypoglycemic drugs. As a rule, the more severe a patient's diabetes, the greater his need for insulin therapy. This includes most juvenile-onset types and some mature-onset diabetics. Since insulin is a protein that is destroyed by digestive enzymes, the drug must be injected into the body.

The last 15 to 20 years have seen the development of various oral hypoglycemic drugs. Of the many that have been tested, there seem to be five that are fairly effective, yet have minimal side effects. The first four—tolbutamide, tolazamide, acetohexamide, and chlorpropamide—contain a sulfonylurea radical as an active portion ($-SO_2-NH-CO-NH-$), and are commonly called the *sulfonylureas*. The last drug, phenformin, differs from the others in that its active portion is a biquanide radical ($-NH-CNH-NH-CNH-NH_2$). Although all of these drugs have hypoglycemic effects, the sulfonylureas differ from phenformin in their mode of action. The sulfonylureas act by stimulating the beta cells to produce insulin. This type of drug is therefore ineffective in the juvenile-onset diabetic whose beta cells are nonfunctional or destroyed. In the mature-onset diabetic, however, the sulfonylureas are usually fairly effective, especially in the milder cases where there are presumably many functioning beta cells.

Like the sulfonylureas, phenformin requires the presence of some insulin to be effective. It does not, however, stimulate the release of insulin from the pancreas (Krall, 1970). The site of action of phenformin appears to be peripheral, and studies have implicated the intestines (Williams, 1968b), as well as the carbohydrate pathways (Meyer, Ipaktchi, & Clauser, 1967; Wick, Larson, & Serif, 1958; Williams, Tanner, & Odell, 1958). Phenformin augments the insulin that is present, and is not effective in the absence of endogenous or exogenous insulin. One of the more successful recent treatments of maturity onset diabetes has been a combination of phenformin plus a sulfonylurea. It has been suggested that 50% of the existing diabetics could be successfully treated with this type of combination (Beaser, 1960).

Hypoglycemia. Hypoglycemia (reduced blood sugar levels) is not nearly as prevalent as diabetic hyperglycemia. Nevertheless, this topic is important because of the possibility of hypoglycemia resulting from an accidental insulin overdose during the treatment of diabetes mellitus. Most of the symptoms of the hypoglycemic state are due to a loss of oxygen in the brain. This oxygen loss, in turn, is due to the lowered blood glucose level, since oxygen utilization is directly tied to carbohydrate metabolism. The untreated hypoglycemic person will lapse into a coma. This fact causes severe problems for the diabetic on insulin treatment. If a known diabetic is found in a coma, the physician must decide if the coma is due to an overdose of insulin (hypoglycemic coma) or to a failure to receive adequate insulin (hyperglycemic coma). In many ways, of course, the treatments would be directly opposite, and a mistake could prove fatal. Fortunately, there are numerous differences between these two types of coma (see Williams, 1968a).

Psychological Considerations

The hormones of the pancreas are not yet used to any great extent in behavioral research. Their primary uses are in persons with clinical problems related to carbohydrate metabolism, especially in diabetes mellitus. The major exception to the above is insulin therapy. Sakel (1936) began using insulin-induced coma therapy to treat schizophrenics during the 1930s. Insulin comas were induced and then terminated after 20 to 40 minutes by the administration of glucose. Sakel reported that the patients seemed to show marked improvement after this type of insulin-induced coma. Insulin coma is no longer in general use in psychiatry. The greatest effectiveness of coma induction seems to be in depression, where ECT or antidepressant drugs are now preferred. Coma therapy is now believed not to be beneficial in schizophrenia.

THE THYROID GLAND

The thyroid affects a wide variety of tissues and organs and has an important role with respect to general metabolism. Thyroxine (the major thyroid hormone) primarily influences protein synthesis. Besides its effect on general metabolism, the thyroid aids in the development and growth of the central nervous system and complements growth hormone with respect to the skeletal and muscular systems.

Structure

The mammalian thyroid gland is a two-lobed structure located bilaterally on the sides of the trachea near the anterior base of the neck. The entire thyroid normally weighs between 20 and 40 grams in the adult human and has an extremely rich vascular supply. The thyroid is composed of closely packed follicles, which are lined with a single layer of secretory epithelial cells, which produce the thyroid hormone.

Physiology

Iodine and the synthesis of thyroxine. The major hormone produced by the thyroid gland is thyroxine (tetraiodothyronine, T_4). Thyroxine is derived from the amino acid, tyrosine, in a series of reactions involving the addition of iodine to the tyrosine molecule (Figure 11.4). Although thyroxine is often designated as thyroid hormone, the various intermediates are also stored within the follicles. There are three stages to the formation of hormone in the thyroid gland: (1) the accumulation or trapping of iodide from the circulation; (2) the iodination of tyrosine; and (3) the proteolysis or breakdown of thyroglobin (this bound form of thyroid hormone is not found in the circulation). The thyroid gland accumulates iodide and converts it to iodine before it binds the iodine to

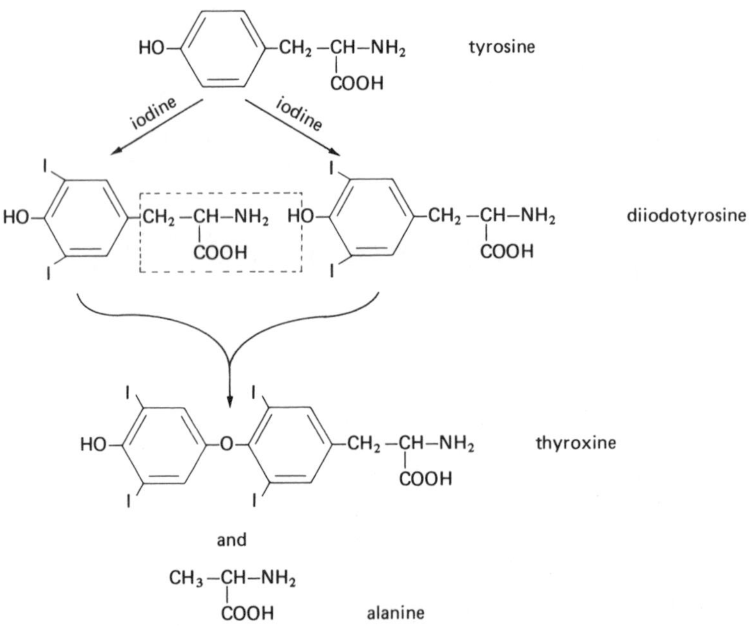

FIGURE 11.4. The synthesis of thyroxine.

tyrosine, forming monoiodotyrosine (T_1) and diiodotyrosine (T_2). Two molecules of diiodotyrosine are then coupled to form thyroxine (tetraiodothyronine). Triiodothyronine is also formed by the binding of one molecule of monoidotyrosine plus one molecule of diiodotyrosine. The stored colloid (thyroglobin), therefore, consists of T_1, T_2, thyroxine, and triiodothyronine (T_3), all bound to other proteins. One of these products, triiodothyronine (T_3), has been found to be as much as seven times as effective as thyroxine, although it exists in much smaller quantities (Turner & Bagnara, 1971). Neither of the other intermediates (T_1 or T_2) are thought to exert biologic activity.

An outstanding feature of the thyroid gland is the ability of its cells to concentrate iodide; the normal thyroid to blood ratio of this substance is at least 20 to 1 (Halmi, 1961), and can, under certain conditions become several hundredfold. The daily intake of iodine is about 150 micrograms. This quantity, plus about 70 micrograms from the daily thyroxine secretion and degradation, form the inorganic pool of iodine. The thyroid gland uses up about 70 micrograms of this iodine a day.

Effects of thyroid hormone.   The most obvious effect of thyroid hormone in the human is an increase in energy production and oxygen usage by the tissues. Thyroid hormone has a pronounced stimulatory effect on protein synthesis. It is possible that the protein metabolic effects of thyroxine may account for many of the physiologic changes produced by this hormone. The effects of thyroxine on carbohydrate and fat metabolism may be quite variable depending on the state of the organism. In general, the thyroid hormones have a greater effect on lipolysis (fat breakdown) than on lipogenesis (fat synthesis) (Ingbar & Woeber, 1974). Thyroxine causes breakdown of glycogen in the liver, and at the same time, an increase in oxidation of glucose by the tissues, partially offsetting the blood sugar rise (Turner & Bagnara, 1971, p. 211).

Thyroid hormone exerts an influential effect on the growing organism. Thyroxine aids pituitary growth hormone in skeletal growth functions. More important than this effect on growth, however, is the role that thyroxine plays with respect to the development of various systems of the organism, especially the nervous system. Without minimum levels of thyroid hormone during early life, both the reproductive development (Turner & Bagnara, 1971) and the neurological development (Brasel & Blizzard, 1974) of the organism will be retarded (see the section on psychological considerations below for further discussion of this subject).

Mechanism of action of thyroxine.   Because thyroxine seems to affect a great many types of tissues, it has been extremely difficult to pin down any one direct action of the hormone. The time lag between administration of thyroxine and its various actions suggests the synthesis of particular proteins, probably enzymes. More specifically, evidence has accumulated suggesting that thyroid hormone stimulates RNA synthesis, which may then direct the production of various proteins (Tata, 1966).

Control of thyroid secretion. The major regulator of thyroid secretion is thyrotropin (TSH) from the anterior pituitary. The TSH itself, however, is in turn regulated by a variety of both internal and external environmental stimuli, including environmental temperature and stress.

Thyrocalcitonin (TCT, Calcitonin)

Thyrocalcitonin, which affects calcium levels, is another hormone isolated from the thyroid gland. When this substance was first discovered, it was believed to originate in the parathyroid glands, and was named *calcitonin* (Rasmussen, 1974). Later work revealed that the cellular origin of this hormone was actually in the thyroid (Hirsch, Voelkel, & Munson, 1964). The parafollicular cells, which are between the actual thyroxine containing follicles, produce this substance. Thus it has often been called *thyrocalcitonin.* This name is probably the more popular and more widely used one at present. Thryocalcitonin is a polypeptide with a molecular weight of less than 5,000 (Rasmussen, 1974; Taylor, 1968). Its principal action is to lower blood calcium, by inhibiting the resorption of this mineral from bone. The only known internal regulator of thyrocalcitonin is plasma calcium level. Hypercalcemia causes a rapid increase in circulating thyrocalcitonin, which will then oppose any rise in calcium, such as that produced by parathyroid hormone.

Pathology of the Thyroid Gland

Hypothyroidism (cretinism, myxedema). Diminished functioning of the thyroid gland results in a series of metabolic disturbances called *cretinism* in infants and *myxedema* in adults. Developmental abnormalities are seen in the cretin due to early onset of the hormonal loss. The cretin is characterized by an inhibition of longitudinal growth, a flattened nose, thickened tongue, and a yellowish complexion. Sexual and neurological development are usually retarded, as is behavioral development. If replacement therapy with thyroid hormone is begun, development of these systems will improve. With early enough treatment, normal height and intelligence are possible, but any developmental defects that occur during an untreated period cannot be corrected by later treatment.

The remaining symptoms in hypothyroidism are similar in cretinism and myxedema and will be discussed with reference to the latter. Because these effects are not related to growth or development, they are reversible with adequate replacement therapy. Several preparations are available when treatment with thyroid hormone is indicated. Thyroid is normally administered orally as the powdered dry thyroid gland obtained from animals. Thyroxine and triiodothyronine are also prepared synthetically and are available commercially for replacement therapy in myxedema and cretinism. These agents have also been used for other conditions in which their indications are questionable, such as in reducing regimens. This use is discouraged, since treatment should probably be directed at reducing the caloric intake rather than at increasing metabolism.

Nervousness and heart palpitations are common side effects of thyroid medication when it is not used for replacement of an existing deficiency.

The most prominent symptoms of the myxedemic patient are a drop in metabolic rate and an accumulation of fluid in the extracellular space (edema; hence the name myx*edema*). The edema is caused by a microprotein, which becomes situated under the skin (but ouside the blood vessels) and raises the osmotic pressure of this space, thereby causing retention of fluid. The lowered metabolic rate also causes the skin to be cold and the surface vessels to be constricted.

Hyperthyroidism (Grave's disease).   An excess secretion of thyroid hormone is called *hyperthyroidism.* Of the various causes of hypersecretion of the thyroid the most prominent is Grave's disease. The classic triad of symptoms of Grave's disease include thyrotoxicosis, goiter, and exophthalmos. The thyrotoxicosis is manifested as a series of symptoms related to the nervous system, skin, and muscles. Nervousness and insomnia are two of the earliest signs of this disease. Later, the person exhibits jerks and tremors, and the tendon reflexes become hyperactive (Pachkis et al., 1967; Woodbury, Hurley, Lewis, McArthur, Copeland, Kirschvink, & Goodman, 1952). Thyrotoxicosis causes the skin to be warm and moist. Finally, general muscle weakness and wasting occur, and are probably a result of a disturbance in energy metabolism.

Goiter (enlargement of the thyroid), averaging two to four times normal size, is characteristic of Grave's disease (Ingbar & Woeber, 1974). *Exophthalmos* refers to an abnormal protrusion of the eyeball such that the lids are retracted, producing a stare, which may cause subsequent injury due to loss of ocular protection. There also may exist a weakness of convergence (the ability to turn the eyes inward to focus on nearby objects) or palsy of one or more of the extraocular muscles.

A substance similar to TSH has been discovered in patients with Grave's disease (Adams & Purves, 1956). This substance differs from TSH principally in its greater duration of effect, and has been named long-acting thyroid stimulator (LATS). Another substance has been isolated from the pituitary (and from the blood of some patients with severe exophthalmos) which seems to have exophthalmos-producing properties (Daughaday, 1974). It has been named EPS (exophthalmos-producing substance). Whether any or all of these three substances (TSH, LATS, or EPS) turn out to be the same remains to be decided by future research.

Psychological Considerations

The thyroid, perhaps more than any other gland, is associated with behavioral disturbances. Behavioral changes indicative of central nervous system malfunctions are found in both the hypothyroid and hyperthyroid conditions (Eayrs, 1968).

Development: Behavior.   Probably the most obvious neurological abnormality seen in the hypothyroid state is the mental retardation of the cretin. In one study of 79 treated cretins, only about one-fifth attained an intelligence quotient of 80 or better, while the others ranged between 10 and 80 with a median of about 50 (Danowski, 1962a). While it is generally agreed that thyroidectomy performed on an adult rat does not have a significant effect on learning capacity, this is not the case for the neonatally thyroidectomized rat (Eayrs & Levine, 1963). Although these cretinoid animals become more readily habituated to a novel setting, they make more errors than normals in a more complex situation (Eayrs & Lishman, 1955). Experiments using a Hebb-Williams closed-field test show that number of errors during a fixed number of trials is directly related to the age at which thyroidectomy takes place (Eayrs, 1961). Thus, it seems clear that intellectual development takes place during early life, and that the influence of thyroid hormone is critical for cerebral maturation during this period.

Development: Neurology.   While it is obvious that congenital (or neonatally induced) hypothyroidism is associated with mental retardation, the nature of the effect on cerebral growth and maturation is less clear. Some recent studies, however, are beginning to clarify this influence. In one study, it was demonstrated that the amplitude of the EEG in conscious, unrestrained animals was reduced in neonatally thyroidectomized animals, as opposed to normals. These cretinic animals also showed a delay or absence in capacity of the cortex to "block" in response to auditory stimuli or to "follow" the frequency of rhythmic visual stimulation (Bradley, Eayrs, & Schmalbach, 1960). These same phenomena were not observed in animals thyroidectomized later in life. Other studies have demonstrated that cretinic rats showed changes in latency, duration, and amplitude of cortical evoked potentials, and that thyroid administration normalized these effects (Bradley, Eayrs, Glass, & Heath, 1961; Bradley, Eayrs, & Richards, 1964). Furthermore, rats thyroidectomized during adult life undergo changes in evoked potential latency and duration.

From an anatomical standpoint, the cretinic brain is both small in size and misshapen. Probably due to a disparity between the growth of the brain and the skull, the cretinic brain grows in height and width, but not in length (Dye & Maughm, 1929). The cell bodies of neurons located in the sensorimotor cortex are reduced in size and very tightly packed in the cretinic rat (Eayrs & Taylor, 1951). Also, both the axons and dendrites of these cells are underdeveloped (Eayrs, 1955).

Adult hypothyroidism.   As with the cretin, the adult hypothyroid patient usually displays behavioral disturbances. In the patient with myxedema, the manifestations range from slowed responses and mood changes to schizo-phrenic-type behaviors including paranoid delusions, hallucinations, and mania (Abrams, 1971; Reichlin, 1974). These latter behaviors are responsible for the phrase *myxedemic madness* which is often seen in the literature (Asher, 1949). Although most patients with myxedema show dramatic improvement in behavior after thyroxine treatment, some do not. Failure to respond is thought to be due to permanent organic brain damage (except for coincidental psychosis of some other origin).

Adult hyperthyroidism. The hyperthyroid patient will almost always manifest some type of behavioral symptom (Abrams, 1971). Typical symptoms include overactiveness, anxiety, tremor, or frank psychosis. A small percentage of the patients become indifferent and apathetic (Hare & Ritchey, 1946). Extreme cases may even show delirium and coma (Reichlin, 1974). In a series of studies comparing hyperthyroid patients with normals, significant differences were found with respect to (1) reaction time, with thyrotoxic patients having slower times; (2) muscular coordination and motor ability, with the hyperthyroid group doing more poorly; and (3) the Minnesota Multiphasic Personality Inventory (MMPI), with the thyrotoxic group showing elevations on the paranoia, depression, and schizophrenic scales (Artunkal & Togrol, 1964).

One factor that might account for the high correlation between hyperthyroidism and behavioral disorders is that personality disturbances and psychoses seem to precipitate the thyrotoxic state (Danowski, 1962a). Levi (1968) has even found that prolonged stress (3 days) in normal human military "volunteers" resulted in blood levels of thyroid hormone usually considered indicative of thyrotoxicosis. However, one might make a case for the reverse (thyrotoxicosis precipitating behavioral disorders) since thyroid treatment often leads to cessation of behavioral symptoms. In some cases, this type of treatment is not successful and it is believed that brain damage may have occurred.

THE PARATHYROID GLANDS

It has been less than 100 years since the parathyroid glands were described. Before the existence of these glands was realized, surgeons would often remove the parathyroids while performing a thyroidectomy. Since the turn of the century, however, researchers have made great strides concerning these tiny glands and their regulation of the body's calcium levels. Calcium itself has been revealed as one of the more essential minerals and is now shown to be a major component of a variety of physiological systems. The body contains more calcium than any other positive ion (1,200–1,400 g); about 99% of the calcium and also 90% of the phosphate in the body are found in the skeleton. Not only is calcium necessary for the formation of the skeletal system, but it also plays critical roles in nerve and muscle excitability and in blood clotting, as well as in the regulation of various enzymes.

Structure

There are usually two pairs of parathyroid glands in the human being, located on the posterior surface of the lateral portions of the thyroid gland. It is not uncommon, however, for the number or location to vary. They are normally very small, having a combined weight of about 120 mg. Looking at the microstructure of these glands, we find that each gland is surrounded by a thin fibrous tissue. Inside the tissue, each gland is mainly composed of a rich vascular system and epithelial secretory cells.

Physiology

Bone and mineral metabolism.   Because the parathyroid glands are so closely associated with bone metabolism, we will deal with this topic first. Although not going into detail, this section should enable the reader to better understand the relationship of parathyroid hormone to bone and mineral metabolism. The two major functions of the human skeletal system are: (1) supporting and protecting the various parts of the body; and (2) aiding in the regulation of essential minerals. These functions cannot really be discussed separately, since each is dependent on the other. We therefore speak of bone and mineral metabolism, and together they constitute a single regulatory system.

Bone is made up of about 35% organic matrix and about 65% inorganic material called *hydroxyapatite.* The organic matrix is practically all collagen, a structural protein similar to that in other connective tissue (i.e., tendon or cartilage). The inorganic or mineral portion (hydroxyapatite) is a crystal surrounded by a water shell. Calcium and phosphorus constitute the major portion of the crystal. In addition to these two main minerals, calcium and phosphorus, the inorganic part of bone also contains small amounts of other minerals including magnesium, potassium, sodium, fluorine, and strontium. In an adult mammal, bone material is constantly changing; old bone is being broken down and is simultaneously being rebuilt.

Parathyroid hormone.   Parathyroid hormone (parathormone, PTH) is a straight-chain polypeptide and is thought to contain from 74 to 80 amino acids (Potts & Aurbach, 1965; Rasmussen, Sze, & Young, 1964). The main regulator of parathormone secretion is plasma calcium level, with a lowered blood calcium level causing increased parathormone release and excess calcium having an inhibitory effect. The normal level of calcium in human blood is about 10 mg per 100 ml.

Parathormone seems to have three basic actions. The first is an effect on bone to cause release of calcium and phosphate into the blood. The second effect is at the kidney tubules to cause a decreased reabsorption (therefore an increased urinary excretion) of phosphate. Finally, parathormone acts on the intestines to cause increased absorption of both calcium and phosphate. Like the other endocrine hormones, parathormone has been linked to the cyclic AMP system (Chase, Fedak, & Aurbach, 1969). The primary mechanism of action of PTH may involve increasing the solubility of calcium in the bloodstream.

Vitamin D.   The D vitamins are chemically classified as *sterols* and have a pronounced effect on calcium metabolism. The naturally occurring D vitamin is formed by the action of ultraviolet light on 7-dehydrocholesterol in the skin. The most common synthetic D vitamin is calciferol, which is made by irradiating ergosterol, a steroid found in plants. The main effect of vitamin D is to promote absorption of calcium from the gastrointestinal tract (Rasmussen, 1974).

A deficiency of vitamin D due to either (1) nutritional factors or (2) lack of sunlight may cause serious problems related to bone metabolism. In children this disease is called *rickets,* and in adults it is termed *osteomalacia.* If not treated, calcium and phosphorus will be removed from bone (via PTH) because of loss of the ability to absorb this mineral. The bones will eventually bend or develop fractures and the lowered blood calcium levels will cause tetanic convulsions (repetitive seizures due to increased neural firing). Treatment consists of giving vitamin D and adding calcium and phosphorus to the diet.

Pathology of the Parathyroid Glands

Hypoparathyroidism. A decrease or loss of parathyroid functioning is due to one of three major causes. The first, idiopathic hypoparathyroidism (of unknown cause), is very rare and very little is known about it. A second cause involves any disease that may partially or totally destroy these glands, for instance, tuberculosis. Also included in this category would be destruction due to hemorrhage or ischemia (blood loss). The final and most common cause is postoperative hypoparathyroidism, which may occur because of accidental removal of the parathyroid glands during thyroidectomy.

The metabolic changes following loss of parathyroid function are: (a) lowered level of blood calcium; (b) reduced urinary excretion of calcium; (c) increased level of blood phosphate; and (d) decreased urinary phosphate excretion. The major clinical manifestation of this state is *tetany*. The decreased calcium will first cause hyperexcitability of the neuromuscular system (termed *latent tetany*). This stage can be demonstrated by muscular responses to mechanical or electrical stimulation of various hyperexcitable nerves (Pachkis et al., 1967). Eventually, involuntary tremors will develop into spasms, followed by violent convulsions and death. Infrequently, mild hypoparathyroidism may occur. The major signs of tetany do not occur, and, if not detected, the disease will cause changes in the hair, skin, and teeth. Also, the person will eventually develop cataracts in the lenses of the eyes. The treatment in either case consists of replacement therapy with parathormone plus adequate amounts of dietary minerals.

Hyperparathyroidism (von Recklinghausen's disease). Hypersecretion of the parathyroids causes von Recklinghausen's disease (osteitis fibrosa), associated with increased plasma levels of calcium and phosphorus and excretion of large amounts of these same substances in the urine. Neuromuscular excitability is decreased and the symptoms include hypotonia and weakness of the muscles, bradycardia (slowed heart rate), and dramatic changes in the bone structure. The majority of patients show a variety of bone related symptoms (bone pain, bone tumors, spontaneous fractures, limp, and bending of long bones or of the vertebral column), due to the excess parathormone which leads to an absorption of calcium and phosphorus from the bones. The treatment for primary hyperparathyroidism is surgical removal of the malfunctioning gland or glands. Postoperative care is very critical and any necessary steps should be taken to prevent tetany.

Psychological Considerations

There have been several reports of behavioral changes related to parathyroid malfunctioning. Central nervous system seizures in hypoparathyroid patients are associated with slow wave EEG activity. These effects are due to the decreased calcium levels that characterize this disease. Usually, if the plasma calcium level is normalized by appropriate treatment, the seizures will cease and the EEG will improve (Woodbury & Vernadakis, 1967).

The most common behavioral changes seen in hyperparathyroidism are drowsiness, stupor, and coma, which are characteristic of most hypercalcemic conditions (Eitinger, 1942; Oliver, 1939). Personality disturbances and psychosis have also been reported (Fitz & Hallman, 1952; Lehrer & Levitt, 1960). In a clinical study of 33 cases of primary hyperparathyroidism, 14 patients (42%) were found to have neuropsychiatric manifestations (Karpati & Frame, 1964), directly related to level of serum calcium (levels of over 17 mg/100 ml were almost always associated with either neurologic or psychiatric problems). In almost all cases, the symptoms improved after the removal of a parathyroid tumor.

Although the exact origin of these behavioral disturbances is not known, central nervous system depression has been produced in animals by parathyroid extracts (Collip, 1926). Data from another study suggested that clinical recovery from depression, produced either by imipramine or electroconvulsive therapy, is associated with decreased urinary calcium levels (Flach, Liang, & Stokes, 1960). This study was followed up by another which showed a significant decrease in urinary calcium excretion in depressed or paranoid schizophrenics who responded to imipramine or ECT treatment; but not in patients with similar symptoms that failed to respond to treatment (Flach, 1964). Finally, it is noteworthy that lithium, which has been found useful in the treatment of manic states, may exert its effects on calcium or some other charged macromolecule (Ban, 1969).

SUMMARY

At this point we would like to make some integrative comments concerning the functioning of the endocrine glands. First and foremost, the student should conceptualize the endocrine glands as component parts of an integrated endocrine system. This system functions to maintain orderly biological processes. This is a metabolic system that serves to mobilize energy resources in stressful emergencies and to maintain homeostatic equilibrium over the long term. The key bodily resources are those that are endocrinologically controlled: water balance and blood pressure by ADH; sodium and potassium by mineralocorticoids; calcium and phosphorus by the parathyroids and by thyrocalcitonin; protein synthesis and growth processes by growth hormone and thyroxine; glucose mobilization by the glucocorticoids, insulin, and glucagon;

autonomic arousal by the adrenal medulla. The gonadotropins, oxytocin, and gonadal hormones, which regulate species survival by controlling reproductive and parental functions, will be the subject of the next chapter.

The second important point to be recognized is that the behavioral manifestations of normal endocrine action and of hormonal impairment are the result of these same basic metabolic alterations, when they occur in the nervous system, and consequently have behavioral concomitants. The idea of the nervous and endocrine systems acting as a unitary neuroendocrine system should be considered. Stimuli impinging on the organism alter endocrine functioning, primarily via hypothalamic control of the anterior and posterior lobes of the pituitary, and also via autonomic arousal of the adrenal medulla. These, and the other endocrine glands, then affect brain function by altering brain metabolism and also by influencing selective hormonal receptors in the brain (for example, those for epinephrine, oxytocin, ADH and the gonadal hormones).

12
SEXUAL BEHAVIOR

Robert A. Levitt and Daniel J. Lonowski*

The sexual behavior of mammals may be viewed as the result of an interaction between several biological and environmental factors. At the most basic level of this interaction are the genetic instructions, which initially define the gender of an organism and subsequently promote the anatomical development and differentiation of the sexes. As this divergence between the sexes begins, certain hormonal factors produced by the pregnant female, but more importantly other hormones produced by the growing fetus itself, carry the physical development of the fetus to a higher level. At this stage of development, hormonal processes directly determine the anatomical status of the organism and are therefore relatively more critical to the organism than its genetic constitution. The combined influences of these genetic and hormonal factors are seen on the structures of copulation and reproduction, and also on such secondary sex-related characteristics as distribution of body hair, body size, and pitch of the voice. There is even evidence that the structure and functioning of the central nervous system is differentiated between the sexes. The impact of these biological processes, however, may be substantially, albeit remarkably, reduced by yet another critical aspect in the sexual development of mammals. This aspect relates to the environment and experiences of the organism. There is considerable human evidence that sexual identity and sex-related behaviors are strongly influenced by learning processes. Such environmental pressures are capable of overriding the biological tableaux by which the sexes are initially differentiated.

*The order of listing of authorship is alphabetical since the two authors made about equal contributions to this chapter.

To attempt an understanding of the interaction of genetics, hormones, the nervous system and experiences in determining sexual functioning is a difficult task indeed. Certain problems in interpreting research and clinical findings are responsible for this situation. Namely, the relative importance and contribution of these factors differs across mammalian species; nor are the determinants of equal importance for males and females within a single species. Thus, the interpretation of research aimed at unraveling the basis of sexual functioning is hampered by a relative inability to generalize results. Yet, critical inroads have been made and tentative theoretical models concerning the basis of sexuality have been advanced. It is our intent, therefore, to explain the progress made in this area and provide a framework through which sexuality may be understood.

GENETICS

By the act of copulation, specialized cells of reproduction called *gametes* are combined in the creation of new organisms. In the male, these cells are the *spermatazoa*, while female gametes are called *ova*. Each of these gametes (called *haploidal* cells) contains only half the number of chromosomes found within the other cells (called *diploidal* cells) of a particular mammalian species.

The haploidal chromosomal nature of gametes is the result of a specialized form of cellular division called *meiosis*. Meiosis involves the separation of the paired chromosomes found in the nucleus of diploidal cells, so that half the total amount of nuclear material, now in an unpaired form, is found in each gamete (a haploidal cell). Meiosis may be more fully illustrated by comparing it to *mitosis*, which involves the separation of a cell into two cells, each of which contains all of the nuclear material in a paired form (see Figure 12.1).

The determination of genetic sex is inextricably related to meiosis within the sex cells. Of the 46 chromosomes found in human cells, two are sex-determining. In the male, there are two forms of the sex-determining chromosome, designated as X and Y. In the female, however, there is only one form of the sex-determining chromosome, designated as X. During meiosis, these sex chromosomes are split apart such that in the male, one gamete may contain an X or a Y sex chromosome. Only X chromosomes, however, are found in the female ova. Upon the fusion of an X-bearing spermatazoa with an ova, therefore, an XX, or female, combination is found, while the fusion of a Y-bearing spermatazoa with an ova will result in an XY or male combination. The full diploidal chromosomal count is restored upon sperm-ova fusion (the fused structure is now referred to as a *zygote*). There is general agreement that the prime sex determinant at fertilization is the male gamete, since the presence of a Y chromosome will direct male development, whereas the presence of an X chromosome will produce female development (Barr, Carr, Pozsonyi, Wilson, Dunn, Jacobson, Miller, Lewis, & Chown, 1963; Grumbach, 1967).

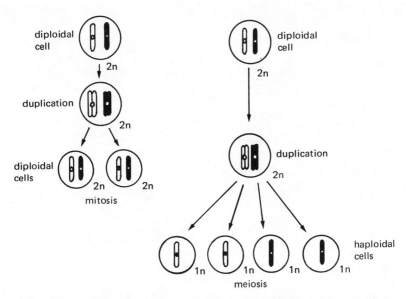

FIGURE 12.1. Meiosis compared to mitosis. During the first division in meiosis, the chromosome pairs separate so that daughter cells have different genetic material.

DEVELOPMENT AND DIFFERENTIATION

As in other species, the human zygote begins a series of mitotic divisions subsequent to fertilization and develops into a multicellular structure (while still in the fallopian tube where fertilization usually occurs). The organism continues to grow for 4 or 5 days while passing through the fallopian tube, and then enters the uterus and eventually implants or burrows into the uterine wall. As mitosis continues, the organism gradually takes on the shape of a human, after which time it is called a *fetus*. The fetus then progressively develops throughout the period of pregnancy until parturition or the birth process occurs.

Until about the seventh or eighth week of embryonic life, genetic males and females show identical anatomical sexual development. The primitive gonad or sex gland shown in Figure 12.2 cannot be distinguished as either an ovary or a testis. At this point in fetal development, therefore, the primitive nondifferentiated gonad possesses the potential for developing into either an ovary or a testis.

The human fetus, at the second month of life, is also equipped with primitive versions of both the male and the female genital duct systems. The *mullerian* or female duct is the embryonic precursor of the uterus and fallopian tubes. The *wolffian* or male duct is the precursor of the male duct system, which consists of the epididymus, vas deferens, seminal vesicle, and ejaculatory duct.

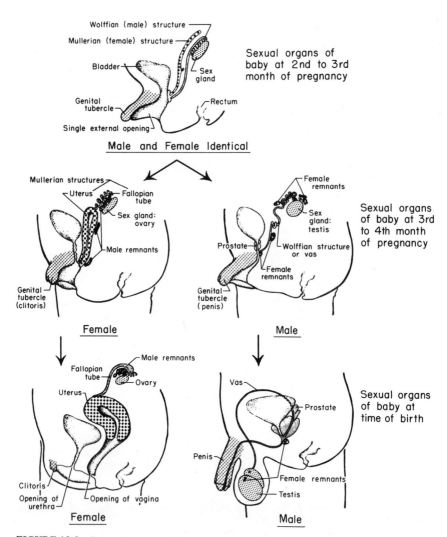

FIGURE 12.2. Internal genital differentiation in the human fetus. (Reprinted by permission from J. Money and A. A. Ehrhardt, *Man and Woman, Boy and Girl*. Copyright 1972 by The Johns Hopkins University Press.)

A third sexual structure is also seen in the fetus during early embryonic life. This external structure, called the *genital tubercle*, is shown in Figures 12.2 and 12.3. It may develop along female lines into the vagina, clitoris, and labia, or may grow in a male fashion with the appearance of a penis and scrotum.

Thus, at the second month of fetal development three bipotential structures common to both males and females are present: (1) the sex gland, (2) the mullerian and wolffian ducts, and (3) the genital tubercle. The integrity of each of these structures is dependent upon a normal genetic constitution and on a

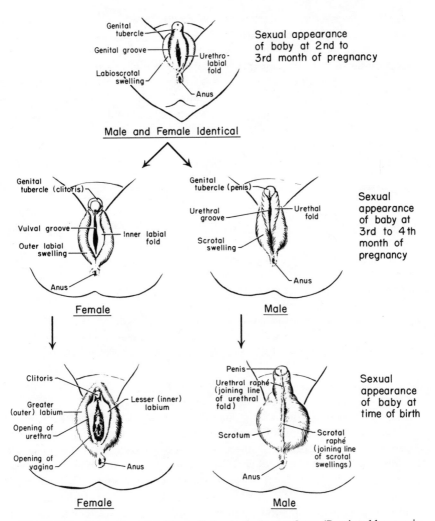

FIGURE 12.3. External genital differentiation in the human fetus. (Reprinted by permission from J. Money and A. A. Ehrhardt, *Man and Woman, Boy and Girl.* Copyright 1972 by The Johns Hopkins University Press.)

proper uterine environment. How each structure develops appropriately in the anatomical sexual differentiation of a growing fetus will require further explanation.

Gonads

The development of the primitive gonad (sex gland) into a testis or an ovary is the first phase of fetal sexual differentiation. At about the second month of fetal life in the human the emergence of the gonad into a testis or an ovary is dependent on whether the inner or outer component of the gonad achieves dominance over the opposite structure (Grumbach & Barr, 1958). Jost (1958) has suggested the theory that the sex-determining genes on the X and Y chromosomes direct appropriate gonadal differentiation by promoting the secretion of certain "inductor substances" from the primitive sex gland. Thus, gonadal differentiation into an ovary would be initiated by an XX chromosome inductor substance. Male development, on the other hand, would result from secretions directed or controlled genetically by an XY chromosomal constitution. Under normal circumstances, from this point of development on to parturition, the testis or ovary will continue to develop along separate lines.

Duct System

About 1 month after gonadal differentiation occurs, the fetus will develop an appropriate accessory duct system. Figure 12.2 illustrates this point. The principal factors involved with this phase of development are chemical substances secreted by the fetal testis (Jost, 1958). There appear to be two such duct-organizing substances. One is an androgen, perhaps testosterone, which induces the wolffian duct system to grow and differentiate into the male duct system. The other duct-organizing substance secreted by the fetal testis has not been identified, but is not an androgen. This substance *inhibits* the development of the mullerian duct system, and is thus called *mullerian-inhibiting substance* (Federman, 1967; Williams, 1968c).

In the presence of functional testes, therefore, the wolffian duct will proceed to full growth while the mullerian duct system atrophies. On the other hand, in the absence of normal testes in the normal female fetus (or in certain abnormal male fetuses) the mullerian duct system develops into a full female duct system and the wolffian system involutes. This fact raises three interesting points. First, since removal or destruction of one testis has been shown to result in mullerian development on that side, with wolffian development on the other (Grumbach, Van Wyk, & Wilkins, 1955), we may see that the effects of the testis duct-organizer substances may be unilateral. Secondly, it is clear that in the complete absence of functional testes a male fetus will differentiate in the female direction. Thirdly, and perhaps most importantly, we now see that female duct differentiation will proceed normally in the absence of any hormonal influence, whereas normal male differentiation requires the addition of two chemical substances secreted by the functional testes.

External Genitalia

At approximately the same time that the fetal duct systems are being organized, the external genital structures are also developing. The external genitals in their primitive fetal state consist primarily of the genital tubercle. The anatomical differentiation of male external genitalia is dependent on the presence of androgenic hormone produced by the fetal testes. The male sex hormone stimulates the genital tubercle to form a penis. Additional androgenic affects include the formation of the scrotum, which houses the testes when they descend from the abdomen, normally before birth.

The source of the fetal androgenic hormone is thought to be a specialized cellular component of the testes called the *interstitial cells of Leydig*. Fetal testes have been shown capable of synthesizing testosterone in vitro from chemical precursors (Avecado, Axelrod, Ishikawa, & Takaki, 1963). A hormone of pregnancy (chorionic gonadotropin) secreted by the mother probably has a cell-stimulating effect on the fetal testes and may thereby aid in androgen production and thus also in the development of external male morphology.

Unlike male differentiation of the primitive genital structures, which is dependent on androgenic hormone and also on maternal hormones secreted during pregnancy, the expression of a female external genital appearance will proceed in the absence of any hormonal influences. In contrast to male external sexual morphogenesis, therefore, the female sexual anatomy will develop without the intervention of any other physiological or chemical entity. Thus, the genital tubercle will transform into the clitoris and the labia characteristic of anatomically normal females.

The Role of Gonadal Hormones

In general terms, it appears that once the gonads have developed in the second month of fetal life, the direction of future anatomical differentiation will be controlled by the presence or absence of functional testes, rather than by the genetic sex of the organism. In mammals, male anatomy is brought about by something added to the system (androgen) by the male gonads and will not be expressed if pathology or experimental manipulations upset the fetal environment provided by the testes (Jost, 1958). Mammalian female anatomy, on the other hand, appears to be a natural expression of fetal growth that will proceed in genetic females despite surgical removal of the gonads. Note, however, that if androgens are added to the intrauterine environment of a female fetus, masculinization of a genetic female may occur.

Critical period. In addition to the presence or absence of particular chemical substances acting as anatomical sex determinants, the timing, or appearance of these substances at various periods in fetal development may also be crucial to normal sexual morphogenesis. Indeed, there appears to be a critical period in the development of male or female sexual anatomy and functioning that will have profound effects on fetal development and later adult sexual physiology and, to a great extent, on sex-related behaviors.

Rabbit: The time of appearance of this critical developmental stage, however, may vary from species to species. In the male rabbit, if removal of the testes (castration) is accomplished before embryonic Day 21, there will be a complete feminization of the duct system and external genitalia. If castration is delayed until embryonic Day 24, however, masculine differentiation will proceed unimpaired; presumably, the critical developmental period for duct system and external genital differentiation in this species has passed (Jost, 1958).

Guinea pig: Similar findings have been obtained from the experimental alteration of the uterine environment of pregnant guinea pigs. If male sex hormone (androgen) is given to pregnant animals during a particular phase of fetal development, masculinization of a female fetus will result. No significant effects are obtained, however, in the male fetus, since androgenic influences are already present. The female guinea pig subjected to male hormone treatment in utero is typically born with male external genitalia, while the gonad and duct systems are female in nature. Of particular interest is the finding that in addition to obvious physiological abnormalities, the sexual behavior of these animals in adulthood may resemble that of normal males more than normal females (Phoenix, Goy, Gerall, & Young, 1959).

Rat: That such a critical period for behavioral organization takes place has also been demonstrated in the rat. The critical period of anatomical sexual differentiation, like that for the rabbit and the guinea pig, begins prenatally. Unlike these two species, however, the process appears to extend into neonatal life, since experimental alterations of the internal hormonal environment of neonate rats (from birth to 10 days of age) may precipitate profound physiological and behavioral abnormalities in adulthood.

Several studies have demonstrated that the normal patterns of sexual behavior in the adult rat may be significantly disturbed by neonatal castration or hormonal treatment. Barraclough and Gorski (1962), for example, found that testosterone, the male sex hormone, if administered to 5-day-old female rats, could permanently impair sexual cycling, rendering them anovulatory, sexually unreceptive, and sterile. Thus, early postnatal hormonal imbalances, such as shown in these animals, can produce a significant disruption of the delicate hormonal regulation of adult animals, and as we shall see in subsequent sections, behavioral aberrations also may be precipitated by upsetting the internal environment of an organism during this important phase of development.

Other studies serve to reinforce the notion that early hormonal dysfunctions can lead to permanent behavioral abnormalities. Whalen and Nadler (1963) injected 4-day-old female rats with estrogen, a female sex hormone. In adulthood, there were no drastic physiological changes in these female rats, but behaviorally they were less sexually receptive and responded less to injections of the female sex hormones, estrogen, and progesterone. The female sex hormones produced a higher frequency of mating when injected in normal adult female rats than in the neonatally treated female rats.

In a similar study, Grady and Phoenix (1963) castrated male rats at various ages ranging from 1 to 90 days. At 120 days they injected all the animals with estrogen and progesterone and then tested for female-type behavior patterns in response to mounting by intact males. As expected, most of the experimental animals displayed some femininelike response characteristics in response to mounting by a male. The most profound effects, however, were seen in those males castrated on or before the fifth day of life. These males, in particular, appeared to develop and permanently retain femalelike response characteristics as opposed to the more transitory effects of the female hormones observed in those rats castrated as late as Day 10.

Implications: The evidence presented above suggests that in addition to the precise and intricate regulation of hormone concentration that must exist in fetal life in order to insure optimal anatomical sexual differentiation, in some species similar requirements must be met in early neonatal life. It has been shown that physiological functions and behavioral characteristics of males and females alike may be manipulated by early disruption of hormonal homeostasis. It is important also to emphasize again the timing of the neonatal critical period phenomenon, since this interesting developmental phase may vary from species to species and may also be relatively brief (i.e., 5 days in the rat).

It seems that in addition to the anatomical sexual differentiation occurring in fetal life, there is also a behavioral differentiation that is dependent on hormonal levels during early neonatal life. Male and female behavioral traits, at least in rodent species (rabbit, guinea pig, rat), appear to be determined very early in life and do not appear to be a function of learning experiences. That the potential for later sex-related behavior patterns is programmed during prenatal or early neonatal life, and is not merely a result of external sexual appearance, is a crucial point. The relative importance of such early programming to the sexual behavior of humans, however, is not so clearly demonstrable.

Sexing (or programming) the hypothalamus. Early hormonal conditions during a specific critical period of nervous system development have been shown to influence various hypothalamic nuclei so that the hypothalamus will function in certain ways that conform either to male or female physiological and behavioral repertoires. It was originally thought that it was the pituitary gland that differed in males and females. Pfeiffer (1936) showed this not to be the case by transplanting pituitaries between male and female animals without altering sexual functioning. Segal and Johnson (1959) have even taken the pituitaries from neonatally androgen-treated female rats who were rendered anovulatory, and transplanted them near the hypothalamus of hypophysectomized female rats. Their procedure completely reinstated the reproductive processes of the female hosts. It has been suggested, therefore, that the early androgen treatments of the donor rats did not disrupt pituitary functioning, but rather had changed the organization of hypothalamic tissue, making it unable to function correctly in the control of the pituitary. Indeed, it appears that the hypothalamus of the androgen-treated females had been "sexed" or programmed inappropriately in terms of pituitary control.

Cyclicity: It has been suggested by Levine and Mullins (1964) that the neural mechanism, i.e., the hypothalamus, controlling gonadotropin release in adulthood will develop in a cyclic manner in the genetic female in the absence of circulating levels of androgens during a critical developmental phase of the CNS. In contrast, in the genetic male the neural processes triggering gonadotropin release will develop acyclically as a consequence of androgen hormones during a critical period of fetal development. Thus, the organization of responsible neural mechanisms for adult sexual functioning appears to be initiated by the presence or absence of androgenic hormones at appropriate times during the development of mammalian organisms.

Behavior: There is now direct evidence from animal studies that sex hormones do, in fact, act on the hypothalamus. By implanting microgram quantities of estrogen directly into the hypothalamus of female cats, Michael (1961) was able to induce sustained sexual receptivity without any other physiological signs of estrus (heat, the period of maximum sexual receptivity in the female). In an experiment similar to that of Michael's, Fisher (1956) injected minute amounts of testosterone directly into the medial preoptic region of the hypothalamus of rats. In males and females alike, central injections of testosterone elicited varying degrees of maternal behavior (pup carrying, pup retrieval, nest building). If, on the other hand, testosterone was injected into the more lateral aspects of the preoptic region, species typical male sexual behaviors could be elicited in male and female rats alike (mounting, intromission, ejaculatory thrust, even by the female). Fisher's results seem to indicate that within the hypothalamus there may be smaller regions that respond along male and female lines. How the neural regions contribute to the behavioral repertoire of adult mammals, however, is not clear.

Gonadotropin release: The control of gonadotropin release by the anterior pituitary has likewise been linked to the integrity of specific regions of the hypothalamus. Flerko and Szentagothai (1951) authographed small ovarian fragments into the anterior hypothamalus of female rats. Their results showed a significant decrease in uterine weight in all animals tested, indicating a decline in production of certain gonadotropins by the pituitary. Similar results have been obtained by placing crystalline estrogens near the arcuate nucleus of the hypothalamus. Flerko and Szentagothai (1957) autographed small ovarian fragments into the anterior hypothalamus of female rats. Their results showed a that circulating sex hormones inhibit the production of releasing factors by the hypothalamus, which otherwise stimulate the production of anterior pituitary gonadotropins; the ovarian graft or hormones would, therefore, appear to be inhibiting RF production (see Chapter 11).

Autoradiography: The results of autoradiographic experimentation also indicate that circulating levels of sex hormones act on various hypothalamic nuclei. Glassock and Michael (1962) injected an estrogenic hormone subcutaneously into ovariectomized cats and found significant and reliable uptake of the compound in the anterior, preoptic, and arcuate nuclei of the hypothalamus (also see Levine & Mullins, 1964). Evidence of this kind indicates that certain neurons of the hypothalamus, that facilitate behavioral estrus, act in response to gonadal hormones, which normally circulate in the bloodstream of adult mammals. When one considers this evidence, as well as that of Sawyer and Robinson (1956) showing permanent anestrus subsequent to anterior hypothalamic lesions, it becomes clear that the hypothalamus functions as a control region for gonadotropin release by the anterior pituitary, and as a mediator for specific sexual behaviors.

Conclusions: The data available on hypothalamic involvement in sexual behavior indicates that the neural substrates for male and female physiological and behavioral processes are present in the hypothalamus of both sexes (Fisher, 1956). Further, certain nuclei in the hypothalamus are highly responsive to circulating levels of sex hormones (Flerko & Szentagothai, 1957; Glassock & Michael, 1962), and may thereby regulate, via RF release, levels of pituitary gland hormones. Other limbic system structures have also been shown by autoradiography to selectively take up sex hormones; these include prepyriform cortex, olfactory tubercle, septal region, preoptic area, amygdala, and stria terminalis (Pfaff, 1968; Stumpf, 1968). These structures may also have a role in the neuroendocrine integration of gonadal and sexual functions.

It may be that the presence of testicular androgens in the male at a critical phase of development programs hypothalamic nuclei in a way that will insure normal male behavior patterns and acyclic hormone secretions in adulthood. In the absence of testicular hormones in the female of the species, these nuclear regions of the hypothalamus may respond in a cyclic manner, thus insuring the expression of female physiology and response characteristics in adulthood. Hormones circulating in a growing organism may interact with neural tissue in specific regions of the hypothalamus. As they interact, the functional responsive thresholds for the hypothalamic nuclei in males and females may come to differ significantly. As a result of varying response characteristics of these nuclear groups, afferent and efferent pathways related to pituitary functioning as well as to other neural regions involved in sexual behavior, i.e., amygdala, septal region, may vary between the two sexes. Such events could thereby represent the neurological bases for sexual dimorphism, or at least, the potential for the observed physiological and behavioral differences in males and females. Consistent with this hypothesis is the recent discovery of differences between the synaptic connections found in the preoptic areas of male and female rats (Raisman & Field, 1971). The percentage of synaptic terminations on different parts of the dendrites of preoptic neurons differed between the sexes. However, the physiological and behavioral implications of this finding remain to be demonstrated.

Reticular formation. The hypothalamus is not the only neural site sensitive to circulating gonadal hormones, nor is it necessarily the only structure sensitized by gonadal hormones during critical developmental periods. Recently, mesencephalic reticular formation placements of progesterone were found most effective for the production of lordosis (the posture assumed by a female animal in heat when she is "presenting" to a male for insertion of the penis) in estrogen-primed rats (Ross, Claybaugh, Clemens & Gorski, 1971). Consistent with this finding is the report that systemically administered radioactive progesterone concentrates in highest levels in the mesencephalon (Whalen &

Luttge, 1971a). However, more recently, progesterone has been found to concentrate in several hypothalamic nuclei of the guinea pig (Sar & Stumpf, 1973).

Spinal cord. Hart (1967) has shown that gonadal hormones potentiate sexual reflexes organized at the level of the spinal cord. The male rat can still display these penile reflexes after spinal cord transection. Following castration, however, the frequency of these responses declines. Precastration levels of these penile reflexes can be reinstated by systemic administration of testosterone or by implantation of testosterone into the spinal cord (Hart & Haugen, 1968).

Male sex hormones appear to have a role in the early organization of spinal sexual reflexes, as well as in the facilitation of these reflexes in adult males. Hart (1968) has found that castration of male rats at 4 days of age results in a deficiency of spinal cord mediated penile reflexes. Moreover, testosterone injection in adulthood did not reinstate these reflexes. In contrast to the data on the male rat, Hart (1969) has failed to find evidence that estrogen and progesterone facilitate lordosislike postural reflexes mediated by the spinal cord in female rats. The frequency of these responses is not altered by castration or by hormone administration.

PUBERTY

Little is known of the basic controlling mechanisms influencing the onset of puberty. Low levels of gonadotropins are found in the blood of children. Then, preceding the clinical signs of puberty, a rise in circulating gonadotropins to postpubertal levels is found. However, the timing mechanism regulating this surge of gonadotropin secretion is not understood. Pathological conditions in the human involving the pineal gland, hypothalamus, or pituitary gland may accelerate or delay pubertal onset, suggesting some involvement of these structures.

It seems likely that the time of puberty is primarily under genetic control. Numerous other influences, however, such as temperature and diet have been shown to have some affect (Money & Ehrhardt, 1972). The release of anterior pituitary gonadotropins is thought to be greatest at the onset of puberty. Gonadotropin release then continues cyclically in females or acyclically in males throughout the reproductive life of the organism. Prior to pubescence, however, the levels of gonadotropic hormones and of sex hormones are quite low (Nathanson, Towne, & Aub, 1942), although detectable traces can be observed when sensitive techniques are employed (Barr, Diczfalusy, & Tillinger, 1961; Fitschen & Clayton, 1965; Frasier & Horton, 1966; Odell, Ross, & Rayford, 1967). The exact role for the gonadotropins and sex hormones in prepubertal life remains somewhat unclear, since the secretion of either may occur in the absence of the rapid growth characteristic of puberty.

Puberty may result from a release from some chemical or higher neural inhibition of the hypothalamic nuclei responsible for gonadotropin secretion.

Since hypogonadal children manifest an earlier rise in gonadotropins than normal children, some investigators have suggested that chemicals produced by prepubertal testes or ovaries exert a restraining influence upon gonadotropic activity (Donovan & Van Der Werff Ten Bosch, 1965). At the onset of puberty in the human, LH (or ICSH) will act directly on the immature cells of the ovaries or testes, ultimately bringing them to an estrogen or androgen secretory capacity.

In the human female, the onset of puberty occurs in Western civilization between about 11 and 15 years of age, with first menstruation at about 13. In males, the average is also about 13 years of age; this is the time of the beginning of penile enlargement, the growth of pubic hair, and the growth spurt in height. Interestingly, the age of puberty has been progressively lowering during the last 150 years (Tanner, 1962). Data from Northern Europe, Great Britain, and the United States show a reduction of the age of pubertal onset from about 17 years of age to 13 years of age between 1830 and 1960. Improvements in nutrition and public health may account for much of this change, since an increase in adult height has paralleled the lowering of the age of puberty. This reduction in the age of puberty is now forcing changes in our political and cultural system. In many countries the voting age and legal age of maturity have been reduced, marriages are taking place earlier, and teenage sexuality is becoming more acceptable, especially with the advent of more effective means of conception control.

ENDOCRINOLOGY OF THE MALE

This discussion of the human male reproductive system will be concerned mainly with those structures closely aligned with hormone and sperm production. The testes, the sites of both hormone and sperm manufacture, are lodged in a pouchlike structure called the *scrotum* (Figures 12.2 and 12.3). The testes normally descend from the abdominal cavity, which serves as the site of testicular development during fetal life. On occasion, however, the testes will fail to descend and thereby remain in the abdominal region. As a consequence of this maldescent, known as *cryptorchidism*, the testes are subjected to the higher body temperature, which eventually creates severe testicular disorganization. Sperm production and hormone secretions are markedly reduced. This then may drastically alter subsequent sexual development (Charney, Conston, & Meranze, 1952).

Each testis is composed of a small number of *seminiferous tubules*, which are the source of sperm manufacture. Once formed, sperm cells empty into a storage are called the *epididymus.* The sperm are then transported through the *vas deferens* to the *ejaculatory duct*, which passes through the prostate gland, and then on through the *penis* in the *urethra* to exit from the body. Along the way, a variety of glands add their secretions to the sperm. These include the seminal vesicles, the prostate gland, and Cowper's gland. These various secretions add bulk and nutritive material to the sperm. The fluid, now containing both sperm and these secretions, is called *semen.*

Penis

The penis, of course, is the organ of intromission that permits the deposition of semen within the reproductive system of the female. The penis also has other reproductive functions, in that it is a source of pleasurable sexual stimulation of the male and female both, thus encouraging sexual congress and fertilization. The penis also aids the male in orienting towards the female as well as providing the pleasurable sexual stimulation to the male that maintains sexual arousal and leads to ejaculation. At least in some mammals, sensory feedback from the penis is critically important, in previously unsuspected ways, to male sexual behavior. For instance, in the cat, severing the dorsal nerves of the penis, which desensitizes the glans penis (the "head" of the penis), but does not interfere with erection, disorients the male, and results in the appearance of a seasonal decline of sexual behavior. The male cats show no observable decrease in sexual motivation during most of the year, but are disoriented. They mount the female at the wrong location and are unable to insert the penis. They also show a pronounced decline in sexual interest in the fall. Such a decline is not found in the unaltered male domestic cat. Thus a latent breeding season appears when penile sensory feedback is interrupted (Aronson & Cooper, 1966). These data point to the more subtle roles played by specific sensory factors in sexual behavior. Castration in the male rat has been shown to result in a loss of the deep folds and papillae from the glans penis. These folds and papillae are presumed to mediate glans sensitivity to sexual stimulation, and this loss after castration may have a role in the decline in sexual behavior seen in castrated animals (Beach & Levinson, 1950). These studies in rats and cats point out the importance of sensory feedback from the penis in maintaining sexual arousal.

Vas Deferens

A vasectomy is a procedure in which the vas deferens is sectioned or tied off bilaterally. This prevents the sperm from traveling in the vas and urethra through the penis. A vasectomized male still emits a seminal discharge at orgasm, but one lacking in sperm. This procedure has acquired considerable popularity as a means of contraception in the human male. It is a relatively simple and inexpensive operation, which can be completed under local anesthesia in a physician's office. The popularity of vasectomy has increased in the last few years; however, questions about the side effects of this procedure are only now being answered. Sexual behavior in vasectomized rhesus monkeys during the first postsurgical month has been found normal (Phoenix, 1973). Androgen levels have also been found normal for the first 18 months following surgery in the rhesus monkey (Resko & Phoenix, 1972), and for one month in humans (Bunge, 1972). However, there is one report of reductions in steroid levels and of gross pathology, including cyst formation, following vasectomy in immature rats

(Alexander & Sackler, 1973; Sackler, Weltman, Pandhli, & Schwartz, 1973). Although the implications of these data on immature rats are unclear, vasectomy does seem to be a simple, effective, safe, and satisfactory means of birth control.

The Testes

The testes are oval organs consisting of one to three coils of seminiferous tubules, each of which is 30-70 cm long and 150-250 micra in diameter. The testes perform two major complementary functions: the proliferation of spermatazoa and the secretion of steroid hormones.

Spermatogenesis. The transformation of a primitive sperm cell (called a *spermatogonium*) through the various stages of development resulting in a mature spermatozoon, is called *spermatogenesis*. During spermatogenesis two processes allow the transformation to occur. The first process involves a reduction by meiosis in the number of chromosomes in each primitive sperm cell from 46 to 23. The second process involves gradual cytoplasmic and structural growth.

The time required for complete spermatogenesis in man is about 74 days (Heller & Clermont, 1963). It has also been shown that the duration of spermatogenesis remains relatively fixed in man, as well as in other species, and that the rate of sperm production is not influenced by steroid or gonadotropic hormones. The overall yield of mature sperm cells, however, is dependent on proper levels of androgenic hormones (Clermont, 1962). There are thus two aspects of spermatogenesis: the rate of sperm formation which appears to remain relatively constant and the yield or number of viable spermatozoa produced from the primitive sperm cells, which is sensitive to hormone levels. By way of evidence, the rate component of spermatogenesis has been shown to be impervious to androgen therapy or hypophysectomy; whereas the yield can be influenced markedly by gonadotropin concentrations and androgenic hormones, as well as by nutritional status, temperature, light cycles, and other physical events (Clermont & Harvey, 1965).

Testicular steroid biochemistry. There is general agreement that the interstitial cells of Leydig, a second major type of cell found in the testes, in addition to the seminiferous tubules, are the major source of testicular androgens. Histochemical tests have confirmed this by showing that the enzyme 3-β-hydroxysteroid-dehydrogenase, which is essential for androgen biosynthesis, is present in the interstitial cells (Shikita & Tamaoki, 1965). Other data, however, show that isolated seminiferous tubules can also accomplish the conversion of progesterone to testosterone (Christenson & Mason, 1965). Whether this hormonal conversion capacity emanates from the seminiferous tubules per se, or from yet a third cell type found within the tubules, called *Sertoli cells*, remains to be shown. Sertoli cells have been found to possess appropriate organelles for steroid biosynthesis (Klinefelter, Reifenstein, & Albright, 1942), and since Sertoli cell tumors have occasionally resulted in high levels of circulating estrogens (Lipsett & Korenman, 1964) these cells may very well constitute an essential part of the hormone production capacity of the testes.

As mentioned in the preceding paragraph, estrogen production has also been associated with testicular functioning. Estrogens have been isolated from the testes of many species including humans, but the total estrogen content in the male is only about one-tenth of that found in the female. The exact locus of estrogen production, however, remains unclear, although the Sertoli cells of the seminiferous tubules seem likely candidates.

Physiological effects of androgens. The androgens are the principal compounds that direct the development of the secondary sexual characteristics in the male and maintain the functional integrity of the internal reproductive structures. The most pronounced general effects of androgenic hormones are the promotion of protein anabolism (cell buildup). The specific physical effects of androgens, which may be described as masculinizing, are the growth of body hair, a deep voice, a large skeletal configuration, and increased activity of sebaceous (oil) glands (Strauss & Pochi, 1963). Additionally, androgens provide a suitable environment for sperm production by the seminiferous tubules.

Androgens also are important for the maintenance of sexual potency. If castration occurs prior to puberty or if the testes fail to mature normally, pubertal development will not take place. When sexual development is curtailed for any reason, a condition known as *eunichoidism* will ensue. Eunichs are said to be characterized by a minimal sex drive, impotence, shyness, and introversion. Physically, they have an absence of pubic hair, no facial hair, and small testes and penis. Despite the fact that the physiological characteristics of eunichs can be linked to androgen deficiencies, it is not certain that the behavioral differences that these individuals also exhibit are directly related to hormonal deficiencies. Again, although it is tempting to make such inferences, one must not dismiss the cultural pressures that tend to create or exaggerate behavioral problems in physically aberrant individuals.

On the other hand, androgen replacement therapy will reinstate normal physical and sexual appearance. For example, daily administration of testosterone will lead to an increase in body weight and muscle bulk, growth of the penis, growth of pubic hair, and a return of sexual interests. Evidence of this sort, available from case histories, points strongly to androgen maintenance of sexual physiology and behavior.

The control of testicular functions. The two principal processes subserved by the testes, namely spermatogenesis and hormone secretion, are under the direct control of gonadotropic hormones from the anterior lobe of the pituitary gland (Chapter 11). Among the most important gonadotropins are follicle-stimulating hormone (FSH) and interstitial-cell-stimulating hormone (ICSH). FSH acts on the seminiferous tubules to promote the proliferation of sperm cells, whereas ICSH induces the Leydig cells to secrete androgens.

A dramatic example of pituitary control over testicular processes is seen upon hypophysectomy of adult mammals. Shortly following the removal or destruction of the anterior pituitary there is a complete absence of circulating levels of FSH and ICSH. As a result of diminished gonadotropins, spermatogenesis and testosterone production are curtailed. ICSH replacement therapy, however, may reinstate complete androgen secretion by the testes (Squire, 1963) and may initiate spermatogenesis, but only marginally. Normal sperm production, unlike androgen secretion, requires the combined action of FSH and ICSH (Lostroh, 1962). Androgens also stimulate the seminiferous tubules. Thus, ICSH and FSH secreted by the anterior pituitary will receive added support in bringing the seminiferous tubules to their full spermatogenic potential.

The continued control and balance of gonadotropins secreted by the anterior pituitary throughout male reproductive life involves a reciprocal relationship with testicular processes. Under normal conditions a negative feedback loop is established between testicular activity and anterior pituitary processes. As testosterone production begins to fall below normal levels, the anterior pituitary releases increased amounts of ICSH. Once a proper testosterone balance is achieved, ICSH levels drop off by a direct inhibitory action of testosterone, thereby decreasing Leydig cell activity. In a similar fashion, a negative feedback mechanism is thought to exist for sperm production and FSH secretion, but the exact nature of the relationship is somewhat unclear at present (see the "inhibin" theory below).

The relationship between the testes and the anterior pituitary in the homeostatic control of reproductive processes may be illustrated by a loss of testicular functioning. In castration, for example, the loss of the testes results in a cessation of both androgen secretion and sperm production. Since a negative feedback loop exists between circulating levels of androgens as well as sperm production and the release of gonadotropins, it should not be surprising that testicular loss is followed by the pituitary production of high levels of FSH and ICSH. The ICSH increase is attributed to a loss of androgen inhibition of the anterior pituitary, causing marked secretion of ICSH in a vain attempt to stimulate the missing Leydig cells and to bring androgen levels back to normal. The increase in FSH release by the pituitary following castration, however, is not so easily explained.

One theory attempting to explain the feedback mechanism operable between sperm production and anterior pituitary release of FSH proposes that the germinal epithelium of the seminiferous tubules secretes a nonsteroidal substance that has been named "inhibin." This substance, it is suggested, then inhibits the gonadotropin, FSH (McCulloch, 1932). Thus, subsequent to castration, loss of the seminiferous tubules involves a loss of inhibin, which then releases the pituitary from a partial state of inhibition, resulting in excessive secretion of FSH.

The Rebound Effect Following Androgen Therapy

When daily injections of testosterone are given to intact males, testicular processes are altered. The testosterone effect is thought to occur by a gradual inhibition of the pituitary gonadotropin, ICSH, which leads to a total suppression of Leydig cell activity and also a partial suppression of seminiferous tubule activity. The knowledge of the pituitary and testicular suppression following large doses of testosterone has been important in treating some cases of male sterility. Where spermatogenesis is subnormal, extensive testosterone therapy may result in a rebound overproduction of mature spermatozoa once the drug is discontinued (Heller, Nelson, Hill, Henderson, Maddock, Jungck, Paulgen, & Mortimore, 1950). Although the physiological events taking place in the rebound phenomenon are not certain, it may be that a temporary suppression of FSH secretion allows the seminiferous tubules to recuperate and regain added spermatogenic power. Similar forms of spermatogenic suppression have been reported with the phenothiazine tranquilizers; Shader and Grinspoon (1967) found a reduction in sperm production in male schizophrenics receiving phenothiazine drugs.

Pharmacological Uses of the Androgens

Androgen therapy is most commonly employed in cases of deficient endocrine functioning by the testes. A failure of the testes to secrete normal levels of androgens at the expected time of pubertal change may necessitate large daily doses of synthetic androgens such as testosterone. Similar justification for androgen replacement therapy would, of course, be applicable to individuals who have been castrated prepubertally.

In recent years androgen therapy has been applied to aging males manifesting the male counterpart to female menopause, the climacteric. Climacteric is suspected in older males when several physical symptoms appear: reduced sexual interest, a lessening of muscular size and strength, an increase in urinary gonadotropins, and a decrease in the volume of semen and total sperm count. Androgen administered to these individuals has, on occasion, been effective in ameliorating many of these physical signs.

Androgen therapy has also been used effectively in the treatment of certain classes of anemia (Gardner & Pringle, 1961), to promote growth in cases of dwarfism (Ray, Kirchuink, Waxman, & Kelley, 1965), and as an agent for treating catabolic states (loss of living cells) which often follow major injuries, surgical operations, and severe illnesses. Androgens are thought to promote recovery by facilitating the incorporation of amino acids into proteins. Currently, there is said to be considerable use of these steroids by athletes (weight lifters, body builders, and others) to increase muscle buildup, and, supposedly, athletic ability. Not surprisingly, considerable controversy surrounds this issue, and evidence of the use of androgens is sufficient to disqualify one from competition (Wade, 1972).

ENDOCRINOLOGY OF THE FEMALE

The female reproductive system is engaged in several different processes. Therefore, a consideration of how the primary, as well as the secondary, sexual organs relate to hormone production, proliferation of mature ova, pregnancy, and lactation will be provided. The main internal structures of the female reproductive system include the ovaries, fallopian tubes, uterus, and vagina. The primary external structures are the clitoris and the labia (Figures 12.2 and 12.3).

The Ovary

The ovary is a complex organ. Figure 12.4 shows the structures commonly observed in the ovary during the monthly cycle of the female. Among these are the growing follicle, the maturing follicle, a recent corpus luteum, a retrogressing corpus luteum and an atretic follicle. Each of these ovarian structures represents an important aspect of female reproductive cycling, as will be shown in the subsequent discussion.

The growing follicle. The ovaries are composed of a central connective portion through which blood vessels enter and a cortical portion concerned mainly with two functions: (1) the development of mature ova or germ cells; and (2) the secretion of ovarian hormones. During fetal life, the primitive ova differentiate from the germinal epithelium on the ovary and migrate to the ovarian cortex. The ova are then surrounded by granulosa cells and become what are known as *primary follicles.*

At birth, a human female may possess up to 300,000 primary follicles, each of which has the potential to expel a mature ovum. As it turns out, however, most of these follicles never reach a sufficient level of maturation; during the entire reproductive life of a human female, only about 375 ova may actually be expelled.

The maturing follicle. At puberty, under the influence of the gonadotropic hormones of the anterior pituitary, the primary follicles begin to grow. The maturation of the follicles is accomplished by the proliferation of two cell types around the outside of the follicle. The granular or granulosa cells first increase in number and are then engulfed by successive layers of *theca cells*. The theca cells

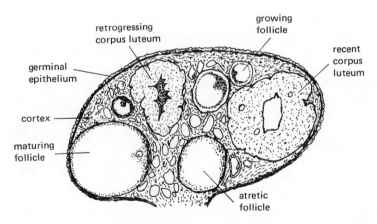

FIGURE 12.4. Structure of the ovary.

eventually begin to secrete a substance called follicular fluid, which gradually fills the internal space of the follicle. The theca and granulosa cells, then, are responsible for the secretion of ovarian steroidal hormones.

Although ovulation has not been observed, it is thought to occur in the following manner: as follicular fluid continues to exude into the follicle, the hydrostatic pressure within progressively reaches a high critical point. This causes the surface of the follicle to necrose, give way, causing a rupture of the follicular wall. The ovum is then forced free and escapes into the peritoneum, eventually finding its way to the adjacent opening of the ipsilateral fallopian tube.

The corpus luteum. Within a few hours after ovulation, the granulosa and theca cells of the ovarian (graffian) follicle take on a yellow color in a process called *luteinization*, which is also under the control of gonadotropic hormones. Henceforth, the remaining ovarian follicle (minus its ova) is referred to as the *corpus luteum*. Under the influence of anterior pituitary gonadotropins, the corpus luteum secretes large amounts of estrogen and also a second gonadal hormone called *progesterone*. A peak stage of development is reached by the corpus luteum about 7 days after ovulation. Afterwards, the corpus luteum regresses and decreases its output of sex hormones. Finally, about 2 weeks following ovulation, the secretory capacity of the corpus luteum is lost and the structure is replaced by connective tissue. The follicular structure is henceforth referred to as an *atretic follicle*. The principal cause of corpus luteum regression is due to a gradual decline in circulating levels of gonadotropic hormones (especially LH, which is the result of an inhibition of LH output by progesterone).

The development of the mature ovum. Coincident with the development of the primary follicle at birth, immature ova develop within the follicle. Beginning at the onset of puberty, under the influence of gonadotropic hormones, the primary follicles periodically mature. During this period, the immature ovum (diploidal) undergoes a developmental process whereby it becomes a mature ovum (haploidal).

The Physiological Actions of the Principal Ovarian Steroids

Estrogen. The physiological effects of estrogen may be divided into two classes: those effects dealing specifically with modifications in the physical characteristics of the reproductive system; and those effects evidenced as generalized physical changes not directly related to reproductive processes. The specific actions of estrogen on the reproductive system of the female are directed at growth and development in preparation for pregnancy. One may speak of estrogen as exerting a building up or anabolic effect on reproductive tissue, especially the uterus and vagina.

The anabolic action of estrogen in the growth of the endometrium or lining of the uterus is typified by an increase in water content, electrolytes, proteins, nucleotides, and enzymes. The vaginal mucosa becomes thicker and cornified or hardened and the vagina becomes more acidic, while the cervix takes on a watery or mucuslike appearance, becoming more susceptible to sperm penetration. The vaginal "sweating phenomenon" also appears to be dependent on estrogenic compounds, since a loss of estrogen secretions tends to decrease the lubricating efficiency of the vagina (Masters & Johnson, 1966).

In addition to the modifications of the primary reproductive anatomy, estrogen also acts on the secondary reproductive anatomy of the female. The initial stimulation of breast growth and subsequent fat deposition in the breasts, for example, are the result of estrogenic action. The priming of the breasts for lactation, too, is partially the work of estrogens.

The generalized results of exposure to estrogen may be described as *feminizing*. The smaller physical size of females, for example, is produced by an estrogen retardation of bone growth in the pubertal female. Estrogen also tends to increase the water content and thickness of the skin creating a skin appearance characteristic of females. The presence of estrogen in the female has a further feminizing effect by simply antagonizing the masculinizing actions of androgens (which are also present in small quantities in the female).

Progesterone. The overall action of progesterone is to antagonize the proliferation of reproductive tissue initiated by estrogens. Therefore, progesterone will inhibit the growth of the uterine endometrium, changing it to a secretory rather than a proliferating structure. The cervix, too, will respond to progesterone and become less mucuslike, thereby decreasing the probability of sperm penetration. Metabolic analyses have shown that progesterone exerts a profound protein catabolic action as evidenced by significant increases in urinary nitrogen secretion (Landau & Lugibih, 1961). Thus, the anabolic effects of estrogen, which promote cell growth, are held in check by subsequent secretions of progesterone, which by catabolic action tends to decrease the growth of reproductive tissue. In this manner a homeostatic balance of reproductive tissue growth may be obtained.

The Menstrual Cycle

Human female sexual physiology is constantly changing in a cyclical manner. This cycle, called the menstrual cycle, averages about 28 days. Figure 12.5 is a diagrammatic representation showing the changes, throughout the menstrual cycle, in levels of ovarian and gonadotropic hormones, as well as the major structural modifications in the most important reproductive tissues.

The follicular phase. Beginning at Day 1 in the menstrual cycle (the first day of menstrual flow) the anterior pituitary releases follicle-stimulating hormone (FSH) in response to depressed levels of estrogen. FSH promotes ovarian follicular proliferation and the maturation of the primary follicle. Soon thereafter the follicle secretes estrogen in progressively increasing amounts reaching a high point at around Day 14. During this proliferative stage, in response to estrogen, the reproductive tissues grow and develop.

As estrogen production reaches a high level, the estrogen inhibits the release of FSH and also promotes the release of a second gonadotropin, called *luteinizing*

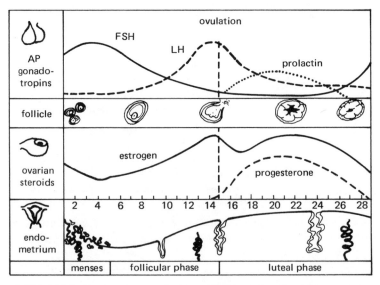

FIGURE 12.5. Hormonal control of menstruation. (Reprinted by permission from G. M. Riley, *Gynecological Endocrinology*. Copyright 1959 by Harper & Row, Publishers.)

hormone (LH). LH secretion thus begins in appreciable amounts around Day 8 and reaches a peak at Day 14. The action of the LH, on an ovary previously "primed" by FSH and estrogen is to "trigger" ovulation (at about day 14), and to promote the creation of the corpus luteum, and the continued growth of reproductive tissues. Therefore, following the follicular phase of the menstrual cycle (Days 1–14), is the onset of the luteal phase, which will extend between Days 14 and 28.

Ovulation and receptivity. In subhuman species, except possibly for a few higher primates, copulation is permitted by the female only around the time of ovulation (estrus). Even in the human female, the time of ovulation appears to coincide with a period of heightened sexual drive. In some species (rabbit, cat) ovulation is actually induced at the time of estrus by copulation. Even in the human, coitus at about the midpoint of the menstrual cycle may actually induce ovulation, and facilitate fertilization. It thus appears that the particular hormonal state existing at ovulation is especially capable of activating neural sex drive mechanisms. Recent data even suggest a role for the hypothalamic releasing factor for LH in this phenomenon. In the female rat, administration of LH-releasing factor has been shown to elicit mating behavior (apparently by a direct action on the nervous system) independently of its actions on LH and estrogen secretion (Moss & McCann, 1973).

The luteal phase. After ovulation has taken place, the ovarian follicle minus the ova is called the corpus luteum. The corpus luteum secretes both progesterone and estrogen. Progesterone will arrest the proliferation of reproductive tissue, add to its stability, and inhibit LH release. The stabilization effect of progesterone is especially marked on the uterine endometrium, since successful implantation of the immature embryo in the uterus is dependent on a stable uterine environment.

The corpus luteum is normally maintained in the ovary for about 2 weeks after ovulation. If pregnancy has not occurred by about Day 23 of the menstrual cycle, the corpus luteum will begin to regress and thereby lose its capacity to secrete progesterone and estrogen (the regression is due to the inhibition of LH by progesterone). When, at this time, the estrogen and progesterone concentrations rapidly fall, two events take place: first, the uterus contracts with sufficient force to dislodge the endometrial tissue, which is then discharged through the vagina (Markee, 1940). This discharge of tissue beginning on about Day 29 (Day 1 of the next cycle) is referred to as *menstruation.* Secondly, the low level of estrogen again allows the anterior pituitary to release FSH and thus the proliferative stage is started once more and the cycle begins anew.

Ovarian-pituitary feedback. From the preceding discussion it should be apparent that the ovarian hormones are somehow determining anterior pituitary processes and vice versa. The overall scheme accounting for this interaction incorporates a negative and positive feedback oscillation within a pituitary-ovary axis, and can be explained in the following manner: the anterior lobe of the pituitary, when not affected by outside hormonal influences, i.e., in the absence of estrogens, will secrete FSH during the first stage of the menstrual cycle. At Day 8, in response to an increasing level of estrogen, LH is released in moderate concentrations, further enhancing the degree of follicular maturation. As estrogen levels reach a critical high point, a positive feedback effect on the pituitary release of LH and a negative feedback on pituitary FSH takes place such that by Day 14, LH concentrations are extremely high; whereas FSH concentrations are now falling progressively from its high point seen at Day 3. The LH surge at Days 8 through 14 will then bring about ovulation. Under the influence of LH at midcycle the corpus luteum begins secreting progesterone and also continuing amounts of estrogen. The progesterone inhibits LH, counteracting the actions of estrogen and leading to corpus luteum degeneration. As the concentration of LH gradually diminishes, a third gonadotropin is released called *prolactin* (luteotropic hormone, LTH). The major role of prolactin in the human is related to the secretory function of the breasts.

In the presence of the waning LH concentrations, the corpus luteum can continue to secrete progesterone and estrogen for only about another 14 days. With the regression of the corpus luteum at about Day 23 as a result of a much reduced LH secretion by the pituitary, estrogen and progesterone levels reach a critical low point, which once again allows the pituitary to increase its output of FSH.

Pregnancy

Subsequent to ovulation, the mature ovum is propelled down the fallopian tube by the ciliary action of the surface epithelium. Most often, fertilization of the ovum by a sperm cell will occur in the upper portions of the fallopian tube

TABLE 12.1

The Hormones of Pregnancy

Period	Uterus	Ovary
First 3 months (ovarian phase)	Chorionic gonadotropin (by trophoblastic cells)	Estrogen and progesterone (corpus luteum)
Last 6 months (placental phase)	Estrogen and progesterone (by placenta)	

and the growing cell mass will spend about 3 days in transit through the fallopian tube prior to entering the uterus (Table 12.1).

Chorionic gonadotropin. Shortly after fertilization, a layer of extra-embryonic tissue (not part of the embryo) on the outside of the embryo, called *trophoblastic cells*, will begin secreting a hormone found only in pregnancy called *chorionic gonadotropin*. A high plasma level of chorionic gonadotropin is found in the pregnant female immediately following fertilization and is sustained for about 12 weeks, at which time the secretory capacity of the trophoblastic cells will begin to gradually decline.

The principal action of chorionic gonadotropin is to mimic the effects of pituitary LH, and it is responsible, therefore, for maintaining the corpus luteum beyond the normal 28-day cycle. Two weeks following ovulation, then, FSH and LH concentrations have dropped as a function of the negative feedback effect from large amounts of estrogen and progesterone, now being secreted by a chorionic gonadotropin-maintained corpus luteum. Sustained production of prolactin, estrogen and progesterone will now interrupt the cyclicity of events normally observed during the human menstrual cycle. Instead, a new pattern of hormonal regulation, one characteristic of pregnancy, will be established.

Implantation.   As the fertilized egg enters the uterus, it will migrate along the uterine wall. After 4 or 5 days the growing organism will attach itself to the uterine endometrium in a process called *implantation*. During the process of implantation, the trophoblastic cells secrete an enzyme which digests the cells on the uterine endometrium. As a result, the organism will become burrowed into the endometrium and will establish a nutritive and circulatory relationship with the uterus.

Placenta.   Immediately after implantation, the trophoblastic cells proliferate. As they do, an endocrine organ, the placenta, found only in pregnant females, is formed. The placenta becomes functional at about the 12th week of pregnancy, at which time it will begin secreting sufficient quantities of estrogen and progesterone to substitute for the corpus luteum. The placenta takes control over maintaining pregnancy at approximately the same time the corpus luteum begins its normal course of regression (due to the regression of the trophoblastic cells in the uterus and a fall in chorionic gonadatropin). Functional problems related to the development of the placenta may, therefore, account for the high incidence of spontaneous abortions which occur around the 12th week of pregnancy.

Phases of pregnancy. Endocrinologically, pregnancy can be divided into two phases: an initial ovarian phase, when the corpus luteum produces the estrogen and progesterone responsible for maintaining pregnancy; and a placenta phase, during which these hormones are produced by the placenta. Towards the end of the ovarian phase (at about 12 weeks postfertilization), the amount of chorionic gonadotropin produced by the trophoblastic cells begins to wane. This leads to a reduction of the steroidal secretory capacity of the now regressing corpus luteum. As chorionic gonadotropin is depleted, the corpus luteum will regress, and the placenta, now functional, will initiate the creation of the essential steroids, as well as continued but smaller amounts of chorionic gonadotropin.

The placental phase of pregnancy is characterized by high levels of placental estrogen, which may reach 300 times the amount found in the nonpregnant female. The overall result of this excess of estrogens during pregnancy is the proliferation of all reproductive tissue. The uterus will enlarge greatly to accommodate the growing fetus, and there will be a significant growth of the external genitalia and of the breasts.

Placental progesterone is also produced in large concentrations during the second phase of pregnancy, reaching a level ten times that seen in nonpregnant females. The progesterone maintains the integrity and secretory capacity of the endometrium by balancing the growth-promoting actions of estrogen. Progesterone, therefore, minimizes the probability of uterine growth and contractions, and also contributes to the preparation of the breasts for lactation (see section on lactation below).

Parturition. As pregnancy approaches the third trimester (the last 3 of the 9 months) the probability rapidly increases that the onset of labor will occur. The mechanisms responsible for the termination of pregnancy and the onset of labor are, however, not well understood. The release of a toxin or metabolic material by the fetus was once thought to signal the occurrence of labor, but the labor process is now known to continue unhampered even after surgical removal of the fetus. The release of the smooth muscle excitant oxytocin, which will initiate uterine contractions, may not even be a prerequisite for the labor process, since its source, the posterior lobe of the pituitary, may be removed without appreciable modification of the events leading to the birth process. What then is responsible for the onset of labor?

The onset of labor is now believed to be triggered by an alteration in the relative levels of the placental hormones, estrogen and progesterone, toward the final phases of pregnancy. From the seventh month onward, estrogen secretion increases at a faster rate than progesterone secretion, such that the ratio of estrogen to progesterone steadily increases up to the onset of labor. It has been demonstrated that progesterone exerts a pregnancy stabilizing effect in the uterus, whereas estrogen promotes uterine excitability and may, therefore, contribute to pregnancy-instability. Thus, a parsimonious theory has been advanced (the progesterone blockage theory) explaining the termination of pregnancy on the basis of hormonal shifts in late pregnancy (Cross, 1959; Csapo, 1959). According to this theory, the blockage of uterine contractions provided by progesterone is gradually removed in late pregnancy, such that at a critical progesterone to estrogen ratio, the uterus begins rhythmic contractions typical of early labor. The contractions then build to a crescendo, promoting the passage of the fetus through the birth canal.

Lactation

Shortly after the birth of the child, the production of milk from the mother's breasts will begin. The preparation of the breasts for the feeding of the young occurs during the course of pregnancy under the influence of a highly complex and synchronized series of hormonal events (Table 12.2). The immature mammary gland found in each female breast is composed of 20 or so lobes that radiate from the nipple. Each lobe consists of a highly branched duct system and terminal alveoli (the secretory structures). The alveoli connect via the duct system to a central pigmented area of each breast, the areola. The alveoli house the epithelial cells that are responsible for milk production. During pregnancy the size of the breasts and the physiological characteristics of the duct and alveolar structures are drastically modified to accomplish milk production.

Breast development. In the human female, development of mammary gland physiology can be divided into two stages: first, the maturation of the glands to a functional state; and second, the formation and secretion of milk. The principal hormones involved in breast maturation are the placental hormones (estrogen and progesterone; Turkington & Topper, 1966) and the pituitary hormone, prolactin (Grosvenor & Turner, 1958, 1959; Lyons, Li, & Johnson, 1958). Estrogen brings about the growth of the duct system to a highly arborized network, whereas progesterone initiates full alveolar development.

Milk production. The initiation of lactation shortly following parturition is thought to be triggered by the rapid decrease in estrogen concentration, which further increases the production of prolactin by the anterior pituitary. Note that estrogen does fall to a very low level immediately after birth, as the placenta is passed out of the uterus. Lactogenesis is induced, therefore, at the termination of pregnancy by the withdrawal of estrogen, coupled with the maintained production of prolactin.

TABLE 12.2

The Hormones of Lactation

Hormone	Function
Estrogen	Duct development
Progesterone	Alveolar development
Prolactin	Milk manufacture
Oxytocin	Milk-let-down reflex

After the mammary glands are capable of secreting milk, the continued secretion of prolactin is necessary for the maintenance of lactation. As milk secretion continues, however, pressure builds up within the glands and the production of milk will be inhibited unless milk is actively evacuated from the breasts. Thus, in addition to a proper hormonal environment, the production of milk for extended periods of time requires active suckling or milking.

Milk-let-down reflex. It can be seen in Figure 12.6 that suckling acts as an effective stimulus for the sensory receptors in the breast, which then transmit impulses along neural pathways to the region of the SON and PVN nuclei of the hypothalamus (see Chapter 11). When the appropriate signals reach the hypothalamus, the posterior lobe of the pituitary is signalled to release oxytocin. The oxytocin is then carried in the bloodstream to the breast, where it causes contractions of the myoepithelial cells surrounding the alveoli. Milk is thereby squeezed out of the alveoli and propelled through the duct system and out the nipple. The *milk-let-down reflex*, as it is called, occurs within 30–90 seconds after suckling begins, and due to the presence of oxytocin in the blood, milk evacuation may persist for a short time after suckling is terminated. This reflex is easily conditionable, however, as evidenced by the fact that nursing human

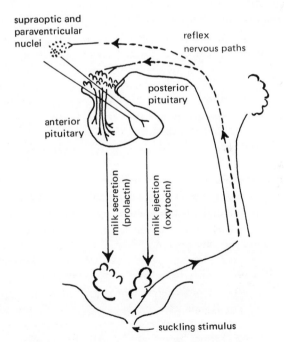

FIGURE 12.6. Milk-let-down reflex. (Reprinted by permission from G. W. Harris, *Neural Control of the Pituitary Gland.* Copyright 1955 by Edward Arnold Publishers, London.)

mothers and milk cows shortly begin to release milk even prior to the actual tactile stimulation of the mammary glands.

The release of oxytocin by the posterior lobe of the pituitary during the milk-let-down reflex has additional effects on the physiology of a lactating female. For example, nursing females frequently experience uterine and vaginal contractions. Oxytocin may, therefore, be promoting a contractile state in the uterine and vaginal smooth musculature. In a similar manner, oxytocin, which is reflexly released during and after copulation, may initiate milk ejection in lactating females in the absence of mechanical stimulation of the breasts.

Estrogen Therapy in the Control of Fertility

Oral contraceptives have been in wide use now for about 15 years, and have generally provided excellent control of fertility. The mechanism of action thought to be at the heart of the effectiveness of the oral contraceptives is an estrogen inhibition of pituitary FSH production, which then prevents follicular maturation and, thus, eliminates ovulation.

Mechanism of action. Most oral contraceptives contain a combination of a synthetic estrogen and progesterone. Progesterone is included since an augmentation of FSH suppression is usually provided with progesterone, and because a more predictable and limited menstruation is attained with the combined form of the pill. Usually, oral preparations are taken for 3 weeks beginning on the 5th day following the last menstrual period, thus providing high levels of estrogen and progesterone at a time when the maturation of the ovarian follicle would normally take place. Instead, in the presence of the high levels of estrogen and progesterone the pituitary responds as though pregnancy had taken place. A normal menstrual period may then be precipitated after ovulation has been prevented, by withdrawing the drugs and thereby causing a sloughing off of the endometrium as a direct result of the progesterone withdrawal.

Side effects. The efficacy of the oral contraceptives is essentially 100%, if the pills are used properly and without omission. The rate of failure has been clearly shown to be a function of the number of tablets skipped or omitted (Pincus, 1965). However, there may be undesirable side effects in some women taking estrogenic compounds. Many women report nausea during the first few days of therapy; headache, breast soreness, and water retention (edema) may also be attributed to estrogenic action.

More serious physiological hazards have also been attributed to oral contraceptives. Recent evidence has shown that some types of thromboembolic disorders (the formation of blood clots which may block circulation) may be precipitated by the pill (Committee on Safety of Drugs, 1967). The rate of mortality, however, is only 3 per 100,000 users per year as contrasted with 12 deaths per 100,000 per year resulting from completed pregnancies.

An undefined number of women taking oral contraceptives may also develop a diabetic type of glucose tolerance curve (Larsson-Conn & Stenram, 1965), which frequently predicts the spontaneous onset of diabetes later in life. Jaundice may also sometimes develop in women with a familial history of liver dysfunction. The incidence of other physiological dysfunctions, although infrequent, points to the problems facing the general application of oral contraceptives. Among these are a suppression of menstruation and the spontaneous flow of milk (Friedman & Goldfien, 1970); an inflammation of connective tissue structures, with pain and stiffness in muscles and joints (Bole, Friedlaender, & Smith, 1969); increased levels of growth hormone (Spellacy, Buhi, & Bendel, 1969); and cutaneous discoloration occurring in patches or spots on the face (Carruthers, 1966).

One influence of oral contraceptives is to produce a profound suppression of endogenous estrogen production (Dafares, 1967). Whether the synthetic estrogens totally compensate for the absent natural estrogens, remains to be shown and is currently the subject of some controversy. In addition, it now appears that prolonged use of the oral contraceptives delays the appearance of the menopause (the cessation of ovarian activity, ovulation, and menstruation that occurs in middle age). However, the effect may be beneficial, since the menopausal changes in a woman's physiology are usually considered unpleasant.

Psychological implications. The behavioral and psychological effects on normal females of sustained high levels of synthetic steroids is also of considerable interest. An evaluation of activity level in women taking oral contraceptives shows a marked depression in physical activity at midcycle in the menstrual period (Morris & Udry, 1969). Since fatigue and depression are widely recognized clinically as side effects of the pill, this result is not surprising. Similar findings have also been obtained with respect to the spontaneous running activity of female rats during the administration of oral contraceptives (Fregly, Hughs, & Cox, 1970).

The sexual behavior of primates is also, of course, significantly affected by circulating hormones. Subsequent to the removal of the ovaries in female rhesus monkeys, the frequency of attempted mountings by male monkeys drops to a minimal level and ejaculations are markedly reduced. If castrated females are given synthetic estrogens, however, mating activity is restored (Michael, 1969). The sexual activity of male rhesus monkeys during the treatment of the female partners with currently used oral contraceptives has also been studied (Michael & Plant, 1969). The findings indicate a marked decrease in the mean number of ejaculations per test session, despite an increased number of thrusts performed by the male.

Other Pharmacological Uses of the Female Sex Hormones

Synthetic estrogenic compounds have received wide use in clinical medicine. Most frequently, estrogens are administered as replacement therapy in cases where deficiencies in endogenous estrogens are evidenced. A classic example of estrogen replacement therapy is seen in the handling of natural or premature menopause. Menopause is associated with a gradual decline in ovarian functioning, and thus decreased levels of endogenous estrogens. Accompanying these physiological changes, menopausal women frequently complain of alternating hot flashes and chills, abnormal swelling, and muscle cramps. Not infrequently, these physical symptoms will give way to overriding feelings of anxiety, palpitation, dizziness, and on occasion, may precipitate severe incapacitation and mental breakdown. Daily doses of estrogenic compounds have been found to be effective in reducing or ameliorating many of these symptoms although in common practice physicians tend to be disinclined to use estrogens on a routine basis.

Estrogen therapy has also been employed in cases where the ovaries fail to develop and, in consequence, where puberty does not occur. In Turner's syndrome (see section later in chapter) or in hypopituitarism, estrogen treatments have been shown to bring about satisfactory pubertal changes in the presence of either dysfunctional ovaries or hypofunctional pituitaries. Therapy, in either case, brings about breast development, growth of pubic hair, and the development of a feminine contour. Estrogens are also often given to antagonize the effects of suspected overproduction of androgens by the ovaries. In females, severe cases of acne and excessive beard growth (hirsutism) may be effectively counteracted by estrogenic treatment.

The relative incidence of certain pathological conditions in men and women has generated interest in the efficacy of estrogens in the treatment of these diseases. For example, the low incidence of occlusive coronary disease in women prior to the menopause has raised interest in the efficacy of estrogen therapy for the treatment of coronary heart disease. Initial experimentation in this area, however, has produced conflicting points of view (Marmorston, Moore, Kuzma, Magidson, & Weiner, 1960; Oliver & Boyd, 1961). Various problems in effective doses, however, leave the general question of efficacy of the estrogen treatment of heart disease unanswered.

ORGASM AND SEXUAL PLEASURE

The Sexual Response Cycle

Sexual stimulation of the human male or female produces quite similar physiological changes. It now appears that sexual pleasure and the orgasmic reaction are very similar in man and woman. Masters and Johnson (1965) have studied the physiological concomitants of the sexual response cycle in the human male and female. They have divided this sexual response cycle into four stages: excitement, plateau, orgasm, and resolution.

The four phases. In both sexes, the *excitement phase* may develop in response to any form of sexual stimulation. If sexual stimulation is maintained, the *plateau phase* is entered in which the degree of sexual tension is intense and marked by vasocongestion of visceral structures throughout the body. From the plateau phase the individual may move relatively easily to orgasmic release of the developed sexual tension. The *orgasmic phase* is accompanied by contractions of the pelvic viscera. There is a marked variation in the intensity of these contractions among different individuals and in the same individual's sexual experiences. However, there is no demonstrable difference in the intensity of these contractions between men and women.

One difference between men and women is that most or all women are capable of multiple orgasms, since there can be an immediate development of another orgasmic experience with continued sexual stimulation. This is not found in men who demonstrate a refractory period before the return of an erection and ejaculatory capacity. The length of this refractory period may only be a few minutes or may be several hours, depending on many factors such as age, health, and recent sexual experience. During the *resolution phase*, with the withdrawal of sexual stimulation, there is a gradual release of sexual tension and a return of the body to its normal state.

Vasocongestion and general bodily reactions. In both the male and female, the primary physiological reaction that occurs during the development of sexual tension from the excitement phase, through the plateau phase, to the orgasmic phase is due to vascongestion of superficial tissues and visceral organs. General bodily reactions in both sexes include nipple erection, hyperventilation, tachycardia, and generalized skeletal muscle tension. A sex-tension flush due to vasocongestion is found in about 25% of males and 75% of females. It is seen as a reddening of the breasts (primarily in females) and of the entire chest wall. The face, head, and neck as well as the lower abdomen, thighs, and lower back may also redden. This flush is more generally distributed and more highly developed in females than in males.

Pelvic reactions. Specific pelvic reactions during the development of sexual tension in the male include the erection of the penis, a purplish discoloration of this organ, and an increase in the circumference of the penis, as well as elevation of the testes. During ejaculation there are repetitive contractions of the accessory organs of reproduction, leading to the pressurized expulsion of about 5 ml of semen from the penis (the volume of semen may be much smaller in the aged or if prior ejaculations have occurred recently).

In the female, the development of sexual excitement is correlated with the lubrication of the vagina, a thickening of its walls, and extension and expansion of the size of the vaginal orifice. Purplish discoloration of the labia and erection of the clitoris are also seen. During orgasm, generalized contractions of the sexual organs occur, including the vagina, uterus, and fallopian tubes. In both male and female the resolution phase may be accompanied by generalized sweating and consists of a relaxation of the sex organs and a return to normalcy (see Table 12.3 and Masters & Johnson, 1965).

TABLE 12.3

Sexual Response Cycle of the Human Male and Female

Phase	Male	Female

Excitement	Penile erection
	Testicular elevation and
	  enlargement
	Nipple erection (30%)
		Vaginal lubrication
		Thickening of vaginal walls
		  and expansion of orifice
		Nipple erection
		Sex-tension flush (75%)

Plateau	Penile enlargement and
	  tumescense; mucoidlike
	  emission (Cowper's gland)
	Sex-tension flush (25%)
	Generalized skeletal muscle
	  tension; hyperventilation
	  and tachycardia
		Full vaginal enlargement
		"Sex-skin" discoloration of
		  labia; sex-tension flush
		  (75%)
		Mucoidlike emission
		  (Batholin's gland)
		Generalized skeletal muscle
		  tension; hyperventilation
		  and tachycardia

Orgasmic	Ejaculation
	Contractions of accessory
	  organs of reproduction
	Generalized skeletal muscle
	  contractions; hyperventilation
	  and tachycardia
		Contractions of uterus, cervix,
		  vagina, labia, clitoris
		Generalized skeletal muscle
		  contractions; hyperventilation
		  and tachycardia

Resolution	Refractory to sexual stimuli
	Loss of penile erection and
	  vasocongestion
	Sweating (40%), hyperventi-
	  lation, and tachycardia
		Ready return to orgasm
		Slow loss of vasocongestion
		  and "sex-skin" color
		Sweating (40%),
		  hyperventilation and
		  tachycardia

Sexual arousal. There are several interesting points about sexuality in the male and female that we would now like to make. They are important especially to dispel certain misconceptions. First, it has been said so many times that the capacity for sexual arousal in women is less than in men. It is quite clear that this is not so. If it ever was, cultural taboos would seem to have been the cause. There is now ample evidence in our freer societies of Northern Europe and

North America that these relatively sexually emancipated women are as easily sexually arousable as are men. Experiments with erotica also show as great a capacity in women for arousal by sexual slides, films, and narrative stores as in men. Although sex differences in psychosexual arousability may exist, they appear relatively slight (Schmidt & Sigusch, 1973).

A Comparison of coitus, birth, and nursing. One interesting finding is the similarity of sexual arousal in the woman during coitus, birth, and breast feeding. It appears that from an anatomical and physiological point of view reactions during these three states are similar. There is evidence that sexual excitement can occur during the birth process (Masters & Johnson, 1966) and that many of the endocrinological and physical reactions that occur during coitus and birth are analogous. The comparison is even more striking for coitus and breast feeding. Contractions of the pelvic viscera similar to those of sexual arousal are found during nursing. Many women report stimulation to orgasm during breast feeding. Likewise, milk expulsion from the breasts is common during coital orgasm in lactating women. Thus, the acts of coitus, parturition, and lactation may be more closely related to each other than has been commonly believed. Oxytocin release (causing contractions of the genital organs) during these three events may be a key to their similarity. One can see how rewards related to sexual pleasure derived from nursing may have a critical role in establishing a positive orientation of the mother toward the infant and be a factor responsible for the so-called maternal instinct (Masters & Johnson, 1966; Newton, 1973).

Orgasmic Pleasure

One can conceive of orgasmic pleasure as resulting from the tactile stimulation of certain erogenous zones. However, visual, auditory, or olfactory stimuli may also be of a sexual nature and there are reports of stimulation to orgasm from visual stimuli or "cognitive stimuli" alone, for example. These stimuli would be carried by neural pathways to CNS regions related to reinforcement processes and physiological homeostasis (MFB and other hypothalamic-limbic system structures). Such pathways and mechanisms appear to be genetically precoded in the mammalian nervous system (Glickman & Schiff, 1967).

The activation of these reinforcement-motivational mechanisms by sexual stimuli appears possible in lower mammals only in the presence of an adequate and appropriate hormonal environment. In humans, however, the orgasmic response may be possible in the absence of sex hormones. This is especially evident in ovariectomized females. In the male it appears that ejaculation and orgasmic pleasure are usually coextensive, suggesting that they result from a unitary process or that one activates the other.

Learning. We might also mention a few points about the reinforcing effect of copulation and the role of learning and experience. Animal studies show that males and females will learn to perform an instrumental response to copulate with a receptive partner, even when ejaculation is prevented by the experimenter who separates the partners in time (Sheffield, Wulff, & Backer, 1951). Copulation itself has been shown to be a reward in several species (Caggiula & Hoebel, 1966), and even in lower mammals without previous copulatory experience. Animal studies have also shown that apparently normal male or female sexual behavior can be directly elicited by electrical stimulation of the medial hypothalamus, even in animals with no previous copulatory experience (Vaughn & Fisher, 1962). Furthermore, sites in the hypothalamus from which sexual behavior is elicitable are invariably sites which will support self-stimulation behavior (Caggiula & Hoebel, 1966).

It is not possible to directly extrapolate from animal data to humans. However, a few interesting suggestions would appear appropriate. Although experience certainly improves sexual behavior in animals, the behavior appears to be primarily genetically precoded and under the rather nonvoluntary control of hormones and lower nervous pathways. One may wonder to what extent human sexual behavior is unlearned. We suspect that in the case of sexual behavior, as for other behaviors, when we compare humans to other species, an increasing independence from precoding and increasing dependence on experience is found. However, perhaps to a previously unsuspected extent, human copulation and sexual behavior may be dependent on unlearned biological processes (Masters & Johnson, 1966; Money & Ehrhardt, 1972; Zubin & Money, 1973).

In order to point out the basic biological nature of sexual behavior we might ask the following question. If a group of young male and female human beings were placed on a desert island and survived to adulthood without the benefit of schooling from our society, and without knowledge of reproductive processes, what is the likelihood that they would independently develop copulatory and parental behavior? Would reproductive processes occur and the group survive, or would the group die out? It seems to us that there is some likelihood that the group would develop its own relatively appropriate patterns of copulation, parturition, nursing, and child care. We believe this is because these behaviors are strongly based on genetic precoding of behavior patterns and rewarding stimuli and responses (Glickman & Schiff, 1967; Valenstein, 1966). That is not to say that learning is not involved in human reproductive behaviors, but that the behaviors develop from strong biological predilections.

Cyclicity in the female. A matter of considerable interest is the cyclicity of sexual arousability in women. In females other than the human, sexual receptivity and arousability is usually confined to a particular period of the hormonal cycle at about the time of ovulation. The hormonal conditions existing at this point of the cycle seem to be necessary for sexual arousal. At other times the female will not submit to sexual advances, but will fight off the male. This is usually found even for many of the higher primates (Jensen, 1973), although there are some reports of females of the great apes permitting copulation outside of the estrus period. In addition, in species other than the human, the female is no longer sexually receptive following ovariectomy.

The findings that human females are sexually arousable to orgasm throughout the menstrual cycle, in older age following menopause, and following ovariectomy emphasize the independence in the human female of sexual motivation and hormonal secretions. There is some cyclicity, however, in the level of sexual arousability in women, with peaks being reported in different women at about the time of ovulation, immediately prior to menstruation, or at both times (Davidson, 1972; Money & Ehrhardt, 1972). There is evidence also for a relative independence of sexual drive from hormonal secretions in adult men. There are several reports of a survival of sexual arousability, erectile capacity, and even ejaculation (of course, not containing sperm) in castrated men.

Clitoral vs vaginal orgasm. Another interesting point is the ability of human females, who have had the vagina, or clitoris, or both excised for cancer, to respond sexually to stimulation of the rebuilt artificial vagina. Clitorectomized patients are capable of reaching orgasm from stimulation of the scar tissue or of the rebuilt vagina. These findings point to the reinnervation of these tissues by the peripheral nerves that are damaged during surgery.

Related to this matter is the question of clitoral vs vaginal orgasms in normal women. The clitoris is clearly most sexually sensitive in women (it also is most highly innervated by tactile sensory nerve endings). The labia also have considerable sensory innervation, but the vaginal wall is only poorly innervated. Orgasm is usually most easily achieved with direct clitoral stimulation, but the nature of the orgasm, its intensity, and its duration is not a function of clitoral vs vaginal stimulation, because the clitoris and labia are stimulated by penile penetration and copulatory movements (see discussion in Masters & Johnson, 1965).

Adrenal Androgens

One question that has been the center of some controversy the last few years is the role of adrenal androgens in human female sexuality. When androgen is given to women, it may have an augmentative effect on sexual desire and it has been suggested that androgen is a "libido" hormone in both sexes. In one study of women undergoing, first, ovariectomy and then, adrenalectomy as a radical treatment for breast cancer, libidinal feeling was said to disappear only after the adrenals had also been removed. However, the validity of these conclusions, which were based on research with cancer patients following serious surgical procedures is open to question (Davidson, 1972; Money & Ehrhardt, 1972). Everitt and Herbert (1969) though, have also found adrenal androgens to have an important role in the sexual arousal of the female rhesus monkey. In disagreement with these studies, experiments in male rats and monkeys suggest that adrenal androgens have little role in male sexual behavior. In these studies, adrenalectomy had no effect on the decline in sexual receptivity following castration (Beach, 1970; Bloch & Davidson, 1968). One possibility is that adrenal androgens or injected androgens in the female produce sexual arousal through their chemical conversion to estrogens.

Aphrodisiacs

Gonadal hormones. Certainly the most potent aphrodisiacs are testosterone in the male and estrogen in the female. Many males whose sexual desire and capacity has declined with aging or following castration, experience a sexual rejuvenation from the administration of testosterone. In menopausal or ovariectomized women, estrogen administration will counteract the atrophic changes and may restore a somewhat declining sexual vigor. The need for these hormones in castrates and the aging is not always found, however, and their effectiveness is not entirely dependable when there is a deficit. As we have already pointed out, in the human, adult sexuality has been somewhat freed from hormonal state and such factors as set and attitude seem to have an important influence on sexual functioning in castrates and in the aging.

Several different related androgenic compounds can be found in the human. Studies in rats have been concerned with the possibility of these substances having different roles in the maintenance of sexual physiology and behavior. While the findings in rats do not have direct bearing on human sexuality, they are at least suggestive of the possibility of analogous relationships. There are three androgenic steroids that can be found in the male rat: androstenedione, testosterone, and dihydrotestosterone. In castrated animals, dihydrotestosterone is the most effective drug for maintaining the weight of the seminal vesicles, while testosterone and androstenedione are most effective for the maintenance of mating behavior (Whalen & Luttge, 1971b). These data suggest that the most effective endogenous compound for the maintenance of peripheral reproductive tissue is different from the most effective compounds for the activation of the nervous system and the maintenance of reproductive behavior.

Consistent with this finding is research with the anaphrodisiac, cyproterone. This compound is thought to be a competitive inhibitor for androgens. However, it may not be equally effective against all of the androgenic compounds. In the male rat, cyproterone reduces seminal vesicle weight almost to castrate size, but does not inhibit mating responses (Whalen & Edwards, 1969). These data suggest that cyproterone is a competitive inhibitor primarily of dihydrotestosterone (Fang & Liao, 1969). However, others have found evidence that cyproterone is a competitive inhibitor for androgen in the hypothalamus of male rats (Block & Davidson, 1967).

It is possible to induce sexual receptivity and lordotic responding in the female rat by treatment with androgenic compounds. Since the metabolic conversion of androgens to estrogens has been demonstrated, the lordosis could result either from androgenic stimulation of from the action of estrogenic metabolites. A competitive inhibitor for estrogen has recently been produced (CI-628; Parke Davis). This agent has been shown to block estrogen-induced lordosis and also to block androgen-induced lordosis. However, this antiestrogen does not inhibit seminal vesicle weight maintenance or male mating response maintenance by testosterone in castrated male rats. Therefore, the lordosis-eliciting action of testosterone would seem to result from conversion to estrogenic compounds (Whalen, 1972), and the sexual-arousing effects in women of adrenal androgens or of administered androgens may likewise result from conversion to estrogens.

Levodopa. A number of substances which are not sex steroids have been suggested as aphrodisiacs. Levodopa has recently enjoyed success in the treatment of Parkinsonian patients. Several incidents of marked increases in sexuality were noted leading to some speculation about aphrodisiac properties. It is now believed, however, that this is simply an indirect effect of the normalization of motor capacity in patients who had been unable to engage in copulation because of the incapacitating nature of the disease (McCary, 1973, p. 175).

PCPA. Another substance that has been suggested as an aphrodisiac in animal studies is the serotonin depleter, PCPA. Several studies have found an increase in mounting behavior by male rats (Tagliamonte, A., Tagliamonte, P., Gessa, & Brodie, 1969) and cats (Ferguson, Hendrikson, Cohen, Mitchell, Barchas, & Dement, 1970) following PCPA administration. Activation of lordotic responding in female rats by PCPA has also been reported (Zemlan, Ward, Crowley, & Margules, 1973). These studies have led to the hypothesis of a serotonergic system that inhibits sexual behavior. However, several investigators have failed to find an activation of sexual responding with PCPA (Whalen & Luttge, 1970; Zitrin, Beach, Barchas & Dement, 1970). Whether PCPA is an aphrodisiac in animals is unclear. Perceptual disorientation (leading to copulation outside of their home territory, for example) and gastrointestinal irritation (producing increased genital canal sensitivity) are two alternatives to the aphrodisiac hypothesis that have been offered as explanations for the observed behavioral changes. However, in clinical trials with PCPA in men, no evidence of increased sexuality has been noted (Zitrin, Dement, & Barchas, 1973).

Other substances. A variety of substances, such as cantheridis (Spanish fly) have been thought of as aphrodisiacs. Cantheridis, however, produces intense urogenital and vaginal irritation and thus may simulate sexual tension, thereby leading to sexual arousal. Other substances, such as oysters, animal horns, etc., have never been shown to have any aphrodisiac power whatsoever, except for that attributable to the power of suggestion. Most of this lore and mythology appears to result from some similarity between the appearance of the supposed aphrodisiac and the appearance of the male or female genital organs themselves.

Anaphrodisiacs

In the male, estrogenic hormone administration will block pituitary production of ICSH and FSH and lead to a regression of reproductive tissues, a loss of sexual interest and a feminization of the body. Likewise, testosterone administration to a female will cause a regression of female reproductive tissue such as the breasts and lead to a masculinization or defeminization of the body, but testosterone may also increase sexual libido (sexual motivation or interest).

A number of drugs that inhibit cell metabolism, such as antibiotics and the barbiturate depressants, have been shown in animals to inhibit masculine development of the male fetus (Gorski, 1971; Kobayashi & Gorski, 1970). Prenatal stress has also been found to be demasculinizing, and leads to femalelike behavior patterns in adult male rats (Ward, 1972). Although it has not been shown in adult animals or in man, it is conceivable that antibiotic drugs, depressant drugs, or prenatal stress, may have a demasculinizing effect on adult male humans (Money & Ehrhardt, 1972).

Cyproterone is a competitive inhibitor of at least some of the actions of androgens. This substance has been tested as a mode of treatment for a variety of sex offenders (Laschet, 1973). Libido, orgasm, and erectile capacity have all been reported to be variably reduced by administration of this drug to men.

SEX-RELATED PATHOLOGIES AND BEHAVIOR

Pathological conditions critically involving reproductive capacity and sexual behavior can have a variety of causes. An initial genetic error can involve an abnormal condition of the sex chromosomes. During fetal and prepubertal development, an abnormal hormonal situation or a surgical or traumatic insult to the body can affect reproductive and sex-related behavioral ability. In addition, sexual psychopathology has been associated with neurological disorders; and lastly, there are cases of aberrant sexual identity and sexual behavior that cannot be related to an organic disorder, but instead appear based on experiential or learning factors (such as seems to be the case with respect to homosexuality).

Genetics

The genetic determination of gender normally proceeds in the manner discussed at the beginning of this chapter, but on occasion genetic mistakes may be observed. Chromosomal errors can arise from faulty meiosis during the development of sperm in the male or during the development of mature ova in the female, or they can occur due to faulty mitosis in the zygote after fertilization. Figure 12.7 illustrates the chromosomal errors that may arise in the zygote from incorrect maternal or paternal meiotic cell divisions.

Turner's syndrome (XO). In this genetic anomaly the sex chromosomal constitution is XO (Ford, Jones, Miller, Mittwoch, Penrose, Ridler, & Shapiro, 1959). In these females, the lack of one X chromosome may result in the basic physical features now recognized as symptomatic of Turner's syndrome. These are a female appearance, very short stature, sexual infantism (failure of secondary sex characteristics to appear), a weblike neck, shieldlike chest, widely separated nipples, and infertility. It should be mentioned that the bodily abnormalities involving stature, neck, chest, and nipple separation are not invariably found, although the failure of sexual maturation is.

The fetus with Turner's syndrome has no functional gonads, the ovaries being only primitive streaks of tissue, and consequently, no gonadal hormones are

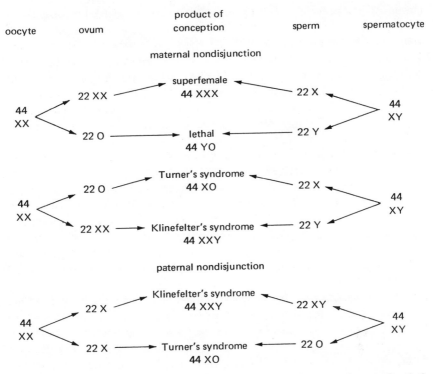

oocyte   ovum   product of   sperm   spermatocyte
                            conception

FIGURE 12.7. Chromosomal errors arising from incorrect maternal and paternal meiotic cell divisions.

secreted during development. However, the neonate will appear female genitally and is assigned and reared as such. The lack of gonadal hormones is not usually realized and is without known effect during childhood. At puberty, the failure to mature due to lack of endogenous hormones brings the disorder to prominence. Hormonal administration of estrogen is usually begun and continued throughout the life of the woman, to first bring on a feminine pubescence and then to maintain the hormone-based sexual characteristics.

Studies of the sexual identification of girls with Turner's syndrome show that they behave and identify as female, just as do normal girls. These conclusions were based on their demonstration of maternalism in choice of toys and types of play behavior, their rehearsal and anticipation of feminine marriage and motherhood roles, aggressivity in behavior, preferences for female or male playmates, athletic interest, propensity for engaging in childhood fights, and preferences and interests as to clothing, jewelry, perfume and hair style. In fact, on some of these measures like athletic interest and skills, behavior in childhood fights, and interest in jewelry, perfume and hair styling, the girls with Turner's syndrome were rated more feminine than the normal girls used as controls. It seems clear from these data that in spite of the absence of one X chromosome and of female sex hormones, girls with Turner's syndrome differentiate an unequivocally feminine gender identity. We may thus infer that the second X chromosome and the female hormones are not necessary for female gender differentiation. In fact, the finding that these girls are "more feminine" than normal may suggest that the second X chromosome disposes females to be psychosexually closer to the male than in its absence (Ehrhardt, 1973; Money & Ehrhardt, 1972). However, an alternative interpretation of the etiology of these psychological characteristics associated with Turner's syndrome is possible. Since their parents had some knowledge of their condition, it may be that differences in the way they reared these girls are responsible for what seems to be a passivity and introversion. We should also mention that these are quite "unliberated" standards of female conduct. However, it appears that the standards conform to the expectations of the girls' parents, which partially validates the use of these criteria.

YO. The counterpart of Turner's syndrome, the YO zygote, is not a viable product of conception and will not mature. This is of interest, since in Turner's syndrome an XO individual is viable and will grow and develop. Thus, although the Y chromosome acts as the major determinant of gender in genetic terms, the X chromosome is even more basic to life since in its absence, life is not possible (comparing the XO and YO genetic constitutions).

Superfemale (XXX). The superfemale, contrary to the implications of the term, is frequently found to suffer from mental retardation, premature onset of menopause, and menstrual difficulties. There are inconsistencies of the clinical picture, however, since XXX females may, on occasion, show none of these classic symptoms (Day, Larson, & Wright, 1964). Thus, there is a normal female body type and the individual is fertile, although ability to conceive may be somewhat diminished. Gender identity differentiation is that of a normal female.

Klinefelter's syndrome (XXY). This disorder is characterized by a 47 XXY chromosomal constitution (Jacobs & Strong, 1959; Ford et al., 1959). It is thought that this anomaly is the result of a failure of an immature ovum or sperm cell to separate successfully during the meiotic divisions in their development. The Y chromosome in Klinefelter's syndrome is, of course, contributed by the male parent. The XX chromosomes may be both contributed by the female or one of the X chromosomes may be contributed by the male parent in addition to the male-contributed Y chromosome.

Due to the influence of the Y or male sex chromosome, which has been shown to initiate male development, the adult individual with Klinefelter's syndrome will manifest a masculine physique (thus they live as males). As a result of the chromosomal error, the individual may be infertile and show poor virilization at puberty.

Supermale (XYY). This chromosomal aberration has recently been discovered and has engendered considerable interest due to the propensity for XYY individuals to get into difficulty with society. The genetic basis of the XYY genotype is not clear. It cannot simply result from nondisjunction (Figure 12.7) since the male parent can only contribute one Y chromosome even in cases of nondisjunction, and the female parent, of course, can contribute none. It may result from fertilization of an ovum by a faulty sperm with a 24 YY chromosomal constitution or from faulty mitosis during the earliest stages of fetal development. Interestingly, the incidence of the XYY genotype in the general population, 1 to 1.5 per 1,000, is about the same as the incidence of Klinefelter's syndrome (XXY).

The XYY chromosomal aberration has been associated with mental retardation, tall stature, unusually aggressive temperament, and a consequent propensity for violent behavior. Individuals with XYY and XXY chromosomal constitutions are both found in mental hospitals at similar frequencies, about 7 to 9 per 1,000, a higher frequency than their incidence in the population. Both genetic defects predispose affected individuals toward mental retardation, epilepsy, and schizophrenic-type behavioral pathology. Therefore, patients in mental hospitals are more prone to have an extra sex chromosome than are individuals in the general population, but the likelihood of the extra chromosome being an X is about the same as the likelihood of it being a Y. In contrast to these data, the incidence of the XYY and XXY aberrations in prison populations is not the same. The incidence of Klinefelter's syndrome among prisoners is elevated (about 9 per 1,000) and about the same as in mental hospitals. However, the incidence of supermales in prison populations (about 19 per 1,000) is even higher than Klinefelter's (about double), higher than the incidence of supermales in mental hospitals (about double), and about 15 times the incidence of supermales in the general population. Since XYY males tend to be both tall in stature and mentally retarded, it has been suggested that perhaps large size and low mentality may be responsible for the propensity to violence. However, studies of XY juvenile offenders have not supported this idea. An association between height and likelihood of institutionalization was not found (Hook & Kim, 1971).

It is clear from these data that an extra sex chromosome, be it an X or a Y, predisposes the individual towards psychological abnormalities leading to hospitalization or imprisonment. Therefore, the biological consequences of these genetic constitutions are critically important to psychological "makeup" and behavior. Either deviation from normal (XXY or XYY) has pathological consequences. Of particular interest are the implications of these findings for our understanding of human aggression and violence. These data suggest that a social or cultural learning explanation of aggression (although certainly having some validity) would be incomplete. Genetic characteristics present on the X and Y chromosomes may have some directing role in the disposition towards aggression, not only in the aberrant XXY and XYY individuals, but also in normal males and females. It seems possible that the single Y chromosome in normal males disposes to violence and that the two Y chromosomes in supermales further increases this tendency by essentially providing a "double dose" of some predisposing genetic basis (Jarvik, Klodin, & Matsuyama, 1973).

Development

There are basically four conditions to be discussed: the adrenogenital syndrome (and progestin-induced hermaphroditism), the androgen-insensitivity syndrome, and microphallus, along with one case of accidental ablation of the penis during circumcision. The most important implication of these cases is that much of what we mean by psychosexual identification as male or female is learned, and not solely based either on genetic predisposition or endocrinological balance (see Ehrhardt, 1973 and Money & Ehrhardt, 1972 for more detailed discussions of these patients).

Hormonally induced fetal masculinization. There is a distinct parallel between early experimental disturbances of the sexual physiology and behavior of animals and several human disorders where a pathological condition contributes to hormonal aberrations. In animal studies it has been shown that increased levels of androgenic hormones occurring prenatally can result in masculinization of a female fetus.

Adrenogenital syndrome: In the clinical disorder called the *congenital adrenogenital syndrome*, excessive androgenic secretions from the fetal adrenal cortex between the third and fifth month of gestation can cause masculinization of the human female fetus. The principal cause of the syndrome is found in a congenital adrenal hyperplasia (excessive growth of the adrenal cortex). There is, in this disorder, an excessive production of adrenal androgens by the hyperplastic fetal adrenal cortex. The adrenal androgens then mimic the actions of testicular androgens secreted normally by the testes of a male fetus. This syndrome may also be seen in the masculinization of a female fetus due to androgenic steroids produced by a hyperplastic maternal adrenal cortex (in this case there is usually a tumor and many of the symptoms will subside shortly after birth due to elimination of the maternal androgens from the fetus).

Because of the androgen hypersecretion during early fetal life, there is an incomplete development of the female external genitals. At birth the clitoris is enlarged, at times resembling a normal penis of the neonatal male. In the first few years of development a phase of precocious male pseudopuberty occurs in which there is growth of axillary (underarm) hair, a high incidence of acne, and a deepening of the voice. At an age where the onset of puberty normally occurs in females and thereafter, there is no breast development, no onset of menstruation, and the body contour evolves into that resembling a young male.

If the presence of the adrenogenital syndrome is recognized at birth, the child will be sexed as a female and cortisone or another similar corticoid (see Chapter 11) will be used throughout life to supply normal adrenal corticoids and also to inhibit adrenal androgen production by blocking ACTH. Surgery may also be required to return a hypertrophied clitoris to normal size. Such individuals develop into normal girls and women, and may even become pregnant (with little more trouble than normal) and breast feed. If the disorder is not recognized at birth (as occurred more frequently in earlier times), the individual might be sexed as male or as female depending on the degree of masculinization of the external genitals and on the judgment of the attending physician. The external genitals may be sufficiently masculinized to form a normal-appearing penis and an empty scrotum. If sexed as a female, the disorder will be discovered when, at puberty, the adrenal androgens induce masculinization. If sexed as a male, the disorder may not be discovered until the married "man" seeks counseling for an inability to conceive.

The degree of masculinization of an XX female by prenatal androgens may be sufficient to produce some development of the wolffian duct system (although the mullerian system also develops since there is no mullerian-inhibiting substance). Furthermore, the genital tubercle may be sufficiently masculinized to become a normally sized penis carrying a urinary canal. Erectile and orgasmic capacity can also be present, with the ejaculation of a seminal fluid at orgasm; however, containing no sperm cells, of course (there are no testes). The scrotum will be empty and ovaries can be found in the peritoneal cavity.

Progestin-induced masculinization: The cases of progestin-induced masculinization resulted from the use of synthetic progestogens in the 1950s to prevent miscarriage. It was not realized that these synthetic agents could also exert an androgenic action on a female fetus. Before this effect was discovered a few women gave birth to daughters with masculinization of the clitoris. In cases where the clitoral hypertrophy was not great, diagnostic evaluation led to sex assignment as a female and only surgery on the hypertrophied clitoris was required. At puberty these girls' own ovaries would bring on feminization. In cases where the masculinization was greater, with a normal-appearing penis and an empty scrotum, the baby would usually be assigned as a boy (with undescended testes) and would be brought up as a boy. At puberty, the error would be discovered when the ovaries induced feminization.

Masculinized XX individuals raised as girls: The first question we might ask is how did the prenatal androgen influence the behavior of genetic females raised as girls? Money and Ehrhardt review the cases of ten genetic females with progestin-induced masculinization, all given early corrective surgery, if needed, and raised as girls. They also review the cases of 15 early treated genetic females with the adrenogenital syndrome. These girls were matched to a group of normal gilrs of suitable age and background. The results were similar for both groups of fetally androgenized girls. They were more likely to regard themselves as tomboys (and to be so regarded by their mothers and playmates) and to engage in active outdoor games and sports. However, the girls were not rated by themselves or their mothers as aggressive children.

The fetally androgenized girls also tended to dress in a more utilitarian and functional fashion, seemed to be less enthusiastic about marriage and motherhood and more interested in a career than the control group of girls. The androgenized girls were also relatively late in beginning to date and in age of marriage. Yet, it must be emphasized that there were no indications of lesbianism in these girls. Rather, they were somewhat "less feminine" than the control girls in their interests and life style and a bit slower in beginning their heterosexual lives.

In the initial studies, the fetally androgenized girls were found to have an average IQ much above normal (about 130) and above that of the matched group of control girls. This finding led to considerable speculation about the IQ-enhancing efficacy of androgen at least in these individuals. However, more recently it has been shown that prenatal androgens do not raise girls' IQ. The androgenized girls have been compared in IQ to their own nonandrogenized sisters, and it has been found that both groups have similar and higher than normal IQs. Therefore, it seems simply that girls from families seeking medical help at Johns Hopkins Hospital have higher IQs than the population average (Maccoby, 1973; Money & Ehrhardt, 1972).

In subhuman species, fetal androgenization may automatically reverse gender dimorphic behavior (any behavior in which differences can be found between males and females). In human beings, however, the data just reviewed show that this is not the case. Some change may have occurred. It is hard to define, but seems related to increased energy expenditure and agressiveness. However, sexuality is by no means reversed. Although Money and Ehrhardt (1972) interpreted these changes as being the result of fetal androgenization, there are at least two equally likely alternative explanations. First, since the control population was not a good match in terms of IQ, maybe they were also not a good psychological match. Perhaps the families of the androgenized girls were also more assertive and success oriented that the control families. The second possibility is that the families of the androgenized girls knew something of the nature of the girls' disorder, and so expected them to be more "masculine" and less "feminine" than their other daughters. This could easily have led the families to treat the androgenized girls in such a manner as to produce these psychological differences.

In the case of androgenized females who are also androgenized postnatally the story is somewhat different. If the girls are raised as female throughout childhood, sexual identity remains as female, although the tomboyism reviewed above is also found. However, in some cases in which early clitoral surgery is not accomplished, the presence of a penis-sized clitoris may lead to confusion as to sexual identity, with a high incidence of ambivalence as to gender identification and of homosexual imagery and experience (Money & Ehrhardt, 1972).

Masculinized XX individuals raised as boys: Several genetic females with the adrenogenital syndrome or progestin-induced masculinization have been raised as boys. They seem to develop normal masculine psychosexual identities. The problem is that they do not masculinize properly at puberty. Gonadal and external genital surgery may be required; however, penile construction cannot be successfully accomplished due to limitations in the ability of plastic surgery. A penis may be constructed and the urinary canal made to pass through the penis, but there will be no erectile or orgasmic capacity.

Conclusions: With these androgenized individuals, psychological develop-ment either as a male or female is possible. Psychopathology with respect to sexual behavior and identification is found only when there is physical ambiguity or when the parents and others are not consistent in treating the child as male or female. Also, if a gender reassignment is attempted after the first year or two of life, by which time gender identification has begun to develop, the child and later the adult is likely to be in conflict as to his or her sexuality and sex role. The important factor appears to be clear, consistent, and unambiguous cues as to sex role, be they male or female, and be they consistent or inconsistent with genetic or gonadal gender.

Androgen-insensitivity syndrome. This human clinical syndrome (also called *testicular feminization*) occurs when there is a failure of androgenization of genetic males. There are two possible causes. The first is a lack of androgen prenatally and neonatally. Without this substance, the gonads differentiate as testes, but the wolffian duct does not develop and the genital tubercle differentiates along female lines. Since in these cases a nonsteroidal mullerian-inhibiting substance is manufactured by the testes, the uterus and fallopian tubes also fail to develop. Actually, in most cases, the defect is not a failure of androgen secretion by the testes, but rather an insensitivity of the tissues of the body to androgen. The defect in androgen utilization is genetically transmitted via the fertile females in the family.

The nature of the biochemical defect responsible for the inability to utilize androgen has not been identified, but is presumed to be enzymatic and to affect all bodily cells. The undescended testes of adults afflicted with androgen insensitivity are usually found to secrete normal masculine amounts of androgen into the bloodstream. However, the cells of the body are incapable of responding to this substance. The cells are, however, sensitive to estrogen, and are feminized by the small amounts of estrogen that are normally secreted by the testes and adrenal cortex. Feminization of body size and contour, hair distribution, and breast development are therefore all induced at puberty.

Most babies so affected are born indistinguishable in genital appearance from normal females, and are sexed and raised as girls. The fact that the vagina is only a dimple, or a shallow cavity and ends blindly, is usually not discovered until medical attention is drawn to the condition by a failure to begin menstruation at puberty.

In a few cases of androgen insensitivity, the clitoral organ is sufficiently enlarged to draw attention to the undescended testes palpable in the groin. If the physician should then decide to declare the baby a boy, a tragic life history is usually begun. Beginning at puberty, these boys find themselves with a body that refuses to masculinize (due to androgen insensitivity), but is nicely feminized due to the small amounts of testicular and adrenal estrogen. The breasts can be surgically removed, but it is impossible to induce deepening of the voice, masculine body appearance, and hair distribution, or development of the immature clitoris-penis into a functional masculine sex organ. The problems of the plastic surgery construction of a simulated penis are presently insurmountable, and are likely to remain so until it becomes possible to successfully transplant a genital organ. It appears much better in these cases to sexually assign the individual as a female, since body appearance is destined to be such, and with the possibility of adopting a child, a normal life can be lived as wife and mother.

As these patients grow up, it is of special interest to determine the effect of genetic and gonadal status as a male on their lives as females (in the absence of hormonal masculinization). Although this condition is rare, Money and Ehrhardt (1972) have evaluated the psychosexual identification and behavior of ten patients, already past puberty, with this condition. All had been sexed and raised as females. Money and Ehrhardt rate them quite normally feminine in terms of marriage, maternalism, and erotic arousal. Money and Ehrhardt (1972, p. 112) conclude that these findings " . . . clearly tell a story of women whose genetic status as males was utterly irrelevant to their psychosexual status as women, as also was the histology of their gonads."

Traumatic loss of the penis or microphallus. Money and Ehrhardt (1972) also review the case of a boy (with an identical twin brother) who was born a normal male, but whose penis was ablated flush with the abdominal wall by an accident during circumcision at seven months of age. The current from the electrocautery was too powerful and burned off the entire penis. Following consultation between the parents and medical experts, a decision was reached to raise the child as a female. The first step of female genital reconstruction has been undertaken. Further vaginoplasty (construction through plastic surgery of a vaginal orifice) will be required later in life and body feminization will be accomplished by estrogenic hormonal replacement beginning at puberty.

Another case is of a genetic male baby born with a hypospadic microphallus (a very small penis). The phallus was so small (about 1 cm long) as to resemble a slightly enlarged clitoris, and like a clitoris, it did not carry a urinary canal. Again, since this child could not function sexually as a male, a decision was eventually reached to raise the child as a girl and initial genital surgery was undertaken.

Money and Ehrhardt review these cases in some detail. The parents have been very careful to treat the children as girls. The fascinating result of all this is that the children appear to be developing psychologically as normal girls.

Hormones

In animals, castration generally reduces sexual behavior. In males, the effects are rapid and strong in lower mammals, such as rabbits, rats, and guinea pigs, but much less predictable and more variable in carnivores (cats, dogs) and primates. In subhuman females, castration rapidly and permanently inhibits estrual receptivity. These deficits can all be eliminated by appropriate hormonal replacement (see Grossman, 1967 and Schwartz, 1973 for details).

We have already alluded to the discrepancy between these findings and those in human beings. Castration in the human male or female may have little effect on sexual behavior and potency, or may completely depress such activities. In the human female, we see only limited manifestations of depression of sexuality as a function of stage in the menstrual cycle, menopause, or ovariectomy. Some physical changes, however, are noted, but these can be blocked with hormonal replacement. It is clear that human sexuality has become relatively emancipated from hormonal control. However, there are few well controlled studies of human sexuality following castration and hormonal replacement. In addition, the problems of expectations and attitudes in these cases are seemingly insurmountable.

Neurology

Several relationships between human psychosexuality and brain function have been suggested. First, demonstrable brain abnormalities have been associated with unusual sexual behavior. There are several cases of patients with brain tumors in the temporal lobes who have engaged in transvestism (wearing clothing of the opposite sex) or fetishism (the use of some object or nongenital part of the body to obtain sexual gratification). For example, there are the well-known cases of a safety pin fetishist and a hair fetishist with temporal lobe epilepsies. These men obtained erotic gratification from the contemplation of a safety pin or women's long hair. Surgical ablation of the left anterior temporal lobe relieved both the epilepsy and the fetish in both patients. There is also the case of a woman who would engage in automatic sexual behavior in association with right temporal lobe seizures. The tissue damage in this case was the result of CNS involvement in advanced syphilis. Additionally, the case of a young man who developed abnormal sexual behavior following partial bilateral temporal lobectomy for epilepsy can be cited. His fetish was for anatomical diagrams and charts. In the last two cases, amelioration of the sexual symptoms was obtained with the use of anticonvulsant medication (see Green, 1972 for a review of this subject).

In a second type of study, there is one report of abnormal EEGs in nearly half of a sample of 26 male transvestites or transexuals (individuals living as the gender opposite to all biological indications). However, in a larger survey of 86 epileptics, only 10% of the men showed any unusual sexual behavior, which may be a proportion no higher than in the general population (Green, 1972).

In West Germany, the ventromedial nucleus of the hypothalamus in the nondominant hemisphere has been destroyed in men found guilty of sex crimes against young boys (pedophillic homosexuality). This hypothalamic nucleus was destroyed in an attempt to reduce sexual behavior by inhibiting pituitary gonadotropin secretion. The investigators report an elimination or reduction in most of the patients of the aberrant sex drive and criminal behavior. The extent to which the apparent improvement is due to gonadotropin inhibition or is the direct result of the brain damage, or is related to the patient's expectations and motivation to change cannot yet be assessed (see Epstein, 1973; Green, 1972; and Money & Ehrhardt, 1972 for more detailed discussions of this subject).

Heath (1964) has reported the elicitation of penile erection and sexual motivation in three male patients with electrical stimulation of the septal region. In a female patient, application of acetylcholine to the septal region or electrical stimulation of this area produced sexual excitement, including orgasmic responses. This case is especially interesting for its "therapeutic" implications. This woman claimed not to have had an orgasmic experience prior to the orgasms elicited by brain stimulation, although she was then in her third marriage. However, after the elicited orgasms she reported regular orgasmic responses with her current husband (Heath, 1964).

The material presented in this section shows that human sexual psychopathology can result from or be associated with neurological pathology and that neurological treatment may be effective in the treatment of sexual psychopathology.

Learning

In this section we wish to discuss homosexuality, as well as fetishism, transvestism, and transsexualism. Although there have been many attempts to implicate organicity in these behavior patterns, these have generally met with failure. We believe the most reasonable working hypothesis is that these patterns of sexual behavior usually result from particular experiences in childhood and young adulthood.

Organicity. This interpretation of homosexuality as being primarily learned should, however, not preclude the search for evidence of organicity. Homosexuality does seem to appear rather frequently in the XXY and XYY genetic disorders (Money & Ehrhardt, 1972, p. 231). Furthermore, although hormonal levels are normal in most homosexuals, there may be a smaller subpopulation with very low plasma testosterone levels and also very low sperm counts (see Money & Ehrhardt, 1972). We might also point out that prenatal and neonatal conditions that are not verifiable in the adult may predispose toward homosexuality by feminizing the behavior of males in some respects, and also masculinizing the behavior of females. These conditions could include the intervention of stress, antibiotic therapy, sedatives, or some temporary physiological condition in a pregnant woman carrying a male fetus. Each of these conditions could inhibit androgenic activity. For a pregnant woman carrying a female fetus, a temporary adrenocortical pathology, sex steroid ingestion, or some other mechanism could temporarily raise androgenic activity above normal. However, we have shown that genetic and early hormonal influences on the patterns of sexual identification and behavior seem rather slight in the human.

Hormone levels. One subject that has received considerable attention is that of sex steroid levels in the male and female homosexual. In the 1940s there were a few studies that compared the urinary output of sex steroids in homosexuals and heterosexuals. The results of these studies were equivocal, which is not so surprising since liver functioning could contribute as much to the variability as could differences in gonadal functioning (Money, 1961). In the 1970s, however, several studies of urine metabolites have also reported different proportions of various steroidal substances in homosexuals and heterosexuals (Loraine, et al., 1970; Margolese, 1970).

In one interesting study, ICSH (LH) secretion in homosexual males was found to be acyclical (as it is in heterosexual males), rather than cyclical (as found in females). In another study, scrotal skin from transsexual or normal males was incubated with radioactively labeled androgen and the quantity of testosterone and its metabolites recoverable was not found to be different between the two groups (Gillespie, 1971, cited by Green, 1972).

More recently, analyses of levels of androgens and estrogens in the plasma have become possible. Most homosexual men and women are found to have blood hormone levels within the normal range for their sex; however, a small number of individuals with aberrantly low homotypical blood hormone levels have been found (perhaps representing a subpopulation with endocrinological organic involvement) (Kolodny et al., 1971). Males with low blood testosterone levels were also found to have sperm counts only about one-half of normal. Some earlier blood plasma studies had reported low androgen levels in the general male homosexual population, but these are now discounted due to poor control for age and stress (Migeon, Rivarola, & Forest, 1969). Since there is evidence that stress lowers androgen production and also reason to believe that some individuals living a homosexual life style are subject to abnormally high stress, low blood androgens are to be expected in homosexuals who have not become well adapted. For instance, low blood androgen levels similar to those found in poorly adapted homosexuals have been found in heterosexual males awaiting surgery in a hospital or in soldiers during basic training or combat (Rose, Bourne, & Poe, 1969).

Strong evidence against the involvement of adult hormones or hormonal levels in sexual orientation can be found when hormones are administered in an attempt to alter the behavior. The effects of sex hormones are that androgen, within limits, increases libido in both sexes, and that estrogen increases libido in females and decreases it in males (Money & Ehrhardt, 1972, p. 232). No change in gender orientation from the homosexual to the heterosexual is produced.

HUMAN PSYCHOSEXUAL IDENTITY

The animal research discussed earlier in this chapter would suggest that aspects of sexual and aggressive behavior are strongly determined by whether androgen is present prenatally and neonatally. However, it appears that this is not the case for the human. For human and animal alike, androgen and the mullerian-inhibiting substance determine, during early critical periods, the development of the duct system and external genitals as masculine or feminine. These critical period hormonal actions operate upon a genetic sex-determining mechanism.

But, what of *psychosexual identity* in the human? We mean by this term whether a human identifies as male or female, and whether the person meets in sexual behaviors and sex-related behaviors, the cultural expectations regarding psychosexual identity and behavior. According to this description of psychosexual identity and considering the human conditions reviewed in this chapter, we are convinced that psychosexual identity is primarily learned. The ease with which psychosexual identity can develop in opposition to genetic sex, endocrine sex, or genital sex simply by raising the infant as a boy or girl (in opposition to these factors) provides convincing evidence that psychosexual identity is the result of learning.

Certainly genetics, critical period and adult hormonal factors must play roles in gender identification, but these influences would seem to be quite limited in the human. The increased "femininity" in women with Turner's syndrome, and the personality differences in androgenized women may suggest roles for genetic and endocrinological factors. However, it is learning and the consistency of the cues provided by parents, peers, and one's own body that lead to psychosexual identification with one or the other gender. The meaning of gender identity can vary greatly in different societies or subcultures; however, consistency is critical. The evidence from children whose gender has been renounced suggests that if this happens after the first few years of life, problems with psychosexual identity are likely. One might also suspect that homosexuality, transvestism, and transsexualism have a major causation in the ambiguous nature of the gender identification provided by parents and siblings.

SUMMARY AND CONCLUSIONS

In the course of the present chapter, several fundamental factors that determine mammalian sexuality have been explored. Throughout this discussion a general notion regarding the principles of sexual dimorphism seems to have emerged: upon a basic genetic constitution that initially separates the sexes, a series of chemical, hormonal, and physiological processes takes place which builds upon genetic sex and subsequently serves to determine future sexual development. As development progresses and new stages of sexual maturation are seen, earlier levels of sexual differentiation become less influential in controlling future growth. Thus, following fertilization, genetic processes direct the growth and development of male and female gonads. After this stage, chemical secretions by the male gonads and an absence of these secretions in female gonads further direct sexual development along male and female lines. Various neurological structures, too, are influenced by early hormonal events setting the framework for the release of gonadotropic hormones at puberty and perhaps, also, general patterns of sex-related behaviors. As a consequence of the further development of the immature reproductive tissue in males and females at puberty, differential levels of sex hormones are secreted by each sex, which further serve to promote the anatomical distinction between males and females. These distinguishing anatomical characteristics then remain throughout the life of the individual, and together with the influence of complex social and cultural factors, establish a sexual identity for that individual. It will be noted that as each level of sexual development is reached, earlier levels will exert less and less of an influence on present or future sexual status. Thus, disorders of sexual biology or behavior in adulthood are more likely to be related to experiential, gonadal or pituitary pathology than to genetic involvement (assuming a normal development up to that point).

The biology of sexuality and the definition of gender must, therefore, be viewed in light of the long range course of sexual development. Although it may be appropriate to identify an embryo in terms of genetic sex, would it likewise be appropriate to sexually classify the same individual in adulthood on genetic grounds? In view of the ramifications of gonadal pathology, such a procedure loses much of its appeal.

Male and female sexuality is thus not simply a biological phenomenon, but necessarily encompasses social and legal mores that impose standards regarding the meaning of sexuality. In the face of new understanding of the biological and cultural bases of psychosexual identity, many of the traditional concepts of sexuality will most assuredly be modified.

REFERENCES

Abbs, E. T. The release of catecholamines by choline 2, 6-XYLYL ether, bretylium and guanethidine. *British Journal of Pharmacology and Chemotherapy,* 1966, **26**, 162–171.

Abbs, E. T., & Robertson, M. I. Selective depletion of noradrenaline: A proposed mechanism of the adrenergic neurone-blocking action of bretylium. *British Journal of Pharmacology,* 1970, **38**, 776–791.

Abrams, R. L. Clinical neuroendocrinology. In D. H. Ford (Ed.), *Influence of Hormones on the Nervous System,* Basel: Karger, 1971.

Adams, D. D., & Purves, H. D. Abnormal responses in the assay of thyrotrophin. *Proceedings of the University of Otago Medical School,* 1956, **34**, 11.

Adey, W. R., Bell, F. R., & Dennis, B. J. Effects of LSD-25, psilocybin and psilocin on temporal lobe EEG patterns in the cat. *Neurology,* 1962, **12**, 591–602.

Adriani, J. *The Chemistry and Physics of Anesthesia.* Springfield, Ill.: Charles C Thomas, 1962.

Adriani, J. (Ed.). *Appraisal of Current Concepts in Anesthesiology.* Vol. 4. Saint Louis: Mosby, 1968.

Adriani, J. *The Pharmacology of Anesthetic Drugs.* (5th ed.) Springfield, Ill.: Charles C Thomas, 1970.

Agranoff, B. W. Molecules and memories. *Perspectives in Biology and Medicine,* 1965, **2**, 13–22.

Agranoff, B. W. Agents that block memory. In G. C. Quarton, T. Melnechuk, and F. O. Schmidt (Eds.), *The Neurosciences.* New York: Rockefeller University Press, 1967.

Agranoff, B. W., Davis, R. E., & Brink, J. J. Memory fixation in the goldfish. *Proceedings of the National Academy of Sciences* (USA), 1965, **54**, 788–790.

Agurell, S., Nilsson, I. M., Ohlsson, A., & Sandberg, F. Elimination of tritium-labeled cannabinols in the rat with special reference to the development of tests for the identification of cannabis users. *Biochemical Pharmacology*, 1969, **18**, 1195-1201.

Agurell, S., Nilsson, I. M., Ohlsson, A., & Sandberg, F. On the metabolism of tritium-labeled delta-l-tetrahydrocannabinol in the rabbit. *Biochemical Pharmacology*, 1970, **19**, 1333-1339.

Ahlquist, R. P. A study of the adrenotropic receptors. *American Journal of Physiology*, 1948, **153**, 586-600.

Ahlskog, J. E., & Hoebel, B. G. Overeating and obesity from damage to a noradrenergic system in the brain. *Science*, 1973, **182**, 166-169.

Akil, H. & Mayer, D. J. Antagonism of stimulation-produced analgesia by p-CPA, a serotonin synthesis inhibitor. *Brain Research*, 1972, **44**, 692-697.

Alexander, N. J. & Sackler, A. M. An exchange of letters—Vasectomy: Long-term effects. *Science*, 1973, **182**, 946-947.

Algeri, E. J., Katsas, G. G., & Zuango, M. A. Determination of ethchlorovynol in biologic mediums, and report of two fatal cases. *American Journal of Clinical Pathology*, 1962, **38**, 125-130.

Anand, B. K., & Brobeck, J. R. Hypothalamic control of food intake in rats and cats. *Yale Journal of Biology and Medicine*, 1951, **24**, 123-128.

Anand, B. K., & Dua, S. Feeding responses induced by electrical stimulation of the hypothalamus in cat. *Indian Journal of Medical Research*, 1955, **43**, 113-122.

Anden, N. E., Carlsson, A., & Haggendal, J. Adrenergic mechanisms. *Annual Review of Pharmacology*, 1969, **9**, 119-134.

Andersson, B. Polydipsia caused by intrahypothalamic injections of hypertonic NaCl solutions. *Experientia*, 1952, **8**, 157-158.

Anlezark, G. M., Crow, T. J., & Greenway, A. P. Impaired learning and decreased cortical norepinephrine after bilateral locus coeruleus lesions. *Science*, 1973, **181**, 682-684.

Antelman, S. M., Lippa, A. S., Fisher, A. E., Bowers, M. B. Jr., Van Woert, M. H., Strauss, J. S., Carpenter, W. T. Jr., Stein, L., & Wise, C. D. 6-hydroxydopamine, noradrenergic reward, and schizophrenia. *Science*, 1972, **175**, 919-923.

Antoniades, H. N., Bougas, J. A., Camerini-Davalos, R., & Pyle, H. M. Insulin regulatory mechanisms and diabetes mellitus. *Diabetes*, 1964, **13**, 230-240.

Aprison, M. H., & Werman, R. A combined neurochemical and neurophysiological approach to identification of central nervous system transmitters. In *Neurosciences Research* Vol. I, 1968.

Arnold, K., & Gerber, N. The rate of decline of diphenylhydantoin in human plasma. *Clinical Pharmacology and Therapeutics*, 1970, **11**, 121-134.

Aronson, L. R., & Cooper, M. L. Seasonal variation in mating behavior in cats after desensitization of glans penis. *Science*, 1966, **152**, 226-230.

Arrigo, A., Savoldi, F., & Tartara, A. The effects of haloperidol and triperidol on behavior, electric activity and cerebral flow of blood in anesthetized rabbits. *Symposium internazionale nell Haloperido e treperidol.* Milan: Inst. Luso Farmaco A'Italia, 1962.

Artunkal, S., & Togrol, B. Psychological studies in hyperthyroidism. In M. P. Cameron and M. O'Connor (Eds.), *Brain-Thyroid Relationships. Ciba Foundation Study Group No. 18.* London: J. & A. Churchill, 1964.

Artusio, J. F., Jr. Di-ethyl ether analgesia: A detailed description of the first stage of ether anesthesia in man. *Journal of Pharmacology and Experimental Therapeutics,* 1954, 111, 343-348.

Artusio, J. F., & Puleo, A. J. Pharmacology. In D. E. Hale (Ed.), *Anesthesiology.* (2nd ed.) Philadelphia: Davis, 1963.

Asher, R. Myxoedematous madness. *British Medical Journal,* 1949, 2, 555-562.

Auerbach, P., & Carlton, P. L. Retention deficit correlated with a deficit in the corticoid response to stress. *Science,* 1971, 173, 1148-1149.

Avecado, H. F., Axelrod, L. R., Ishikawa, E., & Takaki, F. Studies of fetal metabolism. II. Metabolism of progesterone-4-C^{14} and pregnenolone-7α-H^3 in human fetal testes. *Journal of Clinical Endocrinology and Metabolism,* 1963, 23, 885-890.

Aviado, D. M. Ganglionic stimulant and blocking drugs. In J. R. DiPalma (Ed.), *Drill's Pharmacology in Medicine.* (4th ed.) New York: McGraw-Hill, 1971.

Ax, A. F. The physiological differentiation of fear and anger in humans. *Psychosomatic Medicine,* 1953, 15, 433-442.

Axelrod, J. Noradrenalin: Fate and control of its biosynthesis. *Science,* 1971, 173, 598-606.

Axelrod, J. The pineal gland: A neurochemical transducer. *Science,* 1974, 184, 1341-1348.

Axelrod, J., Brady, R. O., Witkop, B., & Evarts, E. V. The distribution and metabolism of lysergic acid diethylamide. *Annals of the New York Academy of Sciences,* 1957, 66, 435-444.

Ayhan, I. H. Effect of 6-hydroxydopamine on morphine analgesia. *Psychopharmacologia,* 1972, 25, 183-188.

Babbini, M., & Davis, W. M. Time-dose relationships for locomotor activity effects of morphine after acute or repeated treatment. *British Journal of Pharmacology,* 1972, 46, 213-224.

Baird, H. W., Szekely, E. G., Wycis, H. T., & Spiegel, E. A. The effect of meprobamate on the basal ganglia. *Annals of the New York Academy of Sciences,* 1957, 67, 873-884.

Baldessarini, R. J., & Kopin, I. J. The effect of drugs on the release of norepinephrine-H^3 from central nervous system tissues by electrical stimulation in vitro. *Journal of Pharmacology and Experimental Therapeutics,* 1967, 156, 31-38.

Ban, T. A. *Psychopharmacology.* Baltimore: Williams & Wilkins, 1969.

Bandler, R. J., Jr. Facilitation of aggressive behavior in the rat by direct cholinergic stimulation of the hypothalamus. *Nature,* 1969, **224**, 1035-1036.

Bandler, R. J., Jr. Cholinergic synapses in the lateral hypothalamus for the control of predatory aggression in the rat. *Brain Research,* 1970, **20**, 409-424.

Bannister, R. *Brain's Clinical Neurology.* (3rd ed.) London: Oxford University Press, 1969.

Banting, F. G., Best, C. H., Collip, J. B., Campbell, W. R., & Fletcher, A. A. Pancreatic extracts in the treatment of diabetes mellitus. *Canadian Medical Association Journal,* 1922, **12**, 141-146.

Barger, G. *Ergot and Ergotism.* London: Gurney and Jackson, 1931.

Barker, J., & Gainer, H. Pentobarbital: Selective depression of excitatory postsynaptic potentials. *Science,* 1973, **182**, 720-722.

Barondes, S. H. Relationship of biological regulatory mechanisms to learning and memory. *Nature,* 1965, **205**, 18-21.

Barondes, S. H., & Cohen, H. D. Puromycin effect on successive phases of memory storage. *Science,* 1966, **151**, 594-595.

Barondes, S. H., & Cohen, H. D. Comparative effects of cycloheximide and puromycin on cerebral protein synthesis and consolidation of memory in mice. *Brain Research,* 1967, **4**, 44-51.

Barondes, S. H., & Jarvik, M. E. Influence of actinomycin-D on brain RNA synthesis and memory. *Journal of Neurochemistry,* 1964, **11**, 187-195.

Barr, M. L., Carr, D. H., Pozsonyi, J., Wilson, R. A., Dunn, H. G., Jacobson, T. S., Miller, J. R., Lewis, M., & Chown, B. The XXY sex chromosome abnormality. *Canadian Medical Association Journal,* 1963, **87**, 891-901.

Barr, M. L., Diczfalusy, E., & Tillinger, K. G. Studies on oestrogen metabolism in infants and children. *Acta Endocrinology,* 1961, **37**, 241.

Barraclough, C. A., & Gorski, R. A. Studies on mating behavior in the androgen-sterilized female rat in relation to the hypothalamic regulation of sexual behavior. *Journal of Endocrinology,* 1962, **25**, 175-182.

Baudelaire, C. *Artificial Paradises, On Hashish and Wine as Means of Expanding Individuality.* New York: Herder and Herder, 1971.

Beach, F. A. Coital behavior in dogs: VI. Long-term effects of castration upon mating behavior in the male. *Journal of Comparative and Physiological Psychology,* 1970, **70**, 1-32.

Beach, F. A., & Levinson, G. Effects of androgen on the glans penis and mating behavior of castrated male rats. *Journal of Experimental Zoology,* 1950, **114**, 159-171.

Beach, G., & Kimble, D. P. Activity and responsivity in rats after magnesium pemoline injections. *Science,* 1967, **155**, 698-701.

Beaser, S. B. Orally given combinations of drugs in diabetes mellitus therapy. *Journal of the American Medical Association,* 1960, **174**, 2137-2141.

Becker, H. S. *Outsiders Studies in the Sociology of Deviance.* New York: Free Press, 1963.

Beecher, H. K. The use of chemical agents in the control of pain. In R. S. Knighton and P. R. Dumke (Eds.), *Pain.* Boston: Little, Brown, 1966.

Beleslin, D., & Polak, R. Depression by morphine and chloralose of acetylcholinesterase release from cat's brain. *Journal of Physiology,* 1965, **177**, 411–419.

Bennett, E. L., Diamond, M. C., Krech, D., & Rosenzweig, M. R. Chemical and anatomical plasticity of brain. *Science,* 1964, **146**, 610–619.

Berger, B. D., Wise, C. D., & Stein, L. Norepinephrine: Reversal of anorexia in rats with lateral hypothalamic damage. *Science,* 1971, **172**, 281–284.

Berger, B. D., Wise, C. D., & Stein, L. Nerve growth factor: Enhanced recovery of feeding after hypothalamic damage. *Science,* 1973, **180**, 506–508.

Berger, F. M. The pharmacological properties of 2-methyl-2-N-propyl-l, 3 propanediol dicarbamate (Miltown), a new interneuronal blocking agent. *Journal of Pharmacology and Experimental Therapeutics,* 1954, **112**, 412–423.

Berger, F. M. The chemistry and mode of action of tranquilizing drugs. *Annals of the New York Academy of Sciences,* 1957, **67**, 685–700.

Berger, F. M., & Bradley, W. The pharmacological properties of L. B. dihydroxy-o-(2-methylphenoxy)-propane (myanisin). *British Journal of Pharmacology and Chemotherapy,* 1946, **1**, 265–272.

Berson, S. A., & Yalow, R. S. Plasma Insulin. In M. Ellinberg and H. Rifkin (Eds.), *Diabetes Mellitus: Theory and Practice.* New York: McGraw-Hill, 1970.

Bishop, M. P., Elder, S. T., & Heath, R. G. Attempted control of operant behavior in man with intracranial self-stimulation. In R. G. Heath (Ed.), *The Role of Pleasure in Behavior.* New York: Harper & Row, 1964.

Bittner, G. D., & Kennedy, D. Quantitative aspects of transmitter release. *Journal of Cell Biology,* 1970, **47**, 585–592.

Bjorkland, A., Ehinger, B., & Falck, B. A method for differentiating dopamine from norepinephrine in tissue sections by microspectrofluorometry. *Journal of Histochemistry,* 1968, **16**, 263–275.

Black, M. B., Woods, J. H., & Domino, E. F. Some effects of (-)-Δ^9-trans-tetrahydro-cannabinol and other cannabis derivatives on schedule-controlled behavior. *Pharmacologist,* 1970, **12**, 258.

Bleuler, E. *Dementia Praecox or the Group of Schizophrenias.* New York: International Universities Press, 1950.

Bloch, G. J., & Davidson, J. M. Antiandrogen implanted in brain stimulates male reproductive system. *Science,* 1967, **155**, 593–595.

Bloch, G. J., & Davidson, J. M. Effects of adrenalectomy and experience on postcastration sex behavior in the male rat. *Physiology and Behavior,* 1968, **3**, 461–465.

Bloom, F. E. The fine structural localization of biogenic monoamines in nervous tissue. *International Review of Neurobiology,* 1970, **13**, 27–66.

Bloom, F. E., & Giarman, N. J. Physiologic and pharmacologic considerations of biogenic amines in the nervous system. *Annual Review of Pharmacology,* 1968, **8**, 229–258.

Bloom, F. E., Oliver, A. P., & Salmoiraghi, G. C. The responsiveness of individual hypothalamic neurons to microelectrophoretically administered endogenous amines. *International Journal of Neuropharmacology*, 1963, **2**, 181-193.

Blough, D. S. New test for tranquilizers. *Science*, 1958, **127**, 586-587.

Bogoch, S. *The Biochemistry of Memory.* New York: Oxford, 1968.

Bohdanecka, M., Bohdanecky, Z., & Jarvik, M. E. Puromycin effect on memory may be due to occult seizures. *Science,* 1967, **157**, 333-336.

Bohdanecky, Z., Kopp, R., & Jarvik, M. E. Comparison of ECS and flurothyl-induced retrograde amnesia in mice. *Psychopharmacologia,* 1968, **12**, 91-95.

Bole, G. G., Jr., Friedlaender, M. H., & Smith, C. K. Rheumatic symptoms and serologic abnormalities induced by oral contraceptives. *Lancet,* 1969, **1**, 323-326.

Booth, D. A. Localization of the adrenergic feeding system in the rat diencephalon. *Science,* 1967, **158**, 515-517. (a)

Booth, D. A. Vertebrate brain ribonucleic acids and memory retention. *Psychological Bulletin*, 1967, **68**, 149-177. (b)

Booth, D. A. Amphetamine anorexia by direct action on the adrenergic feeding system of rat hypothalamus. *Nature*, 1968, **217**, 869-870.

Borrzetti, L., Goldsmith, S., & Ungerleider, J. T. The "great banana hoax." *American Journal of Psychiatry,* 1967, **124**, 678-679.

Boura, A. L. A., & Green, A. F. Adrenergic neurone blocking agents. *Annual Review of Pharmacology,* 1965, **5**, 183-212.

Bradley, K., Easton, D. M., & Eccles, J. C. An investigation of primary and direct inhibition. *Journal of Physiology,* 1953, **122**, 474-488.

Bradley, P. B. Synaptic transmission in the central nervous system and its relevance for drug action. *International Review of Neurobiology*, 1968, **11**, 1-56.

Bradley, P. B., Eayrs, J. T., Glass, A., & Heath, R. W. The maturational and metabolic consequences of neonatal thyroidectomy upon the recruiting response in the rat. *EEG Journal*, 1961, **13**, 577-586.

Bradley, P. B., Eayrs, J. T., & Richards, N. M. Factors influencing potentials in normal and cretinous rats. *EEG Journal*, 1964, **17**, 308-313.

Bradley, P. B., Eayrs, J. T., & Schmalbach, K. The electroencephalogram of normal and hypothyroid rats. *EEG Journal,* 1960, **12**, 467-477.

Bradley, P. B., & Elkes, J. The effects of some drugs on the electrical activity of the brain. *Brain,* 1957, **80**, 77-117.

Brady, J. V. Emotion and sensitivity of psychoendocrine systems. In D. C. Glass (Ed.), *Neurophysiology and Emotion.* New York: Rockefeller Univ. Press, 1967.

Brain, W. R., & Walton, J. N. *Brain's Diseases of the Nervous System.* (7th ed.) London: Oxford, 1969.

Brasel, J. A., & Blizzard, R. M. The influence of the endocrine glands upon growth and development. In R. H. Williams (Ed.), *Textbook of Endocrinology.* (5th ed.) Philadelphia: Saunders, 1974.

Braun, G. A., Poos, G. I., & Soudyn, W. Distribution, excretion, and metabolism of neuroleptics of the butyrophenone type. *European Journal of Pharmacology*, 1967, **1**, 58–62.

Brazeau, P. Oxytocics: Oxytocin and ergot alkaloids. In L. S. Goodman and A. Gilman (Eds.), *The Pharmacological Basis of Therapeutics*. (4th ed.) New York: Macmillan, 1970.

Brecher, E. M. *Licit and Illicit Drugs*. Boston: Little, Brown, 1972.

Breen, R. A., & McGaugh, J. L. Facilitation of maze learning with post trial injections of picrotoxin. *Journal of Comparative and Physiological Psychology*, 1961, **54**, 498–501.

Breggin, P. R. Sedative-like effect of epinephrine: A review. *Archives of General Psychiatry*, 1965, **12**, 255–259.

Bresler, D. E., & Bitterman, M. E. Learning in fish with transplanted brain tissue. *Science*, 1969, **163**, 590–592.

Bridger, W. H., & Gantt, H. W. The effect of mescaline on differentiated conditional reflexes. *American Journal of Psychiatry*, 1956, **113**, 352–360.

Brobeck, J. R., Larsson, S., & Reyes, E. A study of the electrical activity of the hypothalamic feeding mechanism. *Journal of Physiology*, 1956, **132**, 358–364.

Brodie, B. B. Interaction of psychotropic drugs with physiological and biochemical mechanisms in brain. *Modern Medicine*, 1959, **4**, 453–460.

Brodie, B. B., Mark, L. C., Popper, E. M., Lief, P. A., Bernstein, E., & Rovenstein, E. A. The fate of thiopental in man and a method for its estimation in biological material. *Journal of Pharmacology and Experimental Therapeutics*, 1950, **98**, 85–96.

Brodie, B. B., Pletscher, A., & Shore, P. A. Possible role of serotonin in brain function and in reserpine action. *Journal of Pharmacology and Experimental Therapeutics*, 1956, **116**, 9.

Brodie, B. B., & Reid, W. D. Serotonin in brain: Functional considerations. *Advances in Pharmacology*, 1968, **6B**, 97–113.

Brodie, B. B., & Shore, P. A. A concept for the role of serotonin and norepinephrine as chemical mediators in the brain. *Annals of the New York Academy of Sciences*, 1957, **66**, 631–642.

Bromer, W. W., Sinn, L. G., & Behrens, O. K. The amino acid sequence of glucagon. *Journal of the American Chemical Society*, 1957, **79**, 2807–2810.

Brügger, M. Fresstrieb als hypothalmisches Symptom. *Helvetica Physiologica et Pharmacologica*, 1943, **1**, 183–198.

Buerger, P. B., Levitt, R. A., & Irwin, D. A. Chemical stimulation of the brain: Relationship between neural activity and water ingestion in the rat. *Journal of Comparative and Physiological Psychology*, 1973, **82**, 278–285.

Bunge, R. G. Plasma testosterone levels in man before and after vasectomy. *Investigative Urology*, 1972, **10**, 9.

Burn, J. H., & Rand, M. J. Acetylcholine in adrenergic transmission. *Annual Review of Pharmacology*, 1965, **5**, 163–182.

Burt, R. L. Peripheral utilization of glucose in pregnancy. III. Insulin tolerance. *Obstetrics and Gynecology*, 1956, **7**, 658-664.

Butler, T. C., Mahaffee, C., & Waddell, W. J. Phenobarbital: Studies of elimination, accumulation, tolerance and dosage schedules. *Journal of Pharmacology and Experimental Therapeutics*, 1954, **111**, 425-435.

Byrne, W. L., et al. Memory transfer. *Science*, 1966, **153**, 658.

Cade, J. F. J. Lithium salts in the treatment of psychotic excitement. *Medical Journal of Australia*, 1949, **2**, 349-352.

Caggiula, A. R., & Hoebel, B. G. "Copulation-reward site" in the posterior hypothalamus. *Science*, 1966, **153**, 1284-1285.

Cairncross, K. D., Gershon, S., & Gust, I. D. Some aspects of the mode of action of imipramine. *Journal of Neurophysiology*, 1963, **4**, 224-231.

Cameron, D. E., Kral, V. A., Solyom, L., Sved, S., Wainrib, B., Beaulieu, C., & Enesco, H. RNA and memory. In J. Gaito (Ed.), *Macromolecules and Behavior*. New York: Appleton-Century-Crofts, 1966.

Cardo, B. Action of dextrorotatory amphetamine and of eserine on conditioned flight and phenomena of discrimination. *Journal of Physiology* (Paris), 1959, **51**, 845-860.

Carlisle, H. J. Differential effects of amphetamine on food and water intake in rats with lateral hypothalamic lesions. *Journal of Comparative and Physiological Psychology*, 1964, **58**, 47-54.

Carlson, N. J., Doyle, G. A., & Bidder, T. G. The effect of dl-amphetamine and reserpine on runway performance. *Psychopharmacologia*, 1965, **8**, 157-173.

Carlsson, A. On the problem of the mode of action of some psychoactive drugs. *Psychiatry and Neurology*, 1960, **140**, 220.

Carlsson, A. Pharmacology of synaptic monoamine transmission. *Progress in Brain Research*, 1969, **31**, 53-59.

Carlton, P. L. Augmentation of the behavioral effects of amphetamine by scopolamine. *Psychopharmacologia*, 1961, **2**, 377-380. (a)

Carlton, P. L. Potentiation of the behavioral effects of amphetamine by imipramine. *Psychopharmacologia*, 1961, **2**, 364-376. (b)

Carlton, P. L. Cholinergic mechanisms in the control of behavior by the brain. *Psychological Reviews*, 1963, **70**, 14-39.

Carlton, P. L. Brain-acetylcholine and inhibition. In J. T. Tapp (Ed.), *Reinforcement and Behavior*. New York: Academic, 1969.

Carlton, P. L., & Markiewicz, B. Behavioral effects of atropine and scopolamine. In E. Furchtgott (Ed.), *Pharmacological and Biophysical Agents and Behavior*. New York: Academic, 1971.

Carlton, P. L., & Vogel, J. R. Studies of the amnesic properties of scopolamine. *Psychonomic Science*, 1965, **3**, 261-262.

Carpenter, W. T. Jr., Strauss, J. S., & Bartko, J. J. Flexible system for the diagnosis of schizophrenia: Report from the WHO international pilot study of schizophrenia. *Science*, 1973, **182**, 1275-1278.

Carr, L. A., & Moore, K. E. Norepinephrine: Release from brain by d-amphetamine in vivo. *Science,* 1969, **164,** 322–323.

Carrier, O. *Pharmacology of the Peripheral Autonomic Nervous System.* Chicago: Year Book, 1972.

Carruthers, R. Chloasma and oral contraceptives. *Medical Journal of Australia,* 1966, **2,** 17–20.

Cerf, J., & Otis, L. S. Heat narcosis and its effect on retention of a learned behavior in the goldfish. *Federation Proceedings,* 1957, **16,** 20–26.

Chamberlain, T. J., Rothchild, G. H., & Gerard, R. W. Drugs affecting RNA and learning. *Proceedings of the National Academy of Sciences* (USA), 1963, **49,** 918–925.

Chance, M. R. A. Aggregation as a factor influencing the toxicity of sympathomimetic amines in mice. *Journal of Pharmacology,* 1946, **87,** 214–219.

Charney, C. W., Conston, A. S., & Meranze, D. R. Testicular developmental histology. *Annals of the New York Academy of Sciences,* 1952, **55,** 597.

Chase, L. R., Fedak, S. A., & Aurbach, G. D. Activation of skeletal adenyl cyclase by parathyroid hormone in vitro. *Endocrinology,* 1969, **84,** 761–768.

Chen, K. K. *Symposium on Sedative and Hypnotic Drugs.* Baltimore: Williams & Wilkins, 1954.

Cholewiak, R. W., Hammond, R., Seigler, I. C., & Papsdorf, J. D. The effects of strychnine sulphate on the classically conditioned nictitating membrane response of the rabbit. *Journal of Comparative and Physiological Psychology,* 1968, **66,** 77–81.

Chopra, J. C., & Chopra, R. N. The use of cannabis drug in India. *Bulletin of Narcotics,* 1967, **9,** 4–29.

Chorine, V. Action de l'amide nicotiniqué sur les bacilles du gendre mycobacterium. *C. R. Academy of Science* (Paris), 1945, **220,** 150.

Chorover, S. L. Effects of mescaline sulfate on extinction of conditional avoidance response. *Journal of Comparative and Physiological Psychology,* 1961, **54,** 649–652.

Christenson, A. K., & Mason, N. R. Comparative ability of seminiferous tubules and interstitial tissue of rat testes to synthesize androgens from progesterone-4-C^{14} in vitro. *Endocrinology,* 1965, **76,** 646–656.

Clark, F. C., & Steele, B. J. Effects of d-amphetamine on performance under a multiple schedule in the rat. *Psychopharmacologia,* 1966, **9,** 315–335.

Clermont, Y. Quantitative analysis of spermatogenesis in the rat: A revised model for the renewal of spermatogonia. *American Journal of Anatomy,* 1962, **111,** 111–130.

Clermont, Y., & Harvey, S. C. Duration of the cycle of seminiferous epithelium of normal, hypophysectomized and hypophysectomized-hormone treated albino rats. *Endocrinology,* 1965, **76,** 80–89.

Clouet, D. H. The alteration of brain metabolism by narcotic analgesic drugs. In A. Lajtha (Ed.), *Handbook of Neurochemistry*, Vol. VI. New York: Plenum, 1971.

Cochin, J. Role of possible immune mechanisms in the development of tolerance. In D. H. Clouet (Ed.), *Narcotic Drugs: Biochemical Pharmacology*, New York: Plenum, 1971.

Cohen, H. D., & Barondes, S. H. Further studies of learning and memory after intracerebral actinomycin-D. *Journal of Neurochemistry*, 1966, **13**, 207-211.

Cohen, H. D., & Barondes, S. H. Puromycin effect on memory may be due to occult seizures. *Science*, 1967, **157**, 333-334.

Cohen, H. D., Ervin, F. J., & Barondes, S. H. Puromycin and cycloheximide: Different effects on hippocampal electrical activity. *Science*, 1966, **154**, 1557-1558.

Cohen, J. *Secondary Motivation I: Personal Motives*. Chicago: Rand McNally, 1970.

Cohen, P. J., & Dripps, R. D. History and theories of general anesthesia. In L. S. Goodman and A. Gilman (Eds.), *The Pharmacological Basis of Therapeutics*. (4th ed.) New York: Macmillan, 1970.

Cohen, S. Lysergic acid diethylamide side effects and complications. *Journal of Nervous and Mental Disease*, 1960, **130**, 30-40.

Cohen, S., & Ditman, K. S. Prolonged adverse reactions to lysergic acid diethylamide. *AMA Archives of General Psychiatry*, 1963, **8**, 475-480.

Cohn, C. K., Ball, G. G., & Hirsch, J. Histamine: Effect on self-stimulation. *Science*, 1973, **180**, 758-759.

Cole, J. O. Therapeutic efficacy of antidepressant drugs. *Journal of the American Medical Association*, 1964, **190**, 448-455.

Cole, S. O. Experimental effects of amphetamine: A review. *Psychological Bulletin*, 1967, **68**, 81-90.

Cole, S. O. Hypothalamic feeding mechanisms and amphetamine anorexia. *Psychological Bulletin*, 1973, **79**, 13-20.

Collins, W. F., Nuylsen, F. E., & Shealy, C. N. Electrophysiological studies of peripheral and central pathways conducting pain. In R. S. Knighton and P. R. Dumke (Eds.), *Pain*. Boston: Little, Brown, 1966.

Collip, J. B. The parathyroid glands. *Medicine*, 1926, **5**, 1.

Committee on Safety of Drugs. Risk of thromboembolic disease in women taking oral contraceptives. *British Medical Journal*, 1967, **2**, 355-359.

Conney, A. H. Pharmacological implications of microsomal enzyme induction. *Pharmacological Review*, 1967, **19**, 317-366.

Contreras, W., & Tamayo, L. Influence of changes in brain 5-OH tryptamine on morphine analgesia. *Archives of Experimental Medicine and Biology*, 1967, **4**, 69-71.

Cook, L., & Weidley, E. Behavioral effects of some psychopharmacological agents. *Annals of the New York Academy of Sciences*, 1957, **66**, 740-752.

Cook, W. B., & Keeland, W. E. Isolation and partial characterization of a glycoside from *Rivea corymbosa* (L) hallier folius. *Journal of Organic Chemistry*, 1962, 27, 1061-1062.

Cooper, J. R., Bloom, F. E., & Roth, R. H. *The Biochemical Basis of Neuropharmacology*. (2nd ed.) New York: Oxford Press, 1974.

Cooper, J. R., & Kini, M. M. Biochemical aspects of methanol poisoning. *Biochemical Pharmacology*, 1962, 11, 405-416.

Corning, W. C., & John, E. R. Effect of ribonuclease on retention of response in regenerated planarians. *Science*, 1961, 134, 1363-1365.

Corrodi, H., Fuxe, K., Hokfelt, T., & Schou, M. The effect of lithium on cerebral monamine neurons. *Psychopharmacologia*, 1967, 11, 345-353.

Costa, E., & Neff, N. H. Estimation of turnover rates to study the metabolic regulation of the steady state level of neuronal monoamines. In A. Lajtha (Ed.), *Handbook of Neurochemistry*, Vol. 4. New York: Plenum, 1970.

Cotzias, G. C., Tang, L. C., Miller, S. T., & Ginos, J. Z. Melatonin and abnormal movements induced by L-dopa in mice. *Science*, 1971, 173, 450-452.

Coupland, R. E. *The Natural History of the Chromaffin Cell.* Boston: Little, Brown, 1965.

Coury, J. N. Neural correlates of food and water intake in the rat. *Science*, 1967, 156, 1763-1765.

Coyle, J. T., & Axelrod, J. Development of the uptake and storage of L-$[^3H]$ norepinephrine in the rat brain. *Journal of Neurochemistry*, 1971, 18, 2061-2075.

Crancer, A. Jr., Dille, J. M., Delay, J. C., Wallace, V. E., & Haykin, M. D. Comparison of the effects of marijuana and alcohol on simulated driving performance. *Science*, 1969, 164, 851-854.

Crane, G. E. Clinical psychopharmacology in its 20th year. *Science*, 1973, 181, 124-128.

Creaser, E. H. The effect of 8-azaguanine on enzyme formation in staphylococcus aureus. *Biochemical Journal*, 1956, 64, 539-545.

Cross, B. A. Neurohypophyseal control of parturition. In C. W. Loyd (Ed.), *Endocrinology of Reproduction.* New York: Academic, 1959.

Csapo, A. Function and regulation of the myometrium. *Annals of the New York Academy of Sciences*, 1959, 75, 790.

Cullumbine, H. Cholinergic blocking drugs. In J. R. DiPalma (Ed.), *Drill's Pharmacology in Medicine.* New York: McGraw-Hill, 1971.

Curtis, B. A., Jacobson, S., & Marcus, E. M. *An Introduction to the Neurosciences.* Philadelphia: Saunders, 1972.

Curtis, D. R., & Watkins, J. C. The pharmacology of amino acids related to gamma-amino butyric acid. *Pharmacological Reviews*, 1965, 17, 347-392.

Dackin, M. A. Puromycin inhibition of protein synthesis. *Pharmacological Reviews*, 1964, 16, 223-243.

Dafares, J. G. Influence of oral contraceptives on women. *Neder. L. tijdschr. geneesk*, 1967, 111, 1115-1120.

Dahlstrom, A. Influence of colchicine on axoplasmic transport of amine storage granules in rat sympathetic adrenergic nerves. *Acta Physiologica Scandinavica,* 1970, **76**, 33A-34A.

Dahlstrom, A., & Fuxe, K. Evidence for the existence of monoamine-containing neurons in the central nervous system. I. Demonstration of monoamines in the cell bodies of the brain stem neurons. *Acta Physiologica Scandinavica,* 1964, **62**, Suppl. 232, 1-55.

Dahlstrom, A., & Haggendal, J. Studies on the transport and life-span of amine storage granules in a peripheral adrenergic neuron system. *Acta Physiologica Scandinavica,* 1966, **67**, 278-288.

Dale, H. H. Chemical transmission of the effects of nerve impulses. *British Medical Journal,* 1934, **1**, 835-841.

Dale, H. H. The beginnings and the prospects of neurohormonal transmission. *Pharmacological Reviews,* 1954, **6**, 7-13.

D'Amour, F. E., & Smith, D. L. A method for determining loss of pain sensation. *Journal of Pharmacology and Experimental Therapeutics,* 1941, **72**, 74-79.

Danowski, T. S. *Clinical Endocrinology, Vol. II-Thyroid.* Baltimore: Williams & Wilkins, 1962. (a)

Danowski, T. S. *Clinical Endocrinology, Vol. III-Adrenal Cortex and Medulla.* Baltimore: Williams & Wilkins, 1962 (b)

Daughaday, W. H. The Adenohypophysis. In R. H. Williams (Ed.), *Textbook of Endocrinology.* (5th ed.) Philadelphia: Saunders, 1974.

Davidson, J. M. Hormones and reproductive behavior. In S. Levine (Ed.), *Hormones and Behavior.* New York: Academic, 1972.

Davis, W. M., Babbini, M., & Khalsa, J. H. Antagonism by alpha-methyltyrosine of morphine induced motility in non-tolerant and tolerant rats. *Research Communications in Pathological Pharmacology,* 1972, **4**, 267-279.

Davis, W. M., & Smith, B. G. Alpha-methyltyrosine to prevent self-administration of morphine and amphetamine. *Current Therapeutic Research,* 1972, **14**, 814-819.

Davson, H. The blood-brain barrier. In G. H. Bourne (Ed.), *The Structure and Function of Nervous Tissue.* Vol. 4. New York: Academic, 1972.

Day, R. W., Larson, W., & Wright, S. W. Clinical and cytogenic studies on a group of females with XXX chromosome compliment. *Journal of Pediatrics,* 1964, **64**, 24-33.

De Bodo, R. C., & Prescott, K. F. The antidiuretic action of barbiturates (phenobarbital, Amytal, pentobarbital) and the mechanism involved in this action. *Journal of Pharmacology and Experimental Therapeutics,* 1945, **85**, 222-233.

DeFeudis, F. V., Delgado, J. M. R., & Roth, R. H. Content, synthesis and collectability of amino acids in various structures of the brain of rhesus monkeys. *Brain Research,* 1970, **18**, 15-23.

Delay, J., & Deniker, P. Trente-huit cas de psychoses traitées par la une prolongee et continue de 4560 RP. Le Congress des Al. et Neurol. de Langue Fr. In *Compte rendu du Congrés.* Masson et Cie, Paris, 1952.

Delay, J., Deniker, P., & Harl, J. M. Utilisation en thérapeutique psychiatrique d'une phenothiazine d'action centrale élective (4560 RP). *Annals of Medical Psychology* (Paris), 1952, **110**, 112–117.

Delay, J., Laine, B., & Buisson, J. F. Note concernant l'action de l'isonicotinyl-hydrazide dans le traitement des etats dépressifs. *Annals of Medical Psychology* (Paris), 1952, **110**, 689.

Delgado, J. M. R., & Anand, B. K. Increased food intake induced by electrical stimulation of the lateral hypothalamus. *American Journal of Physiology,* 1953, **172**, 162–168.

De Robertis, E. Ultrastructure and cytochemistry of the synaptic region. *Science,* 1967, **156**, 907–914.

De Ropp, R. S. *Drugs and the Mind.* New York: Grove Press, 1957.

Deutsch, J. A. The cholinergic synapse and the site of memory. *Science,* 1971, **174**, 788–794.

Deutsch, S., & Vandam, L. D. General anesthesia I: Volatile agents. In J. R. Dipalma (Ed.), *Drill's Pharmacology in Medicine.* (4th ed.) New York: McGraw-Hill, 1971.

Devor, M. G., Wise, R. A., Milgram, N. W., & Hoebel, B. G. Physiological control of hypothalamically elicited feeding and drinking. *Journal of Comparative and Physiological Psychology,* 1970, **73**, 226–232.

DeWied, D., Bohus, B., & Greven, H. M. Influence of pituitary and adrenocortical hormones on conditioned avoidance behavior in rats. In R. P. Michaels (Ed.), *Endocrinology and Human Behavior,* London: Oxford, 1968.

DeWied, D., van Delft, A. M. L., Gispen, W. H., Weignen, J. A. W. M., & van Wimersma Greidanus, T. I. B. The role of pituitary-adrenal system hormones in active avoidance and conditioning. In S. Levine (Ed.), *Hormones and Behavior.* New York: Academic, 1972.

Dews, P. B. Studies on behavior. IV. Stimulant actions of methamphetamine. *Journal of Pharmacology and Experimental Therapeutics,* 1958, **122**, 137–147.

Dews, P. B., & Morse, W. H. Behavioral pharmacology. *Annual Review of Pharmacology,* 1961, **1**, 145–174.

DiMascio, A., & Barrett, J. Comparative effects of oxazepam in high and low anxious student volunteers. *Psychosomatics,* 1965, **6**, 298–305.

Dingell, J. V., Wilcox, H. G., & Klausner, H. A. Biochemical interactions of delta-9-tetrahydrocannabinol. *Pharmacologist,* 1971, **13**, 296.

Dingman, W., & Sporn, M. B. The incorporation of 8-azaguanine into rat brain RNA and its effect on maze-learning by the rat: An inquiry into the biochemical bases of memory. *Journal of Psychiatric Research,* 1961, **1**, 1–11.

Dole, V. P. Narcotic addiction, physical dependence and relapse. *New England Journal of Medicine,* 1972, **286**, 988–992.

Donovon, B., & Van Der Werff Ten Bosch, J. J. *Physiology of Puberty.* Baltimore: Williams & Wilkins, 1965.

Dorfman, R. I., Forschielli, E., & Gut, M. Androgen biosynthesis and related studies. *Recent Progress in Hormonal Research,* 1963, **19**, 251.

Douglas, W. W. Histamines and antihistamines; 5-hydroxytryptamine and antagonists. In L. S. Goodman and A. Gilman (Eds.), *The Pharmacological Basis of Therapeutics.* (4th ed.) New York: Macmillan, 1970.

Doyle, A. C. *The Complete Sherlock Holmes.* New York: Garden City, 1938.

Drease, A., & DeMeyer, R. Influence of four butyrophenone neuroleptics on rat brain noradrenalin depletory effect of reserpine. *Life Sciences,* 1964, **3**, 759-762.

Dreyfus, P. M. Nutritional disorders of the nervous system. In P. B. Beeson and W. McDermott (Eds.), *Cecil-Loeb Textbook of Medicine.* (13th ed.) Philadelphia: Saunders, 1971.

Dubas, T., Lundy, P., Calhoun, E., & Parker, J. M. Investigation of mechanisms involved in toxic effects of narcotic analgesics. *International Journal of Clinical Pharmacology, Therapy and Toxicology,* 1972, **6**, 397-402.

Dye, J. A., & Maughm, G. H. Further studies of the thyroid gland V. The thyroid gland as a growth-promoting and form-determining factor in the development of the animal body. *American Journal of Anatomy,* 1929, **44**, 331.

Eayrs, J. T. The cerebral cortex of normal and hypothyroid rats. *Acta Anatomy* (Basel), 1955, **25**, 160.

Eayrs, J. T. Age as a factor determining the severity and reversibility of the effects of thyroid deprivation in the rat. *Journal of Endocrinology,* 1961, **22**, 409-419.

Eayrs, J. T. Developmental relationship between brain and thyroid. In R. P. Michaels (Ed.), *Endocrinology and Human Behavior,* London: Oxford, 1968.

Eayrs, J. T., & Levine, S. Influence of thyroidectomy and subsequent replacement therapy upon conditioned avoidance learning in the rat. *Journal of Endocrinology,* 1963, **25**, 505-513.

Eayrs, J. T., & Lishman, W. A. The maturation of behavior in hypothyroidism and starvation. *British Journal of Animal Behavior,* 1955, **3**, 17.

Eayrs, J. T., & Taylor, S. H. The effect of thyroid deficiency induced by methyl thiouracil on the maturation of the central nervous system. *Journal of Anatomy,* 1951, **85**, 350-358.

Eddy, N. B. The search for a potent non-addicting analgesic. In E. L. Way (Ed.), *Pain and its Clinical Management,* Philadelphia: Davis, 1967.

Efron, D. H. (Ed.) *Psychotomimetic Drugs.* New York: Raven Press, 1970.

Ehrhardt, A. A. Maternalism in fetal hormonal and related syndromes. In J. Zubin and J. Money (Eds.), *Contemporary Sexual Behavior: Critical Issues in the 1970s.* Baltimore: Johns Hopkins, 1973.

Eidelberg, E., & Barstow, C. A. Morphine tolerance and dependence induced by intraventricular injection. *Science,* 1971, **174**, 74-76.

Eist, H., & Seal, U. S. The permeability of the blood-brain barrier and blood-CSF barrier to C^{14} tagged ribonucleic acid. *American Journal of Psychiatry,* 1965, **122**, 584-586.

Eitinger, L. Hyperparathyroidism with mental changes. *Nord Medicine,* 1942, **14**, 1581.

Elliot, K. A. C., & Florey, E. Factor I–inhibitory factor from brain. Assay. Conditions in brain. Simulating and antagonizing substances. *Journal of Neurochemistry*, 1956, **1**, 181-191.

Elliot, T. R. The action of adrenalin. *Journal of Physiology*, 1905, **32**, 401-467.

Ellis, H. Mescal: A study of a divine plant. *Popular Science Monthly*, 1902, **61**, 59.

Endroczi, E. Pavlovian conditioning and adaptive hormones. In S. Levine (Ed.), *Hormones and Behavior*. New York: Academic, 1972.

Enesco, H. E. Fate of ^{14}C-RNA injected into mice. *Experimental Cell Research*, 1966, **42**, 640-645.

Epstein, A. N. Reciprocal changes in feeding behavior produced by intra-hypothalamic chemical injections. *American Journal of Physiology*, 1960, **199**, 969-974.

Epstein, A. N., Fitzsimons, J. T., & Simons, B. J. Drinking caused by the intracranial injection of angiotensin into the rat. *Journal of Physiology*, 1969, **200**, 98-100.

Epstein, A. W. The relationship of altered brain states to sexual psycho-pathology. In J. Zubin and J. Money (Eds.), *Contemporary Sexual Behavior: Critical Issues in the 1970s*. Baltimore: Johns Hopkins, 1973.

Ericsson, A. D. Potentiation of the L-DOPA effect in man by the use of catechol-o-methyltransferase inhibitors. *Journal of the Neurological Sciences*, 1971, **14**, 193-197.

Esplin, D. W. Centrally acting muscle relaxants; drugs for Parkinson's disease. In L. S. Goodman and A. Gilman (Eds.), *The Pharmacological Basis of Therapeutics*. (4th ed.) New York: Macmillan, 1970.

Esplin, D. W., & Zablocka-Esplin, B. Central Nervous System Stimulants. In L. S. Goodman and A. Gilman (Eds.), *The Pharmacological Basis of Therapeutics*. (4th ed.) New York: Macmillan, 1970.

Essman, W. B. Effect of tricyanoaminopropene on the amnesic effect of electroconvulsive shock. *Psychopharmacologia*, 1966, **9**, 426-433.

Eugster, C. H. Isolation, structure and synthesis of central-active compounds. In Efron, D. H. (Ed.), *Ethnopharmacologic Search for Psychoactive Drugs*. Washington, D.C.: Dept. of Health, Education and Welfare, 1967.

Everitt, B. J., & Herbert, J. Adrenal glands and sexual receptivity in female rhesus monkeys. *Nature*, 1969, **222**, 1065-1066.

Exton, J. H., Jefferson, L. S. Jr., & Park, C. R. Effects of insulin antiserum and insulin on glucose production and gluconeogenesis in liver. *Federation Proceedings*, 1966, **25**, 584.

Eyzaguirre, C., & Lilienthal, J. L., Jr. Veratrinic effects of pentamethylenetetra-zol (metrazol) and 2, 2-bis (p-chlorophenyl) 1,1,1 trichloroethane (DTT) on mammalian neuromuscular function. *Federation Proceedings*, 1949, **70**, 272-275.

Fahn, S., & Cote, L. J. Regional distribution of gamma-aminobutyric acid (GABA) in the brain of the rhesus monkey. *Journal of Neurochemistry*, 1968, **15**, 209-213.

Fain, J. N., Kovacev, V. P., & Scow, R. O. Antilipolytic effect of insulin in isolated fat cells of the rat. *Endocrinology,* 1966, **78**, 773-778.

Falck, B., Hillarp, N. A., Thieme, G., & Torp, A. Fluorescence of catecholamines and related compounds condensed with formaldehyde. *Journal of Histochemistry and Cytochemistry,* 1962, **10**, 348-354.

Fambrough, F. M., Drachman, D. B., & Satymurty, S. Neuromuscular junction in myasthenia gravis: Decreased acetylcholine receptors. *Science,* 1973, **182**, 293-295.

Fang, S., & Liao, S. Antagonistic action of anti-androgens on the formation of a specific dihydrotestosterone-receptor protein complex in rat ventral prostate. *Molecular Pharmacology,* 1969, **5**, 420-431.

Farnham, A. E., & Dubin, D. T. Studies on the mechanism of action of puromycin aminonucleoside in L cells. *Biochemistry and Biophysics Acta,* 1967, **138**, 35-50.

Federman, D. D. *Abnormal Sexual Development.* Philadelphia: Saunders, 1967.

Feinberg, I. Effects of age on human sleep patterns. In A. Kales (Ed.), *Sleep: Physiology and Pathology.* Philadelphia: Lippincott, 1969.

Feldberg, W. *A Pharmacological Approach to the Brain from its Inner and Outer Surface.* London: E. Arnold, 1963.

Feldberg, W., & Sherwood, S. L. Injections of drugs into lateral ventricle of the cat. *Journal of Physiology,* 1954, **123**, 148-167.

Ferguson, J., Hendrikson, S., Cohen, H., Mitchell, G., Barchas, J., & Dement, W. "Hypersexuality" and behavioral changes in cats caused by administration of p-chlorophenylalanine. *Science,* 1970, **168**, 499-501.

Fink, M. Significance of EEG pattern changes in psychopharmacology. *EEG Journal,* 1959, **11**, 398.

Fink, P. J., Goldman, M. J., & Lyons, I. Morning glory seed psychosis. *Archives of General Psychiatry,* 1966, **15**, 209-213.

Fishbein, W., McGaugh, J. L., & Swarz, J. R. Retrograde amnesia: Electroconvulsive shock effects after termination of rapid eye movement sleep deprivation. *Science,* 1971, **172**, 80-82.

Fisher, A. E. Maternal and sexual behavior induced by intracranial chemical stimulation. *Science,* 1956, **124**, 228-229.

Fisher, A. E., & Coury, J. N. Cholinergic tracing of a central neural circuit underlying the thirst drive. *Science,* 1962, **138**, 691-693.

Fitschen, W., & Clayton, B. E. Urinary excretion of gonadotropins with particular reference to children. *Archives of Disease in Childhood,* 1965, **40**, 16-26.

Fitz, T. E., & Hallman, B. L. Mental changes associated with hyperparathyroidism: Report of two cases. *Archives of Internal Medicine,* 1952, **89**, 547.

Fitzgerald, J. D. Perspectives in adrenergic beta-receptor blockade. *Clinical Pharmacology,* 1969, **10**, 292-306.

Fitzsimons, J. T., & Simons, B. J. The effect on drinking in the rat of intravenous infusion of angiotensin given alone or in combination with other stimuli of thirst. *Journal of Physiology,* 1969, **203,** 45-57.

Flach, F. F. Calcium metabolism in states of depression. *British Journal of Psychiatry,* 1964, **110,** 588-593.

Flach, F. F., Liang, E., & Stokes, P. The effects of electric convulsive treatments on nitrogen, calcium and phosphorus metabolism in psychiatric patients. *Journal of Mental Sciences,* 1960, **106,** 638-647.

Flerko, B., & Szentagothai, J. Oestrogen sensitive nervous structures in the hypothalamus. *Acta Endocrinology,* 1957, **26,** 121-127.

Flexner, L. B., & Flexner, J. B. Intracerebral saline: Effect on memory of trained mice treated with puromycin. *Science,* 1968, **159,** 330-331.

Flexner, L. B., Flexner, J. B., & Roberts, R. B. Memory in mice analyzed with antibiotics. *Science,* 1967, **155,** 1377-1383.

Florio, V., Lipparini, F., Scotti-Decarolis, A., & Longo, V. G. EEG and behavioral effects of DOM (STP). *Archives of International Pharmacodynamics,* 1969, **180,** 81-88.

Floyd, J. C., Jr., Fajane, S. S., Knopf, R. F., Rull, J., & Conn, J. W. Postprandial aminoacidemia and insulin secretion, a physiologic relationship. *Journal of Laboratory and Clinical Medicine,* 1964, **64,** 858-859.

Foldes, F. F. Treatment of acute narcotic intoxication. In F. F. Foldes, M. Swerdlow and E. Spiker (Eds.), *Narcotics and Narcotic Antagonists,* Springfield, Ill.: Charles C Thomas, 1964.

Ford, C. E., Jones, K. W., Miller, O. J., Mittwoch, V., Penrose, L. S., Ridler, M., & Shapiro, A. The chromosomes in a patient showing both mongolism and the Klinefelter syndrome. *Lancet,* 1959, **1,** 709.

Forney, R. B., & Harger, R. N. The alcohols. In J. R. Dipalma (Ed.), *Drill's Pharmacology in Medicine.* (4th ed.) New York: McGraw-Hill, 1971.

Forney, R. B., & Hughs, F. W. *Combined Effects of Alcohol and Other Drugs.* Springfield, Ill.: Charles C Thomas, 1968.

Forsham, P. H. Juvenile Diabetic. In M. Ellenberg and H. Rifkin (Eds.), *Diabetes Mellitus: Theory and Practice,* New York: McGraw-Hill, 1970.

Frank, B., Stein, D. G., & Rosen, J. Interanimal memory transfer: Results from brain and liver homogenates. *Science,* 1970, **189,** 399-402.

Frasier, S. D., & Horton, R. Androgens in the peripheral plasma of prepubertal children and adults. *Steroids,* 1966, **8,** 777-784.

Freedman, I., & Peer, I. Drug addiction among pimps and prostitutes in Israel. *International Journal of the Addictions,* 1968, **3,** 271-300.

Fregly, M. J., Hughs, R. E., & Cox, C. E. Effect of an oral contraceptive on the spontaneous running activity of female rats. *Canadian Journal of Physiology and Pharmacology,* 1970, **48,** 107-114.

Freund, G. Alcohol withdrawal syndrome in mice. *Archives of Neurology,* 1969, **21,** 315-320.

Freund, G. Impairment of shock avoidance learning by prolonged ethanol consumption in mice. *Science,* 1970, **168,** 1599-1601.

Freund, G. Chronic CNS toxicity of alcohol. In H. Elliott (Ed.), *Annual Review of Pharmacology,* Vol. 13. Palo Alto, Calif.: Annual Reviews, 1973.

Freund, G., & Walker, D. Impairment of avoidance learning by prolonged ethanol consumption in mice. *Journal of Pharmacology and Experimental Therapeutics,* 1971, **179,** 284-292.

Friedman, A. H. Circumstances influencing Otto Loewi's discovery of chemical transmission in the nervous system. *Pfugers Archives,* 1971, **325,** 85-86.

Friedman, S., & Goldfien, A. Amenorrhea and galactorrhea following oral contraceptive therapy. In T. B. Schwartz (Ed.), *Yearbook of Endocrinology.* Chicago: Yearbook, 1970.

Funkenstein, D. H. The physiology of fear and anger. *Scientific American,* 1955, **192,** 74-80.

Funkenstein, D. H., Greenblatt, M., & Solomon, H. C. Norepinephrine-like and epinephrine-like substances in psychotic and psychoneurotic patients. *American Journal of Psychiatry,* 1952, **108,** 652-662.

Fuxe, K. The distribution of monoamine nerve terminals in the central nervous system. *Acta Physiologica Scandinavica,* 1965, **64,** 37-85.

Fuxe, K., Hokfelt, T., & Ungerstedt, U. Central monoaminergic tracts. In C. G. Clark and J. del Giudice (Eds.), *Principles of Psychopharmacology.* New York: Academic, 1970. (a)

Fuxe, K., Hokfelt, T., & Ungerstedt, U. Morphological and functional aspects of central monoamine neurons. *International Review of Neurobiology,* 1970, **13,** 93-126. (b)

Gaddum, J. H., & Hameed, K. A. Drugs which antagonize 5-hydroxytryptamine. *British Journal of Pharmacology and Chemotherapy,* 1954, **9,** 240-248.

Gaito, J. DNA and RNA as memory molecules. *Psychological Reviews,* 1963, **70,** 471-480.

Gaito, J., & Zavala, A. Neurochemistry and learning. *Psychological Bulletin,* 1964, **61,** 45-62.

Gall, E. A., & Mostof, F. K. *The Liver.* Baltimore: Williams & Wilkins, 1973.

Gaoni, Y., & Mechoulam, R. Isolation, structure and partial synthesis of an active component of hashish. *Journal of the American Chemical Society,* 1964, **86,** 1646-1647.

Gardner, F. H., & Pringle, J. C. Androgens and erythropoesis. I. Preliminary clinical observations. *Archives of Internal Medicine,* 1961, **107,** 846-862.

Gardner, L. I. Deprivation dwarfism. *Scientific American,* 1972, **1,** 76-82.

Garattini, S., & Ghetti, V. (Eds.), *Psychotropic Drugs.* New York: Elsevier, 1957.

Gautier, T. Le club des hachischins. In *La Revue des Deux Mondes,* Paris, 1846.

Geller, I., & Seifter, J. The effects of meprobamate, barbiturates, d-amphetamine and promazine on experimentally induced conflict in the rat. *Psychopharmacologia,* 1960, **1,** 482-492.

Gerard, R. W. Biological roots of psychiatry. *Science,* 1955, **122,** 225-230.

Gerle, B. Clinical observations on the side effects of Haloperidol. *Acta Psychiatrica Scandinavica,* 1964, **40,** 65-76.

Gessner, P. K., & Cabana, B. E. Chloral alcoholate: Reevaluation of its role in the interaction between the hypnotic effects of chloral hydrate and ethanol. *Journal of Pharmacology and Experimental Therapeutics,* 1967, **156,** 602-605.

Giachetti, A., & Shore, P. A. Permeability changes induced in the adrenergic neurone by reserpine. *Biochemical Pharmacology,* 1970, **19,** 1621-1626.

Girden, E., & Culler, E. Conditioned responses in curarized striate muscle in dogs. *Journal of Comparative Psychology,* 1937, **23,** 261-274.

Glaser, G. H. The epilepsies. In P. B. Beeson and W. McDermott (Eds.), *Cecil-Loeb Textbook of Medicine.* (13th ed.) Philadelphia: Saunders, 1971.

Glasky, A. J., & Simon, L. N. Magnesium pemoline: Enhancement of brain RNA polymerases. *Science,* 1966, **151,** 702-703.

Glassock, R. F., & Michael, R. P. The localization of estrogen in the neurological system in the brain of the female cat. *Journal of Physiology,* 1962, **163,** 38-39.

Glessa, G. L., Krishna, G., Forn, J., Tagliamente, A., & Brodie, B. B. Behavioral and vegetative effects produced by dibutyryl cyclic AMP injected into different areas of the brain. In P. Greengard and E. Costa (Eds.), *Role of Cyclic AMP in Cell Function.* New York: Raven, 1970.

Glick, S. D., Greenstein, S., & Zimmerberg, B. Facilitation of recovery by α-methyl-p-tyrosine after lateral hypothalamic damage. *Science,* 1972, **177,** 534-535.

Glickman, S. E. Perseverative neural processes and consolidation of the memory trace. *Psychological Bulletin,* 1961, **58,** 218-230.

Glickman, S. E., & Schiff, B. B. A biological theory of reinforcement. *Psychological Reviews,* 1967, **74,** 81-109.

Glowinski, J. Storage and release of monoamines in the central nervous system. In A. Lajtha (Ed.), *Handbook of Neurochemistry,* Vol. 4. New York: Plenum, 1970.

Glowinski, J., & Axelrod, J. Effects of drugs on the disposition of H^3-norepinephrine in the rat brain. *Pharmacological Reviews,* 1966, **18,** 775-785.

Glowinski, J., & Baldessarini, R. J. Metabolism of norepinephrine in the central nervous system. *Pharmacological Reviews,* 1966, **18,** 1201-1238.

Glowinski, J., & Iverson, L. L. Regional studies of catecholamine in the rat brain I. Disposition of H^3-norepinephrine, H^3-dopamine, and H^3-DOPA in various regions of the brain. *Journal of Neurochemistry,* 1966, **13,** 655-669. (a)

Glowinski, J., & Iverson, L. L. Regional studies of catecholamines in the rat brain III. Subcellular distribution of endogenous and exogenous catecholamines in various brain regions. *Biochemical Pharmacology,* 1966, **15,** 977-987. (b)

Goldstein, A., Aronow, L., & Kalman, S. M. *Principles of Drug Action: The Basis of Pharmacology.* (2nd ed.) New York: Wiley, 1973.

Goldstein, M., Battista, A. F., Ohmoto, T., Anagnoste, B., & Fuxe, K. Tremor and involuntary movements in monkeys: Effect of L-dopa and of a dopamine receptor stimulating agent. *Science,* 1973, **179**, 816-817.

Goodman, L. S., & Gilman, A. *The Pharmacological Basis of Therapeutics.* (4th ed.) New York: Macmillan, 1970.

Goodwin, D. W., Powell, B., Bremer, D., Haine, H., & Stern, J. Alcohol and recall: State-dependent effects in man. *Science,* 1969, **163**, 1358-1360.

Goridis, C., & Neff, N. H. Monoamine oxidase: An approximation of turnover rates. *Journal of Neurochemistry,* 1971, **18**, 1673-1682.

Gorski, R. A. Gonadal hormones and the perinatal development or neuroendocrine function. In L. Martini and W. F. Ganong (Eds.), *Frontiers in Neuroendocrinology.* New York: Oxford, 1971.

Goth, A. *Medical Pharmacology.* (7th ed.) Saint Louis: Mosby, 1974.

Gothelf, B., & Karczmar, A. G. Distribution of intravenously administered chlorpromazine in cat tissues. *International Journal of Neuropharmacology,* 1963, **2**, 39-49.

Grady, K. L., & Phoenix, C. H. Hormonal determinants of mating behavior; the display of feminine behavior by adult rats castrated neonatally. *American Zoologist,* 1963, **3**, 482-483.

Gray, J. *The Psychology of Fear and Stress.* New York: McGraw-Hill, 1971.

Green, R. Neuroendocrine and neuroanatomic correlates of atypical sexuality. In J. L. McGaugh (Ed.), *The Chemistry of Mood, Motivation, and Memory.* New York: Plenum, 1972.

Greene, R. *Human Hormones.* New York: McGraw-Hill, 1970.

Grinker, R. R., & Saks, A. L. *Neurology.* Springfield, Ill.: Charles C Thomas, 1966.

Grinspoon, L. *Marijuana Reconsidered.* Cambridge, Mass.: Harvard, 1971.

Grollman, A., & Grollman, E. F. *Pharmacology and Therapeutics.* (7th ed.) Philadelphia: Lea and Febiger, 1970.

Groppetti, A., & Costa, E. Tissue concentrations of p-hydroxynorephedrine in rats injected with d-amphetamine: Effect of pretreatment with desipramine. *Life Sciences,* 1969, **8**, 653-665.

Grossman, S. P. Eating or drinking elicited by direct adrenergic or cholinergic stimulation of hypothalamus. *Science,* 1960, **132**, 301-302.

Grossman, S. P. Direct adrenergic and cholinergic stimulation of hypothalamic mechanisms. *American Journal of Physiology,* 1962, **202**, 872-882.

Grossman, S. P. Effect of chemical stimulation of the septal area on motivation. *Journal of Comparative and Physiological Psychology,* 1964, **58**, 194-200. (a)

Grossman, S. P. Some chemical aspects of the central regulation of thirst. In M. J. Wayner (Ed.), *Thirst.* New York: Macmillan, 1964. (b)

Grossman, S. P. *A Textbook of Physiological Psychology.* New York: Wiley, 1967.

Grossman, S. P. Behavioral and electroencephalographic effects of microinjections of neuro-humors into the midbrain reticular formation. *Physiology and Behavior,* 1968, **3**, 777-786.

Grossman, S. P. *Essentials of Physiological Psychology.* New York: Wiley, 1973.

Grossman, S. P., & Grossman, L. Effects of chemical stimulation of the midbrain reticular formation on appetitive behavior. *Journal of Comparative and Physiological Psychology,* 1966, **61**, 333-338.

Grossman, S. P., & Peters, R. H. Acquisition of appetitive and avoidance habits following atropine-induced blocking of the thalamic reticular formation. *Journal of Comparative and Physiological Psychology,* 1966, **61**, 325-332.

Grossman, S. P., Peters, R. H., Freedman, P. E., & Willer, H. I. Behavioral effects of cholinergic stimulation of the thalamic reticular formation. *Journal of Comparative and Physiological Psychology,* 1965, **59**, 57-65.

Grossman, S. P., & Sclafani, A. Sympathomimetic amines. In E. Furchtgott (Ed.), *Pharmacological and Biophysical Agents and Behavior.* New York: Academic, 1971.

Grosvenor, C. E., & Turner, C. W. Pituitary lactogenic hormone concentration and milk secretion in lactating rats. *Endocrinology,* 1958, **63**, 535-539.

Grosvenor, C. E., & Turner, C. W. Thyroid hormone and lactation in the rat. *Federation Proceedings,* 1959, **100**, 162.

Grumbach, M. M. Male reproductive tract development—anatomy physiology, and disorders. In R. E. Cook (Ed.), *Biological Basis of Pediatric Practice.* New York: McGraw-Hill, 1967.

Grumbach, M. M., & Barr, M. L. Cytologic tests of chromosomal sex in sexual anomalies in man. *Recent Progress in Hormone Research,* 1958, **14**, 335.

Grumbach, M. M., Van Wyk, J. J., & Wilkins, L. Chromosomal sex in gonadal dysgenesis (ovarian agenesis): Relationship to male pseudohermaphroditism and theories of human sex differentiation. *Journal of Clinical Endocrinology and Metabolism,* 1955, **15**, 1161-1193.

Guiraud, P., & David, C. Traitment de l'agitation mortice par un antihistiminique. (3277 RP) ou phenergau. XLVIII Congies des Al. et Neurol. de Langue Fr. In, *Compte rendu du Congies.* Paris: Masson et Cie, 1950.

Gunn, C. G., Gogerty, J., & Wolf, S. Clinical pharmacology of anticonvulsant compounds. *Clinical Pharmacology and Therapeutics,* 1961, **2**, 733-749.

Gurowitz, E. M. *The Molecular Basis of Memory.* Englewood Cliffs, N.J.: Prentice-Hall, 1969.

Guyton, A. C. *Textbook of Medical Physiology.* (4th ed.) Philadelphia: Saunders, 1971.

Gyermek, L. 5-Hydroxytryptamine antagonists. *Pharmacological Reviews,* 1961, **13**, 339-440.

Haefliger, F. Chemistry of tofranil. *Canadian Psychiatric Association Journal,* 1959, **4**, 69-74.

Hakim, R. A. Indigenous drugs in the treatment of mental diseases. Sixth Gujret Saurashta Provincial Medical Conference, Baroda, India, 1953.

Halas, E. S., James, R. L., & Knutson, C. S. An attempt at classical conditioning in the planarian. *Journal of Comparative and Physiological Psychology,* 1962, **55**, 969-971.

Halmi, N. S. Thyroidal iodide transport. *Vitamins and Hormones,* 1961, **19**, 133.

Hanson, L. C. Evidence that the central action of amphetamines is mediated via catecholamines. *Psychopharmacologia,* 1967, **10**, 289-297.

Hare, L., & Ritchey, J. O. Apathetical response to hyperthyroidism: Report of two cases. *Annals of Internal Medicine,* 1946, **24**, 634.

Harris, L. S. General and behavioral pharmacology of Δ^9-THC. *Pharmacological Reviews,* 1971, **23**, 285-294.

Harris, S. C., Ivy, A. C., & Searle, L. M. The mechanism of amphetamine-induced loss of weight. *Journal of the American Medical Association,* 1947, **134**, 1468-1475.

Hart, B. L. Testosterone regulation of sexual reflexes in spinal male rats. *Science,* 1967, **155**, 1283-1284.

Hart, B. L. Neonatal castration: Influence on neural organization of sexual reflexes in male rats. *Science,* 1968, **160**, 1135-1136.

Hart, B. L. Gonadal hormones and sexual reflexes in the female rat. *Hormones and Behavior,* 1969, **1**, 65-71.

Hart, B. L., & Haugen, C. M. Activation of sexual reflexes in male rats by spinal implantation of testosterone. *Physiology and Behavior.* 1968, **3**, 735-738.

Hartry, A. L., Keith-Lee, P., & Morton, W. D. Planaria: Memory transfer through cannibalism reexamined. *Science,* 1964, **146**, 274-275.

Hasbrouck, J. D. Morphine anesthesia for open-heart surgery. *Annals of Thoracic Surgery,* 1970, **10**, 364-369.

Haug, J. Pneumoencephalographic evidence of brain damage in chronic alcoholics. *Acta Psychiatry and Neurology Scandinavica,* 1968, **203**, 135-143.

Hays, K. J. Anoxic and convulsive amnesia in rats. *Journal of Comparative and Physiological Psychology,* 1953, **46**, 216-217.

Hearst, E., & Whalen, R. E. Facilitating effect of d-amphetamine on discriminated avoidance performance. *Journal of Comparative and Physiological Psychology,* 1963, **56**, 124-128.

Heath, R. G. Pleasure responses of human subjects to direct stimulation of the brain: Physiological and psychodynamic considerations. In R. G. Heath (Ed.), *The Role of Pleasure in Behavior.* New York: Harper & Row, 1964.

Hebb, D. O. *The Organization of Behavior.* New York: Wiley, 1949.

Heller, A., & Moore, R. Y. Control of brain serotonin and norepinephrine by specific neural systems. *Advances in Pharmacology,* 1968, **6**, 191-206.

Heller, A., Seiden, L. S., & Moore, R. Y. Regional effects of lateral hypothalamic lesions on brain norepinephrine in the cat. *International Journal of Neuropharmacology,* 1966, **5**, 91-101.

Heller, C. G., & Clermont, Y. Spermatogenesis in man: An estimate of its duration. *Science,* 1963, **140**, 184-185.

Heller, C. G., Nelson, W. O., Hill, K. B., Henderson, E., Maddock, W. O., Jungck, E. C., Paulgen, C. A., & Mortimore, G. E. Improvement in spermatogenesis following depression of human testis with testosterone. *Fertility and Sterility,* 1950, **1**, 415-420.

Hendley, C. D. Effect of 2-methyl-2-N-propyl-1,3-propanediol dicarbomate (Miltown) on central nervous system. *Federation Proceedings,* 1954, 87, 608.

Hendley, E. D., & Snyder, S. H. Relationship between the action of monoamine oxidase inhibitors on the noradrenaline uptake system and their antidepressant efficacy. *Nature,* 1968, 220, 1330-1331.

Henkin, R. I. The neuroendocrine control of perception. In D. Hamburg (Ed.), *Perception and its Disorders,* Baltimore: Williams & Wilkins, 1970.

Hernández-Peón, R., & Chávez-Ibarra, G. Sleep induced by electrical or chemical stimulation of the forebrain. *EEG Journal,* 1963, 24, 188-198.

Herz, A., & Metys, J. Inhibition of nociceptive responses by substances acting on central cholinoceptive systems. In A. Soulairac, J. Chan, and J. Charpentier (Eds.), *Pain.* New York: Academic, 1968.

Herz, A., & Teschemacher, J. Activities and sites of anti-nociceptive action of morphine-like analgesics. *Advances in Drug Research,* 1971, 6, 79-119.

Herz, A., Teschemacher, J., Albus, K., & Zieglgansberger, S. Morphine abstinence syndrome in rabbits precipitated by injection of morphine antagonists into the ventricular system and restricted parts of it. *Psychopharmacologia,* 1972, 26, 219-235.

Hess, W. R. *Das Zwischinhiru: Syndrome, Lokalisationeu, Funkzionin.* Basel: Schwaka, 1954.

Hetherington, A. W., & Ranson, S. W. The spontaneous activity and food intake of rats with hypothalamic lesions. *American Journal of Physiology,* 1942, 136, 609-617.

Hillarp, N. A., Fuxe, K., & Dahlström, A. Demonstration and mapping of central neurons containing dopamine, noradrenaline, and 5-hydroxytryptamine and their reactions to psychopharmaca. *Pharmacological Reviews,* 1966, 18, 727-741.

Himwich, H. E. Anatomy and physiology of the emotions and their relation to psychoactive drugs. In J. Marks, and C. M. Pare (Eds.), *The Scientific Basis of Drug Therapy in Psychiatry.* New York: Pergamon, 1965.

Hirsch, P. F., Voelkel, E. F., & Munson, P. L. Thyrocalcitonin: Hypocalcemic-hypophosphatemic principle of the thyroid gland. *Science,* 1964, 146, 412-413.

Hively, R. W., Mosher, W. A., & Hoffman, F. W. Isolation of trans-delta-9-tetrahydrocannabinol from marijuana. *Journal of the American Chemical Society,* 1966, 88, 1832-1833.

Ho, I. K., Lu, S. E., Stolman, S., Loh, H. H., & Way, E. L. Influence of p-chlorophenylalanine on morphine tolerance and physical dependence and regional brain serotonin turnover studies in morphine tolerant-dependent mice. *Journal of Pharmacology and Experimental Therapeutics,* 1972, 182, 155-165.

Ho, I. K., Loh, H. H., & Way, E. L. Influence of 5,6-dihydroxytryptamine on morphine tolerance and physical dependence. *European Journal of Pharmacology,* 1973, 21, 331-336.

Hoffer, A., & Osmond, H. *The Hallucinogens.* New York: Academic, 1967.

Hoffmeister, F. Effects of psychotrophic drugs on pain. In A. Soulairac, J. Chan, and J. Charpentier (Eds.), *Pain.* New York: Academic, 1968.

Hofmann, A. Psychotomimetic agents. In A. Burger (Ed.), *Drugs Affecting the Central Nervous System,* Vol. 2. New York: Marcel Dekker, 1968.

Hofmann, A., & Tscherter, A. Isoliequng von lysergsäure-alkaloiden aus der mexikanischen zauberdroge ololiuqui. *Experimentia,* 1960, **16**, 414.

Höhn, R., & Lasagna, L. Effects of aggregation and temperature on amphetamine toxicity in mice. *Psychopharmacologia,* 1960, **1**, 210-220.

Hökfelt, T., Ljungdahl, Å., Fuxe, K., & Johansson, O. Dopaminergic nerve terminals in the rat limbic cortex: Aspects of the dopamine hypothesis of schizophrenia. *Science,* 1974, **184**, 177-179.

Holden, C. Psychosurgery: Legitimate therapy or laundered lobotomy? *Science,* 1973, **179**, 1109-1112.

Holland, W. C., Klein, R. L., & Briggs, A. H. *Introduction to Molecular Pharmacology.* New York: Macmillan, 1964.

Hollister, L. E., Motzenbecker, F. P., & Degan, R. O. Withdrawal reactions from chlordiazepoxide ("Librium"). *Psychopharmacologia,* 1961, **2**, 63-68.

Hook, E. B., & Kim, D. S. Height and antisocial behavior in XY and XYY boys. *Science,* 1971, **172**, 284-286.

Hordern, A. Psychopharmacology: Some historical considerations. In C. R. B. Joyce (Ed.), *Psychopharmacology: Dimensions and Perspectives.* Philadelphia: Lippincott, 1968.

Hornykiewicz, O. Dopamine (3-hydroxytyramine) and brain function. *Pharmacological Reviews,* 1966, **18**, 925-964.

Houpt, K. A., & Epstein, A. N. The complete dependence of beta-adrenergic drinking on the renal dipsogen. *Physiology and Behavior,* 1971, **7**, 897-902.

Houston, J. Phenomenology of the psychedelic experience. In R. E. Hicks and P. J. Fink (Eds.), *Psychedelic Drugs.* New York: Grune and Stratton, 1969.

Hudspeth, W. J. Strychnine: Its facilitating effect on the solution of a simple oddity problem by the rat. *Science,* 1964, **145**, 1331-1333.

Hunt, H. F. Some effects of meprobamate on conditioned fear and emotional behavior. *Annals of the New York Academy of Science,* 1957, **67**, 712-723.

Hunter, B., Boast, C., Walker, D., & Zornetzer, S. Alcohol withdrawal syndrome in rats: Neural and behavioral correlates. *Pharmacology Biochemistry and Behavior.* (in press)

Hutcheon, D. E. Diuretics. In J. R. DiPalma (Ed.), *Drill's Pharmacology in Medicine.* (4th ed.) New York: McGraw-Hill, 1971.

Huxley, A. *The Doors of Perception.* New York: Harper & Row, 1954.

Hydén, H. The question of a molecular basis for the memory trace. In K. H. Pribram, and D. E. Broadbent (Eds.), *Biology of Memory.* New York: Academic, 1970.

Ingbar, S. H., & Woeber, K. A. The thyroid gland. In R. H. Williams (Ed.), *Textbook of Endocrinology.* (5th ed.) Philadelphia: Saunders, 1974.

Innes, I. R., & Nickerson, M. Drugs acting on postganglionic adrenergic nerve endings and structures innervated by them (sympathomimetic drugs). In L. S. Goodman, and A. Gilman (Eds.), *The Pharmacological Basis of Therapeutics.* (4th ed.) New York: Macmillan, 1970. (a)

Innes, I. R., & Nickerson, M. Drugs inhibiting the action of acetylcholine on structures innervated by postganglionic parasympathetic nerves (antimuscarinic or atropinic drugs). In L. S. Goodman, and A. Gilman (Eds.), *The Pharmacological Basis of Therapeutics.* (4th ed.) New York: Macmillan, 1970. (b)

Isbell, H. Comparison of the reactions induced by psilocybin and LSD-25 in man. *Psychopharmacologia,* 1959, **1**, 29–38.

Isbell, H. Alcohol problems and alcoholism. In P. B. Beeson, and W. McDermott (Eds.), *Cecil-Loeb Textbook of Medicine.* (13th ed.) Philadelphia: Saunders, 1971.

Isbell, H., Altschule, S., Kornetsky, C. H., Eisenman, A. J., Flanary, H. G., & Fraser, H. F. Chronic barbiturate intoxication. *AMA Archives of Neurology and Psychiatry,* 1950, **64**, 1–28.

Isbell, H., & Gorodetsky, G. W. Effect of alkaloids of ololiuqui in man. *Psychopharmacologia,* 1966, **8**, 331–339.

Isbell, H., Gorodetsky, G. W., Jasinski, D., Claussen, V., Spulak, F., & Korte, F. Effects of (-) delta 9-transtetrahydrocannabinol in man. *Psychopharmacologia,* 1967, **11**, 184–188.

Isbell, H., Wolbach, A. B., Wikler, A., & Miner, E. J. Cross tolerance between LSD and psilocybin. *Psychopharmacologia,* 1961, **2**, 147–159.

Iverson, L. L. Neurotransmitters, neurohormones, and other small molecules in neurons. In F. O. Schmitt (Ed.), *The Neurosciences: Second Study Program.* New York: Rockefeller University Press, 1970.

Jacobs, F. A., & Strong, J. A. A case of human intersexuality having a possible XXY sex determining mechanism. *Nature,* 1959, **183**, 302.

Jacobsen, E. The metabolism of ethyl alcohol. *Pharmacological Review,* 1952, **4**, 107–135.

Jacobson, A. C., & Schlecter, J. M. Chemical transfer of training: Three years later. In K. H. Pribram, and D. E. Broadbent (Eds.), *Biology of Memory.* New York: Academic, 1970.

Jacquet, Y. F., & Lajtha, A. Morphine action at central nervous system sites in rat: Analgesia or hyperalgesia depending on site and dose. *Science,* 1973, **182**, 490–492.

Jaffe, J. H. Drug addiction and drug abuse. In L. Goodman and A. Gilman (Eds.), *The Pharmacological Basis of Therapeutics.* (3rd ed.) New York Macmillan, 1965.

Jaffe, J. H. Drug addiction and drug abuse. In L. Goodman, and A. Gilman (Eds.), *The Pharmacological Basis of Therapeutics.* (4th ed.) New York: Macmillan, 1970. (a)

Jaffe, J. H. Narcotic analgesics. In L. Goodman, and A. Gilman (Eds.), *The Pharmacological Basis of Therapeutics.* (4th ed.) New York: Macmillan, 1970. (b)

Jameson, H. D., & Hasbrouck, J. D. Encephalographic signs during cardiac surgery with morphine anesthesia and reversal with naloxone. *Transactions of the American Neurological Association,* 1971, **96**, 256-258.

Janssen, P. A. J. The pharmacology of haloperidol. *International Journal of Neuropsychiatry,* 1967, **3**, 510-518.

Janssen, P. A. J., & Niemegeers, C. J. E. Haloperidol (R3201), a highly potent and selective anti-emetic agent in dogs. *Nature,* 1961, **190**, 911-912.

Jarvik, L. F., Klodin, V., & Matsuyama, S. S. Human aggression and the extra Y chromosome. *American Psychologist,* 1973, **28**, 674-682.

Jarvik, M. E. Drugs used in the treatment of psychiatric disorders. In L. S. Goodman, and A. Gilman (Eds.), *The Pharmacological Basis of Therapeutics.* (4th ed.) New York: Macmillan, 1970.

Jarvik, M. E., & Kopp, R. Transcorneal electricity, convulsions, and retrograde amnesia in mice. *Journal of Comparative and Physiological Psychology,* 1967, **64**, 431-434.

Jensen, G. D. Human sexual behavior in primate perspective. In J. Zubin and J. Money (Eds.), *Contemporary Sexual Behavior: Critical Issues in the 1970s.* Baltimore: Johns Hopkins, 1973.

John, E. R. *Mechanisms of Memory.* New York: Academic Press, 1967.

Johnson, G., & Gershon, S. Controlled evaluation of lithium and chlorpromazine in the treatment of manic states: An interim report. *Comprehensive Psychiatry,* 1968, **9**, 563-573.

Johnson, J. L., & Aprison, M. H. The distribution of glutamic acid, a transmitter candidate, and other amino acids in the dorsal sensory neuron of the cat. *Brain Research,* 1970, **24**, 285-292.

Johnson, P. C., Charalanupous, K. D., & Braun, G. A. Absorption and excretion of tritiated haloperidol in man. (A preliminary report). *International Journal of Neuropsychiatry,* 1967, **3**, 524-525.

Jones, B. E., & Prada, J. A. Relapse to morphine use in dog. *Psychopharmacologia,* 1973, **30**, 1-12.

Jones, Ernest. *The Life and Work of Sigmund Freud,* I. New York: Basic Books, 1953.

Jost, A. Embryonic sexual differentiation (morphology, physiology, abnormalities). In H. W. Jones and W. W. Scott (Eds.), *Hermaphrodites, Genital Anomalies, and Related Endocrine Disorders.* Baltimore: Williams & Wilkins, 1958.

Jouvet, M. Biogenic amines and the states of sleep. *Science,* 1969, **163**, 32-40.

Jungas, R. L. Inhibition by insulin of glucagon phosphorylase activity of adipose tissue. *Federation Proceedings,* 1966, **25**, 584. (Abstract)

Kahnt, F. W., Neher, R., Schmid, K., & Wettstein, A. Bilding von 17αhydroxy A 5-pregnenolone und 3B-hydroxy-17-keto-Δ5-androsten in nebennieren und testes-gewebe. *Experimentia,* 1961, **17**, 19.

Kales, A., Malmstrom, E. J., Scharf, M. B., & Rubin, R. T. Psychophysiological and biochemical changes following uses and withdrawal of hypnotics. In A. Kales (Ed.), *Sleep: Physiology and Pathology*. Philadelphia: Lippincott, 1969.

Kalkhoff, R., Schalch, D. S., Walker, J. L., Beck, P., Kipnis, D. M., & Daughaday, W. H. Diabetogenic factors associated with pregnancy. *Transactions of the Association of American Physicians*, 1964, **77**, 270.

Kaplan, H. S. Psychosis associated with marijuana. *New York State Journal of Medicine*, 1971, **71**, 433-435.

Karpati, G., & Frame, B. Neuropsychiatric disorders in primary hyperparathyroidism. *Archives of Neurology*, 1964, **10**, 387-397.

Katsoyannis, P. G. Synthetic insulins. *Recent Progress in Hormone Research*, 1967, **23**, 505.

Katz, B. Quantal mechanism of neural transmitter release. *Science*, 1971, **173**, 123-126.

Katz, J. J., & Halstead, W. C. Protein organization and mental function. *Comparative Psychology Monographs*, 1950, **20**, 1-38.

Keats, A. S., & Beecher, H. K. Pain relief with hypnotic doses of barbiturates and a hypothesis. *Journal of Pharmacology and Experimental Therapeutics*, 1950, **100**, 1-13.

Keleman, K., & Bovet, D. Effect of drugs upon the defensive behavior of rats. *Acta Physiologica of the Hungarian Academy of Sciences*, 1961, **19**, 143-154.

Kelleher, R. T., & Morse, W. H. Determinants of the specificity of behavioral effects of drugs. *Ergeb Physiologica, Biology, Chemistry and Experimental Pharmacology*, 1968, **60**, 1-56.

Kerr, F. W. L., & Pozuelo, J. Suppression of physical dependence and induction of hypersensitivity to morphine by stereotaxic hypothalamic lesions in addicted rats. *Mayo Clinic Proceedings*, 1971, **46**, 653-665.

Kety, S. S. Biochemical theories of schizophrenia. A two-part review of current theories and the evidence used to support them. *Science*, 1959, **129**, 1528-1532; 1590-1596.

Kety, S. S. Catecholamines in neuropsychiatric states. *Pharmacological Reviews*, 1966, **18**, 787-798.

Kimball, C. P., & Murlin, J. R. Aqueous extracts of pancreas. III. Some precipitation reactions of insulin. *Journal of Biological Chemistry*, 1924, **58**, 337-346.

Kissin, B., & Beglister, H. (Eds.), *The Biology of Alcoholism: Volume I Biochemistry*. New York: Plenum, 1971.

Klausner, H. A., & Dingell, J. V. The metabolism and excretion of Δ^9-tetrahydrocannabinol in the rat. *Life Sciences*, 1971, **10**, 49-59.

Klein, D. F., & Davis, J. M. *Diagnosis and Drug Treatment of Psychiatric Disorders*. Baltimore: Williams & Wilkins, 1969.

Klerman, G. L., DiMascio, A., Havens, L. L., & Snell, J. E. Sedation and tranquilization: A comparison of the effects of a number of psychopharmacologic agents upon normal human subjects. *AMA Archives of General Psychiatry*, 1960, **3**, 4–13.

Kline, N. S. *Psychopharmacology Frontiers.* Boston: Little, Brown, 1959.

Klinefelter, H. F. Jr., Reifenstein, E. C. Jr., & Albright, F. Syndrome characterized by gynecomastia, aspermatogenesis without aleydigism and increased excretion of FSH. *Journal of Clinical Endocrinology*, 1942, **2**, 615–627.

Kling, J. W., & Schrier, A. M. Positive reinforcement. In J. W. Kling and L. A. Riggs (Eds.), *Woodworth and Schlosberg's Experimental Psychology.* (3rd ed.) New York: Holt, 1971.

Knapp, S., & Mandell, A. J. Short- and long-term lithium administration: Effects on the brain's serotonergic biosynthetic systems. *Science,* 1973, **180**, 645–647.

Knights, R. M., & Hinton, G. S. The effects of methylphenidate (Ritalin) on the motor skills and behavior of children with learning problems. *Journal of Nervous and Mental Disease,* 1969, **148**, 643–653.

Kobayashi, F., & Gorski, R. A. Effects of antibiotics on androgenization of the neonatal female tract. *Endocrinology,* 1970, **86**, 285–289.

Koe, B. K. Tryptophan hydroxylase inhibitors. *Federation Proceedings,* 1971, **30**, 886–896.

Koe, B. K., & Weissman, A. The pharmacology of parachlorophenylalanine, a selective depletor of serotonin stores. *Advances in Pharmacology,* 1968, **6**, 29–47.

Koelle, G. B. The histochemical identification of acetylcholinesterase in cholinergic, adrenergic and sensory neurons. *Journal of Pharmacology and Experimental Therapeutics,* 1955, **114**, 167–184.

Koelle, G. B. A new general concept of the neurohormonal function of acetylcholine and acetylcholinesterase. *Journal of Pharmacy and Pharmacology,* 1962, **14**, 65–90.

Koelle, G. B. Cytological distributions and physiological functions of cholinesterases. In G. B. Koelle (Ed.), *Cholinesterases and Anticholinesterases: Handbuch der Experimentellen Pharmacologie.* Berlin: Springer, 1963

Koelle, G. B. Anticholinesterase agents. In L. S. Goodman and A. Gilman (Eds.), *The Pharmacological Basis of Therapeutics.* (4th ed.) New York: Macmillan, 1970. (a)

Koelle, G. B. Neurohumoral transmission and the autonomic nervous system. In L. S. Goodman and A. Gilman (Eds.), *The Pharmacological Basis of Therapeutics.* (4th ed.) New York: Macmillan, 1970. (b)

Koelle, G. B. Neuromuscular blocking agents. In L. S. Goodman and A. Gilman (Eds.), *The Pharmacological Basis of Therapeutics.* (4th ed.) New York: Macmillan, 1970. (c)

Koelle, G. B. Parasympathomimetic agents. In L. S. Goodman and A. Gilman (Eds.), *The Pharmacological Basis of Therapeutics.* (4th ed.) New York: Macmillan, 1970. (d)

Koelle, G. B. Current concepts of synaptic structure and function. *Annals of the New York Academy of Sciences,* 1971, **183**, 5-20.

Kolansky, H., & Moore, W. T. Effects of marijuana on adolescents and young adults. *Journal of the American Medical Association,* 1971, **216**, 486-492.

Kolodny, R. C., Masters, W. H., Hendryx, J., & Toro, G. Plasma testosterone and semen analysis in male homosexuals. *New England Journal of Medicine,* 1971, **285**, 1170-1174.

Kolodny, R. C., Masters, W. H., Kolodner, R. M., & Toro, G. Depression of plasma testosterone levels after chronic, intensive marihuana use. *New England Journal of Medicine,* 1974, **290**, 872-874.

Kopin, I. J. False adrenergic transmitters. *Annual Review of Pharmacology,* 1968, **8**, 377-394.

Kornetsky, C. Effects of meprobamate, phenobarbital, and dextroamphetamine on reaction time learning in man. *Journal of Pharmacology and Experimental Therapeutics,* 1958, **123**, 216-219.

Krall, L. P. The clinical use of oral hypoglycemic agents. In M. Ellenberg and H. Rifkin (Eds.), *Diabetes Mellitus: Theory and Practice.* New York: McGraw-Hill, 1970.

Kravitz, E. A. Acetylcholine, γ-aminobutyric acid: Physiological and chemical studies related to their roles as neurotransmitter agents. In G. C. Quarton, T. Melnechuk and F. O. Schmitt (Eds.), *The Neurosciences.* New York: Rockefeller University Press, 1967.

Krebs, H., Bindra, D., & Campbell, J. F. Effects of amphetamine on neural activity in the hypothalamus. *Physiology and Behavior,* 1969, **4**, 685-691.

Krikstone, B. J., & Levitt, R. A. Interactions between water deprivation and chemical brain stimulation. *Journal of Comparative and Physiological Psychology,* 1970, **71**, 334-340.

Krivanek, J., & McGaugh, J. L. Effects of pentylenetetrazol on memory storage in mice. *Psychopharmacologia,* 1968, **12**, 303-321.

Kuhn, R. The treatment of depressive states with G22355 (imipramine hydrochloride). *American Journal of Psychiatry,* 1958, **115**, 459-464.

Kulkarni, A. S. Facilitation of instrumental avoidance learning by amphetamine: An analysis. *Psychopharmacologia,* 1968, **13**, 418-425.

Kuno, M. Quantum aspects of central and ganglionic synaptic transmission in vertebrates. *Physiological Reviews,* 1971, **51**, 647-678.

Kundstadter, R. H. Experience with benzedrine sulfate in the management of obesity in children. *Journal of Pediatrics,* 1940, **17**, 490-501.

Kuriyama, K., Roberts, E., & Vos, J. Some characteristics of the binding of GABA and ACh to a synaptic vesicle fraction from mouse brain. *Brain Research,* 1968, **9**, 231-252.

Kurland, A. A. Outpatient management of the narcotic addict. In P. Black (Ed.), *Drugs and the Brain.* Baltimore: Johns Hopkins, 1969.

LaBarre, W. *The Peyote Cult.* Hamden, Conn.: The Shoe String Press, 1964.

LaBarre, W., McAllester, D. P., Slotkin, J. S., Stewart, O. C., & Tax, S. Statement on peyote. *Science,* 1951, **114**, 582-583.

Laborit, H., Hugnenard, P., & Allusume, R. Un nouolau stabilsateni negetatif, le 4560 RP. *Presse Mid.,* 1952, **60**, 206-208.

Lake, N., & Jordan, L. M. Failure to confirm cyclic AMP as second messenger for norepinephrine in rat cerebellum. *Science,* 1974, **183**, 663-664.

Landau, R. L., & Lugibih, L. K. The catabolic and natriuretic effects of progesterone in man. *Recent Progress in Hormone Research,* 1961, **17**, 249-292.

Larson, M. D., & Major, M. The effect of hexobarbital on the duration of the recurrent IPSP in cat motoneurons. *Brain Research,* 1970, **21**, 309-311.

Larsson-Conn, U., & Stenram, U. Jaundice during treatment with oral contraceptive agents: A report of two cases. *Journal of the American Medical Association,* 1965, **193**, 422-426.

Lasagna, L. A study of hypnotic drugs in patients with chronic diseases: Comparative efficacy of placebo; methyprylon (Noludar); meprobamate (Miltown, Equanil); pentobarbital; phenobarbital; secobarbital. *Journal of Chronic Diseases,* 1956, **3**, 122-133.

Laschet, U. Antiandrogen in the treatment of sex offenders: Mode of action and therapeutic outcome. In J. Zubin and J. Money (Eds.), *Contemporary Sexual Behavior: Critical Issues in the 1970s.* Baltimore: Johns Hopkins, 1973.

Lashley, K. S. In search of the engram. *Symposium of the Society of Experimental Biology,* 1950, **4**, 454-482.

Laties, V., Weiss, B., Clark, R. L., & Reynolds, M. D. Overt "mediating" behavior during temporally spaced responding. *Journal of the Experimental Analysis of Behavior,* 1965, **8**, 107-116.

Laverty, R., & Taylor, K. M. Effects of intraventricular 2, 4, 5-trihydroxy-phenylethylamine (6-hydroxydopamine) on rat behavior and brain catecholamine metabolism. *British Journal of Pharmacology,* 1970, **40**, 836-846.

Leake, N. H., & Burt, R. L. Insulin-like activity in serum during pregnancy. *Diabetes,* 1962, **11**, 419-421.

Leary, T. *High Priest.* New York: World, 1968.

Le Gros Clark, W. E., Beattie, J., Riddoch, G., & Dott, N. M. *The Hypothalamus.* London: Oliver & Boyd, 1938.

Lehmann, H. E. Depression: Categories, mechanisms and phenomena. In J. O. Cole and W. Henborn (Eds.), *Pharmacotherapy of Depression.* Springfield, Ill.: Charles C Thomas, 1966.

Lehr, D., Mallow, J., & Krukowski, M. Copious drinking and simultaneous inhibition of urine flow elicited by beta-adrenergic stimulation and contrary effect of alpha-adrenergic stimulation. *Journal of Pharmacology and Experimental Therapeutics,* 1967, **158**, 150-163.

Lehrer, G. M., & Levitt, M. F. Neuropsychiatric presentation of hypercalcemia. *Journal of the Mt. Sinai Hospital,* 1960, **27**, 10.

Lennard, H. L., Epstein, L. J., & Rosenthal, M. S. The methadone illusion. *Science,* 1972, **176**, 881–884.

Levi, L. Sympatho-adrenomedullary and related biochemical reactions during experimentally induced emotional stress. In R. P. Michael (Ed.), *Endocrinology and Human Behavior.* London: Oxford, 1968.

Levine, R. Insulin: Its biosynthesis and mode of action. In M. Ellenberg and H. Rifkin (Eds.), *Diabetes Mellitus: Theory and Practice.* New York: McGraw-Hill, 1970.

Levine, S. Stress and behavior. *Scientific American,* 1971, **224**, 26–31.

Levine, S., & Mullins, R., Jr. Estrogen administered neonatally affects adult sexual behavior in male and female rats. *Science,* 1964, **144**, 185–187.

Levitt, R. A. Sleep deprivation in the rat. *Science,* 1966, **153**, 85–87.

Levitt, R. A. Paradoxical sleep: Activation by sleep deprivation. *Journal of Comparative and Physiological Psychology,* 1967, **63**, 505–509.

Levitt, R. A. Biochemical blockade of cholinergic thirst. *Psychonomic Science,* 1969, **15**, 274–276.

Levitt, R. A. Cholinergic substrate for drinking in the rat. *Psychological Reports,* 1971, **29**, 431–448.

Levitt, R. A., & Fisher, A. E. Anticholinergic blockade of centrally induced thirst. *Science,* 1966, **154**, 520–522.

Levitt, R. A., & Fisher, A. E. Failure of central anticholinergic brain stimulation to block natural thirst. *Physiology and Behavior,* 1967, **2**, 425–428.

Levitt, R. A., & O'Hearn, J. Y. Drinking elicited by cholinergic stimulation of CNS fibers. *Physiology and Behavior,* 1972, **8**, 641–644.

Lewin, J., & Esplin, D. W. Analysis of the spinal excitatory action of pentylenetetrazol. *Journal of Pharmacology and Experimental Therapeutics,* 1961, **132**, 245–250.

Lewin, L. *The Therapie Gazette,* 1888, **4**, 231.

Lewis, P. R., & Shute, C. C. D. The cholinergic limbic system: Projections to hippocampal formation, medial cortex, nuclei of the ascending cholinergic reticular system, and the subfornical organ and supra-optic crest. *Brain,* 1967, **40**, 521–540.

Lewy, A. J., & Seiden, L. S. Operant behavior changes norepinephrine metabolism in rat brain. *Science,* 1972, **175**, 454–456.

Lim, R. K. S., & Guzman, F. Manifestations of pain in analgesic evaluation in animals and man. In A. Soulairac, J. Chan and J. Charpentier (Eds.), *Pain.* New York: Academic, 1968.

Lingeman, R. R. *Drugs from A to Z: A Dictionary.* Baltimore: Penguin, 1970.

Lipsett, M. B., & Korenman, S. G. Androgen metabolism. *Journal of the American Medical Association,* 1964, **190**, 757–762.

Lisk, R. D. Estrogen-sensitive centers in the hypothalamus of the rat. *Journal of Experimental Zoology,* 1960, **145**, 197–205.

Lisk, R. D. Testosterone-sensitive centers in the hypothalamus of the rat. *Acta Endocrinology,* 1962, **41**, 195-204.

Lloyd, K., & Hornykiewicz, O. Parkinson's disease: Activity of L-dopa decarboxylase in discrete brain regions. *Science,* 1970, **170**, 1212-1213.

Loewe, S. Cannabis. Wikstoffe und pharmacologie der cannabinole. *Archives of Experimental Pathology and Pharmacology,* 1950, **211**, 175-189.

Loewi, O. An autobiographical sketch. *Perspectives in Biology and Medicine,* 1960, **4**, 3-25.

Loh, H. H., Shen, F., & Way, E. L. Effect of d-actinomycin on the acute toxicity and brain uptake of morphine. *Journal of Pharmacology and Experimental Therapeutics,* 1971, **177**, 327-331.

Longo, V. G. Behavioral and electroencephalographic effects of atropine and related compounds. *Pharmacological Reviews,* 1966, **18**, 965-996.

Longo, V. G. *Neuropharmacology and Behavior.* San Francisco: Freeman, 1972.

Lonowski, D. J., Levitt, R. A., & Larson, S. D. Effects of cholinergic brain injections on mouse killing or carrying by rats. *Physiological Psychology,* 1973, **1**, 341-345.

Loomis, T. A., & West, T. C. Comparative sedative effect of barbiturate and some tranquilizer drugs in normal subjects. *Journal of Pharmacology and Experimental Therapeutics,* 1958, **122**, 525-531.

Loraine, J. A., Ismail, A. A. A., Adamopoulos, D. A., & Dove, G. A. Endocrine function in male and female homosexuals. *British Medical Journal,* 1970, **4**, 406-409.

Lostroh, A. J. Parameters in the biology of spermatogenesis. In R. F. Escamilla (Ed.), *Laboratory Tests of Endocrine Functions.* Philadelphia: Davis, 1962.

Lotti, V. J., Lomax, P., & George, R. Temperature responses in the rat following intra-cerebral microinjection of morphine. *Journal of Pharmacology and Experimental Therapeutics,* 1965, **150**, 135-139.

Luttges, J., Johnson, T., Buck, C., Holland, J., & McGaugh, J. An examination of transfer of learning by nucleic acid. *Science,* 1966, **151**, 834-837.

Lynch, V. D., Aceto, M. D., & Thomas, R. K. Avoidance-escape conditioning. *Journal of the American Pharmaceutical Association: Scientific Edition,* 1960, **49**, 205-210.

Lyons, W. R., Li, C. H., & Johnson, R. E. The hormonal control of mammary growth and lactation. *Recent Progress in Hormone Research,* 1958, **14**, 219.

Maccoby, E. E. Sex in the social order. *Science,* 1973, **182**, 469-471.

Macon, J. B., Sokoloff, L., & Glowinski, J. Feedback control of rat brain 5-hydroxytryptamine synthesis. *Journal of Neurochemistry,* 1971, **18**, 323-331.

MacPhail, E. M., & Miller, N. E. Cholinergic brain stimulation in cats: Failure to obtain sleep. *Journal of Comparative Physiological Psychology,* 1968, **65**, 499-503.

Mahler, R., Tarrant, M. E., Staffard, W. S., & Ashmore, J. Antilipolytic effects of insulin. *Diabetes,* 1963, **12**, 359.

Major, C. T., & Pleuvry, B. J. Effects of α-methyl-p-tyrosine, p-chlorophenyl-alanine, 1- -(3,4-dihydroxyphenyl) alanine, 5-hydroxytryptophan and diethyl-dithiocarbamate on the analgesic activity of morphine and methylamphet-amine in the mouse. *British Journal of Pharmacology,* 1971, **42**, 512–521.

Malmfors, T., & Sachs, C. Degeneration of adrenergic nerves produced by 6-hydroxydopamine. *European Journal of Pharmacology,* 1968, **3**, 89–92.

Malmfors, T., & Thoenen, H. *6-Hydroxydopamine and Catecholamine Neurons.* New York: Elsevier, 1971.

Mandell, A. J., Markham, C. H., Tallman, F. F., & Mandell, M. P. Motivation and ability to move. *American Journal of Psychiatry,* 1962, **119**, 544–549.

Mandell, A. J., & Spooner, C. E. Psychochemical research studies in man. *Science,* 1968, **162**, 1442–1453.

Mardones, J. The alcohols. In W. S. Root and F. G. Hoffman (Eds.), *Physiological Pharmacology: A Comprehensive Treatise Vol. I, Part A.* New York: Academic, 1963.

Margolese, M. Homosexuality: A new endocrine correlate. *Hormones and Behavior,* 1970, **1**, 151–155.

Margules, D. L. Noradrenergic synapses in perifornical hypothalamus for the suppression of feeding behavior by satiety. *Federation Proceedings,* 1969, **28**, 641. (Abstract)

Margules, D. L. Alpha-adrenergic receptors in hypothalamus for the suppression of feeding behavior by satiety. *Journal of Comparative and Physiological Psychology,* 1970, **73**, 1–12.

Margules, D. L., Lewis, M. J., Dragovich, J. A., & Margules, A. S. Hypothalamic norepinephrine: Circadian rhythms and the control of feeding behavior. *Science,* 1972, **178**, 640–643.

Marihuana menaces youth, *Scientific American,* 1936, **154**, 151.

Marinesco, G. *Presse Médicale,* 1933, **74**, 1433.

Markee, J. E. Menstruation in intraocular endometrial implants in the rhesus monkey. *Contributions in Embryology of the Carnegie Institute,* 1940, **28**, 219.

Marley, E. Behavioral and electrophysiological effects of catecholamines. *Pharmacological Reviews,* 1966, **18**, 753–768.

Marley, E., & Key, B. J. Maturation of the electrocorticogram and behavior in the kitten and guinea pig and the effect of some sympathomimetic amines. *EEG Journal,* 1963, **15**, 620–636.

Marmorston, J., Moore, F. J., Kuzma, O. T., Magidson, O., & Weiner, J. Effect of Premarin on survival in men with myocardial infarction. *Biology and Medicine,* 1960, **105**, 618–620.

Martin, W. R., & Jasinski, D. R. Physiological parameters of morphine dependence in man—Tolerance, early abstinence, protracted abstinence. *Journal of Psychiatric Research,* 1969, **7**, 9–17.

Marx, J. L. Cyclic AMP in brain: Role in synaptic transmission. *Science,* 1972, **178**, 1188–1190.

Masters, W. H., & Johnson, V. E. The sexual response cycles of the human male and female: Comparative anatomy and physiology. In F. A. Beach (Ed.), *Sex and Behavior.* New York: Wiley, 1965.

Masters, W. H., & Johnson, V. E. *Human Sexual Response.* Boston: Little, Brown, 1966.

Maugh, T. H. Narcotic antagonists: The search accelerates. *Science,* 1972, **177**, 249-250.

Mayer, D. J., Wolfle, T. L., Akil, H., Carder, B., & Liebeskind, J. C. Analgesia from electrical stimulation in the brainstem of the rat. *Science,* 1971, **174**, 1351-1354.

Maynert, E. W. Sedatives and hypnotics I: Nonbarbiturates. In J. R. DiPalma (Ed.), *Drill's Pharmacology in Medicine.* (4th ed.) New York: McGraw-Hill, 1971. (a)

Maynert, E. W. Sedatives and hypnotics II: Barbiturates. In J. R. DiPalma (Ed.), *Drill's Pharmacology in Medicine.* (4th ed.) New York: McGraw-Hill, 1971. (b)

McBay, A. J., & Katsas, G. G. Glutethimide poisoning. *New England Journal of Medicine,* 1957, **257**, 97-100.

McCary, J. L. *Human Sexuality.* (2nd ed.) New York: Van Nostrand, 1973.

McConnell, J. V. Memory transfer through cannibalism in planarians. *Journal of Neuropsychiatry,* 1962, **3**, 42-48.

McConnell, J. V., Jacobson, A. L., & Kimble, D. P. Effects of regeneration upon retention of a conditioned response in the planarian. *Journal of Comparative and Physiological Psychology,* 1959, **52**, 1-5.

McConnell, J. V., Shigehisa, T., & Salive, H. Attempts to transfer approach and avoidance responses by RNA injections in rats. In K. H. Pribram and D. E. Broadbent (Eds.), *Biology of Memory.* New York: Academic, 1970.

McCulloch, D. R. Dual endocrine activity of testis. *Science,* 1932, **76**, 19.

McEwen, B. S., Zigmond, R. E., & Gerlach, J. Sites of steroid binding and action in the brain. In G. H. Bourne (Ed.), *Structure and Function of the Nervous System,* Vol. 4. New York: Academic, 1972.

McGaugh, J. L. Facilitative and disruptive effects of strychnine sulphate on maze learning. *Psychological Reports,* 1961, **8**, 99-104.

McGaugh, J. L. Time-dependent processes in memory storage. *Science,* 1966, **153**, 1351-1358.

McGaugh, J. L. Effects of analeptics on learning and memory in infrahumans. In P. Black (Ed.), *Drugs and the Brain.* Baltimore: Johns Hopkins, 1969.

McGaugh, J. L. Memory storage processes. In K. H. Pribram and D. E. Broadbent (Eds.), *Biology of Memory.* New York: Academic, 1970.

McGaugh, J. L., & Herz, M. J. *Memory Consolidation.* San Francisco: Albion, 1972.

McGaugh, J. L., & Petrinovich, L. F. Effects of drugs on learning and memory. *International Review of Neurobiology,* 1965, **8**, 139-196.

McGaugh, J. L., Thompson, C. W., Westbrook, W. H., & Hudspeth, W. J. A further study of learning facilitation with strychnine sulfate. *Psychopharmacologia*, 1962, **3**, 352-360.

McGeer, P. L. The chemistry of mind. *American Scientist*, 1971, **59**, 221-229.

McIsaac, W. M., Fritchie, G. E., Idänpään-Heikkilä, G. E., Ho, B. T., & Englert, L. F. Distribution of marihuana in monkey brain and concomitant behavioral effects. *Nature*, 1971, **230**, 593-594.

McKenzie, R. E., & Elliott, L. L. Effects of secobarbital and d-amphetamine on performance during a simulated air mission. *Aerospace Medicine*, 1965, **36**, 774-779.

McLennan, H. *Synaptic Transmission.* Philadelphia: Saunders, 1970.

McMillan, D. E. Effects of d-amphetamine on performance under several parameters of multiple fixed ratio, fixed interval schedules. *Journal of Pharmacology and Experimental Therapeutics*, 1969, **167**, 26-33.

McMillan, D. E., Harris, L. S., Frankenheim, J. M., & Kennedy, J. S. (1)-Δ^9-trans-tetrahydrocannabinol in pigeons: Tolerance to the behavioral effects. *Science*, 1970, **169**, 501-503.

Meek, J. L., & Fuxe, K. Serotonin accumulation after monoamine oxidase inhibition. *Biochemical Pharmacology*, 1971, **20**, 693-706.

Meier, G. W. Hypoxia. In E. Furchtgott (Ed.), *Pharmacological and Biophysical Agents and Behavior.* New York: Academic, 1971.

Melges, F. T., Tinklenberg, J. R., Hollister, L. E., & Gillespie, H. K. Temporal disintegration and depersonalization during marijuana intoxication. *Archives of General Psychiatry*, 1970, **23**, 208-209.

Mellin, G. W., & Katzenstein, M. The saga of thalidomide. *New England Journal of Medicine*, 1962, **267**, 1184-1238.

Melzack, R., & Wall, P. D. Pain mechanisms: A new theory. *Science*, 1965, **150**, 971-979.

Mendels, J., Frazer, A., Fitzgerald, R. G., Ramsey, T. A., & Stokes, J. W. Biogenic amine metabolites in cerebrospinal fluid of depressed and manic patients. *Science*, 1972, **175**, 1380-1381.

Merritt, H. H. *Textbook of Neurology.* (4th ed.) Philadelphia: Lea & Febiger, 1967.

Metys, J., Wagner, N., Metysova, J., & Herz, A. Studies on the central antinociceptive action of cholinomimetic agents. *International Journal of Neuropharmacology*, 1969, **8**, 413-425.

Meyer, F., Ipaktchi, M., & Clauser, H. Specific inhibition of gluconeogenesis by biguanides. *Nature*, 1967, **213**, 203.

Meyers, F. H., Jawetz, E., & Goldfien, A. *Review of Medical Pharmacology.* (3rd ed.) Los Altos, Calif.: Lange, 1972.

Michael, R. P. An investigation of the sensitivity of circumscribed neurological areas to hormonal stimulation by means of application of oestrogens directly into the brain of a cat. In S. S. Kety and J. Elkes (Eds.), *Regional Neurochemistry.* New York: Pergamon, 1961.

Michael, R. P. Behavioral effects of gonadal hormones and contraceptive steroids in primates. In H. A. Salhanick, D. M. Kipnis, & R. Vandewiele (Eds.), *Metabolic Effects of Gonadal Hormones and Contraceptive Steroids.* New York: Plenum, 1969.

Michael, R. P., & Plant, T. M. Contraceptive steroids and sexual activity. *Nature,* 1969, **222**, 579–581.

Migeon, C., Rivarola, M., & Forest, M. Studies of androgens in male transsexual subjects. In R. Green and J. Money (Eds.), *Transsexualism and Sex Reassignment.* Baltimore: Johns Hopkins, 1969.

Miller, N. E. Experiments on motivation. *Science,* 1957, **126**, 1271–1278.

Miller, N. E. Motivational effects of brain stimulation and drugs. *Federation Proceedings,* 1960, **19**, 846–854.

Miller, N. E. Chemical coding of behavior in the brain. *Science,* 1965, **148**, 328–338.

Miller, N. E. Learning of visceral and glandular responses. *Science,* 1969, **163**, 434–445.

Millichap, J. G., & Fowler, G. W. Treatment of "minimal brain dysfunction" syndromes: Selection of drugs for children with hyperactivity and learning disabilities. *Pediatric Clinics of North America,* 1967, **14**, 767–777.

Milner, B. Memory and the medial temporal regions of the brain. In K. H. Pribram and D. E. Broadbent (Eds.), *Biology of Memory.* New York: Academic, 1970.

Miras, C. J. Experience with chronic hashish smokers. In J. R. Wittenborn, H. Brill, J. P. Smith, and S. A. Wittenborn (Eds.), *Drugs and Youth.* Springfield, Ill.: Charles C Thomas, 1969.

Misra, A. L., Mitchell, C. T., & Woods, L. A. Persistence of morphine in central nervous system of rats after a single injection and its bearing on tolerance. *Nature,* 1971, **232**, 48–50.

Mize, D., & Isaac, W. Effects of sodium pentobarbital and d-amphetamine on latency of the escape response in the rat. *Psychological Reports,* 1962, **10**, 643–645.

Molinoff, P. B., Weinshilboum, R., & Axelrod, J. A sensitive enzymatic assay for dopamine-β-hydroxylase. *Journal of Pharmacology and Experimental Therapeutics,* 1971, **178**, 425–431.

Money, J. Components of eroticism in man: I. The hormones in relation to sexual morphology and sexual desire. *Journal of Nervous and Mental Disease,* 1961, **132**, 239–248.

Money, J., & Ehrhardt, A. A. *Man & Woman, Boy & Girl.* Baltimore: Johns Hopkins, 1972.

Monnier, M., & Krupp, P. Classification electro-physiologique des stimulants ou systeme nerveux central. *Archives of International Pharmacodynamics,* 1960, **127**, 337–360.

Monti, J. M., Rance, A. J., & Killam, K. F. CNS effects of haloperidol. *Federation Proceedings*, 1966, **25**, 229.

Moore, K. Toxicity and catecholamine releasing actions of d- and l-amphetamine in isolated and aggregated mice. *Journal of Pharmacology and Experimental Therapeutics*, 1963, **142**, 6-12.

Moore, K. E. Biochemical correlates of the behavioral effects of drugs. In R. H. Rech and K. E. Moore (Eds.), *An Introduction to Psychopharmacology*. New York: Raven, 1971.

Moreau, J. J. *Du Hachish et de L'Alienation Mentale: Etudes Psychologiques 34*. Paris: Libraire de Fortin, Masson, 1845.

Morrell, F., Bradley, W., & Ptashne, M. Effect of drugs on discharge characteristics of chronic epileptogenic lesions. *Neurology*, 1959, **9**, 492-498.

Morris, N. M., & Udry, J. R. Depression of physical activity by contraceptive pills. *American Journal of Obstetrics and Gynecology*, 1969, **104**, 1012-1014.

Morris, N. R., Aghajanian, G. K., & Bloom, F. E. Magnesium pemoline: Failure to affect in vivo synthesis of brain RNA. *Science*, 1967, **155**, 1125-1126.

Moss, R. L., & McCann, S. M. Induction of mating behavior in rats by luteinizing hormone-releasing factor. *Science*, 1973, **181**, 177-179.

Mowrer, O. H. On the dual nature of learning: A reinterpretation of "conditioning" and "problem solving." *Harvard Education Review*, 1947, **17**, 102-148.

Moyer, K. E. Kinds of aggression and their physiological basis. *Communications in Behavioral Biology*, 1968, **2**, 65-87.

Moyer, K. E., & Bunnell, B. N. Effect of injected adrenalin on an avoidance response in the rat. *Journal of Genetic Psychology*, 1958, **92**, 247-251.

Moyer, K. E., & Bunnell, B. N. Effect of adrenal demedullation on an avoidance response in the rat. *Journal of Comparative and Physiological Psychology*, 1959, **52**, 215-216.

Mrosovsky, N. Retention and reversal of conditioned avoidance following severe hypothermia. *Journal of Comparative and Physiological Psychology*, 1963, **56**, 811-813.

Muehlberger, C. W. The physiological action of alcohol. *Journal of the American Medical Association*, 1958, **167**, 1842-1845.

Müller, G. E., & Pilzecker, A. Experimentalle beitrage zur lehre vom gedachtnis. *Z. Psychol. Suppl.*, 1900, **1**, 1-288. (Germany)

Muller, H. F., & Warnes, H. Electrophysiological effects of butyrophenone drugs. In N. E. Lehmann and T. A. Ban (Eds.), *The Butyrophenones in Psychiatry*. Montreal: Quebec Psychopharmacological Research Assoc., 1964.

Murphree, H. B. Narcotic analgesics I: Opium alkaloids. In J. R. DiPalma (Ed.), *Drill's Pharmacology in Medicine*. (4th ed.) New York: McGraw-Hill, 1971.

Myer, J. S., & White, R. T. Aggressive motivation in the rat. *Animal Behavior*, 1965, **13**, 430-433.

Myers, R. D., & Sharpe, L. G. Chemical activation of ingestive and other hypothalamic regulatory mechanisms. *Physiology and Behavior,* 1968, **3**, 987-995.

Myschetzky, A. The significance of Megimide in the treatment of barbiturate poisoning. *Danish Medical Bulletin,* 1961, **8**, 33-36.

Nachmansohn, D. Proteins in excitable membranes. *Science,* 1970, **168**, 1059-1066.

Nagle, D. R. Anesthetic addiction and drunkenness. *International Journal of the Addictions,* 1968, **3**, 23-36.

Nahas, G. G. *Marihuana–Deceptive Weed.* New York: Raven, 1973.

Nathans, D. Puromycin inhibition of protein synthesis: Incorporation of puromycin into peptide chains. *Proceedings of the National Academy of Sciences* (USA), 1964, **51**, 585-592.

Nathanson, M. H. The central action of beta-aminopropylbenzene (benzedrine). *Journal of the American Medical Association,* 1937, **108**, 528-531.

Nathanson, I. T., Towne, L. E., & Aub, J. C. Normal excretions of sex hormones in childhood. *Endocrinology,* 1942, **28**, 851.

Newton, N. Interrelationships between sexual responsiveness, birth, and breast feeding. In J. Zubin and J. Money (Eds.), *Contemporary Sexual Behavior: Critical Issues in the 1970s.* Baltimore: Johns Hopkins, 1973.

Nickerson, M. Drugs inhibiting adrenergic nerves and structures innervated by them. In L. S. Goodman and A. Gilman (Eds.), *The Pharmacological Basis of Therapeutics.* (4th ed.) New York: Macmillan, 1970.

Nicoll, R. The effects of anesthetics on synaptic excitation and inhibition in the olfactory bulb. *Journal of Physiology,* 1972, **223**, 803-814.

Norton, S. Behavioral patterns as a technique for studying psychotropic drugs. In S. Garattini and V. B. Ghetti (Eds.), *Psychotropic Drugs.* Amsterdam: Elsevier, 1957.

Novales, R. R. Melanocyte-stimulating hormone and the intermediate lobe of the pituitary: Chemistry, effects, and mode of action. In L. Martini and W. F. Ganong (Eds.), *Neuroendocrinology.* New York: Academic, 1967.

Oberst, F. W., & Crook, J. W. Behavioral, physical, and pharmacodynamic effects of haloperidol in dogs and monkeys. *Archives of International Pharmacodynamics,* 1967, **167**, 450-464.

Ochs, S. *Elements of Neurophysiology.* New York: Wiley, 1965.

Odell, W. D., Ross, G. T., & Rayford, P. L. Radioimmunoassay for luteinizing hormone in human plasma or serum: Physiological studies. *Journal of Clinical Investigations,* 1967, **46**, 248-255.

Ohneda, A., Parada, E., Eisentraut, A., & Unger, R. H. Control of pancreatic glucagon secretion by glucose. *Diabetes,* 1968, **17**, 312.

Olds, J. Pleasure centers in the brain. *Scientific American,* 1956, **195**, 105-117.

Olds, J. Hypothalamic substrates of reward. *Physiological Reviews,* 1962, **42**, 554-604.

Olds, J., & Olds, M. E. The mechanisms of voluntary behavior. In R. G. Heath (Ed.), *The Role of Pleasure in Behavior.* New York: Harper & Row, 1964.

Oliver, M. F., & Boyd, G. S. The influence of reduction of serum lipids on prognosis of coronary heart disease, a five year study using oestrogens. *Lancet,* 1961, 2, 499-505.

Oliver, W. A. Acute hyperparathyroidism. *Lancet,* 1939, 2, 240.

Osmond, H. Ololiuqui: The ancient Aztec narcotic. *Journal of Mental Sciences,* 1955, 101, 526-537.

Osmond, H. A review of the clinical effects of psychotomimetic agents. *Annals of the New York Academy of Sciences,* 1957, 66, 418-434.

Osmond, H. Discussion. In D. H. Efron (Ed.), *Psychotomimetic Drugs.* New York: Raven, 1970.

Oswald, I., Berger, R. J., Jaramillo, R. A., Keddie, K. M. G., Olley, P. C., & Plunkett, G. B. Melancholia and barbiturates: A controlled EEG, body and eye movement study of sleep. *British Journal of Psychiatry,* 1963, 109, 66-78.

Oswald, I., & Priest, R. G. Five weeks to escape the sleeping-pill habit. *British Medical Journal,* 1965, 2, 1093-1099.

Overton, D. A. Drugs and learning. In J. A. Harvey (Ed.), *Behavioral Analysis of Drug Action.* Glenview, Ill.: Scott, Foresman, 1971.

Paalzow, L., & Paalzow, G. Studies on the relationship between morphine analgesia and the brain catecholamines in mice. *Acta Pharmacology et Toxicology,* 1971, 30, 104-114.

Pachkis, K. E., Rakoff, A. E., Cantarow, A., & Rupp, J. J. *Clinical Endocrinology.* (3rd ed.) New York: Harper & Row, 1967.

Panksepp, J. Effects of hypothalamic lesions on mouse-killing and shock-induced fighting in rats. *Physiology and Behavior,* 1971, 6, 311-316.

Park, C. R. The transport of glucose and other sugars across cell membranes and the effect of insulin. In G. E. W. Wolstenholme and C. M. O'Connor (Eds.), *Ciba Foundation Colloquia on Endocrinology, Vol. 9, Internal Secretion of the Pancreas.* Boston: Little, Brown, 1956.

Paterson, A. S. *Electrical and Drug Treatments in Psychiatry.* New York: Elsevier, 1963.

Patton, R. G., & Gardner, L. I. *Growth Failure in Maternal Deprivation.* Springfield, Ill.: Charles C Thomas, 1963.

Pearlman, C. A. Jr., Sharpless, S. K., & Jarvik, M. E. Retrograde amnesia produced by anesthetic and convulsant agents. *Journal of Comparative and Physiological Psychology,* 1961, 54, 109-112.

Pepler, R. D. Ambient temperature. In E. Furchtgott (Ed.), *Pharmacological and Biophysical Agents and Behavior.* New York: Academic, 1971.

Pert, C. B., Pasternak, G., & Snyder, S. H. Opiate agonist and antagonist discriminated by receptor binding in brain. *Science,* 1973, 182, 1359-1361.

Pert, C. B., Snowman, A. M., & Snyder, S. H. Localization of opiate receptor binding in synaptic membranes of rat brain. *Brain Research,* 1974, 70, 184-188.

Pert, C. B., & Snyder, S. H. Opiate receptor: Demonstration in nervous tissue. *Science*, 1973, **179**, 1011-1014.

Peters, J. M. Caffeine-induced hemorrhagic automutilation. *Archives of International Pharmacodynamics*, 1967, **169**, 139-146. (a)

Peters, J. M. Factors affecting caffeine toxicity. *Journal of Clinical Pharmacology*, 1967, **7**, 131-141. (b)

Pevzner, Z. Nucleic acid changes during behavioral events. In J. Gaito (Ed.), *Macromolecules and Behavior*. New York: Appleton-Century-Crofts, 1966.

Pfaff, P. W. Autoradiographic localization of radioactivity in rat brain after injection of tritiated sex hormones. *Science*, 1968, **161**, 1355-1356.

Pfaff, P. W., Silva, M. T. A., & Weiss, J. M. Telemetered recording of hormone effects on hippocampal neurons. *Science*, 1971, **172**, 394-395.

Pfeiffer, C. A. Sexual differences of the hypophyses and their determination by the gonads. *American Journal of Anatomy*, 1936, **58**, 195-226.

Pfeiffer, E. F., Schoffling, K., Ditschuneit, H., Ziegler, R., & Gepts, W. Pharmacology and mode of action of the hypoglycemic sulfonylureas. In G. D. Campbell (Ed.), *Oral Hypoglycemic Agents*. New York: Academic, 1969.

Phoenix, C. H. Sexual behavior in rhesus monkeys after vasectomy. *Science*, 1973, **179**, 493-494.

Phoenix, C. H., Goy, R. W., Gerall, A. A., & Young, W. C. Organizing action of prenatally administered testosterone proprionate on the tissue mediating mating behavior in the female guinea pig. *Endocrinology*, 1959, **65**, 369-382.

Pincus, G. *The Control of Fertility*. New York: Academic, 1965.

Plotnikoff, N. Magnesium pemoline: Enhancement of learning and memory of a conditioned avoidance response. *Science*, 1966, **151**, 703-704.

Plotnikoff, N. Enhancement of EEG conditioning with pemoline and magnesium hydroxide. In P. Black (Ed.), *Drugs and the Brain*. Baltimore: Johns Hopkins, 1969.

Porte, D., Jr., & Williams, R. H. Inhibition of insulin release by norepinephrine in man. *Science*, 1966, **152**, 1248-1250.

Poschel, B. P. H., & Ninteman, F. W. Norepinephrine: A possible excitatory neurohormone of the reward system. *Life Sciences*, 1963, **2**, 782-788.

Poschel, B. P. H., & Ninteman, F. W. Excitatory (antidepressant?) effects of monoamine oxidase inhibitors on the reward system of the brain. *Life Sciences*, 1964, **3**, 903-910.

Poschel, B. P. H., & Ninteman, F. W. Hypothalamic self-stimulation: Its suppression by blockade of norepinephrine biosynthesis and reinstatement by methamphetamine. *Life Sciences*, 1966, **5**, 11-16.

Post, R. M., Gordon, E. K., Goodwin, F. K., & Bunney, W. E., Jr. Central norepinephrine metabolism in affective disease: MHPG in the cerebrospinal fluid. *Science*, 1973, **179**, 1002-1003.

Potts, J. T., Jr., & Aurbach, G. D. The chemistry of parathyroid hormone. In P. J. Gaillard, R. V. Talmage, and A. M. Budy (Eds.), *The Parathyroid Glands*. Chicago: The University of Chicago Press, 1965.

Powell, G. F., Brasel, J. A., & Blizzard, R. M. Emotional deprivation and growth retardation simulating idiopathic hypopituitarism. I. Clinical evaluation of the syndrome. *New England Journal of Medicine,* 1967, **276**, 1271-1278.

Price, H. L., & Dripps, R. D. General anesthetics I: Gas anesthetics. In J. R. DiPalma (Ed.), *Drill's Pharmacology in Medicine.* (4th ed.) New York: McGraw-Hill, 1971. (a)

Price, H. L., & Dripps, R. D. General anesthetics II: Volatile anesthetics. In J. R. DiPalma (Ed.), *Drill's Pharmacology in Medicine.* (4th ed.) New York: McGraw-Hill, 1971. (b)

Price, H. L., Kovnak, P. H., Safer, J. N., Conner, E. H., & Price, M. L. The uptake of thiopental by body tissues and its relation to the duration of narcosis. *Clinical Pharmacology and Therapeutics,* 1960, **1**, 16-22.

Purpura, D. Electrophysiological analysis of psychotogenic drug action. *Archives of Neurology and Psychiatry,* 1956, **75**, 132-143.

Quetsch, R. M., Achol, R. W. P., Litin, E. M., & Faucett, R. L. Depressive reactions in hypertensive patients: A comparison of those treated with rauwolfia and those receiving no specific antihypertensive treatment. *Circulation,* 1959, **19**, 366-375.

Raben, M. S. Growth hormone, 1. Physiological aspects. *New England Journal of Medicine,* 1962, **266**, 31-35.

Rabinowitz, D., Merimec, T. J., Maffezzoli, R., & Purgess, J. A. Patterns of hormonal release after glucose, protein, and glucose plus protein. *Lancet,* 1966, **2**, 454-456.

Rado, S. Hedonic self-regulation of the organism. In R. Heath (Ed.), *The Role of Pleasure in Behavior.* New York: Harper & Row, 1964.

Raisman, G., & Field, P. M. Sexual dimorphism in the preoptic area of the rat. *Science,* 1971, **173**, 731-733.

Randall, L. O., Schallek, W., Heise, G. A., Kieth, E. F., & Bagdon, R. E. The psychosedative properties of methaminodiezepoxide. *Journal of Pharmacology and Experimental Therapeutics,* 1960, **129**, 163-171.

Randt, C. T., Quartermain, D., Goldstein, M., & Anagnoste, B. Norepinephrine biosynthesis inhibition: Effects on memory in mice. *Science,* 1971, **172**, 498-499.

Ransmeier, R. E., & Gerard, R. W. Effects of temperature, convulsion and metabolic factors on rodent memory and EEG. *American Journal of Physiology,* 1954, **179**, 663-664.

Rasmussen, H. Parathyroid hormone, calcitonin, and the calciferols. In R. H. Williams (Ed.), *Textbook of Endocrinology.* (5th ed.) Philadelphia: Saunders, 1974.

Rasmussen, H., Sze, Y. L., & Young, R. Further studies on the isolation and characterization of parathyroid polypeptides. *Journal of Biological Chemistry,* 1964, **239**, 2852-2857.

Ray, A., Mukherj, M., & Ghosh, J. Adrenal catecholamines and related changes during different phases of morphine administration: A histochemical study. *Journal of Neurochemistry,* 1968, **15**, 875-881.

Ray, C. G., Kirchvink, J. P., Waxman, S. H., & Kelley, V. C. Studies of anabolic steroids. III. The effect of oxandrolone on height and skeletal maturation in mongoloid children. *American Journal of the Diseases of Children*, 1965, **110**, 618-623.

Ray, O. S. *Drugs, Society, and Human Behavior.* St. Louis: Mosby, 1972.

Ray, O. S., & Barrett, R. J. Disruptive effects of electroconvulsive shock as a function of current level and mode of delivery. *Journal of Comparative and Physiological Psychology*, 1969, **67**, 110-116.

Ray, O. S., & Bivens, L. W. Reinforcement magnitude as a determinant of performance decrement after electroconvulsive shock. *Science*, 1968, **160**, 330-332.

Ray, O. S., & Hochhauser, S. Growth hormone and environmental complexity effects on behavior in the rat. *Developmental Psychology*, 1969, **1**, 311-317.

Redmond, D. E., Jr., Hinrichs, R. L., Maas, J. W., & Kling, A. Behavior of free-ranging macaques after intraventricular 6-hydroxydopamine. *Science*, 1973, **181**, 1256-1258.

Regush, N. M. *The Drug Addiction Business.* New York: Dial Press, 1971.

Reich, E. Biochemistry of actinomycins. *Cancer Research*, 1963, **23**, 1428-1441.

Reichlin, S. Neuroendocrinology. In R. H. Williams (Ed.), *Textbook of Endocrinology.* (5th ed.) Philadelphia: Saunders, 1974.

Reimann, H. A. Caffeinism. *Journal of the American Medical Association*, 1967, **202**, 1105-1106.

Reiter, L. Effects of amphetamine on lateral hypothalamic activity in response to amygdaloid stimulation. *Federation Proceedings*, 1970, **29**, 383. (Abstract)

Remmien, E. *Psychochemotherapy.* Los Angeles: Western Medical Publications, 1962.

Resko, J. A., & Phoenix, C. H. Sexual behavior and testosterone concentrations in the plasma of Rhesus monkey before and after castration. *Endocrinology*, 1972, **91**, 499-503.

Rethy, C. R., Smith, C. B., & Villarreal, J. E. Effects of narcotic analgesics upon the locomotor activity and brain catecholamine content of the mouse. *Journal of Pharmacology and Experimental Therapeutics*, 1971, **176**, 472-479.

Reynolds, D. V. Surgery in the rat during electrical analgesia induced by focal brain stimulation. *Science*, 1969, **164**, 444-445.

Reynolds, R. W. The effect of amphetamine on food intake in normal and hypothalamic hyperphagic rats. *Journal of Comparative and Physiological Psychology*, 1959, **52**, 682-684.

Richards, C. On the mechanism of barbiturate anesthesia. *Journal of Physiology*, 1972, **227**, 749-767.

Richels, K., & Bass, H. A comparative, controlled clinical trial of seven hypnotic agents in medical and psychiatric in-patients. *American Journal of Medical Science*, 1963, **245**, 142-152.

Ritchie, J. M. The aliphatic alcohols. In L. S. Goodman and A. Gilman (Eds.), *The Pharmacological Basis of Therapeutics.* (4th ed.) New York: Macmillan, 1970. (a)

Ritchie, J. M. "Central Nervous System Stimulants: II The Xanthines." In L. S. Goodman and A. Gilman (Eds.), *The Pharmacological Basis of Therapeutics.* (4th ed.) New York: Macmillan, 1970. (b).

Ritchie, J. M., Cohen, P. J., & Dripps, R. D. Cocaine, procaine and other local anesthetics. In L. S. Goodman and A. Gilman (Eds.), *The Pharmacological Basis of Therapeutics.* (4th ed.) New York: Macmillan, 1970.

Ritvo, M. Drugs as an aid in roentgen examination of the gastrointestinal tract: The use of mecholyl, physostigmine, and benzedrine in overcoming atonicity, sluggishness or peristalsis spasm. *American Journal of Roentgenology,* 1936, **36**, 868-879.

Robbins, J., & Van der Kloot, W. G. The effect of picrotoxin on peripheral inhibition in the crayfish. *Journal of Physiology,* 1958, **143**, 541-552.

Roberts, E., & Kuriyama, K. Biochemical-physiological correlations in studies of the γ-aminobutyric acid system. *Brain Research,* 1968, **8**, 1-35.

Robinson, B. W. Forebrain alimentary responses: Some organizational principles. In M. J. Wayner (Ed.), *Thirst.* New York: Pergamon, 1964.

Robinson, V. *An Essay on Hasheesh.* (2nd ed.) New York: E. H. Ringer, 1925.

Rodahl, K., & Issekutz, B. (Eds.), *Nerve as a Tissue.* New York: Harper & Row, 1966.

Rose, R. M., Bourne, P., & Poe, R. Androgen responses to stress. *Psychosomatic Medicine,* 1969, **31**, 418-436.

Rosenblatt, F., Farrow, J. T., & Herblin, W. F. Transfer of conditioned responses from trained rats to untrained rats by means of a brain extract. *Nature,* 1966, **209**, 46-48.

Rosenblatt, F., Farrow, J. T., & Rhine, S. Transfer of learned behavior from trained to untrained rats by means of brain extracts. I, II. *Proceedings of the National Academcy of Science* (USA), 1966, **55**, 548-555; 787-792.

Rosenthal, R. A. *Experimenter Effects in Behavioral Research.* New York: Appleton-Century-Crofts, 1966.

Rosenzweig, M. R. Evidence for anatomical and chemical changes in the brain during primary learning. In K. H. Pribram and D. E. Broadbent (Eds.), *Biology of Memory.* New York: Academic, 1970.

Rosenzweig, M. R., Krech, D., & Bennett, E. L. A search for relations between brain chemistry and behavior. *Psychological Bulletin,* 1960, **57**, 476-492.

Ross, J., Claybaugh, C., Clemens, L. G., & Gorski, R. A. Short latency induction of estrous behavior with intracerebral gonadal hormones in ovariectomized rats. *Endocrinology,* 1971, **89**, 32-38.

Rossum, J. M., & Janssen, P. A. The pharmacology of haloperidol. *International Journal of Neuropsychiatry,* 1967, **1**, 510-518.

Rothballer, A. B. Studies on the adrenaline-sensitive component of the reticular activating system. *EEG Journal,* 1956, **8**, 603-621.

Rothballer, A. B. The effect of phenylephrine, methamphetamine, cocaine, and serotonin upon the adrenaline-sensitive component of the reticular activating system. *EEG Journal,* 1957, **9**, 409–417.

Rothballer, A. B. The effects of catecholamines on the central nervous system. *Pharmacological Reviews,* 1959, **11**, 494–547.

Routtenberg, A. Intracranial chemical injection and behavior: A critical review. *Behavioral Biology,* 1972, **7**, 601–641.

Rubenstein, E. *Intensive Medical Care.* New York: McGraw-Hill, 1971.

Rubin, E., & Lieber, C. S. Experimental alcoholic hepatitis: A new primate model. *Science,* 1973, **182**, 712–713.

Rubin, R. P. The role of calcium in the release of neurotransmitter substances and hormones. *Pharmacological Reviews,* 1970, **22**, 389–428.

Russek, H. I., Naegele, C. F., & Ragan, F. D. Alcohol in the treatment of angina pectoris. *Journal of the American Medical Association,* 1950, **143**, 355–357.

Russell, W. R., & Nathan, P. W. Traumatic amnesia. *Brain,* 1946, **69**, 280–300.

Rutledge, L. T., & Doty, R. W. Differential action of chlorpromazine on reflexes conditioned to central and peripheral stimulation. *American Journal of Physiology,* 1957, **191**, 189–192.

Sackler, A. M., Weltman, A. S., Pandhi, V., & Schwartz, R. Gonadal effects of vasectomy and vasoligation. *Science,* 1973, **179**, 293–294.

Sakel, M. Zur Methodik der Hypoglykamie-behandlung von Psychosen. *Wien. Klin. Wschr.,* 1936, **49**, 1278.

Salmoiraghi, G. C. Central adrenergic synapses. *Pharmacological Reviews,* 1966, **18**, 717–726.

Salmoiraghi, G. C., & Bloom, F. E. Pharmacology of individual neurons. *Science,* 1964, **144**, 493–499.

Samanin, R., & Bernasconi, S. Effects of intraventricular injected 6-OH-dopamine or midbrain raphe lesion on morphine analgesia in rats. *Psychopharmacologia,* 1972, **25**, 175–182.

Samanin, R., Gumulka, W., & Valzelli, L. Reduced effect of morphine in midbrain raphe lesioned rats. *European Journal of Pharmacology,* 1971, **16**, 298–302.

Sanger, F. Chemistry of insulin. *British Medical Bulletin,* 1960, **16**, 183–188.

Santi, R., & Guiliana, F. Dexamphetamine and lipid mobilization in obesity. *Journal of Pharmacy and Pharmacology,* 1964, **16**, 130–131.

Sar, M., & Stumpf, W. Neurons of the hypothalamus concentrate [3-H] progesterone or its metabolites. *Science,* 1973, **182**, 1266–1268.

Sawyer, C. H., & Robinson, B. Separate hypothalamic areas controlling pituitary gonadotropin functions and mating behavior in female cats and rabbits. *Journal of Clinical Endocrinology,* 1956, **16**, 914–915.

Sawyer, W. H. Neurohypophyseal secretions and their origin. In A. V. Nalbandov (Ed.), *Advances in Neuroendocrinology,* Urbana, Illinois: The University of Illinois Press, 1963.

Schacter, S., & Singer, J. E. Cognitive, social, and physiological determinants of emotional state. *Psychological Review,* 1962, **69**, 374–399.

Schacter, S., & Wheeler, L. Epinephrine, chlorpromazine and amusement. *Journal of Abnormal and Social Psychology,* 1962, **45**, 121-128.

Schallek, W., & Kuehn, A. Effects of psychotropic drugs on limbic system of cat. *Federation Proceedings,* 1960, **105**, 115-117.

Schallek, W., & Kuehn, A. Effects of benzodiazepines on spontaneous EEG and arousal responses of cats. *Progress in Brain Research,* 1965, **18**, 231-238.

Schally, A. V., Arimura, A., & Kastin, A. J. Hypothalamic regulatory hormones. *Science,* 1973, **179**, 341-350.

Schapiro, S. Influence of hormones and environmental stimulation on brain development. In D. H. Ford (Ed.), *Influence of Hormones on the Nervous System,* Basel: Kargem, 1971.

Schaumann, W. A hypothesis of a cholinergic mechanism for the action of morphine. *Naunyn-Schmiedburg Archives Pharmacology and Experimental Pathology,* 1959, **247**, 229-240.

Schechter, M. J., & Rosencrans, J. A. Behavioral evidence for two types of cholinergic receptor in the C.N.S. *European Journal of Pharmacology,* 1971, **15**, 375-378.

Schildkraut, J. J. The catecholamine hypothesis of affective disorders—A review of supporting evidence. *American Journal of Psychiatry,* 1965, **122**, 509-522.

Schildkraut, J. J., & Kety, S. S. Biogenic amines and emotion. *Science,* 1967, **156**, 21-30.

Schmidt, G., & Sigusch, V. Women's sexual arousal. In J. Zubin and J. Money (Eds.), *Contemporary Sexual Behavior: Critical Issues in the 1970s.* Baltimore: Johns Hopkins, 1973.

Schou, M. Treatment of manic psychoses by administration of lithium salts. *Journal of Neurology, Neurosurgery and Psychiatry,* 1954, **17**, 250-260.

Schulte, J. W., Reif, E., Bacher, J. A., Lawrence, W. S., & Tainter, M. L. Further study of central stimulation from sympathomimetic amines. *Journal of Pharmacology and Experimental Therapeutics,* 1941, **71**, 62-74.

Schultes, R. E. Hallucinogens of plant origin. *Science,* 1969, **163**, 246-254.

Schumer, W., & Nyhus, L. *Corticosteroids in the Treatment of Shock.* Urbana, Ill.: The University of Illinois Press, 1970.

Schur, M. *Freud Living and Dying.* New York: International University Press, 1972.

Schwartz, M. *Physiological Psychology.* New York: Appleton-Century-Crofts, 1973.

Scott, J. M. *The White Poppy: A History of Opium.* New York: Funk & Wagnalls, 1969.

Scrafani, J. T., & Hug, C. Active uptake of dihydromorphine and other narcotic analgesics by cerebral cortex slices. *Biochemical Pharmacology,* 1968, **17**, 1557-1566.

Searle, L. V., & Brown, C. W. Effect of variation in the dose of benzedrine sulfate on the activity of white rats. *Journal of Experimental Psychology,* 1938, **22**, 555-563. (a)

Searle, L. V., & Brown, C. W. Effects of subcutaneous injections of benzedrine sulfate on the activity of white rats. *Journal of Experimental Psychology,* 1938, **22**, 480–490. (b)

Seaton, D. A., Rose, K., & Duncan, L. J. P. A comparison of the appetite suppressing properties of dexamphetamine and phentermine. *Scottish Medical Journal,* 1964, **9**, 482–485.

Seeman, P. The membrane actions of anesthetics and tranquilizers. *Pharmacological Reviews,* 1972, **24**, 583–655.

Seevers, M. H. Laboratory evaluation for drug dependence. In E. L. Way (Ed.), *New Concepts in Pain and its Clinical Management.* Philadelphia: Davis, 1967.

Segal, S. J., & Johnson, D. C. Inductive influence of steroid hormones on the neural system: Ovulation controlling mechanisms. *Archives of Anatomy,* 1959, **48**, 261–273.

Seiden, L. S., & Peterson, D. D. Reversal of the reserpine-induced suppression of the conditioned avoidance response by L-dopa: Correlation of behavioral and biochemical differences in two strains of mice. *Journal of Pharmacology and Experimental Therapeutics,* 1968, **159**, 422–428.

Sen, G., & Bose, K. C. *Rauwolfia serpentina* a new Indian drug for insanity and high blood pressure. *Indian Medical World,* 1931, **2**, 194–201.

Setter, G. J., Maher, J. F., & Schreiner, G. E. Barbiturate intoxication: Evaluation of therapy including dialysis in a large series selectively referred because of severity. *Archives of Internal Medicine,* 1966, **117**, 224–236.

Shader, R. I., & Grinspoon, L. Schizophrenia, oligospermia, and phenothiazines. *Diseases of the Nervous System,* 1967, **28**, 240–244.

Sharp, J. C., Nielson, H. C., & Porter, P. B. The effect of amphetamine upon cats with lesions in the ventro-medial hypothalamus. *Journal of Comparative and Physiological Psychology,* 1962, **55**, 198–200.

Sharpless, S. K. Hypnotics and sedatives I: The barbiturates. In L. S. Goodman and A. Gilman (Eds.), *The Pharmacological Basis of Therapeutics.* (4th ed.) New York: Macmillan, 1970. (a)

Sharpless, S. K. Hypnotics and sedatives II: Miscellaneous agents. In L. S. Goodman and A. Gilman (Eds.), *The Pharmacological Basis of Therapeutics.* (4th ed.) New York: Macmillan, 1970. (b)

Sheffield, P. D., Wulff, J. J., & Backer, R. Reward value of copulation without sex drive reduction. *Journal of Comparative and Physiological Psychology,* 1951, **44**, 3–8.

Shen, F. H., Low, H. H., & Way, E. L. Reserpine antagonism of morphine analgesia in tolerant mice. *Federation Proceedings,* 1969, **28**, 793. (Abstract)

Shikita, M., & Tamaoki, B. -I. Testosterone formation by subcellular particles of rat testes. *Endocrinology,* 1965, **76**, 563–569.

Shore, P. A. Release of serotonin and catecholamines by drugs. *Pharmacological Reviews,* 1962, **14**, 531–550.

Shute, C. C. D., & Lewis, P. R. The ascending cholinergic reticular system: Neocortical, olfactory and subcortical projections. *Brain,* 1967, **40**, 497–520.

Sigg, E. B. Neuropharmacologic assessment of tofranil (imipramine) a new antidepressant agent. *Federation Proceedings*, 1959, **18**, 144. (Abstract)

Simpson, J. B., & Routtenberg, A. The subfornical organ and carbachol-induced drinking. *Brain Research*, 1972, **45**, 135–152.

Simpson, J. B., & Routtenberg, A. Subfornical organ: Dipsogenic site of action of angiotensin-II. *Science*, 1973, **181**, 1172–1175.

Simpson, L. L. The role of calcium in neurohumoral and neurohormonal extrusion processes. *Journal of Pharmacy and Pharmacology*, 1968, **20**, 889–910.

Singer, J. E. Sympathetic activation, drugs and fear. *Journal of Comparative and Physiological Psychology*, 1963, **56**, 612–615.

Sjoerdsma, A. Clinical implication of unnatural amino acids and amines. *Federation Proceedings*, 1971, **30**, 908–911.

Slusher, M. A. Influence of adrenal steroids on self-stimulation rates in rats. *Federation Proceedings*, 1965, **120**, 617–620.

Smith, D. E., King, M. B., & Hoebel, B. G. Lateral hypothalamic control of killing: Evidence for a cholinoceptive mechanism. *Science*, 1970, **167**, 900–901.

Smith, D. E., & Mehl, C. An analysis of marijuana toxicity. In D. E. Smith (Ed.), *The New Social Drug*. Englewood Cliffs, N.J.: Prentice-Hall, 1970.

Smith, O. A., Jr. Food intake and hypothalamic stimulation. In D. E. Sheer (Ed.), *Electrical Stimulation of the Brain*. Austin: University of Texas Press, 1961.

Smith, R. G. Magnesium pemoline: Lack of facilitation in human learning, memory and performance tests. *Science*, 1967, **155**, 603–605.

Smith, R. G., & Baker, W. J. Drug effects on learning and memory in man: Approaches, problems and suggestions. In P. Black (Ed.), *Drugs and the Brain*. Baltimore: Johns Hopkins, 1969.

Snyder, J. J., & Levitt, R. A. Neural activity changes correlated with central anticholinergic blockade of cholinergically-induced drinking. *Pharmacology, Biochemistry and Behavior*, in press.

Snyder, S. H. Catecholamines, brain function, and how psychotropic drugs act. In C. G. Clark and J. del Giudice (Eds.), *Principles of Psychopharmacology*. New York: Academic, 1970.

Snyder, S. H., Banerjee, S. P., Yamamura, H. I., & Greenberg, D. Drugs, neurotransmitters and schizophrenia. *Science*, 1974, **184**, 1243–1253.

Snyder, S. H., Faillace, L., & Hollister, L. 2,5-Dimethoxy-4-methyl-amphetamine (STP): A new hallucinogenic drug. *Science*, 1967, **158**, 669–670.

Sokal, J. E. Glucagon: An essential hormone. *American Journal of Medicine*, 1966, **41**, 331–341.

Sokal, J. E. Glucagon. In M. Ellenberg and H. Rifkin (Eds.), *Diabetes Mellitus: Theory and Practice*, New York: McGraw-Hill, 1970.

Solomon, D. (Ed.) *The Marihuana Papers*. New York: New American Library, 1966.

Somjen, G. Effect of anesthetics on spinal cord of mammals. *Anesthesiology,* 1967, **28**, 135-143.

Soueif, M. I. Hashish consumption in Egypt with special reference to psychological aspects. *Bulletin of Narcotics,* 1967, **19**, 1-12.

Speck, L. B. Toxicity and effects of increasing doses of mescaline: *Journal of Pharmacology and Experimental Therapeutics,* 1957, **119**, 78-84.

Speck, L. B. EEG changes in the rat with mescaline intoxication. *Journal of Pharmacology and Experimental Therapeutics,* 1958, **122**, 201-206.

Spellacy, W. N., Buhi, W. C., & Bendel, R. P. Growth hormone and glucose level after one year of combination-type oral contraceptive treatment. *International Journal of Fertility,* 1969, **14**, 51-55.

Spooner, C. E., & Winters, W. D. Evidence for a direct action of monoamines on the chick nervous sytem. *Experientia,* 1965, **21**, 256-258.

Spragg, S. D. S. Morphine addiction in chimpanzees. *Comparative Psychology Monographs,* 1938, **15**, 79.

Squire, P. G. Intratesticular injections of ICSH in hypophysectomized rats. *International Journal of Fertility,* 1963, **8**, 531-537.

Staub, A., Sinn, L., & Behrens, O. K. Purification and crystallization of hyperglycemic glycogenolytic factor (HGF). *Science,* 1953, **117**, 628-629.

Stein, G. W., & Levitt, R. A. Lesion effects on cholinergically elicited drinking in the rat. *Physiology and Behavior,* 1971, **7**, 517-522.

Stein, L. Reciprocal action of reward and punishment mechanisms. In R. G. Heath (Ed.), *The Role of Pleasure in Behavior,* New York: Harper & Row, 1964.

Stein, L. Psychopharmacological substrates of mental depression. In S. Garattini (Ed.), *Antidepressant Drugs.* Amsterdam: Excerpta Medica, 1967.

Stein, L. Chemistry of purposive behavior. In J. T. Tapp (Ed.), *Reinforcement and Behavior,* New York: Academic, 1969.

Stein, L. Neurochemistry of reward and punishment: Some implications for the etiology of schizophrenia. *Journal of Psychiatric Research,* 1971, **8**, 345-361.

Stein, L., & Seifter, J. Possible mode of antidepressive action of imipramine. *Science,* 1961, **134**, 286-287.

Stein, L., & Seifter, J. Muscarinic synapses in the hypothalamus. *American Journal of Physiology,* 1962, **202**, 751-756.

Stein, L., & Wise, C. D. Release of norepinephrine from hypothalamus and amygdala by rewarding medial forebrain bundle stimulation and amphetamine. *Journal of Comparative and Physiological Psychology,* 1969, **67**, 189-198.

Stein, L., & Wise, C. D. Behavioral pharmacology of central stimulants. In W. G. Clark and J. Del Giudice (Eds.), *Principles of Psychopharmacology.* New York: Academic, 1970.

Stein, L., & Wise, C. D. Possible etiology of schizophrenia: Progressive damage to the noradrenergic reward system by 6-hydroxydopamine. *Science,* 1971, **171**, 1032-1036.

Sternbach, L. H., Randall, L. O., & Gustafson, S. R. 1, 4-Benzodiazepines (Chlordiazepoxide and related compounds). In M. Gordon (Ed.), *Psychopharmacological Agents*, New York: Academic, 1964.

Stewart, C. N., & Brookshire, K. H. Shuttle box avoidance learning and epinephrine. *Psychonomic Science*, 1967, **9**, 419-420.

Stewart, C. N., & Brookshire, K. H. Effect of epinephrine on acquisition of conditioned fear. *Physiology and Behavior*, 1968, **3**, 601-604.

St. Jean, A. The psychophysical effects of the butyrophenones in male schizophrenics. In H. E. Lehmann and T. A. Ban (Eds.), *The Butyrophenones in Psychiatry*. Montreal: Quebec Psychopharmacological Research Association, 1964.

Storm, T., Caird, W. K., & Korbin, E. The effects of alcohol on rote verbal learning and retention. *Psychonomic Science*, 1967, **9**, 43-44.

Strauss, J. S., & Pochi, P. E. The human sebaceous gland: Its regulation by steroidal hormones and its use as an end organ for assaying androgenicity in vivo. *Recent Progress in Hormone Research*, 1963, **19**, 385-435.

Streit, P., Akert, K., Sandrl, C., Livingston, R., & Moor, H. Dynamic ultrastructure of presynaptic membranes at nerve terminals in the spinal cord of rats. Anesthetized and unanesthetized preparations compared. *Brain Research*, 1972, **48**, 11-26.

Stumpf, W. E. Estradiol-concentrating neurons: Topography in the hypothalamus by dry-mount autoradiography. *Science*, 1968, **162**, 1001-1003.

Sturgeon, R. D., Brophy, P. D., & Levitt, R. A. Drinking elicited by intracranial microinjection of angiotensin in the cat. *Pharmacology Biochemistry and Behavior*, 1973, **1**, 353-355.

Sturtevant, F. M., & Drill, V. A. Effects of mescaline in laboratory animals and influence of ataraxics on mescaline-response. *Federation Proceedings*, 1956, **92**, 383-387.

Suits, E., & Isaacson, R. L. The effects of scopolamine hydrobromide on one-way and two-way avoidance learning in rats. *International Journal of Neuropharmacology*, 1968, **7**, 441-446.

Sulser, F., & Sanders-Bush, E. Effect of drugs on amines in the CNS. *Annual Review of Pharmacology*, 1971, **11**, 209-230.

Sutherland, E. W. Studies on the mechanism of hormone action. *Science*, 1972, **177**, 401-408.

Sved, S. The metabolism of exogenous ribonucleic acid injected into mice. *Canadian Journal of Biochemistry*, 1965, **43**, 949-958.

Tagliamonte, A., Tagliamonte, P., Gessa, G. L., & Brodie, B. B. Compulsive sexual activity induced by p-chlorophenylalanine in normal and pinealectomized male rats. *Science*, 1969, **166**, 1433-1435.

Tainter, M. L. Actions of benzedrine and propadrine in the control of obesity. *Journal of Nutrition*, 1944, **27**, 89-105.

Talbott, J. A., & Teague, J. W. Marijuana psychosis: Acute toxic psychosis associated with the use of cannabis derivatives. *Journal of the American Medical Association*, 1969, **210**, 299-302.

Talland, G. A. *Deranged Memory.* New York: Academic, 1965.

Talland, G. A. Improvement of sustained attention with Cylert. *Psychonomic Science,* 1966, **6**, 493–494.

Talland, G. A. Drug enhancement of human memory and attention: Experiments with pemoline and magnesium hydroxide. In P. Black (Ed.), *Drugs and the Brain.* Baltimore: Johns Hopkins, 1969.

Talland, G. A., Hagen, D. Q., & James, M. Performance tests of amnesic patients with Cylert. *Journal of Nervous and Mental Disease,* 1967, **144**, 421–429.

Talwar, G. P., Goel, B. K., Chopra, S. P., & D'Monte, B. Brain RNA: Some information on its nature and metabolism as revealed by studies during experimentally induced convulsions and its response to sensory stimulation. In J. Gaito (Ed.), *Macromolecules and Behavior.* New York: Appleton-Century-Crofts, 1966.

Tanner, J. M. *Growth at Adolescence.* (2nd ed.) Oxford: Blackwell Scientific Publications, Ltd., 1962.

Tart, C. T. (Ed.), *Altered States of Consciousness.* New York: Wiley, 1969.

Tart, C. T. Marijuana intoxication: Common experiences. *Nature,* 1970, **226**, 701–704.

Tata, J. R. Requirement for RNA and protein synthesis for induced regression of the tadpole tail in organ culture. *Developmental Biology,* 1966, **13**, 77–94.

Taylor, K. M., & Snyder, S. H. Amphetamine: Differentiation by d and l isomers of behavior involving brain norepinephrine or dopamine. *Science,* 1970, **168**, 1487–1489.

Taylor, S. Calcitonin. In S. Taylor (Ed.), *Symposium on Thyrocalcitonin and C Cells.* London: Heineman, 1968.

Teitelbaum, P., & Derks, P. Amphetamine and forced drinking. *Journal of Comparative and Physiological Psychology,* 1958, **51**, 801–810.

Theobald, W. Pharmakologische und experimentalpsychologische Untersuchungen mit zwei Inhaltsstoffen des Fliegenpilzes. *Arzneiniettel-Forsch* (Drug Research), 1968, **18**, 311–315.

Thiele, J., & Holzinger, O. Uber O-Sianidodibenzyl. *Annals of Chemistry,* 1899, **305**, 96.

Thompson, J., & Schuster, C. R. *Behavioral Pharmacology.* New York: Prentice-Hall, 1968.

Thompson, R., & Pryer, R. S. The effect of anoxia on the retention of a discrimination habit. *Journal of Comparative and Physiological Psychology,* 1956, **149**, 297–300.

Tormey, J., & Lasagna, L. Relation of thyroid function to acute and chronic effects of amphetamine in the rat. *Journal of Pharmacology and Experimental Therapeutics,* 1960, **128**, 201–209.

Towman, J. E. P., & Davis, J. The effects of drugs upon the electrical activity of the brain. *Pharmacological Review,* 1949, **1**, 425–492.

Tranzer, J. P., & Thoenen, H. An electron microscopic study of selective, acute degeneration of sympathetic nerve terminals after administration of 6-hydroxydopamine. *Experientia*, 1968, **24**, 155–156.

Triggle, D. J. *Chemical Aspects of the Autonomic Nervous System.* New York: Academic, 1965.

Triggle, D. J. *Neurotransmitter–Receptor Interactions.* New York: Academic, 1971.

Truitt, E. B., Jr. Pharmacological activity in a metabolite of (1)-trans-delta-8-hydrocannabinol. *Federation Proceedings*, 1970, **29**, 619.

Truitt, E. B., Jr., & Anderson, S. M. Biogenic amine alterations produced in the brain by tetrahydrocannabinols and their metabolites. *Annals of the New York Academy of Sciences*, 1971, **191**, 68–72.

Tsou, K., & Jang, C. S. Studies on the site of analgesic action of morphine by intracerebral microinjection. *Scientia Sinica*, 1964, **13**, 1099–1109.

Tumarkin, B., Wilson, J., & Snyder, G. Cerebral atrophy due to alcoholism in young adults. *U.S. Armed Forces Medical Journal*, 1955, **6**, 64–74.

Turkington, R. W., & Topper, Y., Jr. Stimulation of casein synthesis and histological development of mammary gland by human placental lactogen *in vitro*. *Endocrinology*, 1966, **79**, 175–181.

Turner, C. D., & Bagnara, J. T. *General Endocrinology*, Philadelphia: Saunders, 1971.

Ungar, G., & Cohen, M. Induction of morphine tolerance by material extracted from brain of tolerant animals. *International Journal of Neuropharmacology*, 1965, **5**, 1–10.

Ungar, G., & Irwin, L. N. Transfer of acquired information by brain extracts. *Nature*, 1967, **214**, 453–455.

Ungar, G., & Oceguera-Navarro, C. Transfer of habituation by material extracted from brain. *Nature*, 1965, **207**, 301–302.

Ungerstedt, U. Histochemical studies on the effect of intracerebral and intraventricular injections of 6-hydroxydopamine on monoamine neurons in the rat brain. In T. Malmfors and H. Thoenen (Eds.), *6-Hydroxydopamine and Catecholamine Neurons.* New York: Elsevier, 1971. (a)

Ungerstedt, U. Stereotaxic mapping of the monoamine pathways in the rat brain. *Acta Physiologica Scandinavica*, 1971, Supplement 367, 1–48. (b)

Ungerstedt, U. Use of intracerebral injection of 6-hydroxydopamine as a tool for morphological and functional studies on central catecholamine neurons. In T. Malmfors and H. Thoenen (Eds.), *6-Hydroxydopamine and Catecholamine Neurons.* New York: Elsevier, 1971. (c)

Ungerstedt, U., & Arbuthnott, G. W. Quantitative recordings of rotational behavior after 6-hydroxy-dopamine lesions of the nigrostriatal dopamine system. *Brain Research*, 1970, **24**, 485–493.

U.S., Department of Health, Education and Welfare. *Marihuana and health.* Washington, D.C.: U.S. Government Printing Office, 1971.

Utena, H. Behavior aberrations in methamphetamine-intoxicated animals and chemical correlates in the brain. *Progress in Brain Research,* 1966, **21,** 192–207.

Valenstein, E. S. The anatomical locus of reinforcement. In E. Stellar and J. M. Sprague (Eds.), *Progress in Physiological Psychology, Volume 1.* New York: Academic, 1966.

Valenstein, E. S. *Brain Control.* New York: Wiley, 1973.

Vandam, L. D. The physiology and clinical pharmacology of anesthetic administration. In J. R. DiPalma (Ed.), *Drill's Pharmacology in Medicine.* (4th ed.) New York: McGraw-Hill, 1971. (a)

Vandam, L. D. Uptake and transport of anesthetics and stages of anesthesia. In J. R. DiPalma (Ed.), *Drill's Pharmacology in Medicine.* (4th ed.) New York: McGraw-Hill, 1971. (b)

van Dyke, H. B., Adamsons, K., Jr., & Engel, S. L. The storage and liberation of neurohypophyseal hormones. In H. Heller (Ed.), *The Neurohypophysis.* Washington, D.C.: Butterworth, 1957.

van Dyke, H. B., Chow, B. F., Greep, R. O., & Rothen, A. The isolation of a protein from the pars neuralis of the ox pituitary with constant oxytocic, pressor, and diuresis-inhibiting effects. *Journal of Pharmacology and Experimental Therapeutics,* 1942, **74,** 190–209.

Vaughn, E., & Fisher, A. E. Male sexual behavior induced by intracranial electrical stimulation. *Science,* 1962, **137,** 758–760.

Verhave, T. The effect of d-methamphetamine on avoidance and operant level. *Journal of Experimental Analysis of Behavior,* 1958, **1,** 207–220.

Volicer, L. Correlation between behavioral and biochemical effects of p-chlorophenylalanine in mice and rats. *International Journal of Neuropharmacology,* 1969, **8,** 361–364.

Volle, R. L. Modification by drugs of synaptic mechanisms in autonomic ganglia. *Pharmacological Reviews,* 1966, **18,** 839–870.

Volle, R. L. Cholinomimetic Drugs. In J. R. DiPalma (Ed.), *Drill's Pharmacology in Medicine.* (4th ed.) New York: McGraw-Hill, 1971. (a)

Volle, R. L. Introduction to the Autonomic Nervous System. In J. R. DiPalma (Ed.), *Drill's Pharmacology in Medicine.* (4th ed.) New York: McGraw-Hill, 1971. (b)

Volle, R. L., & Koelle, G. B. Ganglionic stimulating and blocking agents. In L. S. Goodman and A. Gilman (Eds.), *The Pharmacological Basis of Therapeutics.* (4th ed.) New York: Macmillan, 1970.

von Euler, U. S. Quantitation of stress by catecholamine analysis. *Clinical Pharmacology and Therapy,* 1964, **5,** 398–404.

von Euler, U. S. Adrenergic transmitter functions. *Science,* 1971, **173,** 202–206.

Von Mering, J., & Minkowski, O. Diabetes Mellitus nach Pankreas Extirpation. *Archives of Experimental Pathology and Pharmacology,* 1889, **26,** 371–387.

Wade, N. Anabolic steroids: Doctors denounce them, but athletes aren't listening. *Science,* 1972, **176,** 1399–1403.

Walker, D., & Freund, G. Impairment of shuttlebox avoidance learning following prolonged alcohol consumption in rats. *Physiology and Behavior,* 1971, **7**, 773-778.

Walker D., & Freund, G. Impairment of timing behavior following prolonged alcohol consumption in rats. *Science,* 1973, **182**, 597-599.

Walker, D., & Zornetzer, S. Alcohol withdrawal in mice: Electroencephalographic and behavioral correlates. *EEG Journal.* (in press)

Wang, J. H., & Takemori, A. E. Studies on the transport of morphine out of the perfused cerebral ventricles of rabbits. *Journal of Pharmacology and Experimental Therapeutics,* 1972, **181**, 46-52.

Wapner, I., Thurston, D. L., & Holowach, J. Phenobarbital: Its effect on learning in epileptic children. *Journal of the American Medical Association,* 1962, **182**, 937.

Ward, I. L. Prenatal stress feminizes and demasculinizes the behavior of males. *Science,* 1972, **175**, 82-84.

Waser. P. G., & Bersin, P. Turnover of monoamines in brain under the influences of muscimol and ibotenic acid, two psychoactive principles of amanita muscaria. In Efron, D. H. (Ed.), *Psychotomimetic Drugs.* New York: Raven, 1970.

Wasson, R. G. Fly agaric and man. In D. H. Efron (Ed.), *Ethnopharmacologic Search for Psychoactive Drugs.* Washington, D.C.: National Institue of Mental Health, 1967.

Watson, J. D. *Molecular Biology of the Gene.* (2nd ed.) New York: Benjamin, 1970.

Waud, D. R., & Waud, B. E. Agents acting on the neuromuscular junction and centrally acting muscular relaxants. In J. R. DiPalma (Ed.), *Drill's Pharmacology in Medicine.* (4th ed.) New York: McGraw-Hill, 1971.

Way, E. L. Brain uptake of morphine: Pharmacologic implications. *Federation Proceedings,* 1967, **26**, 1115-1118.

Way, E. L. Distribution and metabolism of morphine and its surrogates. In A. Winkler (Ed.), *The Addictive States.* Baltimore: Williams & Wilkins, 1968.

Way, W. L., Costle, E. C., & Way, E. L. Respiratory sensitivity of the newborn infant to meperidine and morphine. *Clinical Pharmacology and Therapeutics,* 1965, **6**, 454-461.

Wei, E., Loh, H. H., & Way, E. L. Neuroanatomical correlates of morphine dependence. *Science,* 1972, **177**, 616-617.

Weil, A. T. Adverse reactions to marijuana: Classification and suggested treatment. *New England Journal of Medicine,* 1970, **282**, 997-1000.

Weil, A. T., Zinberg, N. E., & Nelson, J. M. Clinical and psychological effects of marijuana in man. *Science,* 1968, **162**, 1234-1242.

Weiner, N. Regulation of norepinephrine biosynthesis. *Annual Review of Pharmacology,* 1970, **10**, 273-290.

Weiss, B., & Laties, V. G. Enhancement of human performance by caffeine and the amphetamines. *Pharmacological Reviews,* 1962, **14**, 1-36.

Weissman, A., Koe, B. K., & Tenen, S. Anti-amphetamine effects following inhibition of tyrosine hydroxylase. *Journal of Pharmacology and Experimental Therapeutics*, 1966, **151**, 335-352.

Welch, B. L., Hendley, E. D., & Turek, I. Norepinephrine uptake into cerebral cortical synaptosomes after one fight or electroconvulsive shock. *Science*, 1974, **183**, 220-221.

Wells, B. *Psychedelic Drugs.* Baltimore: Penguin, 1973.

Wender, P. H. *Minimal Brain Dysfunction in Children.* New York: Wiley, 1971.

Wentink, E. A. Effects of certain drugs and hormones upon conditioning. *Journal of Experimental Psychology*, 1938, **22**, 150-163.

West, L. J. On the marijuana problem. In D. Efron (Ed.), *Psychotomimetic Drugs.* New York: Raven, 1970.

West, L. J., Pierce, C. M., & Thomas, W. D. Lysergic acid diethylamide: Its effect on a male asiatic elephant. *Science,* 1962, **138**, 1100-1102.

Westerfeld, W. W. The intermediary metabolism of alcohol. *American Journal of Clinical Nutrition*, 1961, **9**, 426-431.

Whalen, R. E. Gonadal hormones, the nervous system and behavior. In J. L. McGaugh (Ed.), *The Chemistry of Mood, Motivation, and Memory.* New York: Plenum, 1972.

Whalen, R. E., & Edwards, D. A. Effects of the anti-androgen cyproterone acetate on mating behavior and seminal vesicle tissue in male rats. *Endocrinology*, 1969, **84**, 155-156.

Whalen, R. E., & Luttge, W. G. P-chlorophenylalanine methyl ester: An aphrodisiac? *Science,* 1970, **169**, 1000-1001.

Whalen, R. E., & Luttge, W. G. Differential localization of progesterone uptake in brain: Role of sex, estrogen pretreatment and adrenalectomy. *Brain Research*, 1971, **33**, 147-155. (a)

Whalen, R. E., & Luttge, W. G. Testosterone, androstenedione and dihydrotestosterone: Effects on mating behavior of male rats. *Hormones and Behavior*, 1971, **2**, 117-125. (b)

Whalen, R. E., & Nadler, R. D. Suppression of the development of female mating behavior by estrogen administered in infancy. *Science,* 1963, **141**, 273-274.

White, A., Handler, P., & Smith, E. L. *Principles of Biochemistry.* (4th ed.) New York: McGraw-Hill, 1968.

Whitehead, R. W., & Virtue, R. W. General anesthesia III: Intravenous agents. In J. R. DiPalma (Ed.), *Drill's Pharmacology in Medicine.* (4th ed.) New York: McGraw-Hill, 1971.

Whitehouse, J. M. Effects of atropine on discrimination learning in the rat. *Journal of Comparative and Physiological Psychology*, 1964, **57**, 13-15.

Wick, A. N., Larson, E. R., & Serif, G. S. A site of action of phenethylbiguanide, a hypoglycemic compound. *Journal of Biological Chemistry*, 1958, **233**, 296-298.

Wikler, A. Relationship between clinical effects of barbiturates and their neurophysiological mechanisms of action. *Federation Proceedings*, 1952, **11**, 647-652.

Wilk, S., Shopsin, B., Gershon, S., & Suhl, M. Cerebrospinal fluid levels of MHPG in affective disorders. *Nature,* 1972, **235**, 440-441.

Williams, E. E. Effects of alcohol on workers with carbon disulfide. *Journal of the American Medical Association,* 1937, **109**, 1472-1473.

Williams, M. Memory studies in electric convulsion therapy. *Journal of Neurology, Neurosurgery and Psychiatry,* 1950, **13**, 30-35.

Williams, R. H. Hypoglycemia and hypoglycemoses. In R. H. Williams (Ed.), *Textbook of Endocrinology.* (4th ed.) Philadelphia: Saunders, 1968. (a)

Williams, R. H. The pancreas. In R. H. Williams (Ed.), *Textbook of Endocrinology.* (4th ed.) Philadelphia: Saunders, 1968. (b)

Williams, R. H. *Textbook of Endocrinology.* (4th ed.) Philadelphia: Saunders, 1968. (c)

Williams, R. H., Tanner, D. C., & Odell, W. D. Hypoglycemic actions of phenethyl-, amyl-, and isoamyl-biguanide. *Diabetes,* 1958, **7**, 87-92.

Wilson, C., & Linken, A. *The Use of Cannabis in Adolescent Drug Dependents.* New York: Pergamon, 1968.

Winter, C. A. The physiology and pharmacology of pain and its relief. In G. De Stevens (Ed.), *Analgetics.* New York: Academic, 1965.

Wise, C. D., Berger, B. D., & Stein, L. Benzodiazepines: Anxiety-reducing activity by reduction of serotonin turnover in the brain. *Science,* 1972, **177**, 180-183.

Wise, C. D., & Stein, L. Facilitation of brain self-stimulation by central administration of norepinephrine. *Science,* 1969, **163**, 299-301.

Wise, C. D., & Stein, L. Dopamine-β hydroxylase deficits in the brains of schizophrenic patients. *Science,* 1973, **181**, 344-347.

Wolf, G., & Miller, N. E. Lateral hypothalamic lesions: Effects on drinking elicited by carbachol in preoptic area and posterior hypothalamus. *Science,* 1964, **143**, 585-587.

Wolf, S., & Wolff, H. G. *Human Gastric Function.* New York: Oxford, 1947.

Wollman, H., & Dripps, R. D. Uptake, distribution, elimination and administration of inhalational anesthetics. In L. S. Goodman and A. Gilman (Eds.), *The Pharmacological Basis of Therapeutics.* (4th ed.) New York: Macmillan, 1970.

Woodbury, D. M. Mechanism of action of anticonvulsants. In H. H. Jasper, A. A. Ward Jr., and A. Pope (Eds.), *Basic Mechanisms of The Epilepsies.* Boston: Little, Brown, 1969.

Woodbury, D. M., Hurley, R. E., Lewis, N. G., McArthur, M. W., Copeland, W. W., Kirschvink, J. F., & Goodman, L. S. Effect of thyroxine, thyroidectomy and 6-N-propyl-2-thiouracil on brain function. *Journal of Pharmacology and Experimental Therapeutics,* 1952, **106**, 331-340.

Woodbury, D. M., & Vernadakis, A. Influence of hormones on brain activity. In L. Martini and W. F. Ganong (Eds.), *Neuroendocrinology, Vol. 2.* New York: Academic, 1967.

Wool, I. G., & Krahl, M. E. Incorporation of ^{14}C-amino acids into protein of isolated diaphragms, an effect of insulin independent of glucose entry. *American Journal of Physiology*, 1959, **196**, 961-964.

Wunsch, E. Die Totalsynthese des pankreas-hormons Glucagon. *Z. Naturforsch.*, 1967, **22b**, 1269-1276.

Wurtman, R. J., Axelrod, J., & Phillips, L. S. Melatonin synthesis in the pineal gland: Control by light. *Science*, 1963, **142**, 1071-1073.

Wurtman, R. J., Frank, M. M., Morse, W. H., & Dews, P. B. Studies on behavior, V. Actions of l-epinephrine and related compounds. *Journal of Pharmacology and Experimental Therapeutics*, 1959, **127**, 281-287.

Wynn, L. C., & Solomon, R. L. Traumatic avoidance learning: Acquisition and extinction in dogs, deprived of normal peripheral autonomic functioning. *Genetic Psychology Monographs*, 1955, **52**, 241-284.

Yahr, M. D. Drugs in the treatment of convulsive disorders. In J. R. DiPalma (Ed.), *Drill's Pharmacology in Medicine*. (4th ed.) New York: McGraw-Hill, 1971.

Yamaguchi, N., Ling, G. M., & Marczynski, T. J. The effects of chemical stimulation of the preoptic region, nucleus centralis medialis, or brain stem reticular formation with regard to sleep and wakefulness. *Recent Advances in Biological Psychiatry*, 1964, **6**, 9-20.

Yamaguchi, N., Marczynski, T. J., & Ling, G. M. The effects of electrical and chemical stimulation of the preoptic region and some nonspecific thalamic nuclei in unrestrained, waking animals. *EEG Journal*, 1963, **15**, 154.

Yarmolinski, M. B., & de la Haba, G. L. Inhibition by puromycin of amino acid incorporation into protein. *Proceedings of the National Academy of Science (USA)*, 1959, **45**, 1721-1729.

Youmans, W. Control of breathing. In J. Brobeck (Ed.), *Best and Taylor's Physiological Basis of Medical Practice*. (9th ed.) Baltimore: Williams & Wilkins, 1973.

Zamenof, S., van Marthens, E., & Grauel, L. Prenatal cerebral development: Effect of restricted diet, reversal by growth hormone. *Science*, 1971, **174**, 954-955.

Zbinden, G., Bagdon, R. E., Keith, E. F., Phillips, R. D., & Randall, L. O. Experimental and clinical toxicology of chlordiezepoxide ("Librium"). *Toxicology and Applied Pharmacology*, 1961, **3**, 619-637.

Zeller, E. A. Influence of isonicotinic acid hydrazine (INH) and 1-isonicotinyl-2-isopropyl hydrazine (IIH) on bacterial and mammalian enzymes. *Experientia*, 1952, **8**, 349-350.

Zemlan, F. P., Ward, I. L., Crowly, W. R., & Margules, D. L. Activation of lordotic responding in female rats by suppression of serotonergic activity. *Science*, 1973, **179**, 1010-1011.

Zerbolio, D. J. Within-strain facilitation and disruption of avoidance learning by picrotoxin. *Psychonomic Science*, 1967, **9**, 411-412.

Zierler, K. L., & Rabinowitz, D. Effect of very small concentrations of insulin on forearm metabolism: Persistence of its action on potassium and free fatty acids without its effect on glucose. *Journal of Clinical Investigations,* 1964, **43,** 950-962.

Zieve, L. Effects of benzedrine on activity. *Psychological Record,* 1937, **1,** 393-396.

Zigmond, M. J., & Stricker, E. M. Deficits in feeding behavior after intraventricular injection of 6-hydroxydopamine in rats. *Science,* 1972, **177,** 1211-1213.

Zitrin, A., Beach, F. A., Barchas, J. D., & Dement, W. C. Sexual behavior of male cats after administration of parachlorophenylalanine. *Science,* 1970, **170,** 868-870.

Zitrin, A., Dement, W. C., & Barchas, J. D. Brain serotonin and male sexual behavior. In J. Zubin and J. Money (Eds.), *Contemporary Sexual Behavior: Critical Issues in the 1970s.* Baltimore: Johns Hopkins, 1973.

Zubin, J., & Barrera, S. E. Effect of convulsive therapy on memory. *Federation Proceedings,* 1941, **48,** 596-597.

Zubin, J., & Money, J. *Contemporary Sexual Behavior: Critical Issues in the 1970s.* Baltimore: Johns Hopkins, 1973.

AUTHOR INDEX

Numbers in italics refer to the pages on which the complete references are listed.

SUBJECT INDEX